Massachusetts General Hospital Illustrated Tips and Tricks in Thoracic Surgery

Editors

Yolonda L. Colson, MD, PhD
Chief, Division of Thoracic Surgery
Hermes C. Grillo Professor of Surgery in the Field of Thoracic Surgery
Harvard Medical School
Massachusetts General Hospital
Boston, Massachusetts

Christopher R. Morse, MD
Division of Thoracic Surgery
Department of Surgery
Harvard Medical School
Massachusetts General Hospital
Boston, Massachusetts

Wolters Kluwer

Philadelphia • Baltimore • New York • London
Buenos Aires • Hong Kong • Sydney • Tokyo

Acquisitions Editor: Keith Donnellan
Senior Development Editor: Ashley Fischer
Editorial Coordinators: Sean Hanrahan and Marisa Solorzano-Taylor
Marketing Manager: Kirsten Watrud
Production Project Manager: Kirstin Johnson
Manager, Graphic Arts & Design: Stephen Druding, Leslie Caruso
Senior Manufacturing Coordinator: Margie Orzech-Zeranko
Prepress Vendor: TNQ Tech

9 8 7 6 5 4 3 2 1

Printed in Mexico

Library of Congress Cataloging-in-Publication Data

ISBN-13: 978-1-975171-93-3

Cataloging in Publication data available on request from publisher.

shop.lww.com

QUADM0824

Contributors

James S. Allan, MD, MBA
Associate Professor of Surgery
Division of Thoracic Surgery
Department of Surgery
Harvard Medical School
Massachusetts General Hospital
Boston, Massachusetts

Hugh G. Auchincloss, MD
Assistant Professor of Surgery
Department of Surgery
Harvard Medical School
Surgeon
Division of Thoracic Surgery
Department of Surgery
Massachusetts General Hospital
Boston, Massachusetts

Andrea L. Axtell, MD, MPH
Assistant Professor
Division of Cardiothoracic Surgery
Department of Surgery
University of Wisconsin School of Medicine and Public Health
Madison, Wisconsin

Ioana Baiu, MD, MPH
Fellow
Department of Cardiothoracic Surgery
Stanford University School of Medicine
Stanford, California

Justin D. Blasberg, MD MPH
Associate Professor
Division of Thoracic Surgery
Yale School of Medicine
New Haven, Connecticut

Brett L. Broussard, MD, FACS
Thoracic Surgeon
Division of Surgical Oncology
Banner M.D. Anderson Cancer Center
Gilbert, Arizona

Sarah A. Brownlee, MD
Physician
Department of Surgery
Massachusetts General Hospital
Boston, Massachusetts

Corbin Cleary, MD
Surgeon
Henry Ford Health
Detroit, Michigan

Yolonda L. Colson, MD, PhD
Chief, Division of Thoracic Surgery
Hermes C. Grillo Professor of Surgery in the Field of Thoracic Surgery
Harvard Medical School
Massachusetts General Hospital
Boston, Massachusetts

Christina L. Costantino, MD
Fellow
Department of Surgery
Massachusetts General Hospital
Boston, Massachusetts

Pierre de Delva, MD
Professor of Surgery
Department of Surgery
University of Mississippi School of Medicine
University of Mississippi Medical Center
Jackson, Mississippi

David S. Demos, MD
Surgeon
Aurora Health Care
Milwaukee, Wisconsin

Aaron Dinerman, MD
Resident
Department of Surgery
Baylor University Medical Center
Dallas, Texas

Dean Donahue, MD
Director, Thoracic Outlet Syndrome Program
Division of Thoracic Surgery
Department of Surgery
Massachusetts General Hospital
Boston, Massachusetts

Daniel P. Doody, MD
Surgeon
Department of Pediatric Surgery
Massachusetts General Hospital
Boston, Massachusetts

Danielle Ellis, MD, MTS
Resident
Department of Surgery
Massachusetts General Hospital
Boston, Massachusetts

J. Mark Erfe, MD, MPH
Resident
Division of Cardiothoracic Surgery
Department of Surgery
Northwestern University Feinberg School of Medicine
Chicago, Illinois

Nathaniel R. Evans III, MD
Professor
Director of Thoracic and Esophageal Surgery
Department of Surgery
Sidney Kimmel Medical College, Thomas Jefferson University
Philadelphia, Pennsylvania

Matthew P. Fox, MD
Associate Professor
Department of Cardiovascular and Thoracic Surgery
University of Louisville School of Medicine
Louisville, Kentucky

Paul W. Furlow, MD
Instructor
Division of Thoracic Surgery
Department of Surgery
Harvard Medical School
Massachusetts General Hospital
Boston, Massachusetts

Henning A. Gaissert, MD
Associate Professor
Division of Thoracic Surgery
Department of Surgery
Harvard Medical School
Visiting Surgeon
Division of Thoracic Surgery
Department of Surgery
Massachusetts General Hospital
Boston, Massachusetts

Zane T. Hammoud, MD
Professor of Surgery
Wayne State University School of Medicine
Chief of Thoracic Surgery
John Dingell VA Medical Center
Detroit, Michigan

Chinmay Haridas, MBBS
Researcher
Division of Thoracic Surgery
Department of Surgery
Massachusetts General Hospital
Boston, Massachusetts

Kenneth T. Holt, MD
Resident
Department of Surgery
Brookwood Baptist Health
Birmingham, Alabama

Eliza D. Hompe, MD
Fellow
Department of Surgery
Massachusetts General Hospital
Boston, Massachusetts

Mark R. Katlic, MD, MMM
Chair
Department of Surgery
Director
Center for Geriatric Surgery
LifeBridge Health System
Baltimore, Maryland

Colleen M. Keyes, MD, MPH
Instructor
Division of Pulmonary & Critical Care Medicine
Department of Medicine
Massachusetts General Hospital
Boston, Massachusetts

Samuel S. Kim, MD
Associate Professor
Department of Surgery
Northwestern University Feinberg School of Medicine
Chicago, Illinois

Austin Kluis, MD
Resident
Department of Surgery
Baylor University Medical Center
Dallas, Texas

Kate Krause, MD
Resident
Department of Surgery
Harvard Medical School
Boston, Massachusetts

Antonia Kreso, MD, PhD
Instructor
Division of Cardiac Surgery
Department of Surgery
Massachusetts General Hospital
Boston, Massachusetts

Kumar Krishnan, MD
Assistant Professor of Medicine
Department of Medicine
Massachusetts General Hospital
Boston, Massachusetts

Elbert Kuo, MD, MPH, MMS, FACS
Section Chief of Thoracic Surgery
Division of Surgical Oncology
Banner M.D. Anderson Cancer Center
Gilbert, Arizona

Michael Lanuti, MD
Associate Professor of Surgery
Division of Thoracic Surgery
Department of Surgery
Harvard Medical School
Director of Thoracic Oncology
Division of Thoracic Surgery
Department of Surgery
Massachusetts General Hospital
Boston, Massachusetts

Natalie S. Lui, MD, MAS
Assistant Professor
Department of Cardiothoracic Surgery
Stanford University School of Medicine
Stanford, California

Maria Lucia L. Madariaga, MD
Assistant Professor
Department of Surgery
Section of Thoracic Surgery
The University of Chicago Medicine & Biological Sciences
Chicago, Illinois

Chase C. Marso, MD
Resident in General Surgery
Department of Surgery
Massachusetts General Hospital
Boston, Massachusetts

Jessica L. Masch, MD
Resident Physician
Department of Surgery
University of Louisville School of Medicine
Louisville, Kentucky

Camille A. Mathey-Andrews, MD
Cardiovascular Resident
Department of Cardiothoracic Surgery
Massachusetts General Hospital
Boston, Massachusetts

Douglas J. Mathisen, MD
Professor of Surgery
Division of Thoracic Surgery
Department of Surgery
Massachusetts General Hospital
Boston, Massachusetts

Robert E. Merritt, MD, MBA
Professor of Surgery
Division of Thoracic Surgery
The Ohio State University College of Medicine
The Ohio State Wexner Medical Center
Columbus, Ohio

Cynthia L. Miller, MD
Fellow
Department of Surgery
Harvard Medical School
Massachusetts General Hospital
Boston, Massachusetts

Timothy M. Millington, MD
Assistant Professor
Department of Surgery
Geisel School of Medicine at Dartmouth
Dartmouth-Hitchcock Medical Center
Lebanon, New Hampshire

Douglas J. Minnich, MD
Surgeon
Alabama Thoracic Surgery, LLC
Birmingham, Alabama

Daniela Molena, MD
Professor of Thoracic Surgery
Department of Surgery
Memorial Sloan Kettering Cancer Center
New York, New York

Philicia Moonsamy, MD, MPH
Surgeon
Cedars-Sinai Medical Center
Los Angeles, California

Christopher R. Morse, MD
Division of Thoracic Surgery
Department of Surgery
Harvard Medical School
Massachusetts General Hospital
Boston, Massachusetts

Ashok Muniappan, MD
Assistant Professor
Department of Surgery
Harvard Medical School
Massachusetts General Hospital
Boston, Massachusetts

Lucy Nam, MD, AB
Resident
Department of Surgery
Massachusetts General Hospital
Boston, Massachusetts

James T. Nawalaniec, MD
Resident
Department of Surgery
Harvard Medical School
Massachusetts General Hospital
Boston, Massachusetts

Harald C. Ott, MD, MBA
Vice President, Kidney Manufacturing
IVIVA Medical
United Therapeutics
Medford, Massachusetts

Nikhil Panda, MD, MPH
Resident
Division of Thoracic Surgery
Department of Surgery
Harvard Medical School
Massachusetts General Hospital
Boston, Massachusetts

Numa P. Perez, MD
Fellow
Department of Surgery
Cincinnati Children's Hospital
Cincinnati, Ohio

Eitan Podgaetz, MD, MPH, FACS
Director of Minimally Invasive Thoracic Surgery
Department of Thoracic Surgery
Baylor University Medical Center
Dallas, Texas

Jarrod D. Predina, MD
Assistant Professor of Surgery
Department of Surgery
Perelman School of Medicine at the University of Pennsylvania
Philadelphia, PA

Uzma Rahman, BSc, MD
Resident
Department of General Surgery
Thomas Jefferson University Hospital
Philadelphia, Pennsylvania

Michael F. Reed, MD
Professor
Department of Surgery
Penn State College of Medicine
Penn State Health Milton S. Hershey Medical Center
Hershey, Pennsylvania

Jonathan Rice, MD, PhD
Assistant Professor of Surgery
Division of Cardiothoracic Surgery
Department of Surgery
University of Arizona College of Medicine – Tucson
Tucson, Arizona

Uma M. Sachdeva, MD, PhD
Assistant Professor of Surgery
Department of Surgery
Harvard Medical School
Massachusetts General Hospital
Boston, Massachusetts

Lana Y. Schumacher, MD
Department of Surgery
Tufts University School of Medicine
Tufts Medical Center
Boston, Massachusetts

Elliot L. Servais, MD, FACS
Associate Professor
Department of Cardiothoracic Surgery
UMass Chan School of Medicine
Burlington, Massachusetts

K. Robert Shen, MD
Professor of Surgery
Division of General Thoracic Surgery
Department of Surgery
Mayo Clinic
Rochester, Minnesota

Joseph B. Shrager, MD
Professor and Chief
Division of Thoracic Surgery
Department of Cardiothoracic Surgery
Stanford University School of Medicine
Stanford, California
Veterans Affair Palo Alto Healthcare System
Palo Alto, California

Smita Sihag, MD, MPH
Assistant Professor of Thoracic Surgery
Department of Surgery
Memorial Sloan Kettering Cancer Center
New York, New York

S. Ansley Smith, MD
Resident
Department of Surgery
University of Louisville School of Medicine
Louisville, Kentucky

Philip J. Spencer, MD
Assistant Professor
Department of Cardiovascular Surgery
Mayo Clinic
Rochester, Minnesota

Cameron T. Stock, MD, FACS
Assistant Professor
Department of Cardiothoracic Surgery
UMass Chan School of Medicine
Burlington, Massachusetts

Leonidas Tapias, MD
Assistant Professor
Division of Thoracic and Esophageal Surgery
Case Western Reserve University School of Medicine
University Hospitals Cleveland Medical Center
Cleveland, Ohio

Luis F. Tapias, MD
Assistant Professor of Surgery
Division of General Thoracic Surgery
Department of Surgery
Mayo Clinic
Rochester, Minnesota

Danny Wang, MD
Resident
Department of Surgery
Massachusetts General Hospital
Boston, Massachusetts

James L. West, MD
Fellow
Department of Surgery
University of Alabama at Birmingham Marnix E. Heersink School of Medicine
Birmingham, Alabama

Cameron D. Wright, MD
Professor of Surgery
Division of Thoracic Surgery
Department of Surgery
Harvard Medical School
Massachusetts General Hospital
Boston, Massachusetts

Chi-Fu Jeffrey Yang, MD
Associate Professor of Surgery
Department of Surgery
Harvard Medical School
Surgeon
Department of Surgery
Massachusetts General Hospital
Boston, Massachusetts

Olivia Ziegler, MD
Resident
Department of Surgery
Penn State College of Medicine
Penn State Health Milton S. Hershey Medical Center
Hershey, Pennsylvania

Preface

"We are what we repeatedly do. Excellence, then, is not an act, but a habit."

Will Durant

Although clinical excellence and resident education have always been central to the core mission of Thoracic Surgery at Massachusetts General Hospital, the importance of these teachings and the legacy they represent have never been more important than in our rapidly changing field. It is in the setting of increasing clinical complexity, financial pressures to increase clinical productivity and shorten length of stay, the increasing tendency to become distracted from the tenets central to an operation, and the subsequent normalization of "cutting corners" in the guise of care efficiency that we need to call on our years of training and make excellence our habit every time. It is during these times that our teachings of the surgical principles of gentle tissue handling with minimization of tension, precise suture placement, attention to detail, and excellence in postoperative management are critical to practice as they can truly mean the difference between success and failure, life and death for our patients.

From a lobectomy for bronchiectasis by Samuel Robinson in 1909, to defining segmental anatomy and advocating for lobectomy as the treatment of lung cancer by Edward Churchill, to the unsurpassed technical excellence of esophagectomy in the hands of Richard Sweet, the creation of the field of tracheal surgery by Hermes Grillo, the focus on the thymus by Earle Wilkins, and advances in airway surgery and neoadjuvant approaches for thoracic malignancies by Doug Mathisen, the legendary surgeons at MGH have created, advanced, and refined the field of thoracic surgery—all with an unwavering commitment to excellence in patient outcomes and a steadfast dedication to education of the trainee. Therefore, it is in honor of those master surgeons from whom we have had the privilege of learning, the patients who have entrusted us with their lives, and the talented, inspiring residents whom we have had the privilege of training, that we have written this surgical textbook that uniquely highlights the importance of attention to detail in every aspect of the operation and shares the pearls of thoracic surgical training at MGH with our colleagues around the world.

Yolonda L. Colson, MD, PhD
Chief, Division of Thoracic Surgery
Hermes C. Grillo Professor of Surgery in the Field of Thoracic Surgery
Harvard Medical School
Massachusetts General Hospital
Boston, Massachusetts

Christopher R. Morse, MD
Division of Thoracic Surgery
Department of Surgery
Harvard Medical School
Massachusetts General Hospital
Boston, Massachusetts

Acknowledgments

It is an honor and a privilege to be part of a surgical legacy of excellence and education as notable and as celebrated as that of the Massachusetts General Hospital. However, this legacy is about the people, our surgical and clinical partners, and the unbreakable bond between mentee and mentor, generation after generation, that is the true strength of this remarkable institution and of the Thoracic Surgery Division. The authors' dedication to patient care and the next generation is clearly evident in the unwavering efforts put forward in the completion of this textbook despite the challenges of the COVID-19 pandemic, and to the unrelenting fortitude of my co-editor to make this gift to our resident trainees a reality.

Contents

LUNG/AIRWAY

Video Contents

LUNG/AIRWAY

ESOPHAGEAL

ENDOSCOPY

SECTION I Lung/Airway

Chapter 1
Massive Hemoptysis

KENNETH T. HOLT
JAMES L. WEST
DOUGLAS J. MINNICH

Background

Key Definitions

- Hemoptysis—bleeding from the respiratory tract below the vocal cords
- Pseudohemoptysis—bleeding from another source, such as the upper respiratory or GI tract, mimicking hemoptysis
- Massive hemoptysis (MH)—no longer defined by quantity or briskness of bleeding but rather any hemoptysis causing respiratory failure or hypotension
  - MH, although rare, is a true medical emergency that requires quick diagnosis and treatment. Even small to moderate amounts of blood in the airway can rapidly impair ventilation and oxygenation, leading to death.
  - Most fatal cases of MH are due to respiratory failure from blood in airways rather than hemorrhagic shock.
  - Even with modern advancements in the diagnosis and treatment of MH, mortality has still been reported to be 13% to 17%.

Diagnosis

- When able, a detailed history and physical examination will often provide clues to the source of bleeding.
- Labs should be obtained including type and screen, complete blood count (CBC), comprehensive metabolic panel, and coagulation profile or thromboelastogram.
- Chest x-ray is often performed early in the workup of MH but is a poor diagnostic tool, identifying the laterality of bleeding in less than 50% of cases in some studies.
- A noncontrasted CT can be helpful in identifying masses as a source of hemoptysis. However, given the emergent nature of MH, CT angiography (CTA) is a better choice.
- CTA is a superior imaging modality for evaluating hemoptysis and identifying laterality and cause of bleeding in greater than 70% of cases.
- Bronchoscopy is less effective at localizing bleeding than CTA. However, it can be easily performed at bedside, can aid with difficult intubations, and allows for therapeutic interventions.
- In a case of true MH in an unstable patient, bronchoscopy should be performed first to aid with intubation and assist with temporizing measures.

Etiology

- Etiology of MH can be divided into eight major categories: cardiac, pulmonary, infectious, rheumatologic, traumatic, hematologic, vascular, and miscellaneous (Table 1.1).

TABLE 1.1 | Etiologies of Massive Hemoptysis

Cardiac: Aortic aneurysm Congenital heart disease Congestive heart failure Mitral stenosis
Pulmonary: Bronchiectasis Broncholithiasis Lymphangioleiomyomatosis Malignancy Pulmonary embolism/infarction
Infectious: Aspergillosis Bacterial/viral pneumonia Flukes and other parasites Lung abscess Necrotizing pneumonia Tuberculosis
Rheumatologic: Alveolar hemorrhage secondary to vasculitis (ie, Behçet disease, Goodpasture syndrome, granulomatous polyangiitis, systemic lupus)
Traumatic: Blunt injuries Penetrating injuries
Hematologic: Disseminated intravascular coagulation Platelet disorders (thrombotic thrombocytopenic purpura, inherited platelet disorders, etc.)
Vascular: Arteriovenous malformations Pulmonary artery aneurysm
Miscellaneous: Blast injury Cocaine abuse Foreign body Iatrogenic (anticoagulants, endobronchial brachytherapy, instrumentation, radiation therapy, etc.)

- The most common cause varies within different patient populations. The most common cause worldwide remains tuberculosis (TB), though much less likely in regions where TB is not endemic.
- In developed countries, the most common cause is malignancy.

Perioperative Considerations

General Management

- Large-bore IVs for rapid transfusion
- Transfer to the ICU
- Early notification of a multidisciplinary team consisting of:
  - Thoracic surgery
  - Anesthesia
  - Interventional radiology
  - Interventional pulmonology
  - Respiratory therapist and bronchoscopy equipment
- Correct any coagulopathy
- Transfuse as needed
- The patient should be transferred to a center with interventional radiology once stabilized, if not available.

Airway Management

- Death from MH is most often a result of asphyxiation rather than hemorrhagic shock. The total conducting airway volume is on average only 150 mL, thus making airway control and isolation critical for stabilization.
- Placing the patient in a lateral decubitus position with the bleeding side down can help isolate blood to the dependent lung.
- Multiple approaches can be used based on availability and proficiency of care team and providers (Figure 1.1).

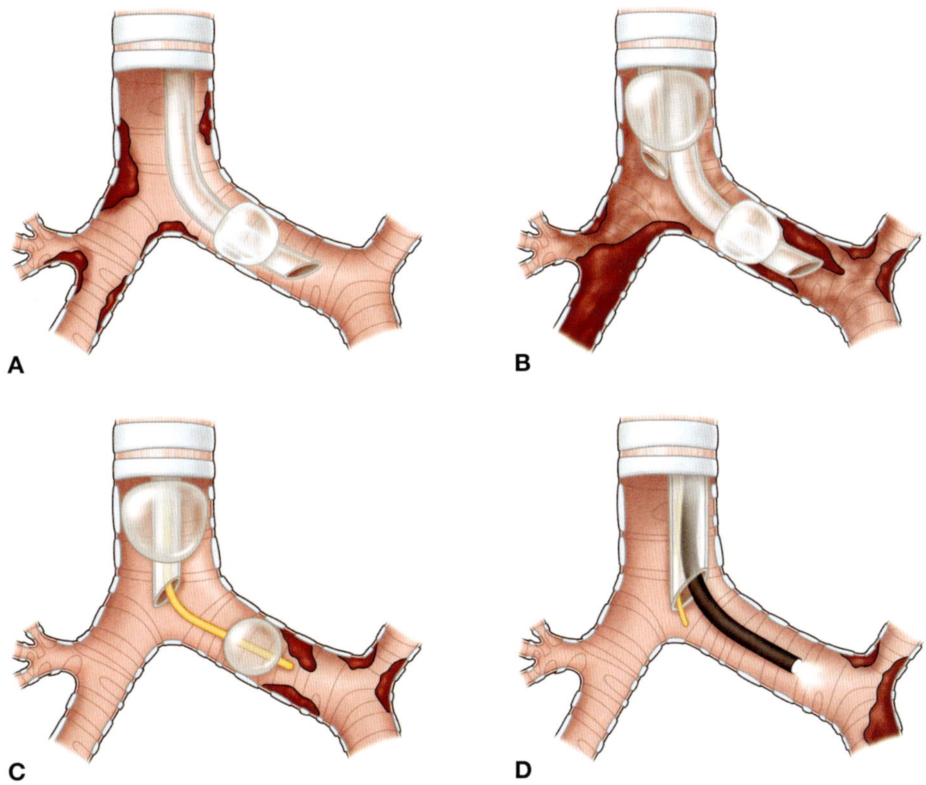

FIGURE 1.1 | A-D. Airway control in massive hemoptysis. **A.** A large endotracheal tube is used to secure the left-sided mainstem. **B.** A double-lumen tube is the least optimal choice for massive hemoptysis. **C.** A bronchial blocker can be positioned to prevent spillage of blood to the contralateral side. **D.** Left-sided mainstem is intubated with rigid bronchoscope safeguards to the right-sided airways, whereas blood can be suctioned efficiently with the use of a rigid suction catheter and therapeutic flexible bronchoscope simultaneously.

- A standard endotracheal tube (ETT) gives the ability to ventilate but does not isolate the hemorrhaging lung from the other.
  - Use an 8.0 ETT or larger to allow for easier instrumentation.
- Bronchial blocker allows for selective isolation of the bleeding lobe while ventilating the remaining lobes bilaterally. The blocker can also aid in tamponade and hemostasis of the bleeding lesion. Blocker placement should be aided by and confirmed with flexible bronchoscopy. Fogarty balloons can also be used as a blocker.
- Main stem ETT isolates the left and right lung from one another but only allows for ventilation of one lung.
  - Recommend a bronchial blocker rather than a main stem ETT. However, if a blocker or Fogarty balloon is not available, then an ETT can be placed in the nonbleeding main bronchus. This will allow for clearance of the blood in the unaffected side and also ventilation of this lung, which will serve as temporizing measures prior to further interventions.

- Rigid bronchoscope—particularly effective with central airway lesions. A rigid bronchoscopy is likely the optimal technique for diagnosis and essential intervention, although it is more technically difficult to use compared to a flexible bronchoscopy.
  - A rigid bronchoscope can be advanced to the bleeding side, then a flexible bronchoscope can be placed in the affected side, providing working ports for interventions while the rigid scope maintains a patent airway.

TIPS

- *Though particularly useful in thoracic surgery, a double-lumen ETT has little to no role in the management of MH. Due to their lumen size, only smaller bronchoscopes may be used, making suctioning large clots difficult.*

Technique

Bronchoscopy

- The main role of bronchoscopy should be to localize the bleeding and temporize the hemorrhage prior to more definitive treatment, such as interventional radiology.
- Depending on the airway obtained, endoscopic options for control of hemorrhage vary.
- Often the initial intervention used after suctioning is cold saline lavage, which may provide temporary control until further interventions can be undertaken.
- Similarly, dilute epinephrine lavage is thought to promote vasoconstriction. Epinephrine should be avoided in patients with arrhythmias or coronary artery disease.
- Intravenous and nebulized tranexamic acid have been described as adjuncts in treating hemoptysis, although studies proving their effectiveness are limited.
- Cautery and argon plasma can both be effective though they do rely on adequate visualization of the source of bleeding, which is rare.
- Lastly, if the hemorrhage cannot be controlled, bronchial blockers or Fogarty balloons can be placed to isolate the hemorrhaging segment, allowing for ventilation while moving to interventional radiology or the operating room.

Interventional Radiology

- The lungs are perfused by two different blood supplies: the pulmonary arteries (mean pulmonary artery pressures 12-16 mm Hg) and the bronchial arteries at much higher systemic pressures.
- The majority of bleeds are attributed to the bronchial arterial systems, with some studies estimating upward of 90%.
- Bronchial artery embolization (BAE) was first described in the 1970s and has risen in popularity as the availability of interventional radiologists has increased.
- Bronchial arteries typically originate from the T5 or T6 thoracic aorta, although they can have collateral flow from several additional sources such as the intercostal, inferior phrenic, internal mammary, or the subclavian arteries.
- Many different embolization techniques are used by interventional radiologists, for example, polyvinyl alcohol, gelatin sponges, and metal coils.
- BAE is not without risk, as a few major complications are secondary to inadvertent embolizations.
  - Neurologic deficits from embolization of the anterior spinal artery
    - Spinal cord ischemia has been reported in 1% to 6% of BAE.
  - Esophageal necrosis
  - Bronchial-esophageal fistula
  - Intimal dissection of the aorta
- The above major complication rates have all decreased with improvements in the field of interventional radiology and highly selective embolization techniques.
- The most common complaints following embolization are pain at the cannulation site, self-limiting chest/back pain, and dysphagia.
- BAE initial success rates are between 70% and 99%, though the 30-day rebleeding rate is approximately 60%.

Surgical Management

- When all other modalities of intervention fail, surgery is an option for hemorrhage control.
- Ideally, a particular lobe will have been identified as the source of hemorrhage while securing the airway.
- A left or right posterolateral thoracotomy at the level of the 5th rib allows for optimal exposure of the hilum for pneumonectomy or lobectomy.
- If the bleeding lobe has been identified, a lobectomy will control the hemorrhage.
- In the worst-case scenario, a pneumonectomy can be performed with a much higher mortality and morbidity.
- Part of the difficulty with surgical resections in the emergent setting is the lack of preoperative pulmonary function testing.

Postoperative Care

- Regardless of the technique used for control of hemorrhage, the postoperative care is similar.
- Key points post operation
  - Continue close monitoring of hemodynamics in the ICU.
  - Trend arterial blood gas analysis and CBC.
  - Wean ventilator settings with the goal to extubate when appropriate.
  - Monitor closely for signs of recurrence (estimated to be over 50% at 30 days).
  - Once stable, further workup for source of bleeding can be beneficial especially if the cause has definitive surgical management, which can be performed electively to prevent recurrence.

PEARLS AND PITFALLS

- Obtaining airway control is key to managing MH.
- Though once considered the only treatment for MH, surgery is no longer the first-line therapy. In fact, surgery should be reserved as a last resort with a few exceptions.
- In the acute setting, nonsurgical control of hemoptysis is superior. One study looking at hospital mortality showed better outcomes in those with initial nonsurgical control followed by an elective outpatient procedure when compared to urgent surgery initial control.
- Despite the advances in endoscopic and angiographic control of hemorrhage, there are several scenarios where surgery remains the treatment modality of choice: MH from iatrogenic pulmonary artery rupture, complex arteriovenous malformations, or refractory hemoptysis secondary to trauma, lung abscess, or aspergillomas.

Suggested Readings

1. Chun Y, Morgan R, Belli AM. Radiological management of hemoptysis: a comprehensive review of diagnostic imaging and bronchial arterial embolization. *Cardiovasc Intervent Radiol*. 2010:33(2):240-250.
2. Davidson K, Shojaee S. Managing massive hemoptysis. *Chest*. 2020:157(1):77-88.
3. Kathuria H, Hollingsworth HM, Vilvendhan R, Reardon C. Management of life-threatening hemoptysis. *J Intensive Care*. 2020;8:23.
4. Radchenko C, Alraiyes AH, Shojaee S. A systematic approach to the management of massive hemoptysis. *J Thorac Dis*. 2017;9(suppl 10):S1069-S1086.

Chapter 2

Lung Volume Reduction Surgery

ANDREA L. AXTELL
HENNING A. GAISSERT

Introduction

- Among the many patients with parenchymal destruction and progressive loss of lung elastic recoil due to chronic obstructive pulmonary disease, there exists a subgroup in whom: (1) large volumes of trapped air in hyperinflated lung increase the total lung volume; (2) generalized emphysema is heterogeneously distributed, leaving substantial, relatively well-preserved regions of unexpanded lung; and (3) respiratory diaphragmatic excursion is reduced or nonexistent as a result.
- Lung volume reduction surgery (LVRS) refers to an operation that selectively removes nonfunctioning lung to improve or restore diaphragmatic function and to reduce ventilation-perfusion mismatch. While the concept of LVRS was first introduced in the 1950s, the clinical success of LVRS was demonstrated four decades later when applied to both lungs using sternotomy. The most precise selection of patients in whom all three of the above-noted conditions are observed yields a small group of candidates, often only 10% to 20% of those referred for evaluation, who require a supervised exercise program to reverse physical deconditioning before the ultimate decision is made to proceed with LVRS.
- Upper lobe–predominant smoking-associated emphysema constitutes the preferred indication for LVRS. Selected patients with lower lobe–predominant disease, usually α_1-antitrypsin deficiency (ATD) emphysema, may undergo this procedure; however, this type of emphysema does not spare any region of the lung, and postoperative results are inferior.
- Careful selection of each candidate and a rigorous preoperative physical preparation are key to a successful outcome. The operative technique consists of standard nonanatomic resection conforming the contour of the remaining lung to pleural space.

Perioperative Considerations

Patient Selection

- LVRS may be considered in patients with the obligatory triad of:
  1. heterogeneously distributed, upper lobe–predominant emphysema (Figure 2.1)
  2. compression of the most preserved lung regions by hyperinflated, functionless lung
  3. impaired diaphragmatic excursion
- While lower lobe–predominant disease (α_1 ATD) may be treated, the best results are obtained with upper lobe–predominant disease.
- Operations on patients with preserved diaphragmatic excursion are futile.
- Exercise deconditioning is accepted at the initial evaluation if pulmonary rehabilitation is possible and improvement is documented prior to operation.
- The preoperative evaluation should include the following:
  - Complete history and physical examination
  - Pulmonary function tests
  - Arterial blood gas analysis (at rest on room air)
  - 6-minute walk test

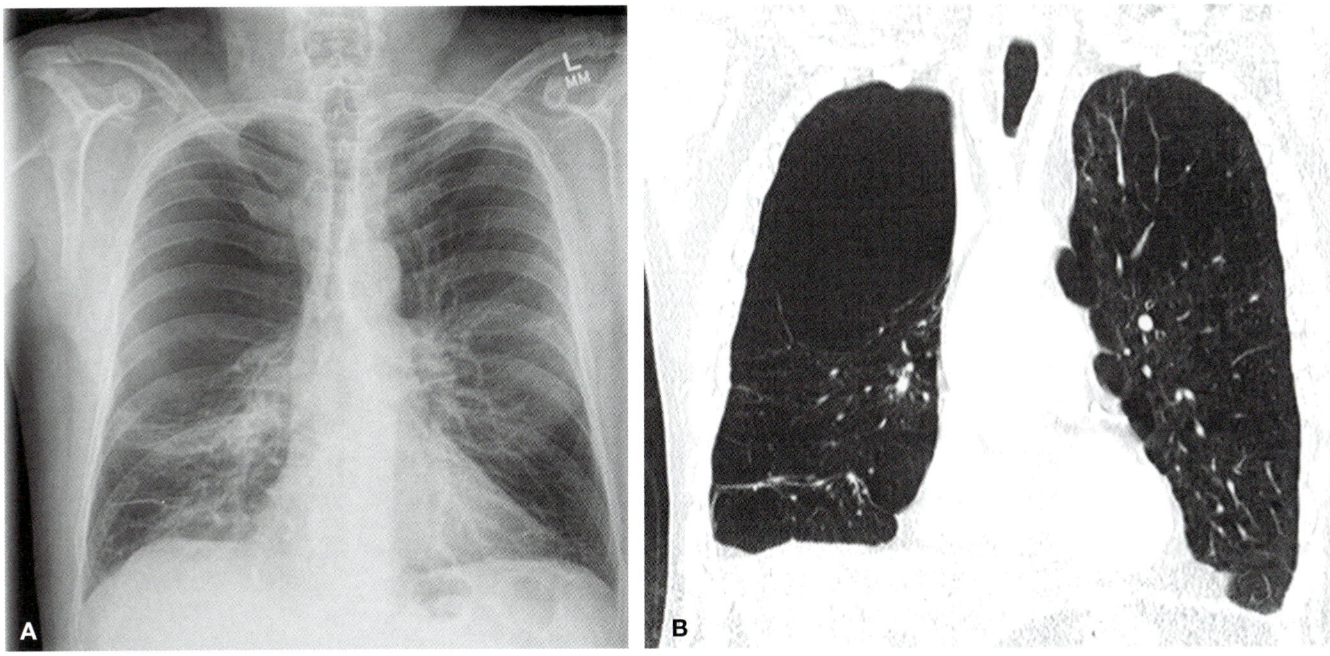

FIGURE 2.1 | Heterogeneous emphysema. **A.** CXR and **B.** CT scan demonstrating a patient with heterogeneous, upper lobe–predominant emphysema.

- Questionnaires assessing quality of life and dyspnea (ex: Nottingham Health Profile or the Medical Outcomes Study 36-Item Short-Form Health Survey)
- Inspiratory and expiratory chest x-ray to assess diaphragmatic excursion (Figure 2.2)
- High-resolution CT chest
- Quantitative V/Q scan
- Evaluation of diaphragmatic excursion by inspiratory and expiratory chest radiographs, magnetic resonance imaging, or fluoroscopy (even though this requirement is not listed in the Centers for Medicare & Medicaid Services [CMS] Coverage Decision Memorandum for LVRS)

- Careful attention should be paid to the evaluation of potential cardiac comorbidities, and all patients should undergo an EKG and echocardiogram. For patients who require stress testing, a dobutamine echo may be difficult to interpret due to hyperinflation and a multiple-gated acquisition scan may be more meaningful.
- CMS "eligibility" criteria for LVRS are summarized in Table 2.1.
- The treatment of giant bullae, defined as loss of any pulmonary architecture involving greater than one-third of one hemithorax in the absence of generalized emphysema, may borrow from the principles of LVRS. Patients selected for bullectomy should demonstrate impaired diaphragmatic excursion, compression of adjacent lung, and symptoms or complication attributable to the bullae such as dyspnea, recurrent pneumothorax, or hemoptysis. The two conditions require careful separation because LVRS is strictly regulated by CMS criteria and conditions, whereas the indication for bullectomy may be determined by the surgeon.

Patient Preparation

- Candidates for surgery should be enrolled in a preoperative pulmonary rehabilitation program, until their walking distance improves. Up to 3 months may be dedicated to this effort, and operation is not assured until preconceived exercise targets are reached.
- Specific components of a pulmonary rehabilitation program include the following:
  - Comprehensive evaluation of medical, psychosocial, and nutritional needs
  - Setting of goals for education and exercise training
  - Exercise training (lower extremity, flexibility, strengthening, and upper extremity)
  - Education about emphysema and medical and surgical treatments
  - Psychosocial counseling
  - Nutritional counseling, with the goal of adjusting body weight to within 20% of the calculated ideal value

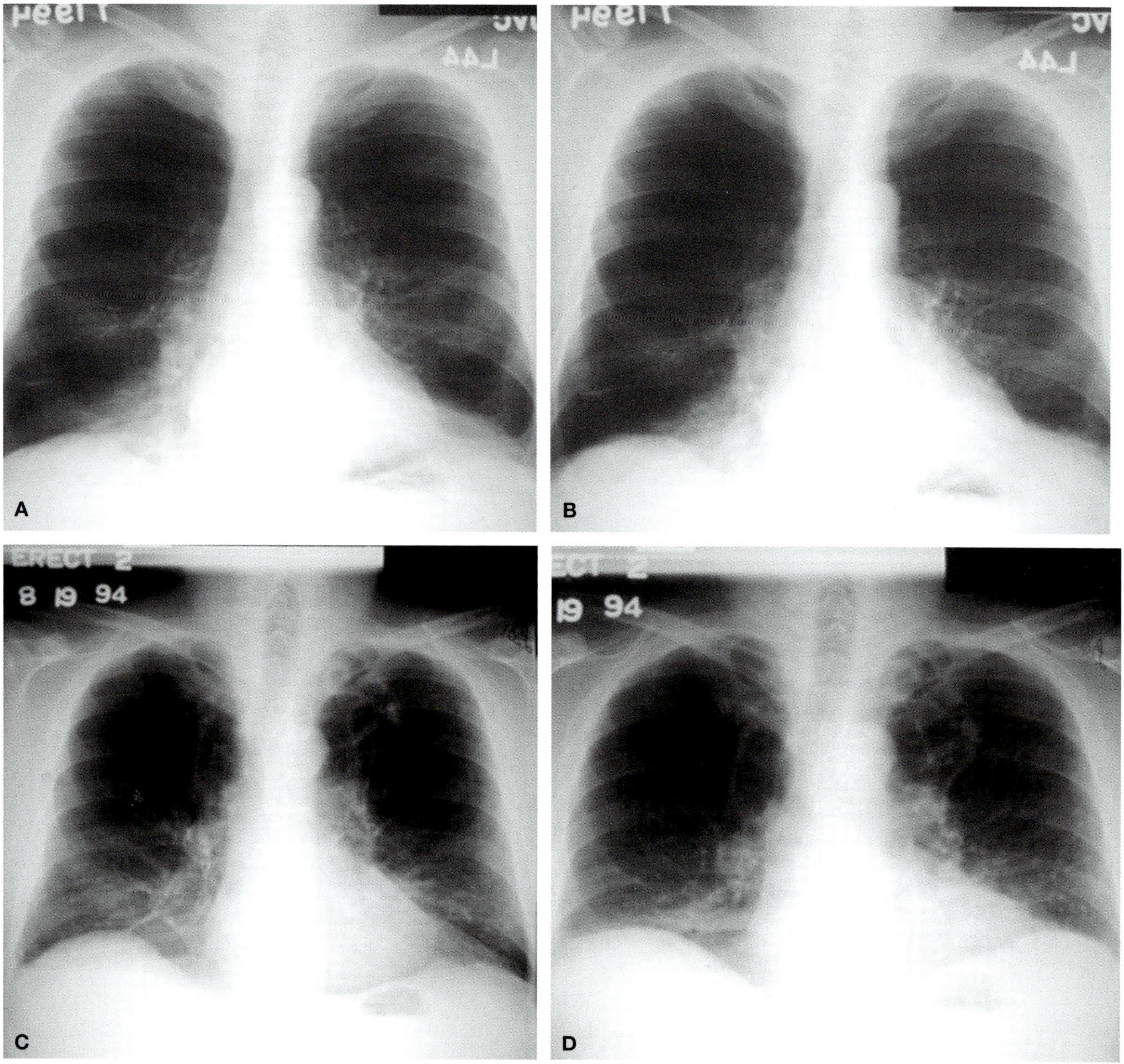

FIGURE 2.2 ▮ Inspiratory and expiratory CXR. **A.** Preoperative inspiratory and **(B)** expiratory CXR compared with **(C)** postoperative inspiratory and **(D)** expiratory CXR in a patient who underwent lung volume reduction surgery.

- At the completion of pulmonary rehabilitation, patients should be assessed with an interval history and physical examination, chest radiography, complete pulmonary function tests, arterial blood gas measurement, 6-minute walk test, and quality-of-life questionnaires.
- Oral steroid therapy is preferably weaned off or at least decreased to a dose below 10 mg/d during pulmonary rehabilitation.
- Lack of improvement results in deferment of operation.

TIPS

- *LVRS improves dyspnea, the need for supplemental oxygen, exercise capacity, lung volumes, and health status in carefully selected patients.*
- *LVRS improves survival in patients with upper lobe–predominant emphysema with low exercise capacity at baseline.*
- *The authors favor bilateral over unilateral LVRS unless a unilateral approach is dictated by anatomy or prior operation.*

TABLE 2.1 | Eligibility Criteria for Lung Volume Reduction Surgery

	Inclusion Criteria	Exclusion Criteria
General	• Dyspnea despite maximal medical therapy and pulmonary rehabilitation • Smoking cessation >6 mo • Completion of pulmonary prehabilitation program	• Current smoking • Surgical considerations (previous thoracic procedures, pleurodesis, chest wall deformity)
Comorbidities		• Pulmonary hypertension (PA systolic pressure >45 mm Hg) • Clinically significant bronchiectasis • Clinically significant CAD • Ejection fraction <45% • Obesity (BMI > 32 kg/m^2)
Respiratory Physiology	• FEV_1 after bronchodilator <45% predicted • Hyperinflation (TLC > 100% predicted or RV > 150% predicted) • Postrehabilitation 6-min walk distance >140 m	• FEV_1 < 20% predicted with either DLCO < 20% or homogenous emphysema • PaO_2 < 45 mm Hg on room air • $PaCO_2$ > 60 mm Hg • Oxygen requirement >6 L/min at rest to maintain O_2 saturation >90% • High functional capacity (maximum workload >25W for women and >40 W for men while cycling for 3 min)
Imaging	• High-resolution CT confirming severe emphysema, ideally with upper lobe predominance	• Heterogeneous emphysema with FEV_1 < 20% predicted • Significant pleural or interstitial changes

BMI, body mass index; CAD, coronary artery disease; DLCO, diffusing capacity of the lungs for carbon monoxide; FEV_1, forced expiratory volume in 1 second; PA, pulmonary artery; RV, residual volume; TLC, total lung capacity.

Technique

Instruments and Equipment for Thoracoscopic LVRS

- 10-mm 30° or 45° thoracoscopic camera
- Ring forceps or atraumatic lung grasper
- Endoscopic GIA stapler with buttressing strips. Where preconfigured buttressed staple cartridges (example: Endo GIA Tri-Staple technology with Reinforced Reload [Medtronic] or Peri-Strips Dry [Baxter]) are not available, strips of bovine pericardium may be tailored and tied to each cartridge and anvil.

Positioning

- For the open technique, patients are positioned for median sternotomy—supine with the arms tucked and a shoulder roll placed under the scapula.
- For the video-assisted thoracic surgery (VATS) technique, patients are positioned in sequential right and left lateral decubitus positions.
- In both cases, patients should be intubated with a double-lumen endotracheal tube. A thoracic epidural should be placed for postoperative analgesia before median sternotomy and may be considered in minimally invasive approaches. All patients should have an arterial catheter placed for serial blood gas analysis.

TIPS

- *LVRS is performed either with open exposure using median sternotomy or by minimally invasive methods assisted with handheld video (VATS) or robotic technique (RATS).*
- *VATS and RATS are preferred due to improved postoperative pain control and enhanced postoperative recovery.*
- *Best results are obtained with bilateral LVRS. The combined morbidity of two unilateral LVRS procedures exceeds that of bilateral LVRS. Unilateral LVRS should only be performed if individual patient findings suggest a one-lung procedure.*

Video-Assisted (VATS) Technique

- As soon as the patient is placed in the lateral decubitus position, single-lung ventilation is instituted because poor elastic recoil and trapped air in the most emphysematous regions cause the isolated lung to decompress very slowly.
- The camera port is placed in the 9th or 10th intercostal space in the mid-axillary line. The position of the utility incision depends on the targeted region or lobe: upper lobe 3rd interspace and lower and middle lobe 4th interspace.
- Entry into the pleural space must occur with caution to avoid immediate injury to the visceral pleura. Adhesions between the lung and any part of the chest wall demand meticulous attention as even small entries into the visceral pleura may result in marked air leaks.
- When destroyed lung tissue fails to collapse, areas of visceral pleura to be removed may be incised to hasten collapse. A single, continuous excision of destroyed lung using sequentially placed cartridges is preferred. In upper lobe–predominant disease and when the minor fissure is incomplete, the staple line may begin on the outer surface of the middle lobe, aiming the direction of excision over the cephalad and posterior portions of the upper lobe so that no part of the staple line touches the phrenic nerve. Complete excision of destroyed lung is avoided; rather, the staple line is placed to preclude excessive tension on the visceral pleura following reinflation.
- The purpose of the operation is to fully expand the relatively compressed middle and lower lobes and to restore the diaphragmatic position to a more normal position.
- Excessive volume reduction creates space problems and may prolong air leak.
- The exact location of the tissue to be resected depends on the preoperative CT scan, ventilation-perfusion scans, and total displacement of volume by the most diseased lobe.
- Reduction of the upper lobe leaves roughly one-third to one-fourth of its volume.
- Staple lines are applied in a continuous line of excision with successive applications of the Endo GIA stapler. The course of the staple line should permit the residual upper lobe to expand fully (rarely if ever should one leave only a stump of the reduced lobe).
- Emphysematous lung tissue does not hold sutures or staples well, and even small defects may generate large air leaks. The staple lines are therefore buttressed with bovine pericardium or Gore-Tex.
- Since some patients require lung transplantation in the future, the staple line should be placed remote from the phrenic nerve.
- The resected lung is removed through the utility incision.
- Two large-bore chest tubes should be placed under direct vision into each pleural space.
- Reexpanding the lung after reduction must be done with the greatest care to avoid creating air leaks and requires close cooperation between the anesthesiologist and surgeon. Because of destroyed architecture, small pleural holes may easily result in the loss of one-third of the entire tidal volume into the pleural space. Such holes must be either avoided or closed when found.
- Ideal reexpansion results in a lung filling the pleural space, a diaphragm regaining near-normal excursion, and staple lines opposing the chest wall.
- If a sizable apical space remains at the end of the procedure, an apical pleural tent may be fashioned so that the parietal and visceral pleura are in apposition, even if the residual lung fails to fill the apex of the pleural space.

Open Technique

- Following incision and prior to sternal division, the retrosternal space is dissected with a sponge stick, sweeping the pleura away from the midline on either side to avoid injury to the lung from the sternal saw.
- Disconnect the endotracheal tube and wait as long as the patient can tolerate to allow the lungs to decompress prior to sternal division.
- Place a sternal retractor and carefully incise the mediastinal pleura, taking care to avoid injury to the phrenic nerve.
- Divide the pulmonary ligament up the inferior pulmonary vein.
- Identify the target lung for reduction and select a long projected path for the staple line beginning medially and coursing laterally and posteriorly, staying away from the mediastinal pleura.
- Great care should be taken to avoid extending the staple line across the major or a complete minor fissure as this often causes significant air leaks.
- All staple lines are buttressed to decrease the incidence of postoperative air leak.

- Two large-bore chest tubes are placed on either side and brought out through the upper abdomen in a subxiphoid position.
- The parietal pleura is closed bilaterally and then the sternotomy is closed in layers.
- A pleural tent maneuver is employed as needed. Pleurodesis is rarely considered during the initial operation.

TIPS

- *The goal of the operation is to wedge the most hyperinflated segment of the lung, not completely excise all emphysematous disease—all you want to accomplish is to improve the V/Q mismatch and expand the lower lobe. As Brantigan and colleagues noted in their initial report in 1959, "It is an operation directed at restoring a physiologic principle, it is not concerned with the removal of pathologic tissue."*
- *Excessive air leaks prolong hospital stay. Thus, a leak-free staple line is of paramount importance, and buttressing the staple line is the usual method to minimize air leaks.*

Postoperative Care

- Extubation in the operating room must be the stated goal, and any deviation from this goal should be considered between the surgeon and the anesthesiologist before the operation is commenced. Any elements facilitating extubation, particularly additional observation and patience, must be employed before overnight intubation is accepted. A patient with advanced emphysema who remains intubated during the first postoperative night is at far greater risk of postoperative complications.
- Anesthetic techniques to avoid coughing against the endotracheal tube, first and foremost removal of the endotracheal tube before the patient is aroused, should be employed in the prevention of sudden air leaks. The process of awakening may take an hour or more, and patience is advised.
- Often, the awakening patient complains of air hunger and inability to breathe; this sensation has two potential causes: inadequate pain control or excessive narcotic administration. Careful attention is required to strike the appropriate balance.
- The most common arterial blood gas abnormality is hypercapnia, and initial values in excess of 90 mm Hg are not uncommon. Close bedside observation with adjustment of pain medications or assisted breaths, either in the operating room or in the postanesthesia care unit, is advised. With correct management, pCO_2 will usually decline over time. Reintubation should be avoided.
- Chest tubes are immediately placed to water seal. Gentle suction is applied only if there is massive subcutaneous emphysema or a large pneumothorax that limits inflation of the remaining lung.
- Three problems predominate in the early postoperative period: sputum retention, air leaks, and lingering effects of preoperative deconditioning. Inadequate preoperative preparation and marginal operative candidacy are exposed mercilessly early after operation.
  1. Sputum retention—consider early bronchoscopy or minitracheostomy for tracheal suction in patients with thick secretions and a feeble cough.
  2. Air leaks—may lead to a loss of total vital capacity. In refractory cases with large loss, reexploration may be needed to close even small pleural holes. For modest leaks that persist beyond the first 4 to 5 postoperative days, the chest tube can be connected to a Heimlich valve to facilitate patient mobility and discharge from the hospital. All chest tubes should remain until the last air leak closes. After bilateral **open** LVRS and closure of air leaks on one side, a single chest tube should remain until the last air leak closes as both pleural spaces are connected.
  3. Deconditioning—a team of specialized chest physiotherapists and experienced thoracic surgical nurses should provide vigorous chest physiotherapy and encourage early ambulation. A "step-down unit" is the preferred location for early postoperative management, since ambulation may be challenging to organize in an intensive care unit.
- Early involvement of a pulmonologist, ideally the one who has met the patient before the operation, is helpful.

PEARLS AND PITFALLS

- Appropriate patient selection is the most important factor for successful LVRS.
- LVRS improves survival in patients with upper lobe–predominant emphysema with low exercise capacity at baseline.
- High-risk patients with an FEV_1 < 20% predicted with either DLCO < 20% or homogenous emphysema have an increased risk of mortality and should not be offered LVRS.
- Involved lung should be resected with a single continuous line of excision with successive applications of a buttressed stapler.
- Postoperatively chest tubes should be placed to water seal and patients encouraged to participate in vigorous chest physiotherapy and early ambulation.

Suggested Readings

1. Ciccone AM, Meyers BF, Guthrie TJ, et al. Long-term outcome of bilateral lung volume reduction in 250 consecutive patients with emphysema. *J Thorac Cardiovasc Surg*. 2003;125(3):513-525.
2. Cooper J. Lung volume reduction surgery. *Operat Tech Thorac Cardiovasc Surg*. 2007;12(2):150-159.
3. Cooper JD, Patterson GA, Sundaresan RS, et al. Results of 150 consecutive bilateral lung volume reduction procedures in patients with severe emphysema. *J Thorac Cardiovasc Surg*. 1996;112(5):1319-1330.
4. Fishman AP, Bozzarello BA, Al-Amin A, et al. Safety and efficacy of median sternotomy versus video-assisted thoracic surgery for lung volume reduction surgery. *J Thorac Cardiovasc Surg*. 2004;127(5):1350-1360.
5. Gaissert HA, Trulock EP, Cooper JD, et al. Comparison of early functional results after volume reduction or lung transplantation for chronic obstructive pulmonary disease. *J Thorac Cardiovasc Surg*. 1996;111(2):296-307.
6. Geddes D, Davies M, Koyama H, et al. Effect of lung-volume-reduction surgery in patients with severe emphysema. *N Engl J Med* 2000;343(4):239-245.
7. Gierada DS, Yusen RD, Villanueva IA, et al. Patient selection for lung volume reduction surgery: an objective model based on prior clinical decisions and quantitative CT analysis. *Chest*. 2000;117(4):991-998.
8. McCarthy DP, Taylor LJ, DeCamp MM. Analysis of recent literature on lung volume reduction surgery. *Thorac Surg Clin*. 2021;31(2):119-128.
9. McKenna RJ. Thoracoscopic lung volume reduction surgery. *Operat Tech Thorac Cardiovasc Surg*. 2007;12(2):141-149.
10. Meyers BF, Yusen RD, Guthrie TJ, et al. Outcome of bilateral lung volume reduction in patients with emphysema potentially eligible for lung transplantation. *J Thorac Cardiovasc Surg*. 2001;122(1):10-17.
11. Meyers BF, Yusen RD, Guthrie TJ, et al. Results of lung volume reduction surgery in patients meeting a National Emphysema Treatment Trial high-risk criterion. *J Thorac Cardiovasc Surg*. 2004;127(3):829-835.
12. National Emphysema Treatment Trial Research Group; Fishman A, Fessler H, Martinez F, et al. Patients at high risk of death after lung-volume-reduction surgery. *N Engl J Med*. 2001;345(15):1075-1083.
13. Naunheim KS, Wood DE, Krasna MJ, et al. Predictors of operative mortality and cardiopulmonary morbidity in the national emphysema treatment trial. *J Thorac Cardiovasc Surg*. 2006;131(1):43-53.
14. Piantadosi S, Rodarte J, Miller C, et al. Rationale and design of the National Emphysema Treatment Trial (NETT): a prospective randomized trial of lung volume reduction surgery. *J Thorac Cardiovasc Surg*. 1999;118(3):518-528.
15. Stanifer PB, Ginsburg ME. Lung volume reduction surgery in the post-National Emphysema Treatment Trial era. *J Thorac Dis*. 2018;10(suppl 23):S2744-S2747.

Chapter 3

Image-Guided Minimally Invasive Wedge Resection of Small Lung Nodules

CAMERON D. WRIGHT
MICHAEL LANUTI

Perioperative Considerations

- Small incidentally discovered suspicious lung nodules are increasingly found on CT scans done for other purposes or for lung cancer screening.
  - Clinical factors determine which lung nodules should be resected based upon their probability of being a lung cancer. Important prognostic factors that favor lung cancer include a history of smoking, age, history of progressive growth, a spiculated margin, a semisolid lesion with a solid more central component, positron emission tomography avidity, and size.
  - Suspicious nodules that are big enough can often be pathologically diagnosed either with a CT-guided fine-needle aspiration or a navigation-guided transbronchial lung biopsy if appropriate. Alternatively wedge resection for both diagnosis and again if appropriate for therapeutic reasons can be performed.
- There are many possible imaging techniques used in different centers for localization of lung nodules to be resected. These include CT-guided placement of a hookwire, injection of dyes either by CT guidance or by bronchoscopic techniques, CT-guided or bronchoscopic placement of microcoils, injection of contrast agents, and injection of radiotracers. Our institution favors CT-guided placement of fiducials for nodule marking.
- In general, minimally invasive wedge resection techniques are useful for nodules present in the outer one-third of the lung. Anatomic segmentectomy is often required for more central nodules.

Patient Positioning

- Patients are positioned in a standard lateral decubitus position with single-lung ventilation.
- All pressure points are padded and care is taken not to overextend the arms to prevent stretching of the brachial plexus.
- The table is typically slightly flexed to open up the rib spaces and separate the chest from the anterior superior iliac spine.
- The operating room table must be positioned such that the fluoroscopy machine can be positioned under the table.

Instruments and Equipment

- If a video-assisted thoracoscopic surgery (VATS) approach is used, standard ports and long instruments are used.
- If a robotic approach is used, standard ports and robotic instruments are used. We typically use CO_2 insufflation with robotic lung surgery and a 15-mm assistant port.
- If a VATS approach is used, standard endoscopic staplers are used. If a robotic approach is used, either the robotic staplers can be used if desired or alternatively standard endoscopic staplers can be used through the assistant port.

- Fluoroscopy equipment should be brought into the operating room by the radiology technicians, but typically the final setup is not done until all ports are placed and the surgeon is ready to localize the nodule and carry out the resection.
- It is very helpful to have the CT scan images up in the operating room typically with both the axial and either the coronal or sagittal views to guide the surgeon performing a localization wedge resection.

Technique

TIPS

Nodules that are essentially subpleural and nodules on an acute angle of the lung are easiest to remove by wedge resection.

Using the suspected location based on the preoperative imaging, a long narrow instrument is placed over the suspected site of the nodule. Thereafter, the fluoroscopy equipment is brought in and centered over the suspected nodule position and fluoroscopy performed to localize the fiducials. The fluoroscopy machine can be rotated if necessary to better identify the fiducials in a 3D fashion (Figures 3.1-3.3).

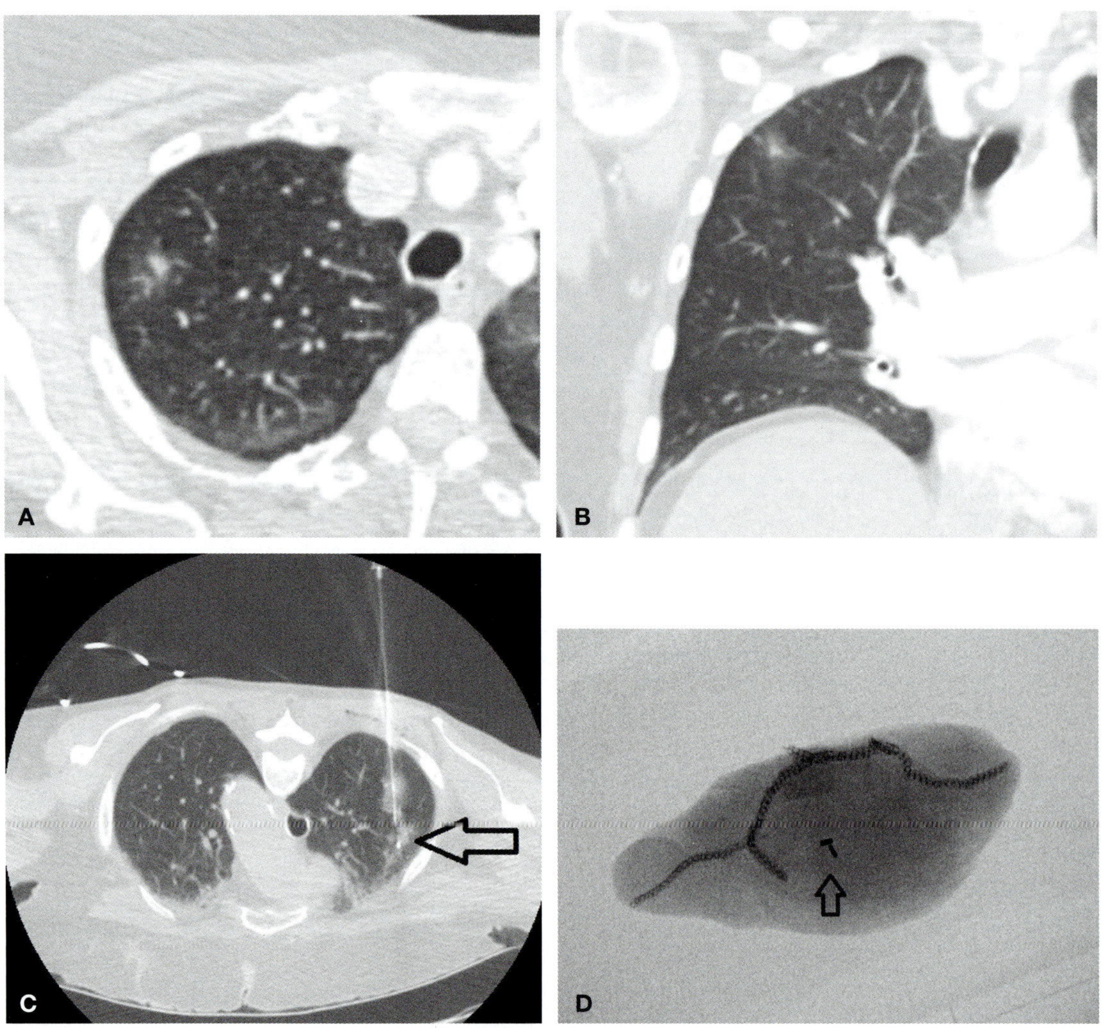

FIGURE 3.1 ▌ A. Axial CT image from a 72-year-old woman with a slowly growing semisolid right upper lobe lung nodule. **B.** Coronal view of the same nodule. **C.** Thoracic interventional radiology needle placement of two small gold fiducials (arrow). **D.** Radiograph of wedge resection specimen demonstrating fiducials (marked by an arrow) in the center of specimen. The nodule was a T1a 1.1-cm adenocarcinoma with a 9-mm area of an invasive component, 65% acinar, 20% lepidic, 10% papillary, and 5% solid.

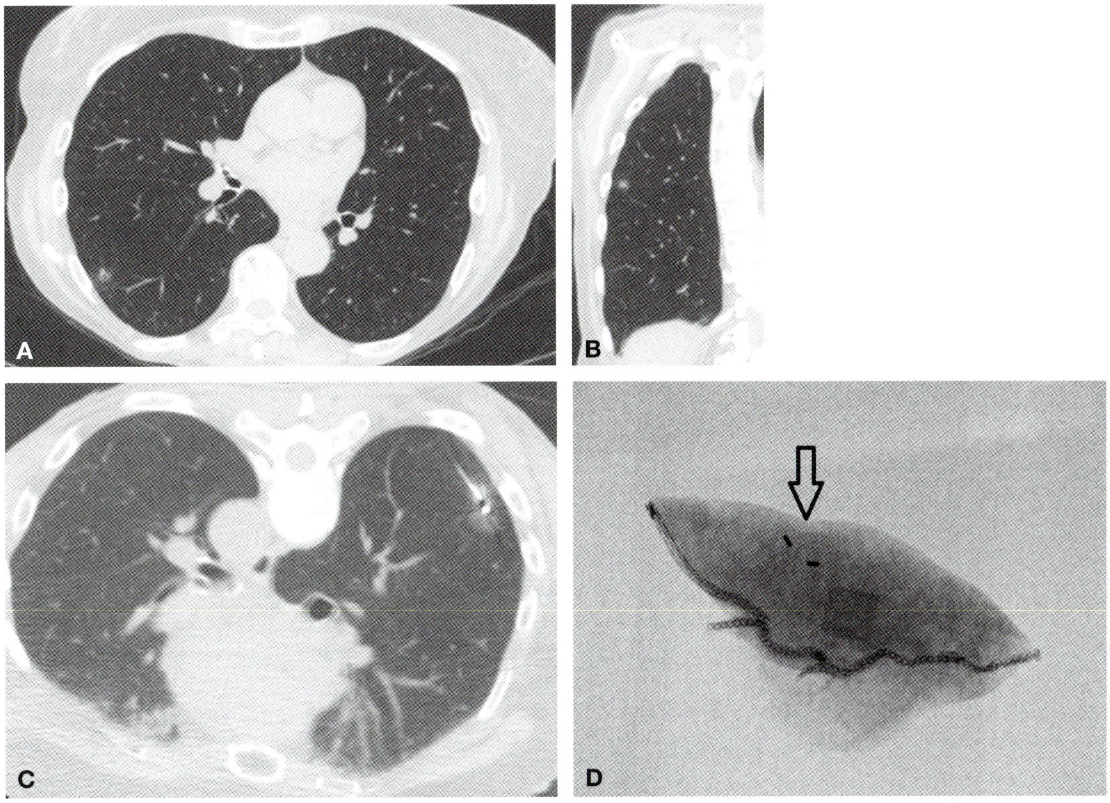

FIGURE 3.2 ▌ **A.** Axial CT image from a 65-year-old woman with a slowly growing partly cystic right lower lobe lung nodule. **B.** Coronal view of the same nodule. **C.** Thoracic interventional radiology needle placement of two small gold fiducials. **D.** Radiograph of wedge resection specimen demonstrating fiducials (marked by an arrow) in the center of the specimen. The nodule was T1mi 8-mm adenocarcinoma with a 4-mm invasive component, 60% lepidic and 40% acinar.

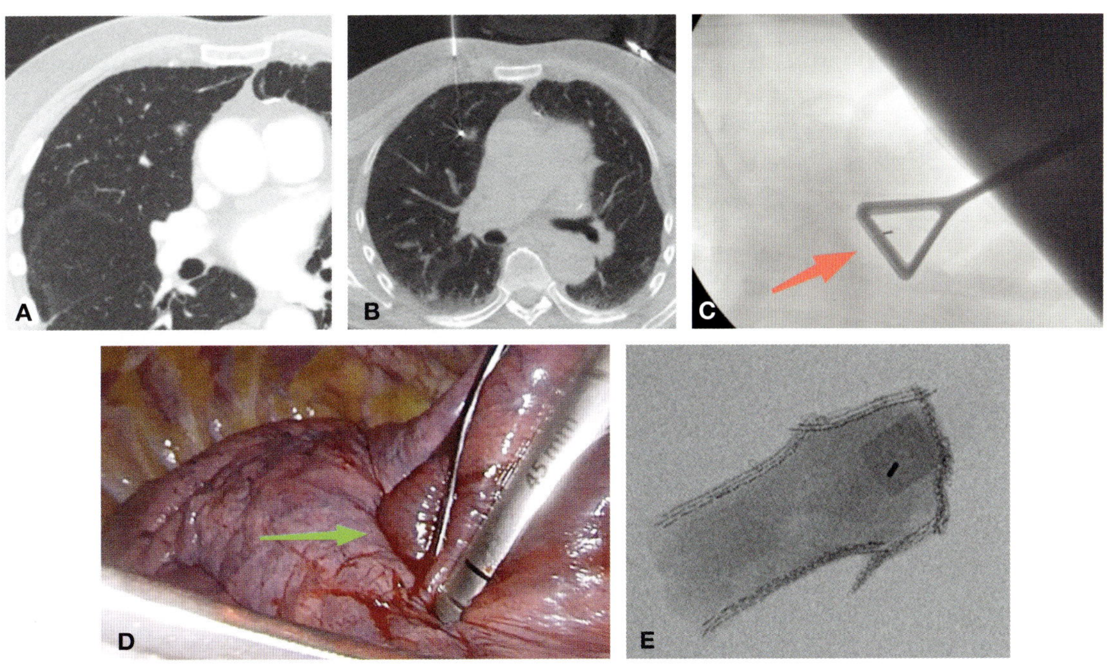

FIGURE 3.3 ▌ **A.** Axial CT image from a 76-year-old man with a history of a previous resection of a left T1a adenocarcinoma many years ago with a slowly growing right upper lobe semisolid 9-mm lung nodule that was mildly PET avid. **B.** Thoracic interventional radiology needle placement of gold fiducials adjacent to the lesion at the proposed deep resection margin. **C.** Intraoperative image from fluoroscopy unit demonstrating a lung clamp grasping the right upper lobe lung nodule with fiducial guidance (arrow). **D.** Intraoperative picture of an endostapler being applied to begin wedge resection of small lung nodules. **E.** Radiograph of wedge resection specimen demonstrating fiducials in the specimen. The nodule was a mucosa-associated lymphoid tumor (MALToma).

- The closest pleural surface to the nodule can be marked with one or two cautery applications to help guide the wedge resection.
- Depending upon the location of the nodule, two atraumatic lung grasping forceps are used to present the lung in such a fashion to allow easy stapler application as well as continuous monitoring of the location of the fiducials with fluoroscopy.
- The appropriate length and size of stapler is then introduced with the aid of both the cauterized pleural markings, ensuring the fiducials are well beyond the staple line to ensure a complete resection of the nodule is performed. Fiducials are placed typically at the deep margin of the nodule such that resection more central to the fiducials ensures a complete resection.
- Intermittent spot fluoroscopy is typically done to minimize total radiation dose.
- Once the resection is done, the specimen is placed in a bag and withdrawn through the largest port.
- The wedge resection specimen is then immediately x-rayed by the radiology technician to ensure the fiducials are in the resected specimen.
- The specimen is then typically sent for frozen section analysis for both the histology on the lesion and to check the margin status.
- The surgeon should have a preoperative plan that was previously discussed with the patient as to what extent resection should be performed based upon patient and pathology characteristics.
  - If an anatomic segmentectomy or formal lobectomy needs to be performed, the fluoroscopy equipment can be removed and the surgeon can carry on with the formal resection.
  - Mediastinal and hilar lymph node sampling or dissection should be done as appropriate.
- Multiple intercostal nerve blocks are done with a long needle with a long-acting local anesthetic at the conclusion of the resection.
- A chest tube is placed and the lung reexpanded under direct vision followed by closure of the port sites.

PEARLS AND PITFALLS

- Nodules that are essentially subpleural and nodules on an acute angle of the lung are easiest to remove by wedge resection.
- Deeper nodules underlying the broad surface of the lung are often very challenging to remove and often require anatomic segmentectomy to remove.
- The ports should be sized and placed such that the stapler can be introduced either anteriorly or posteriorly depending upon the exact location of the nodule. Sometimes stapling needs to start from one port position and then be transferred over to a different port position to optimize resection margins.
- An advantage of the CT-guided fiducial placement approach is that if the nodule is large enough and accessible, a biopsy of the nodule can be performed by the radiologist at the same time as the fiducial placement. This can help guide preoperative decision-making with the patient as well as intraoperative decision-making.

Suggested Readings

1. Cornella KN, Repper DC, Palafox BA, et al. A surgeon's guide for various lung nodule localization techniques and the newest technologies. *Innovations*. 2021;16(1):26-33.
2. Hung CT, Chen CK, Chang YY, et al. Electromagnetic navigation-guided versus computed tomography-guided percutaneous localization of small lung nodules before uniportal video-assisted thoracoscopic surgery: a propensity scored matched analysis. *Eur J Cariothorac Surg*. 2020;58(suppl 1):S185-S191.
3. Lin MW, Chen JS. Image guided techniques for localizing pulmonary nodules in thoracoscopic surgery. *J Thorac Dis*. 2016;8(suppl 9):S749-S755.
4. Nagi K, Kuriyama K, Inoue A, et al. Computed tomography-guided preoperative localization of small lung nodules with indocyanine green. *Acta Radiol*. 2018;59:830-835.
5. Sharma A, McDermott S, Mathisen D, Shepard JAO. Preoperative localization of lung nodules with fiducial markers: feasibility and technical considerations. *Ann Thorac Surg*. 2017;103(4):1114-1120.

Chapter 4

Segmentectomy: Robotic, Video-Assisted Thoracoscopic Surgery, and Thoracotomy

IOANA BAIU
DAVID S. DEMOS
NATALIE S. LUI

Perioperative Considerations

- Segmentectomy is a sublobar lung resection defined as removing a segment or segments by individually dividing the segmental branches of the pulmonary artery, pulmonary vein, and bronchus, as well as the parenchyma in the intersegmental plane.
- The established indication for segmentectomy is an American Joint Committee on Cancer eighth edition T1a-bN0M0 (diameter 2 cm or smaller) peripheral lung cancer in a patient with impaired lung function who is not a candidate for lobectomy. More recently, segmentectomy has been used even in patients who are eligible for lobectomy, particularly for slowly growing, part solid tumors. Other indications include multiple primary lung cancers or metastases in which sparing parenchyma is an important goal, as well as infectious or inflammatory processes.
- Preoperative chest CT with IV contrast with thin cuts is performed to delineate the segmental anatomy. Reviewing axial, coronal, and sagittal images is helpful to confirm that the tumor is located well within a segment and identify anatomic variations.
- Lymph node involvement precludes segmentectomy. Preoperative CT chest with IV contrast and PET/CT are reviewed, and pathologic lymph node staging with endobronchial ultrasound or mediastinoscopy is considered if any lymph nodes have a short-axis diameter more than 1 cm or maximum standardized uptake value more than 2.5.
- Bronchoscopy is performed in the operating room to evaluate the bronchial anatomy for any variations that may affect single-lung ventilation or the surgical plan.
- The right lung has 10 segments, and the left lung has 8 segments (Figure 4.1). The most commonly performed segmentectomies are of the apical (S1), superior (S6), basilar (S7-10), left upper division (S1-3), and lingular segments (S4-5). We review the steps of these procedures here.

Instruments and Equipment

- Segmentectomy is usually performed with a minimally invasive approach, either video-assisted thoracoscopic surgery or robot-assisted surgery. Open segmentectomy is generally performed only when additional lung resections requiring an open approach are planned, such as in metastasectomy.
- The instruments and equipment used in segmentectomy are similar to those used in lobectomy. Smaller pulmonary artery branches may warrant the use of smaller staplers or vessel-sealing devices.

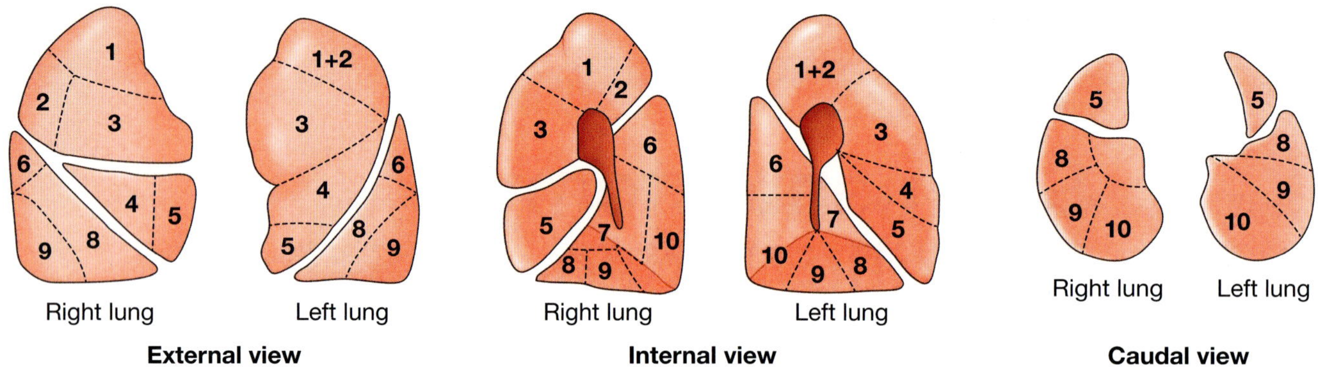

FIGURE 4.1 ▮ Classification of segments.

Positioning

- Single-lung ventilation is obtained using a double-lumen endotracheal tube or bronchial blocker. The double-lumen endotracheal tube allows intraoperative bronchoscopy while maintaining single-lung ventilation.
- Patients are positioned in lateral decubitus with the operating table flexed to widen the intercostal spaces.

TIPS

- *There are several ways to confirm that the correct segmental bronchus is identified. Intraoperative bronchoscopy through the double-lumen endotracheal tube is used to verify the anatomy. Alternatively, the lung is ventilated after the stapler is closed on the segmental bronchus to ensure the remaining segments are ventilated before firing.*
- *The parenchymal margin must be adequate, ideally at least 2 cm or the diameter of the tumor. For tumors near the edge of a segment, the parenchyma can be divided to include tissue from an adjacent segment, making sure to preserve its segmental vessels and bronchi. Preoperative CT-guided or bronchoscopic localization may be helpful to ensure an adequate parenchymal margin. If the margin is not adequate, conversion to lobectomy is considered.*
- *Lymph node staging of segmental, hilar, and mediastinal lymph nodes is performed. If there is any lymph node involvement, conversion to lobectomy is considered.*
- *There are several methods to identify the intersegmental plane when dividing the lung parenchyma. Indocyanine green is given intravenously after the segment has been devascularized; near-infrared cameras show fluorescence in the surrounding segments but not in the target segment. Alternatively, the lung is ventilated after the bronchus is divided; the surrounding segments inflate, but the target segment remains collapsed. Sometimes there are clefts or accessory fissures that help in identification.*

Technique

Right Apical (S1) Segmentectomy

- The right upper lobe contains the apical (S1), posterior (S2), and anterior (S3) segments (Figure 4.1). Right apical (S1) segmentectomy is the most commonly performed procedure and usually completed from anterior to posterior (Figure 4.2).
- The lung is retracted posteriorly, and the apical (V1) vein is isolated and divided. It is the most superior branch of the superior pulmonary vein and lies anterior to the truncus anterior branch of the pulmonary artery (Figure 4.2A).
- The lung is retracted inferiorly, and the station 10R lymph node between the azygos vein and right main bronchus is excised. The truncus anterior artery is dissected until the apical (A1) and anterior (A3) arteries are exposed (Figure 4.2B).

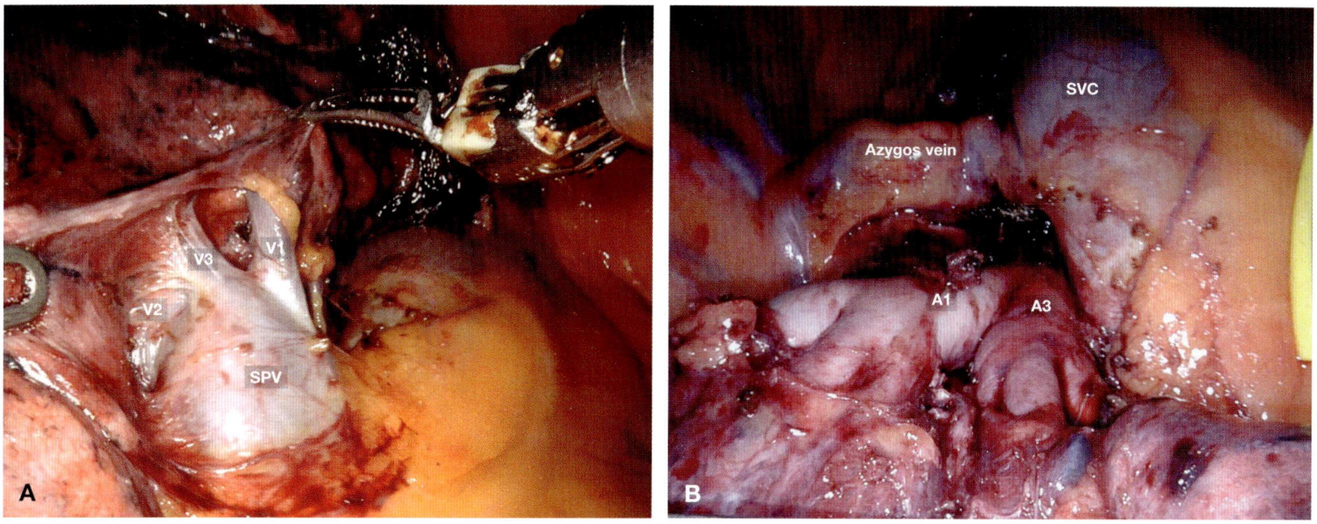

FIGURE 4.2 ▌ Right apical (S1) segmentectomy. **A.** The apical (V1) vein is dissected anteriorly. **B.** The apical (A1) artery is dissected superiorly. SPV, superior pulmonary vein. SVC, superior vena cava.

- The apical (B1) bronchus is isolated and divided. It is the most superior branch of the right upper lobe bronchus, and dissection from a posterior approach is often helpful.
- The lung parenchyma is divided in the intersegmental plane.

Superior (S6) Segmentectomy

- The lower lobes contain the superior (S6) and basilar (S7-10) segments (Figure 4.1). Superior segmentectomy is usually straightforward, with the vein dissected inferiorly and the artery then bronchus dissected in the fissure. A right superior (S6) segmentectomy is described here (Figure 4.3).
- Lymph node dissection, particularly removal of station 11RS lymph nodes between the right upper lobe bronchus and bronchus intermedius, facilitates subsequent division of the posterior fissure and dissection of the superior segmental (B6) bronchus. Care must be taken because the superior segmental (A6) artery lies deep to these lymph nodes.
- The lung is retracted superiorly, and the inferior pulmonary ligament is divided. The inferior pulmonary vein is dissected distally, and the superior segmental (V6) vein is distinguished from the basilar (V7-10) vein and divided. It is the most superior branch of the inferior pulmonary vein (Figure 4.3A).
- The pulmonary artery is identified in the fissure, and the superior segmental (A6) artery is identified and divided (Figure 4.3B). It usually originates across from the middle lobe (A4-5) artery.
- The posterior aspect of the major fissure is divided, connecting the space between the superior segmental (A6) artery and the posterior segmental (A2) artery to the space between the right upper lobe bronchus and bronchus intermedius where station 11RS lymph nodes were removed earlier.
- The superior segmental (B6) bronchus is identified and divided (Figure 4.3C). It is often easier to identify posteriorly rather than in the fissure.
- The lung parenchyma is divided in the intersegmental plane. Indocyanine green is used to identify the plane between the superior segment (S6) and basilar segments (S7-10) (Figure 4.3D).

Basilar (S7-10) Segmentectomy

- The basilar segments include the medial (S7) (only on the right side), anterior (S8), lateral (S9), and posterior (S10) segments (Figure 4.1). They are most commonly resected together. A left basilar (S7-10) segmentectomy is described here (Figure 4.4).
- The pulmonary artery is identified in the fissure. The basilar (A7-10) artery is distinguished from the superior segmental (A6) artery and divided (Figure 4.4A). The superior segmental (A6) artery usually originates opposite the lingular (A4-5) artery.
- The lung is retracted superiorly, and the inferior pulmonary ligament is divided. The inferior pulmonary vein is dissected distally, and the basilar (V7-10) vein is distinguished from the superior segmental (V6) vein and divided. It is the inferior branch of the inferior pulmonary vein (Figure 4.4B).
- The basilar (B7-10) bronchus is distinguished from the superior segmental (B6) bronchus and divided (Figure 4.4C).
- The lung parenchyma is divided in the intersegmental plane.

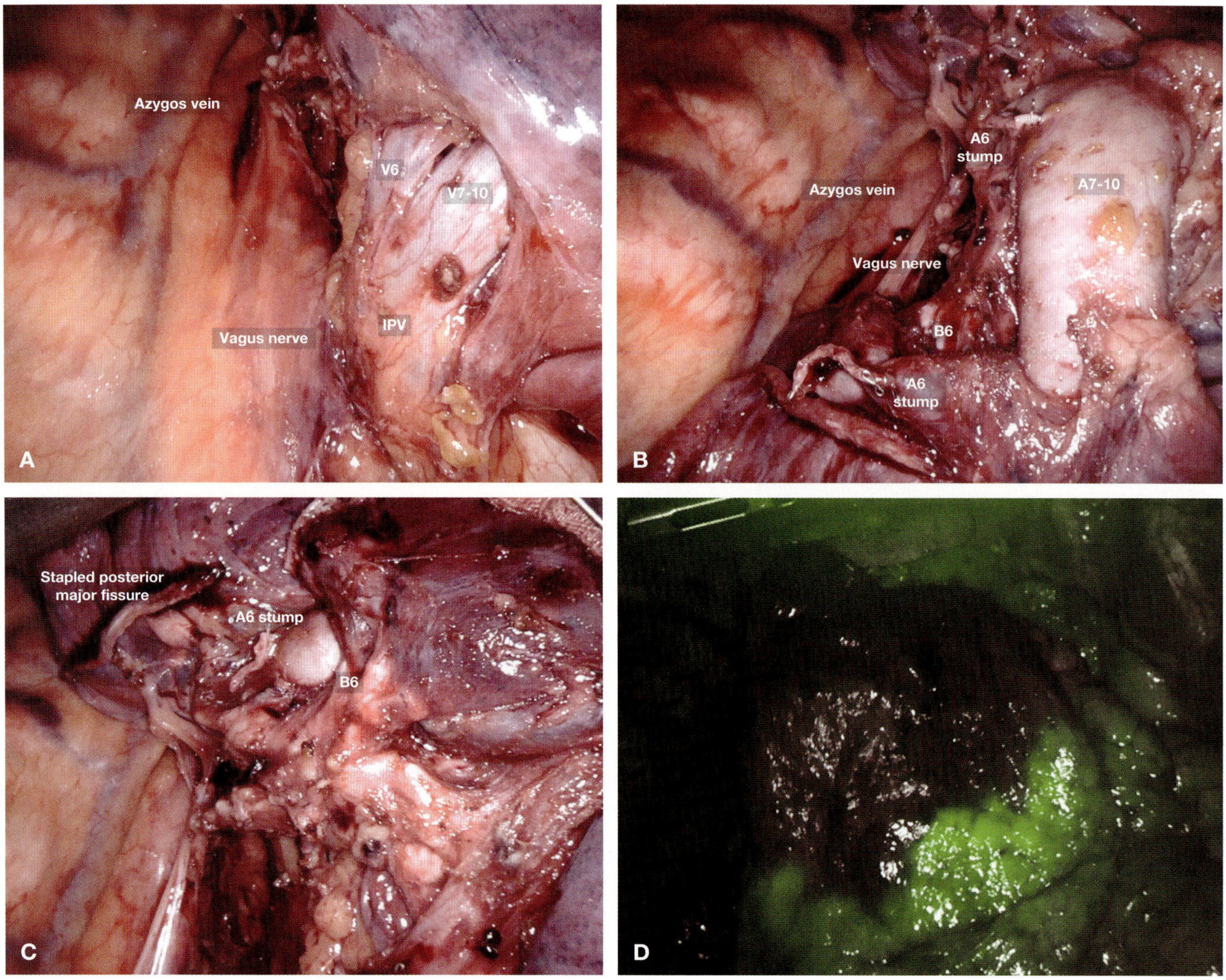

FIGURE 4.3 | Right superior (S6) segmentectomy. **A.** The superior segmental (V6) vein is dissected inferiorly. **B.** The superior segmental (A6) artery is divided in the fissure. **C.** The superior segmental (B6) bronchus is identified posteriorly. **D.** Intravenous indocyanine green is given after the superior segment is devascularized to identify the intersegmental plane between the superior (S6) segment and the basilar (S7-10) segments. IPV, inferior pulmonary vein.

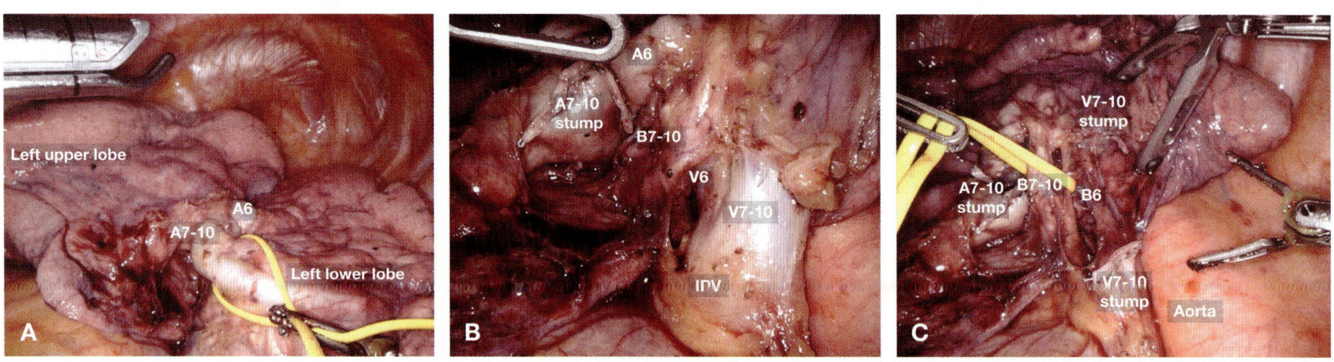

FIGURE 4.4 | Left basilar (S7-10) segmentectomy. **A.** The basilar (A7-10) artery is dissected in the fissure and encircled with a vessel loop. **B.** The basilar (V7-10) vein is identified inferiorly. **C.** Basilar bronchus is dissected inferiorly and encircled with a vessel loop. IPV, inferior pulmonary vein.

Left Upper Division (S1-3) Segmentectomy

- The left upper lobe contains the upper division, which contains the apicoposterior (S1+2) and anterior (S3) segments, and the lingula, which contains the superior (S4) and inferior (S5) segments (Figure 4.1). Left upper division (S1-3) segmentectomy is also known as left apical trisegmentectomy or lingula-sparing left upper lobectomy (Figure 4.5). This procedure is more common than individual left upper lobe segmentectomies, which are more challenging.

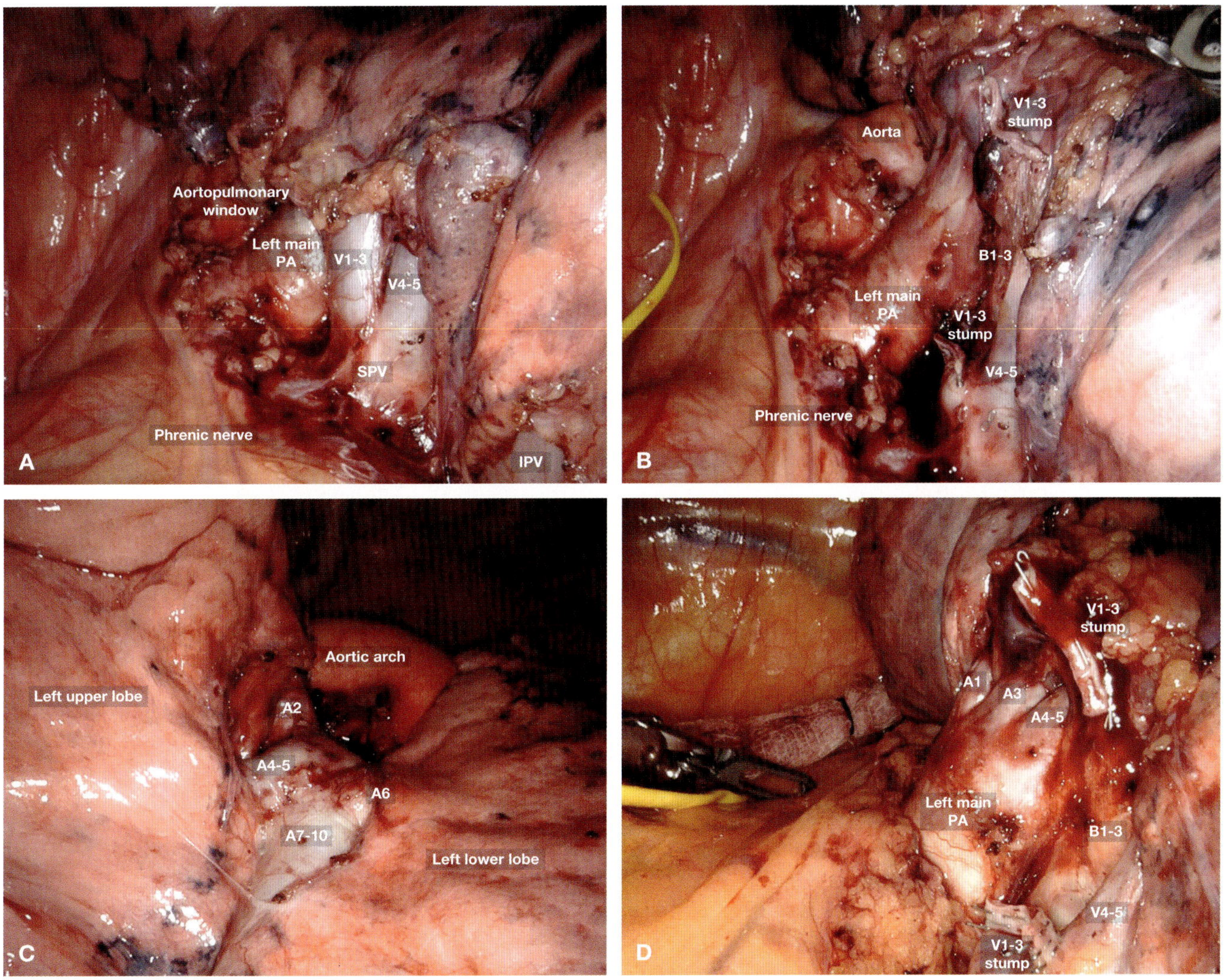

FIGURE 4.5 ‖ Left upper division (S1-3) segmentectomy. **A.** The upper division (V1-3) vein is distinguished from the lingular (V4-5) vein anteriorly. **B.** V1-3 is divided, exposing more of the pulmonary artery. **C.** The pulmonary artery branches are identified in the fissure. **D.** Arterial anatomic variant with lingular (A4-5) artery originating proximally adjacent to upper division (A4-5) arteries. PA, pulmonary artery. SPV, superior pulmonary vein. IPV, inferior pulmonary vein.

- The lung is retracted posteriorly, and the superior pulmonary vein is identified and dissected distally until the upper division (V1-3) veins are separated from the lingula (V4-5) veins (Figure 4.5A). The upper division (V1-3) veins are divided, exposing the left main pulmonary artery (Figure 4.5B).
- The pulmonary artery is identified in the fissure, as well as the upper division (A1-3) from the lingular (A4-5) branches. The lingular (A4-5) arteries usually originate opposite the superior segmental (A6) artery (Figure 4.5C).
- The upper division (B1-3) bronchus is delineated from the lingular (B4-5) bronchus and divided.
- The lung parenchyma is divided in the intersegmental plane.
- One anatomic variation is the lingular (A4-5) artery originating at the same level as the upper division (A1-3) arteries from the proximal left main pulmonary artery (Figure 4.5D). This variant can

make this lingula-sparing approach difficult to complete as the A4-5 artery courses anterior to the origin of the B1-3 bronchus. In this instance, dissection of the bronchus from a cephalad view is usually necessary and challenging to complete as the view is suboptimal.

Lingular (S4-5) Segmentectomy

- Lingulectomy is another common segmentectomy (Figure 4.6).

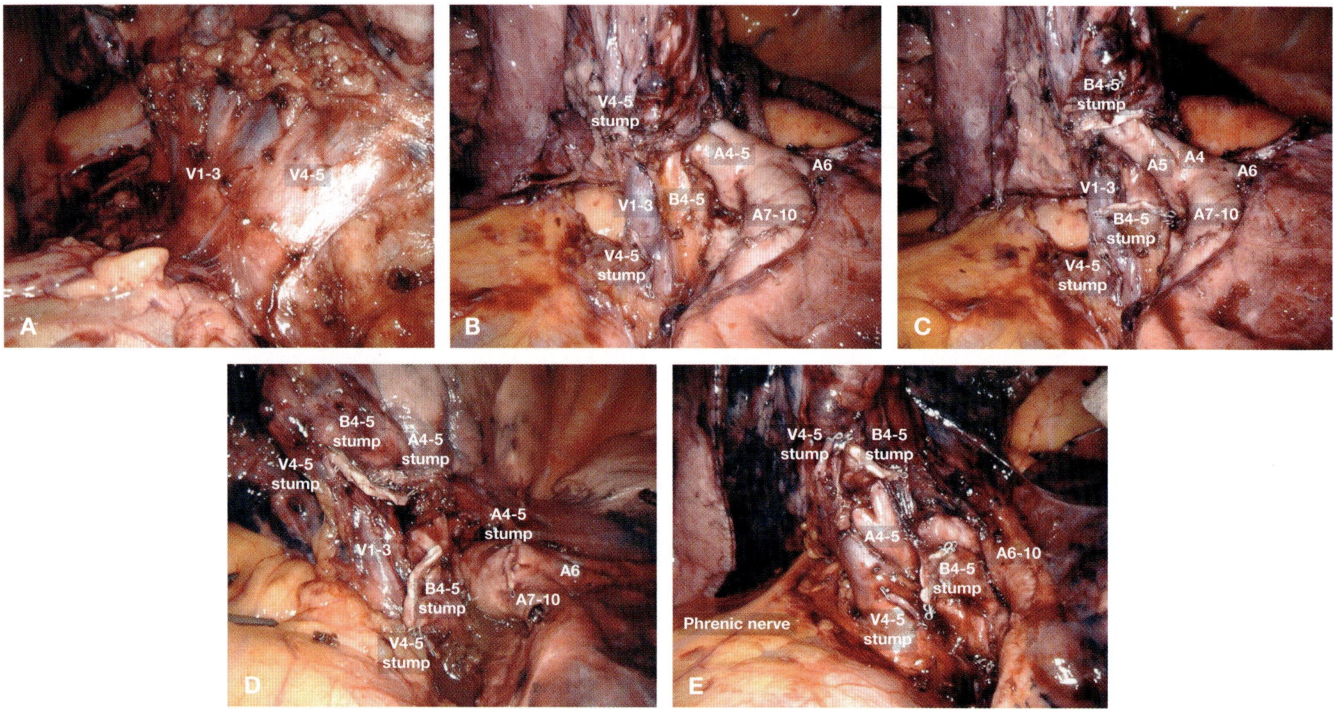

FIGURE 4.6 Left lingular (S4-5) segmentectomy. **A.** The upper division (V1-3) and lingular (V4-5) veins are identified anteriorly. **B.** The lingular (V4-5) vein is divided, and the lingular (B4-5) bronchus and (A4-5) artery are dissected. **C.** B4-5 is divided. **D.** A4-5 is divided. **E.** Arterial anatomic variant with lingular (A4-5) artery originating proximally and located superior to lingular (B4-5) bronchus.

- The lung is retracted posteriorly, and the anterior pleura is opened to expose the pulmonary vein. The superior and inferior pulmonary veins are distinguished, especially if there is a common vein. The superior pulmonary vein is dissected distally, identifying the upper division (V1-3) and lingular (V4-5) branches (Figure 4.6A), keeping in mind that the upper division (A1-3) arteries run behind them. The lingular (V4-5) vein is divided.
- The pulmonary artery is identified in the fissure, identifying the lingular (A4-5), superior segment (A6), and basilar (A7-10) arteries. Dividing the fissure and removing station 11L lymph nodes is helpful in identifying the pulmonary artery branches. Again, the lingular (A4-5) and superior segmental (A6) arteries usually originate across from each other (Figure 4.6B).
- The left upper lobe bronchus is identified and dissected distally to its bifurcation into the upper division (B1-3) and lingular (B4-5) bronchi. The station 12L lymph node between them is removed. The lingular (B4-5) bronchus runs parallel to and between the lingular (V4-5) vein and (A4-5) artery (Figure 4.6B).
- The lingular (B4-5) bronchus (Figure 4.6C) and then the lingular (A4-5) artery (Figure 4.6D) are divided.
- One anatomic variation is a proximal origin of the lingular (A4-5) artery, which runs anterior to the upper lobe bronchus (Figure 4.6E). Dissection of the lingular (V4-5) vein must be performed carefully since the lingular (A4-5) artery runs behind it instead of the lingular (B4-5) bronchus.

Postoperative Care

- The postoperative management following a segmentectomy is similar to that after lobectomy. Chest tubes are placed intraoperatively and removed when there is no air leak, and fluids are used judiciously.
- Pain management and pulmonary hygiene remain important parts of the postoperative care following any lung resection.
- Patients are at higher risk of prolonged air leak and pulmonary complications if segmentectomy was performed due to underlying lung disease.

PEARLS AND PITFALLS

- Segmentectomy is technically more challenging than a lobectomy. Dissection must be gentle since the vasculature is smaller and more fragile, and the distances between the segmental bronchi are very short.
- Segmental arteries and bronchi run parallel to each other to supply each segment; if one structure is identified, then the other is found alongside it. The segmental veins are located between segments in the intersegmental plane.
- Removing lymph nodes reveals critical anatomy.

Suggested Readings

1. Blasberg JD, Pass HI, Donington JS. Sublobar resection: a movement from the lung cancer study group. *J Thorac Oncol*. 2010;5(10):1583-1593.
2. Bryant AK, Mundt RC, Sandhu AP, et al. Stereotactic body radiation therapy versus surgery for early lung cancer among US Veterans. *Ann Thorac Surg*. 2018;105(2):425-431.
3. Crabtree T, Puri V, Timmerman R, et al. Treatment of stage I lung cancer in high-risk and inoperable patients: comparison of prospective clinical trials using stereotactic body radiotherapy (RTOG 0236), sublobar resection (ACOSOG Z4032), and radiofrequency ablation (ACOSOG Z4033). *J Thorac Cardiovasc Surg*. 2013;145(3):692-699.
4. Ginsberg RJ, Rubinstein LV. Randomized trial of lobectomy versus limited resection for T1 N0 non-small cell lung cancer. Lung Cancer Study Group. *Ann Thorac Surg*. 1995;60(3):615-623.
5. Koike T, Koike T, Yamato Y, Yoshiya K, Toyabe S. Prognostic predictors in non-small cell lung cancer patients undergoing intentional segmentectomy. *Ann Thorac Surg*. 2012;93(6):1788-1794.
6. Moroga T, Yamashita S, Tokuishi K, et al. Thoracoscopic segmentectomy with intraoperative evaluation of sentinel nodes for stage I non-small cell lung cancer. *Ann Thorac Cardiovasc Surg*. 2012;18(2):89-94.
7. Nakamura K, Saji H, Nakajima R, et al. A phase III randomized trial of lobectomy versus limited resection for small-sized peripheral non-small cell lung cancer (JCOG0802/WJOG4607 L). *Jpn J Clin Oncol*. 2010;40(3):271-274.
8. Nomori H, Okada M. *Illustrated Anatomical Segmentectomy for Lung Cancer*. Springer; 2012.
9. Schuchert MJ, Abbas G, Awais O, et al. Anatomic segmentectomy for the solitary pulmonary nodule and early-stage lung cancer. *Ann Thorac Surg*. 2012;93(6):1780-1787.
10. Stiles BM, Altorki NK. Segmentectomy versus lobectomy for stage I lung cancer in patients with good pulmonary function. In: Ferguson M, ed. *Difficult Decisions in Thoracic Surgery*. 2nd ed. Springer-Verlag; 2011:125-133.
11. Yang CF, D'Amico TA. Thoracoscopic segmentectomy for lung cancer. *Ann Thorac Surg*. 2012;94(2):668-681.

Chapter 5

Right Upper Lobectomy: Robotic/Video-Assisted Thoracic Surgery/Thoracotomy

PHILICIA MOONSAMY
LANA Y. SCHUMACHER

Introduction

- Operative approach for early stage (I-IIIA) non-small-cell lung cancer is dependent on patient factors and surgeon preference.
- Relative contraindications to a minimally invasive approach include the presence of lymphadenopathy or tumor involvement that would complicate vascular dissection and control. However, these select cases can be performed based on surgeon experience and discretion.
- We favor minimally invasive approaches whenever feasible given the benefits of decreased length of stay, reduced postoperative pain, and decreased postoperative mortality without compromise to oncologic outcomes.
- While endobronchial lesions, a history of prior surgery, and the administration of induction chemotherapy were previously regarded as contraindications to minimally invasive approaches, many studies have shown that video-assisted thoracic surgery (VATS) and robotic-assisted approaches can be used safely and effectively in these cases without an increase in the rate of complications. Furthermore, there are numerous published accounts of thoracoscopic and robotic sleeve resections.

Perioperative Considerations

Anesthesia and Positioning

- If an open approach is planned, we prefer to place a preoperative thoracic epidural. If a minimally invasive approach is planned, we plan to place intercostal nerve blocks at the end of the operation.
- Bronchoscopy is performed to establish anatomy and especially in cases that are concerning for endobronchial extension of the tumor.
- The use of a double-lumen endotracheal tube or bronchial blockers for lung isolation is the standard of care.
- After induction of general anesthesia and intubation, the patient is repositioned from the supine to the left lateral decubitus position for both minimally invasive and open approaches.
- Visual confirmation of placement of the double-lumen endotracheal tube with bronchoscopy is imperative for effective lung isolation especially after the patient has been positioned since the tube can move during positioning.
- For both open and minimally invasive techniques, two rolled up blankets are used on either side of the patient. The patient is secured to the table by applying heavy cloth tape over their greater trochanter. Three pillows are placed between the legs. We no longer use a bean bag positioner as this can limit access to the patient.

- It is important to assure adequate padding to prevent the development of pressure points, and to ensure that the cervical spine is in a neutral position.
- An arterial line is used if the patient has appropriate risk factors (eg, history of heart failure, valvular disease, coronary disease, stroke, carotid stenosis, etc.).
- We do not routinely use a Foley catheter for minimally invasive lung resections.

Instruments and Equipment

- Open
  - Standard thoracotomy instrument tray. A thoracotomy tray should also be readily available for minimally invasive approaches.
- VATS
  - 10-mm angled (30°) thoracoscope
  - Large right-angled clamp
  - Long curved ring clamp
  - Long Metzenbaum scissors
  - Range of 5-mm thoracoscopic instruments (grasping forceps, DeBakey forceps, endopeanuts, metal tip suction)
  - Range of endostaplers, preferably with a curved tip
- Robotic-assisted approach with the Xi robot
  - We prefer to perform a four-arm right upper lobectomy with three 8-mm ports (arms 1-3), one anterior 12-mm port that can accommodate a stapler (arm 4), and an additional assistant port.
  - Suggested instruments
    - Arm 1: Tip-up fenestrated grasper
    - Arm 2: Cadiere grasper
    - Arm 3: Camera
    - Arm 4: Maryland bipolar (with energy) or robotic stapler

Technique

Open

- If the lesion is not amenable to a minimally invasive approach, we prefer to perform a muscle-sparing posterolateral thoracotomy through the fifth intercostal space.

Video-Assisted Thoracic Surgery

- We prefer to use three ports (Figure 5.1)
  - A camera port in the seventh intercostal space place just anterior to the mid-axillary line
  - A posteriorly placed retraction port in the seventh or eighth intercostal space
  - A 4-cm utility incision in the fourth intercostal space anteriorly

Robotic-Assisted

- Port placement with Xi robot (Figure 5.2)
  - Robot arm ports are placed and lined up in the eighth or ninth intercostal space.
  - The assistant port is placed in the 10th intercostal space and it is important to triangulate this port between the anterior port and the camera port.

TIPS

- *The camera port should be positioned along the posterior axillary line anterior to the scapular tip in the eighth intercostal space.*
- *The camera can be moved to any of the ports for better visualization if needed. This is especially useful when inserting and docking new instruments into the chest cavity.*
- *The anterior stapler port is placed as anterior as possible just inferior to the cardiophrenic recess. If performing an anterior approach, a second staple port is needed posteriorly.*

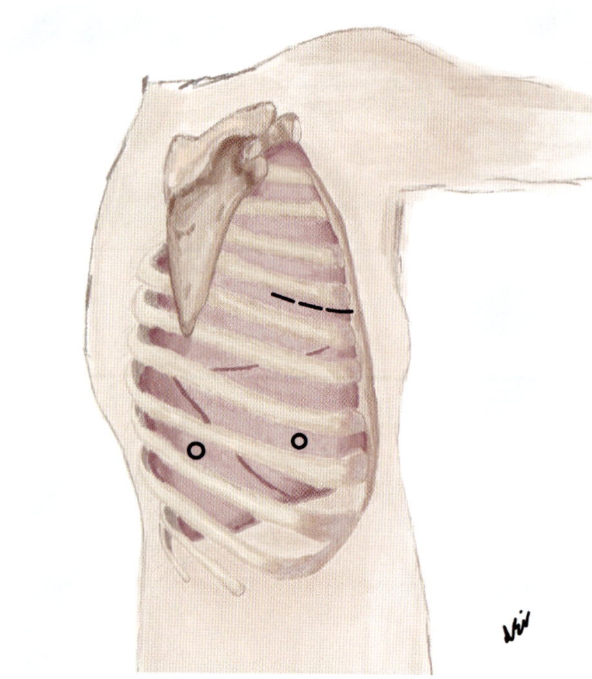

FIGURE 5.1 ▮ Port placement for the video-assisted approach. (Illustration by Danielle Ellis.)

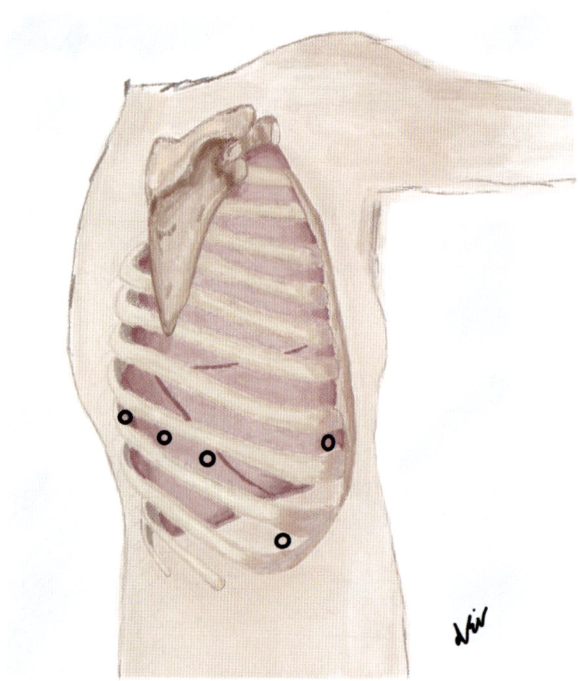

FIGURE 5.2 ▮ Port placement for robotic-assisted approach. (Illustration by Danielle Ellis.)

Operative Approach—Posterior to Anterior

- Dissection of inferior pulmonary ligament and removal of level 8 and 9 nodes
  - The operation commences by retracting the lower lobe cranially and laterally in order to release the inferior pulmonary ligament. Level 8 and 9 lymph node packets are harvested.
- Dissection of level 7 subcarinal lymph nodes (Figure 5.3)
  - The lung is then retracted anteriorly to identify the right upper lobe bronchus and bronchus intermedius from the vantage point of the posterior mediastinum.
  - Level 7 lymph nodes are then harvested from the subcarinal space. To ensure complete resection of the level 7 nodes, the posterior aspect of the pericardium should be visible.
  - Care is taken to ensure hemostasis, which is best achieved by removing the entire lymph node packet.

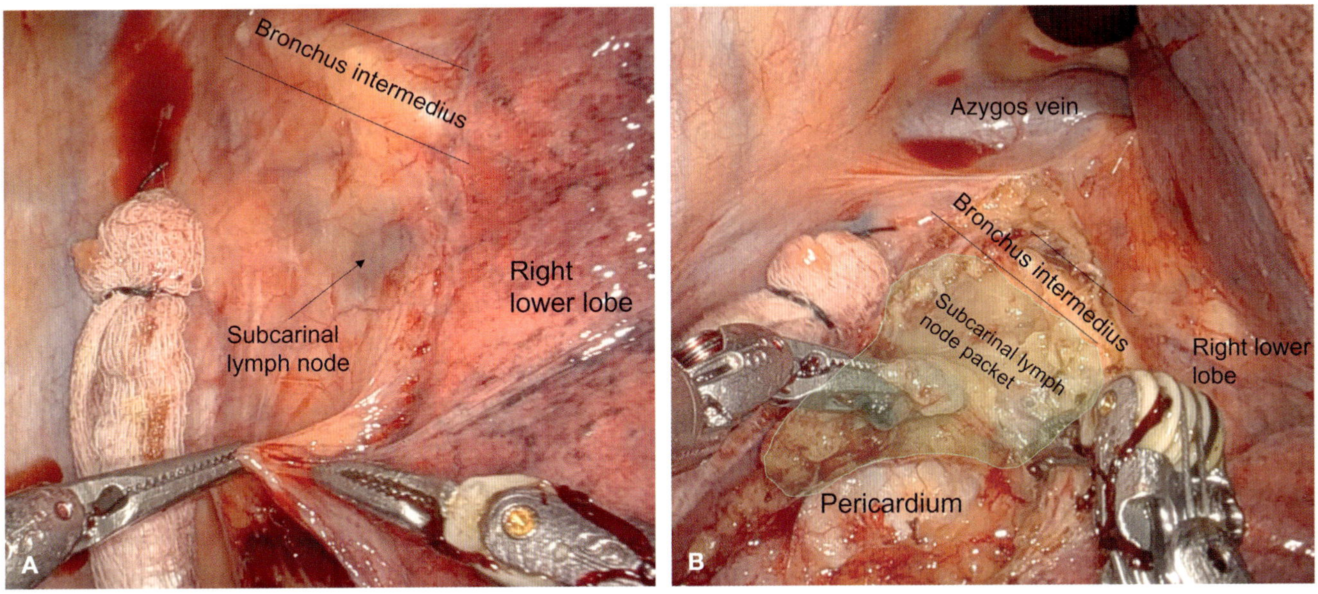

FIGURE 5.3 ‖ **A.** Subcarinal level 7 lymph node before dissection. **B.** Subcarinal lymph node packet dissection revealing the pericardium.

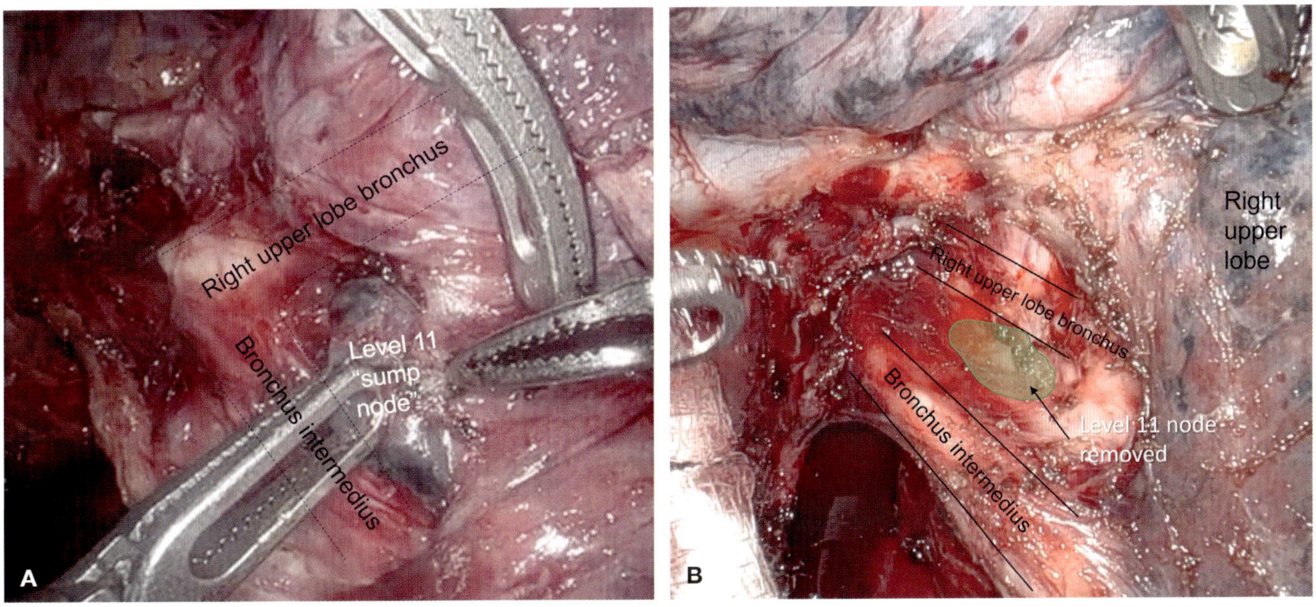

FIGURE 5.4 ‖ **A.** Posterior hilar resection revealing the level 11R "sump" node. **B.** Posterior hilum after level 11R node is resected.

- Posterior hilar dissection and level 11R "sump" node (Figure 5.4)
  - Dissection of the posterior hilar and suprahilar space reveals the pulmonary artery (PA) and bronchial anatomy. The space between the PA and bronchus is dissected.
  - The level 11 "sump" node is identified under the caudal surface of the right upper lobe bronchus. This node is usually quite flat and is removed with extra caution since it lies directly on the PA and the posterior ascending PA branching to the upper lobe resides adjacent to this node.
  - The level 10R node, which lies on the upper border of the right mainstem bronchus, can be harvested at this time or later with the division of the right mainstem bronchus (Figure 5.5).
- Posterior fissure (Figure 5.6)
  - In a patient with a near-complete fissure, the posterior aspect of the fissure can be opened to dissect out the posterior ascending PA and any aberrant veins crossing the fissure.
  - The posterior ascending PA can then be encircled and divided with a vascular stapler from this approach.
  - In an incomplete fissure, we first attempt to identify and divide the PA within the fissure and proceed by completing the posterior fissure. If this is not possible, then we proceed by dividing

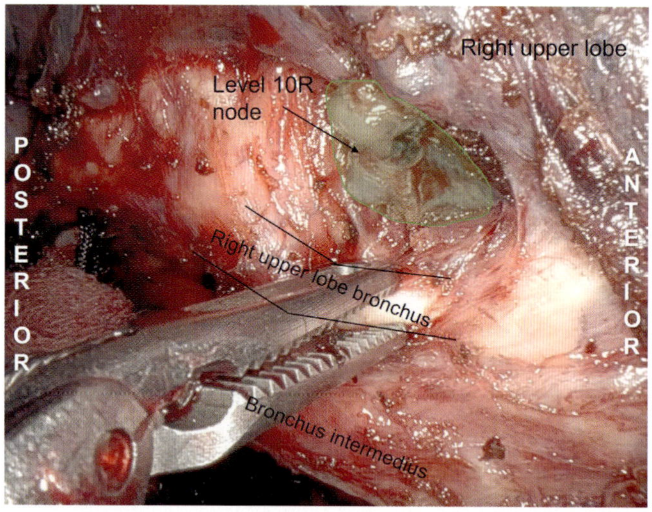

FIGURE 5.5 ▮ Retraction of the right upper lobe bronchus revealing level 10R nodes on the cranial aspect of the bronchus.

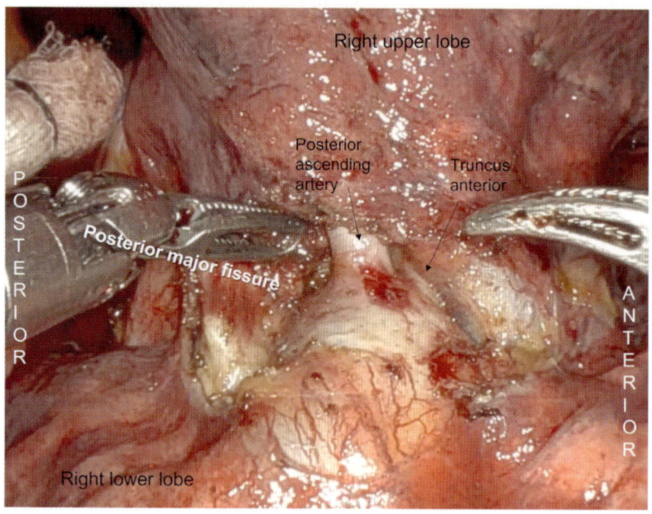

FIGURE 5.6 ▮ Dissection of the major fissure revealing the posterior ascending artery and truncus anterior.

the right upper lobe bronchus first to facilitate identification of the posterior ascending PA and the truncus anterior.

- Dissection and division of the right upper lobe bronchus (Figure 5.7)
  - The right upper lobe bronchus can be carefully dissected off the underlying 10R lymph nodes and the truncus anterior. The bronchus itself is safe to retract to facilitate dissection from underlying structures. It is then divided with an endoscopic stapler.

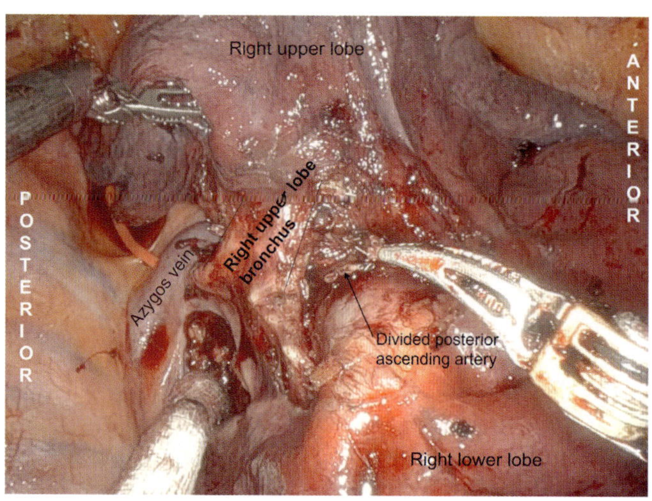

FIGURE 5.7 ▮ Dissection and division of the right upper lobe bronchus.

- It is important to divide the bronchus near the takeoff so that there is not a long stump.
- The 10R lymph node packet can be harvested at this time.
- Dissection and division of the truncus anterior branches
  - The apical and anterior arteries are then dissected and can be divided together or separately with a vascular stapler.
- Dissection and division of the upper lobe pulmonary vein (Figure 5.8)

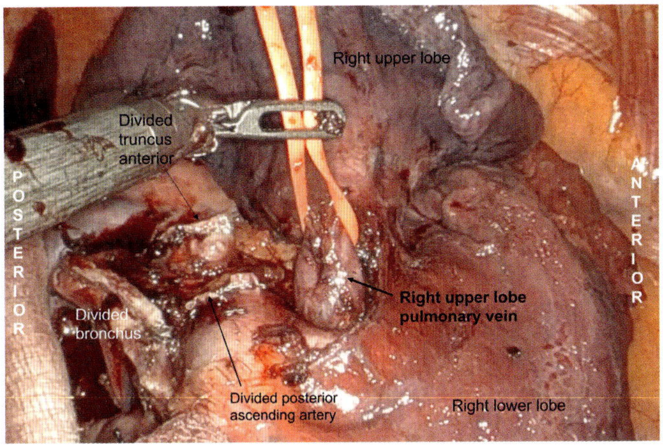

FIGURE 5.8 | Right upper lobe pulmonary vein encircled by a vessel loop from the aspect of the posterior hilum.

  - The upper lobe vein can also be taken from a posterior approach, which allows for less repositioning of the lung and increased in efficiency.
  - The lung continues to be retracted anteriorly and the pulmonary vein is dissected off any remaining 10R lymph nodes.
  - Care is taken to identify and avoid the phrenic nerve, which will be behind the vein in this position.
  - The pulmonary vein is isolated and divided with a vascular stapler.
- Division of the fissure
  - The fissure can also be divided with an endovascular stapler via a posterior approach by continuing to retract the lung anteriorly.
  - It is important to ensure that the divided hilar structures are clear of the staple line as the fissure is transected.
- Level 4R lymph node dissection
  - Level 4R nodes are harvested by clearing the space between the superior vena cava anteriorly, the trachea posteriorly, and the azygos vein inferiorly. It is important to remove the nodal packet in its entirety by dissecting it off the underlying pericardium.
- Intercostal nerve block
  - We perform an intercostal nerve block using 0.25% Marcaine with epinephrine introduced with a long mediastinoscopy needle (Figure 5.9).

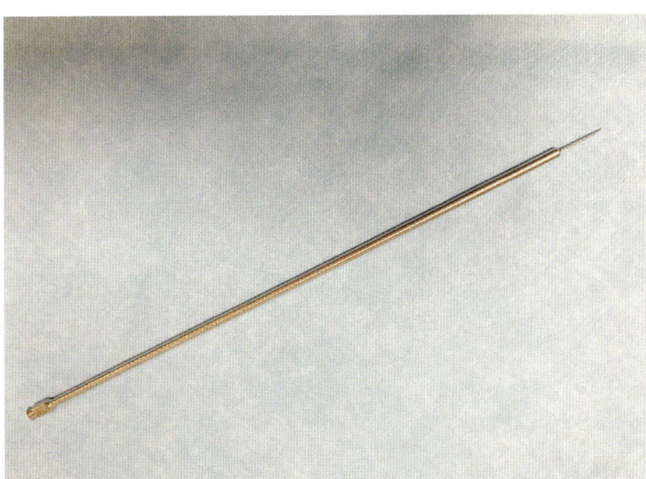

FIGURE 5.9 | Mediastinoscopy needle for intercostal nerve block.

Operative Approach—Anterior to Posterior or "fissureless" Approach

- This approach is often used in VATS cases.
- The fissureless approach is felt to minimize complications of air leak, which may be associated with dissection within an incomplete fissure.
- Pulmonary vein dissection and division (Figure 5.10)

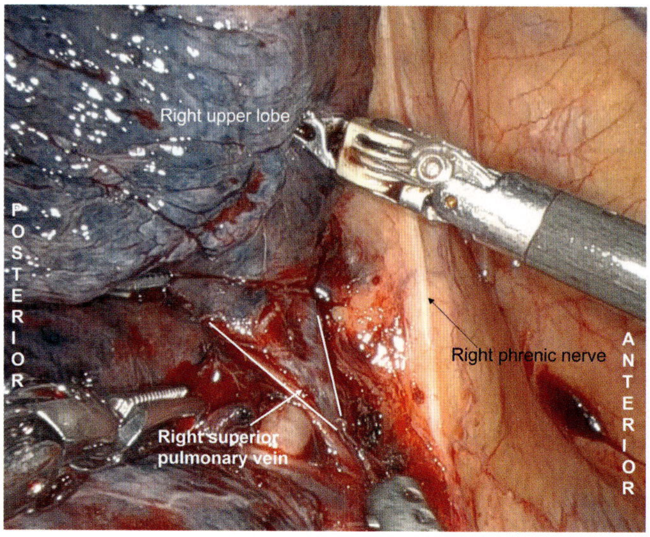

FIGURE 5.10 ▮ Right upper lobe pulmonary vein from the aspect of the anterior hilum.

  - The lung is retracted posteriorly and the pleura overlying the pulmonary vein is dissected, taking care to avoid the phrenic nerve which is medial. This can be accomplished with blunt dissection with a metal suction device or a peanut, but occasionally, the pleura must be lifted and sharply incised.
  - The bifurcation between the middle and upper lobe veins is dissected. Care is taken to identify and preserve the middle lobe pulmonary vein since it can have one of the most common anatomic variants in vein anatomy—the right middle lobe vein usually drains to the right superior pulmonary vein in 60% to 70% of the population; however, an accessory vein draining the middle lobe can be seen in up to 26% of patients.
  - The upper lobe vein is then encircled, elevated off the underlying PA, and transected with a vascular stapler, which is usually introduced through the posterior trocar site in VATS approaches.
- PA and right upper lobe bronchus dissection and division
  - Division of the pulmonary vein generally reveals the right main PA, which lies deep to the vein. It is important to avoid excessive retraction of the lung posteriorly during this dissection since this can lead to pulmonary arterial injury.
  - The truncus anterior is dissected out widely and transected with a vascular stapler through a posterior port.
  - Division of the truncus anterior allows improved retraction of the upper lobe posteriorly, which exposes the right upper lobe bronchus and the posterior ascending PA branch.
  - Either the bronchus or the posterior ascending branch can be divided next, depending on the local anatomy.
- Fissure
  - The fissure between the middle and upper lobes is divided with an endoscopic stapler.
- Division of inferior pulmonary ligament, lymph node dissection (4R, 7, 8, 9), and intercostal nerve block
  - As outlined in the previous section

Postoperative Care

- Patients are usually extubated in the operating room and are cared for on regular inpatient floors.
- With minimally invasive approaches, we have moved toward using just one chest tube, which is kept to water seal and removed when all air leaks subside, and the drainage of pleural fluid is less than 200 cc over a 24-hour period.

- Our enhanced recovery after surgery protocol includes early preoperative administration of Tylenol and Celebrex. Postoperatively, early ambulation on the same day as the operation is encouraged. We assess all chest tubes for removal on postoperative day 1 if possible and minimize narcotics by utilizing toradol, tylenol, and gabapentin as needed.
- Aggressive pulmonary toilet is always encouraged for all approaches.
- The average stay for robotic and VATS approaches at our institution is one to two nights.

PEARLS AND PITFALLS

- Obtaining airway control is key to managing massive hemoptysis.
- Although once considered the only treatment for massive hemoptysis, surgery is no longer the first-line therapy. In fact, surgery should be reserved as a last resort with a few exceptions.
- For a VATS approach, the important hilar structures (vein, truncus PA and posterior ascending PA) can all be dissected out from anterior to posterior.
- It is sometimes necessary to ligate the superior pulmonary vein in order to increase exposure around the truncus PA.
- For very proximal tumors that are close to the truncus PA, the bronchus can also be cut or ligated before dissecting around the truncus PA in order to improve exposure.
- For a robotic approach, the posterior hilar dissection is completed first and it is important to remove the sump 11R node which lies on the posterior ascending PA.

Suggested Readings

1. Balsara KR, Balderson SS, D'Amico TA. Surgical techniques to avoid parenchymal injury during lung resection (fissureless lobectomy). *Thorac Surg Clin*. 2010;20(3):365-369.
2. Hanna JM, Berry MF, D'Amico TA. Contraindications of video-assisted thoracoscopic surgical lobectomy and determinants of conversion to open. *J Thorac Dis*. 2013;5(suppl 3):S182-S189.
3. Ke H, Liu Y, Zhou X, Xue Q. Anterior fissureless uniport *vs.* posterior intra-fissure triple-port thoracoscopic right upper lobectomy: a propensity-matched study. *J Thorac Dis*. 2017;9(10):3866-3874.
4. Mahtabifard A, Fuller CB, McKenna RJ Jr. Video-assisted thoracic surgery sleeve lobectomy: a case series. *Ann Thorac Surg*. 2008;85(2):S729-S732.
5. Marom EM, Herndon JE, Kim YH, McAdams HP. Variations in pulmonary venous drainage to the left atrium: implications for radiofrequency ablation. *Radiology*. 2004;230(3):824-829.
6. Mitchell JD. Techniques of VATS lobectomy. *J Thorac Dis*. 2013;5(suppl 3):S177-S181.
7. Petersen RP, Pham D, Toloza EM, et al. Thoracoscopic lobectomy: a safe and effective strategy for patients receiving induction therapy for non-small cell lung cancer. *Ann Thorac Surg*. 2006;82(1):214-219.
8. Sasankan P, Chang S, Cerfolio R. Robotic right upper lobectomy: twelve Steps. *JTCVS Tech*. 2021;7:280-282.
9. Stamenovic D, Bostanci K, Messerschmidt A, Jahn T, Schneider T. Fissureless fissure-last video-assisted thoracoscopic lobectomy for all lung lobes: a better alternative to decrease the incidence of prolonged air leak? *Eur J Cardio Thorac Surg*. 2016;50(1):118-123.
10. Taioli E, Lee DS, Lesser M, Flores R. Long-term survival in video-assisted thoracoscopic lobectomy vs open lobectomy in lung-cancer patients: a meta-analysis. *Eur J Cardio Thorac Surg*. 2013;44(4):591-597.
11. Yang CFJ, Kumar A, Klapper JA, et al. A national analysis of long-term survival following thoracoscopic versus open lobectomy for stage I non-small-cell lung cancer. *Ann Surg*. 2019;269(1):163-171.

Chapter 6

Right Middle Lobectomy: Minimally Invasive and Open Techniques

DANIELLE ELLIS
HUGH G. AUCHINCLOSS

Perioperative Considerations

- Anatomic resection of the right middle lobe can be approached in a minimally invasive—robot-assisted thoracoscopic surgery (RATS) or video-assisted thoracoscopic surgery (VATS)—or open fashion.
- The right middle lobe is composed of a lateral and a medial segment and is the smallest of the lobes. It is often appropriate to perform a diagnostic resection of the middle lobe in situations where, for another lobe, a preoperative diagnosis would be required.
- Unlike upper and lower lobectomies where access to the posterior pulmonary hilum is critical, the working space required to perform a middle lobectomy can be restricted to the anterior hilum and the major fissure. This allows one to limit the size of the incision for open operations and the general scope of minimally invasive operations. Some access to the posterior hilum is needed to perform a complete lymphadenectomy (ie, station 7 and 11 nodes).
- The pulmonary arterial supply to the middle lobe is variable. Duplicate and recurrent branches should be expected.
- The minor/horizontal fissure is seldom complete. Judgment is required in separating the middle lobe from the upper lobe. The use of indocyanine green (ICG) dye after division of the vascular structures can be helpful in defining this fissure but is usually unnecessary.

Instruments and Equipment

- Flexible bronchoscope
- Three 8-mm robotic ports, one 12-mm robotic stapling port, one 12-mm assistant port (RATS)
- Camera port (VATS)
- 30-degree thoracoscope (RATS and VATS)
- Small chest spreader and soft-tissue retractor (open)
- Wound protector (optional for VATS and open)
- Energy source: Monopolar, bipolar, ultrasonic
- Blunt dissector (pediatric suction, endoscopic Kittner)
- Lung retractors: Duval or ring clamps (open, VATS), tip-up fenestrated grasper (RATS)
- Vessel loops
- Stapling device with tissue (thin and thick) and vascular loads
- ICG dye (optional)

Positioning and Anesthesia

- The patient is intubated in supine position with either a left-sided double-lumen endotracheal tube (ETT) or a single-lumen ETT with bronchial blocker. Bronchoscopy confirms positioning of the tube and normal bronchial anatomy.

- Large-bore IV access is recommended given the potential for blood loss in any anatomic lung resection. The use of continuous blood pressure monitoring with an arterial line is at the discretion of the surgical and anesthesia teams.
- Patient is placed in left lateral decubitus position with the right chest elevated.
- Operating table is flexed with flexion point between the patient's xiphoid and anterior superior iliac spine.
- An axillary roll is optional. Table flexion typically is sufficient to avoid compression of the brachial plexus on the nonoperative side.
- Right arm is supported without hyperextension of the elbow.
- Legs: Bottom straight, top bent
- The surgical field should include the spine posteriorly, the nipple anteriorly, and the costal margin inferiorly. The superior border is draped off obliquely to expose most of the axilla and posterior spine of the scapula almost to the base of the neck. This facilitates performing a posterolateral thoracotomy in the event of an emergency.

Technique

- Although particularly useful in thoracic surgery, a double-lumen ETT has little to no role in the management of massive hemoptysis. Due to their lumen size, only smaller bronchoscopes may be used, making suctioning large clots difficult.

Robot-Assisted Thoracoscopic Surgery

TIPS

- *RATS middle lobectomy typically proceeds in "bottom-up" fashion, with the creation of the major fissure, division of the bronchovascular structures from inferior to superior (vein, bronchus, artery), and then division of the minor fissure.*
- *Understanding the location of the middle lobe bronchus is critical.*
- *Variable pulmonary arterial and venous anatomy should be expected.*

Port Placement and Entry (Figure 6.1)

- The camera port (Arm 3) is placed first. It is an 8-mm port in the seventh or eighth interspace along the mid-axillary line.

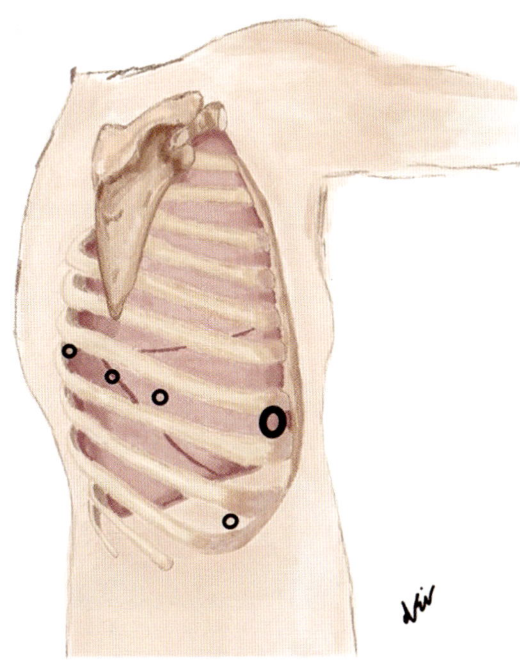

FIGURE 6.1 ▌ Robotic approach port placement. (Illustration by Danielle Ellis.)

- After inspection of the pleural space to confirm safe entry and the absence of factors that would prohibit proceeding, the chest is insufflated to 8 mm Hg. Hemodynamic monitoring and communication with the anesthesia team during insufflation is important. Insufflation shifts the mediastinum, flattens the diaphragm, and collapses the lung, creating more space for additional ports.
- The remaining ports can be placed in any order.
  - An 8-mm working port (Arm 2) is placed in the eighth or nth intercostal space at the posterior axillary line. This is typically a Cadiere forceps.
  - A 12-mm working and stapling port (Arm 4) is placed just lateral to the costal margin in the seventh or eighth interspace. This port should be as far anterior as possible to facilitate stapling and to provide working space for the assistant port. The dissecting/energy instrument (Maryland bipolar, monopolar spatula, harmonic scalpel) works through Arm 4.
  - An 8-mm retracting port (Arm 1) is placed in the fourth or fifth intercostal space just medial to the paraspinal ligament. A lung retractor (tip-up fenestrated grasper) is used in Arm 1 and is most effective when working from above the posterior major fissure.
- All robot ports must be 5 cm or more from each other to prevent collisions. For a patient with a small chest, it may be necessary to move Arm 2 inferior and lateral to create separation between it and both the retractor port (Arm 1) and the camera port (Arm 3).
- An assistant port of 12 to 15 mm is placed in the inferior chest above the diaphragm, triangulated between Arms 3 and 4 (or 2 and 3).
- The robot is docked and the instruments are inserted under direct visualization.

Lymphadenectomy/Opening the Mediastinal Pleura

- The lower lobe is elevated with the retractor arm/assistant and the inferior pulmonary ligament is incised to the level of the inferior pulmonary vein. Station 9 lymph nodes are removed.
- The lung is retracted medially and the posterior mediastinal pleura is opened to reveal the bronchus intermedius and the station 7 lymph nodes, which are dissected completely. Station 11 intralobar nodes between the bronchus intermedius and the right upper lobe bronchus may be sampled/dissected as well.
- The pleura separating the upper lobe bronchus and the azygos vein is dissected. With the lung retracted inferiorly, the station 4 lymph nodes superior to the azygos vein and posterior to the superior vena cava are dissected completely.
- Finally, the lung is retracted posteriorly and mediastinal pleura overlying the anterior aspect of both pulmonary veins is incised. The phrenic nerve marks the anterior extent of this dissection. The middle lobe vein is dissected at its origin from the superior pulmonary vein (Figure 6.2). Space between the inferior pulmonary vein and the middle lobe vein is created. The middle lobe vein is not yet divided to prevent engorgement of the middle lobe.

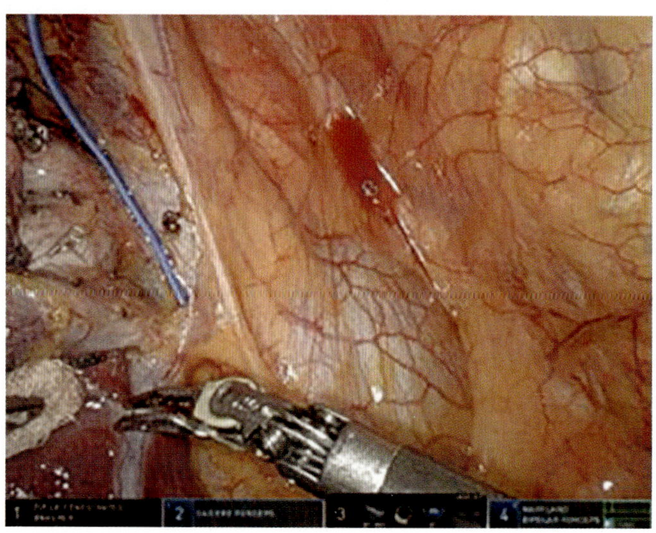

FIGURE 6.2 ▌ The origin of the middle lobe pulmonary vein from the superior pulmonary vein, and its relationship to the phenic nerve.

Developing the Major Fissure

- The upper and middle lobes are elevated and the lower lobe is allowed to drop inferiorly.
- The main pulmonary artery is identified in the fissure and dissection down to the adventitia of the artery is performed. Dissection is continued antegrade and retrograde until a reasonably distance of the pulmonary artery is visible. Ideally, the posterior ascending artery to the upper lobe, the superior and basilar segment arteries to the lower lobe, and the origin of the artery to the middle lobe are visible (Figure 6.3).

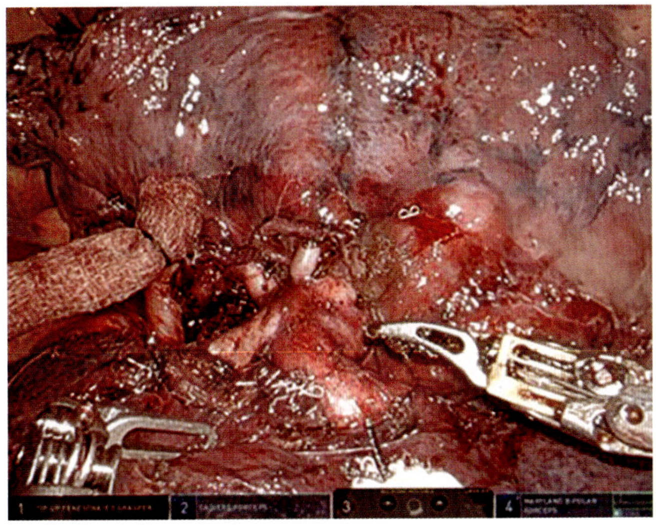

FIGURE 6.3 | Main pulmonary artery (PA) in the major fissure.

- Dissection of the pulmonary artery at this level is best accomplished by performing a complete lymphadenectomy of station 10 and 12 nodes from around the origin of these pulmonary artery branches. Doing so is both oncologically important and creates separation between the vascular structures and the bronchial structures immediately deep to them.
- Deep to the anteromedial aspect of the basilar pulmonary artery lies the middle lobe bronchus. The trifurcation of the bronchus intermedius into the middle lobe bronchus, lower lobe basilar bronchus, and lower lobe superior segment bronchus is obscured by the pulmonary artery and the anatomy is best appreciated during a right lower lobectomy after that pulmonary artery has been divided (Figure 6.4). Understanding the location of the middle lobe bronchus at this stage is critical because all of the tissues anterior and medial to it represent the major fissure separating the lower lobe from the middle lobe. This can all be divided.

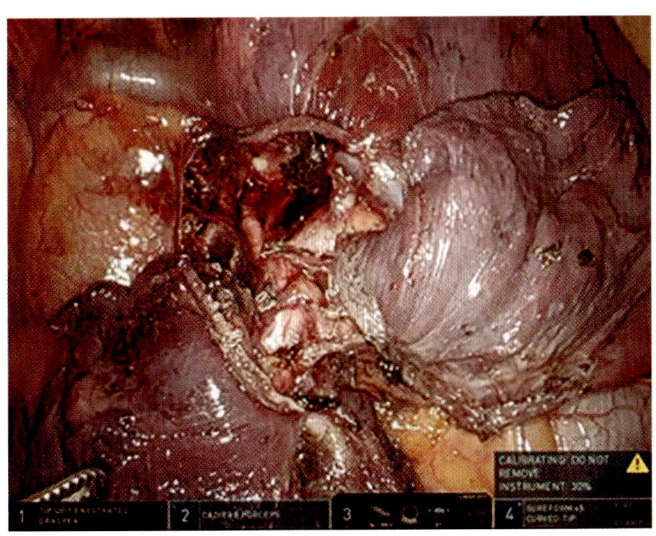

FIGURE 6.4 | The origin of the middle lobe bronchus shown during a lower lobectomy with the pulmonary artery divided.

- Separation of the major fissure can be performed with energy if the fissure is well developed. When using this technique, it is common to encounter small branches of the basilar pulmonary artery that recur to the middle lobe and cross the fissure. These can be stapled, clipped, or taken with a vessel sealer. If the fissure is not well developed, it is best to divide it with a stapler. A tunnel between the anterior aspect of the middle lobe bronchus and the anterior hilum is created by dissecting from the fissure into the space created during separation of the inferior pulmonary vein and middle lobe vein. The tract can be marked with a vessel loop and then a stapler from Arm 4 is passed through it. For a totally incomplete fissure, it is sometimes necessary to improve visualization of the anterior hilum by first firing a stapler beginning at the anterior aspect of the major fissure, thus creating partial separation of the lower and middle lobes (Figure 6.5). The stapling port is located close to the anterior aspect of the fissure and positioning the stapler may require that the port is partially withdrawn from the patient by the bedside assistant. The port should be immediately returned to its starting position to prevent torque on the patient's chest wall during the rest of the case.

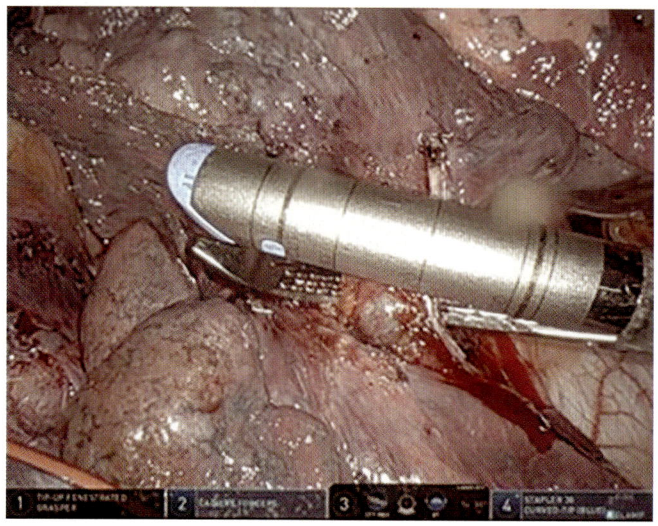

FIGURE 6.5 ▌Division of the major fissure with a stapler.

Division of the Bronchovascular Structures

- Division of the major fissure allows for elevation of the middle lobe and exposure of the critical structures.
- The middle lobe vein can now be divided at its origin using a vascular stapler load. Common variations of middle lobe venous anatomy include multiple branches, a single branch with an intrapericardial origin, or a single branch draining to the inferior pulmonary vein.
- The inferior and anteromedial aspect of the middle lobe bronchus is now visible. Circumferential dissection of the bronchus completes its separation from the middle lobe pulmonary arterial supply, which typically lies posterior and superior (Figure 6.6). Once the bronchus is circumferentially dissected, it may be divided. Test inflation is seldom necessary because the bronchus is reliable in location and appearance, and it would be difficult to narrow the lower lobe bronchus with the application of the stapler. Given the small caliber of the middle lobe bronchus, a thin tissue load is usually sufficient.
    - Pulmonary artery branches to the middle lobe should now be well-visualized. A single dominant artery arising opposite the posterior ascending artery (to the upper lobe) is the expected anatomy (Figure 6.7). However, duplicate or even triplicate middle lobe branches are common, including some that may originate from the distal pulmonary artery, and require division prior to dividing the bronchus.
    - In the case of multiple middle lobe pulmonary artery branches, it may be unclear if the more proximal of the branches is in fact supplying the upper lobe rather than the middle lobe. This ambiguity can be resolved with a one-time dose of ICG dye.

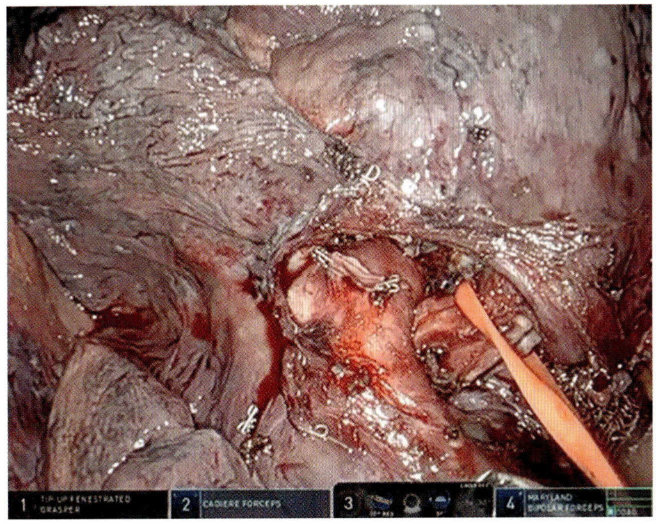

FIGURE 6.6 | The middle lobe bronchus encircled with a vessel loop. The middle lobe pulmonary artery (PA) lies immediately posterior and superior and is partially obscured.

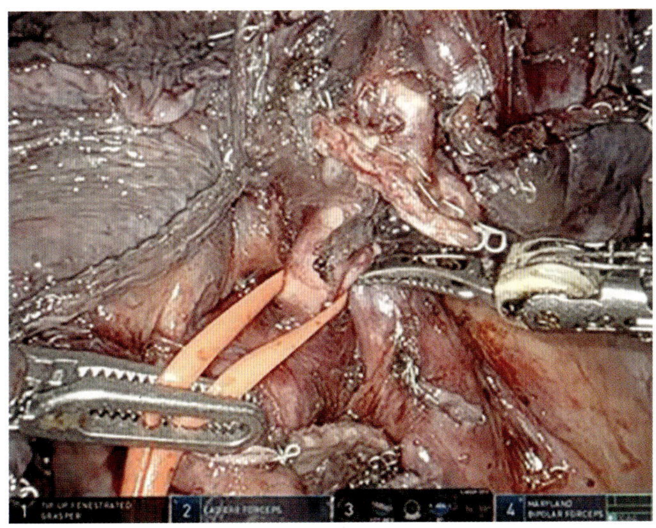

FIGURE 6.7 | View with the anterior major fissure completed, upper lobe to the left, middle lobe up, and the right lower lobe out of frame; the middle lobe pulmonary artery (PA) encircled with a vessel loop after division of the vein and bronchus.

Completion

- After division of the bronchovascular structures, the middle lobe remains connected to the upper lobe by the poorly defined minor fissure. Typically, some demarcation between the upper lobe and middle is present, but the fissure cannot be completed with energy dissection alone without causing significant parenchymal disruption, bleeding, and air leaks.
- It is wise to spend a few extra minutes separating the middle lobe from the upper lobe vascular structures prior to attempting to staple the fissure. Dissecting distally along the underside of the upper lobe branch of the superior pulmonary vein and proximally along the main pulmonary artery (toward its hilar origin) allows the middle lobe to further elevate and the fissure to be visualized on both sides. The lobe becomes more mobile and a stapler is more easily positioned to create the fissure without the theoretical concern of narrowing the upper lobe arterial or venous structures.
- Arm 4—the anterior stapling port—is not optimally located for division of the minor fissure. This difficulty can be resolved with gentle torsion of the lung parenchyma and angulation of the stapler. The fissure can be stapled from anterior to posterior. Occasionally, it may be necessary to upsize Arm 2 to a 12-mm stapling port. Arm 2 provides a straight shot at the minor fissure, which is then divided in a posterior-to-anterior direction (Figure 6.8).
- Once separated, the lobe is set aside and all residual lymph node material now exposed is dissected. Hemostasis is confirmed.

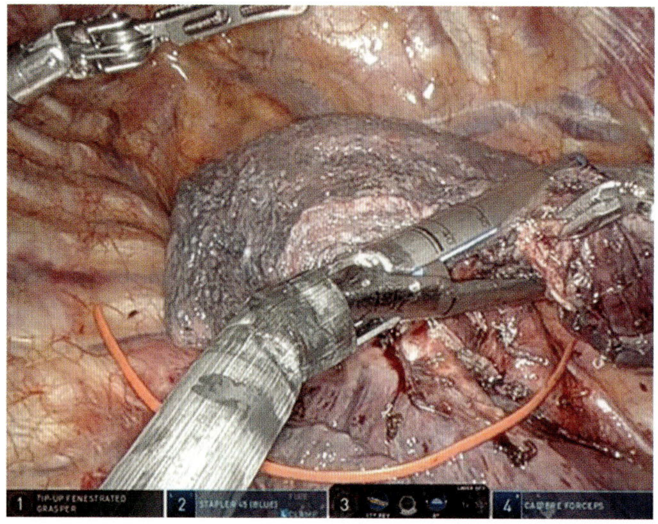

FIGURE 6.8 | Division of the minor fissure.

- The lobe is placed into a large specimen retrieval bag and withdrawn through the assistant port. The port may need to be extended to permit extraction. We usually undock the robot at this juncture to prevent undue traction on the patient's chest wall caused by forceful manipulation of the bag. Similarly, the anesthesia team should be mindful of the security of the ETT.
- Posterior intercostal nerve blocks are administered. A posterior pleural tube is positioned through one of the ports and the lung is reinflated under direct vision.

Video-Assisted Thoracoscopic Surgery

TIPS

- *The access port in a VATS middle lobectomy ideally overlies the superior pulmonary vein and provides excellent exposure to the anterior hilum.*
- *A consequence of this anterior hilar exposure is VATS middle lobectomy typically proceeds in an "anterior-to-posterior" direction, with dissection of the anterior mediastinal pleura, separation and division of the middle lobe vein, division of the middle lobe bronchus, and then isolation and division of the arterial blood supply. The fissures can be created at any point once the location of the middle lobe bronchus is established.*

Port Placement and Entry (Figure 6.9)

- The operating surgeon stands on the patient's left (anterior).
- The camera port is placed in the eighth intercostal space between the anterior and mid-axillary line. The port should be large enough to accommodate a 5- or 10-mm thoracoscope as well as a second 5-mm instrument. This port is usually used later as a chest tube entry site. Thoracoscopic inspection of the hemithorax is performed to exclude metastatic disease or other prohibitive factors.
- An assistant port is placed in the posterior axillary line. This port functions both as a retractor and as an entry site for the stapler.
- An access incision of 3 cm is created overlying the anterior hilum at the level of the superior pulmonary vein. It is helpful to use a finder needle prior to entry into the chest in order to ensure that the port is optimally located. The skin and soft tissue are divided and the serratus anterior muscle is separated in the direction of its fibers. The intercostal muscle and parietal pleura along the superior aspect of the rib (typically the fourth or fifth) are cauterized to prevent nuisance bleeding. We use a small wound protector. The majority of dissection takes place through this access incision and so it must be large enough to permit the surgeon to use both forceps and electrocautery simultaneously and with precision.

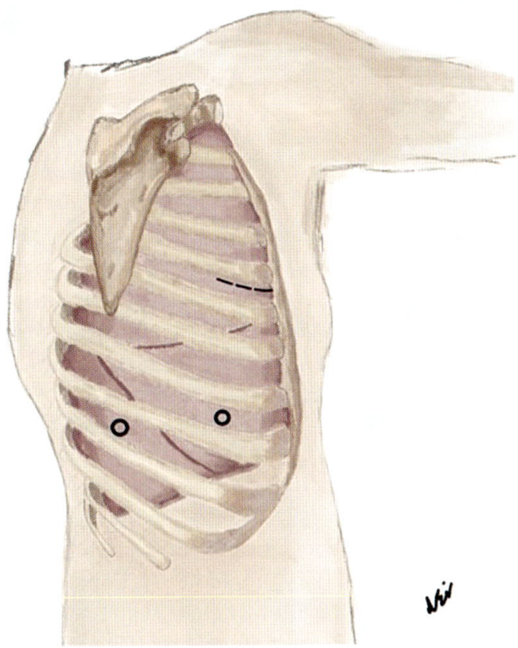

FIGURE 6.9 ▮ Video-assisted thoracoscopic surgery approach port placement. (Illustration by Danielle Ellis.)

Lymphadenectomy/Opening the Mediastinal Pleura

- Similar to RATS, we begin each lobectomy by incising the inferior pulmonary ligament—working from inferior to superior—excising station 9, 7, 11, and 4 lymph nodes from the posterior and superior hilum.
- If a complete lymphadenectomy is not needed (as in the case of benign disease) this step may be omitted and the surgeon may begin by widely opening the anterior mediastinal pleura. The pleura is opened posterior to the phenic nerve to completely expose the superior pulmonary vein and the soft tissue, which separates the superior vein from the inferior vein.
- Much of the anterior major fissure can be developed at this juncture. In the case of a complete major fissure, the investing visceral pleura may be excised entirely with cautery and the middle lobe separated from the lower lobe.

Division of the Bronchovascular Structures

- The middle lobe branch of the superior vein is circumferentially dissected and divided using a vascular load stapler. Like most staple fires in this operation, the stapler is passed through the posterior assistant port and angulated cephalad such that it is parallel with the phrenic nerve.
- The middle lobe is then retracted posteriorly revealing the soft tissue and lymph nodes investing the middle lobe bronchus. These lymph nodes are excised and the bronchus is circumferentially dissected, separating it from the main pulmonary artery located posteriorly and from the middle lobe pulmonary artery located posteriorly and superiorly and following the same course as the bronchus. Once dissected, the bronchus is divided with a thin tissue load.
- Further posterior retraction of the middle lobe reveals the pulmonary arterial supply. Large branches are divided with a vascular load stapler. Small accessory vessels may be clipped or taken with an energy device.

Completion

- After division of the bronchovascular structures, the middle lobe is further separated from the main pulmonary artery and from structures associated with the upper lobe. A stapler passed through the access port is well positioned to create the minor fissure in a posterior-to-anterior direction.
- The lobe is withdrawn through the assistant port. It may be necessary to place the specimen into a specimen retrieval bag to prevent disruption during extraction.
- Any residual lymph nodes are removed. Posterior intercostal nerve blocks are administered. Hemostasis is confirmed. A posterior pleural tube is positioned and the lung is reinflated.
- The port sites—particularly the access incision—are closed in layers.

Open

TIPS

- *An open approach to the middle lobe is necessary only in the face of extenuating circumstances as reoperative surgery, radiation fibrosis, calcified lymphadenopathy, or extensive pleural adhesive disease. The nature of these extenuating circumstances dictates the size and location of the thoracotomy.*
- *Such circumstances may also dictate additions or modifications to the standard operative approach, including performing a handsewn bronchoplasty or pulmonary arterioplasty, or harvesting an intercostal muscle or pericardial fat flap to buttress a bronchial closure.*
- *An epidural catheter for intra- and postoperative analgesia should be placed in all patient's undergoing thoracotomy unless contraindications exist.*

Incision and Entry

- The operating surgeon stands on the patient's right (posterior) for a posterolateral thoracotomy and on the patient's left (anterior) for an axillary thoracotomy. In both cases, it is advisable to first create a 1-cm thoracoscopy port in the anterior inferior chest wall and perform a diagnostic thoracoscopy to exclude metastatic disease. This port is often useful later as access for a stapler or positioning a chest tube.
- A posterolateral thoracotomy begins midway between the spine and the posterior aspect of the scapula. The incision crosses the scapula tip and curves to follow the orientation of the ribs. The latissimus dorsi muscle is divided. The posterior border of the serratus anterior muscle is identified and mobilized. The muscle is retracted anteriorly while the scapula is elevated. The chest is entered above the sixth rib, which is transected posteriorly to improve access. A rib spreader and soft-tissue retractor facilitate exposure.
- An axillary, muscle-sparing thoracotomy is performed by dividing the skin and soft tissue in the axilla, mobilizing the anterior border of the latissimus dorsi muscle and retracting the preserved muscle posteriorly. The serratus anterior muscle is split in the direction of its fibers. The intercostal muscle above the fifth or sixth rib is opened, preserving the long thoracic nerve. The rib is transected anteriorly and a rib spreader and soft-tissue retractor or large wound protector complete the exposure. This incision is associated with less pain and shorter recovery than a posterolateral thoracotomy but does limit working space and exposure to the posterior hilum. In an emergency, an access port created for a VATS approach can be enlarged to an axillary thoracotomy.

General Conduct

- There is no precise order of operations for an open middle lobectomy. Excellent exposure to the fissures and the anterior and posterior hilum allows for the operation to proceed in any order. Given that extenuating circumstances exist by definition, flexibility in approach is a distinct asset.
- Generally, the operation begins with a complete lymphadenectomy and mobilization of the mediastinal pleura on all sides.
- If the major fissure is complete or mostly complete, identifying the main pulmonary artery in the fissure is an expeditious way to determine the location of all the critical structures. The middle lobe artery can be circumferentially dissected sharply or with judicious use electrocautery and then divided, revealing the bronchus and allowing for division of the anterior major fissure.
- If the major fissure is incomplete or a centrally located tumor/lymphadenopathy obscures the pulmonary artery in this location, the operation may instead proceed anterior-to-posterior as with the VATS approach.
- In the case of a central tumor or fixed central lymphadenopathy for which concern exists about the ability to achieve a negative bronchial or pulmonary arterial margin, it may be necessary to perform a bronchoplasty or arterioplasty.
- Bronchoplasty is performed by sharply dividing the middle lobe bronchus, confirming a negative bronchial margin with frozen section, and then hand sewing the bronchial stump. We use interrupted 4-0 Vicryl suture. If the resulting stump is too short to permit closure, a sleeve lobectomy

with creation of a right lower lobe–to–bronchus intermedius anastomosis should be performed. A bronchial sleeve resection is preferable to a bronchial stump closed with excessive tension. The latter is likely to result in stump breakdown and a bronchopleural fistula. All complex bronchial stump closures should be buttressed with well-vascularized tissue such as intercostal muscle.

- Middle lobe pulmonary arterioplasty can be challenging because vascular isolation is difficult to achieve. The main pulmonary artery is encircled either at the hilum or intrapericardially and clamped for proximal control. Distal control typically requires clamping both inferior and superior pulmonary veins and is often imperfect. Back bleeding can be brisk. If heparin is given, the accepted dose is 20 U/kg and should be administered 5 minutes before clamping. There is no consensus about the need for heparin, however. Once isolated, the involved portion of the pulmonary artery can be sharply excised beginning proximal to the tumor or fixed lymph nodes. This is done in a tangential fashion to avoid compromising the posterior ascending or superior segmental arteries. The resulting defect is then closed primarily using a running 5-0 or 6-0 Prolene suture. An autologous or bovine pericardial patch can be used to avoid narrowing the pulmonary artery if a large defect is present. The clamps are removed and repair stitches are placed. A tissue flap should always be interposed between the vascular suture line and the bronchial stump to prevent bronchovascular fistula.

Postoperative Care

- A single chest tube is placed to water seal and removed on the first postoperative day unless an air leak or excessive fluid drainage is present.
- Pain control is achieved with nonsteroidal anti-inflammatory drugs, Tylenol, neuromodulators such as gabapentin, and judicious use of narcotics. An epidural catheter should be used for patients undergoing posterolateral thoracotomy.
- Early mobilization and chest physiotherapy contribute to early recovery. We aim to discharge patients on the first or second day after minimally invasive lobectomy.
- Common complications include persistent air leak, cardiac arrhythmia, and pneumonia. Seldom are these complications life threatening.
- Patients should expect to recover over a period of 3 to 6 weeks and to regain essentially all of their preoperative function. It is common for patients to complain of persistent mild intercostal neuralgia or dry cough for several weeks or months after surgery.

PEARLS AND PITFALLS

- An expectation of abnormal pulmonary arterial and venous anatomy will prevent the surgeon from being surprised. Duplicate and recurrent branches with unusual pathways are the rule in pulmonary surgery.
- Understanding the location of the middle lobe bronchus is critical to middle lobectomy. Once the bronchus is identified and partially dissected, the extent of the major fissure and the location of the middle lobe artery are apparent.

Suggested Readings

1. Hawn MT, Mulholland MW. In: Hawn M, ed. *Operative Techniques in Thoracic and Esophageal Surgery*. 1st ed. Lippincott Williams & Wilkins (LWW); 2015.
2. Mathisen DJ, Morse CR. *Master Techniques in Surgery: Thoracic Surgery—Lung Resections, Bronchoplasty*. Wolters Kluwer; 2015.
3. Zwischenberger BA, D'amico TA, Tong BC. *HOW I TEACH IT How I Teach a Thoracoscopic Lobectomy*; 2016.

Chapter 7

Right Lower Lobectomy: Robotic/Video-Assisted Thoracic Surgery/ Thoracotomy

PAUL W. FURLOW
HARALD C. OTT

Perioperative Considerations

- As for any lobectomy, when right lower lobectomy is considered for the treatment of a patient's lung disease, preoperative evaluation aims to identify those patients in which the risk of surgery is unacceptably high.
- Assessment of cardiopulmonary function and overall functional status should be performed for all patients undergoing lung resection.
- Pulmonary function tests, including measurement of diffusion capacity (DLCO), provide quantitative data on pulmonary status.
- The Six-Minute Walk and Stair Climb tests provide qualitative information regarding a patient's overall cardiopulmonary status.
- In patients with marginal pulmonary function, quantitative perfusion scanning allows for more precise predictions of postoperative pulmonary function.
- All preoperative lung resection patients will undergo a baseline electrocardiogram to assess cardiac function.
- Patients with cardiac risk factors undergo myocardial stress testing to evaluate for cardiac ischemia and echocardiogram for assessment of ventricular function, valve function, and pulmonary arterial pressures.
- Other important preoperative considerations include smoking history, use of supplemental oxygen, nutritional status, and the degree of social support.

TIPS

Aim to have patients quit smoking at least 2 weeks before most pulmonary resections. Lung volume reduction surgery requires a longer duration of smoking cessation (≤3 months).

- Contrast-enhanced computed tomography (CT) scan of the chest is critical for reviewing tumor size and location, involvement of adjacent structures, anatomy of the local airways and vasculature, fissural anatomy, and the presence of infection or lung destruction.
- Previous thoracic operations, including those of the breast, and history of lung infections should also be considered when preparing for any pulmonary resection.

Instruments and Equipment

- Depending on the approach, standard robotic, thoracoscopic, or thoracotomy instruments are required—the specifics of which will be dictated by the operative surgeon.
- For any robotic or thoracoscopic pulmonary resection, a chest tray should be available in case conversion to an open operation is necessary.

Anesthesia and Patient Positioning

- For lung resection via thoracotomy or thoracoscopy with an increased likelihood of open conversion, a thoracic epidural catheter is placed preoperatively.
- The use of deep venous thrombosis (DVT) prophylaxis with subcutaneous heparin or low-molecular-weight heparin (LMWH) is dependent upon surgeon preference and risk of postoperative bleeding.
- General anesthesia with a double-lumen endotracheal tube (or single-lumen tube with bronchial blocker) to allow for single lung ventilation contralateral to the tumor.

TIPS

Left-sided double-lumen endotracheal tubes placed in the left mainstem bronchus are commonly used for both right- and left-sided pulmonary resections.

- Complex cases necessitate a Foley catheter for intraoperative fluid management and postoperative hemodynamic monitoring.
- The need for arterial line and central venous line placement should be made with the thoracic anesthesia team and is dependent upon the patient's clinical status, location of the tumor, extent of the operation, and expected difficulty of dissection.
- Patients should receive perioperative antibiotics (30-60 minutes before incision) suitable to the patient's allergies and clinical history.

TIPS

The operative side is verified with the patient awake and marked preoperatively.

- The patient is placed in the left lateral decubitus position on a padded mattress (Figure 7.1).
  - While supine, the patient's xiphoid is aligned with the break in the bed to allow for maximal rib separation with bed flexion.

TIPS

If the break in the bed is too low, the rib spaces will remain narrow and the elevated iliac crest can interfere with VATS/RATS instrumentation.

- With the head, airway, and legs stabilized, the patient is drawn toward the right side of the bed and then rotated into the left lateral decubitus position.
- The anterior and posterior thorax is supported by a vacuum mattress, gel pads, or shoulder rolls.
- The left arm is straight and extended 90° at the shoulder with padded support at the joints.
- The right arm is extended 90° at the shoulder and flexed to just under 90° at the elbow supported through the elbow and forearm by an elevated cushioned bar.
- The bed is maximally flexed while the head and hips are supported and, once in optimal position, the patient is secured to the bed with a safety strap over the anterior superior iliac spine.

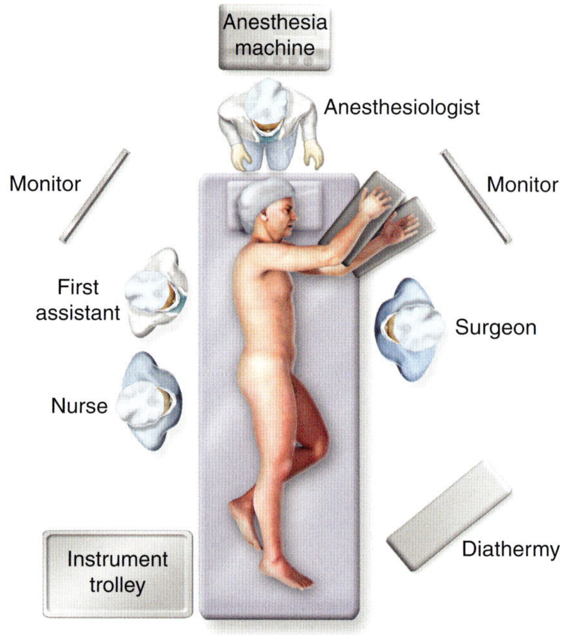

FIGURE 7.1 ▮ Positioning for right lower lobectomy. Schematic description of standard left-lateral decubitus positioning and of operating room configuration for most right video-assisted thoracoscopic surgery pulmonary procedures. (From Weyan MJ. Right lower lobe: VATS. In: Mathisen DJ, Morse C, eds. *Master Techniques in Surgery: Thoracic Surgery—Lung Resections, Bronchoplasty*. Wolters Kluwer; 2015:143-152. Figure 14.1B.)

TIPS

With the bed flexed, ensure that the head is supported with blankets or pillows to ensure the cervical spine remains in a neutral position.

- For minimally invasive cases, when bleeding may require conversion to thoracotomy, the plan for a swift hemostasis and an orderly transition to an open procedure is discussed with the entire team prior to incision.

Technique

Robot-Assisted Thoracoscopic Surgery

- The techniques of robot-assisted thoracoscopic surgery (RATS) right lower lobectomy generally mimic those of video-assisted thoracoscopic surgery (VATS) right lower lobectomy apart from port placement and robotic instrumentation. The key differences are outlined in the section that follows.

Robotic Port Site Placement

- A total of five ports are most commonly utilized in robotic lobectomy—four robotic ports and one assistant (Figure 7.2).

TIPS

A four-port RATS method employing three robotic ports and an assistant port can also be used, where the most posterior robotic port is brought more anteriorly and there is no additional port between that and the camera port.

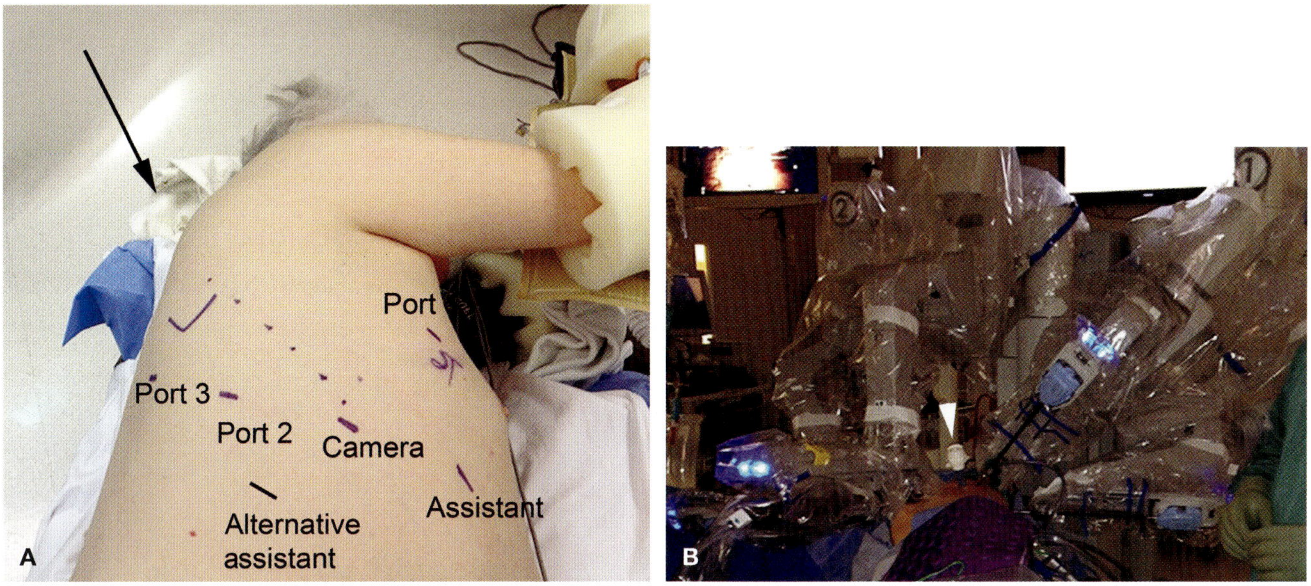

FIGURE 7.2 | Port placement and robotic positioning for robotic-assisted thoracoscopic surgery right lower lobectomy. **A.** The patient is placed in the lateral decubitus position standard port placement for a right-sided robotic lobectomy. **B.** The robot it brought in perpendicular to the patient and the boom is rotated in line with the major fissure. The robotic arms are then docked to the ports. (From Grenda T, Lin J. Lobectomy: robotic. In: Mulholland MW, Albo D, Dalman R, Hawn M, Hughes S, Sabel M, eds. *Operative Techniques in Surgery*. Wolters Kluwer; 2015:52-64. Figure 1.7.3BC.)

- In lower lobectomy all robotic ports are placed in the 8th intercostal space.
- The 12-mm camera port is placed first just above the diaphragm at the posterior axillary line and the correct placement is visualized CO_2 insufflation with a pressure of 10 mm Hg is initiated.
- The remaining ports are placed under direct visualization using the camera.
- Robotic arm 3 (8-mm port) is then placed 12 cm lateral to the vertebral spinous process.
- Robotic arm 2 (8-mm port) is placed 10 cm lateral to robotic arm 3.
- Robotic arm 1 (8-mm port) is placed above the diaphragm anteriorly superiorly ~10 cm from the camera port.
- The assistant port (12 mm) is placed at least two rib spaces lower between the camera port and robotic arm 1.

TIPS

The camera is moved to different ports for optimal visualization during port placement.

- The robot is docked perpendicular to the bed and the boom is rotated at 15° toward the patient's face, off the long axis of the operating table.
- The robotic arms are connected to the ports and the separation between arms is maximized manually by joint rotation.
- The instruments are loaded as follows: (1) 8-mm curved bipolar dissector, (2) 8-mm fenestrated bipolar (Cadiere) forceps, and (3) 8-mm Tip-up grasper.

General Concepts for Robotic Lobectomy

- If dense adhesions are encountered upon chest entry, they can be lysed by typical VATS methods through the assistant port.
- Pre-rolled sponges, introduced though the assistant port, are used for lung retraction and localized hemostasis.
- To encircle the vein, artery, and bronchus safely, we employ a soft blunt-tip vessel loop that can be attached to the lower jaw of the linear stapling device.
- The stapler can be placed though the assistant port, or any of the 8-mm incisions once the robotic trocar is removed.

TIPS

A robotic stapler (EndoWrist) can also be used through robotic arm two if a 12-mm port is created.

Key Steps for RATS vs VATS Right Lower Lobectomy

- With gentle upward traction of the right lower lobe, the inferior pulmonary ligament is divided and the station 9 lymph node is removed (Figure 7.3).

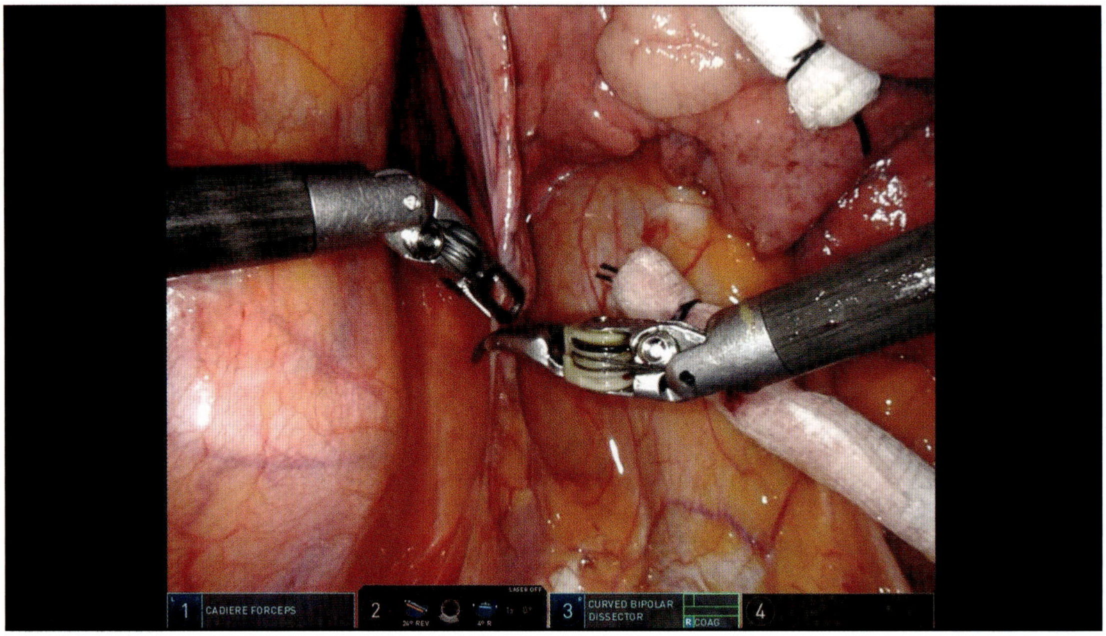

FIGURE 7.3 ▌ Division of the inferior pulmonary ligament with upward retraction on the right lower lobe. The station 9 lymph node, if present, lies adjacent to the right inferior pulmonary vein.

- The inferior pulmonary vein is dissected circumferentially (Figure 7.4).

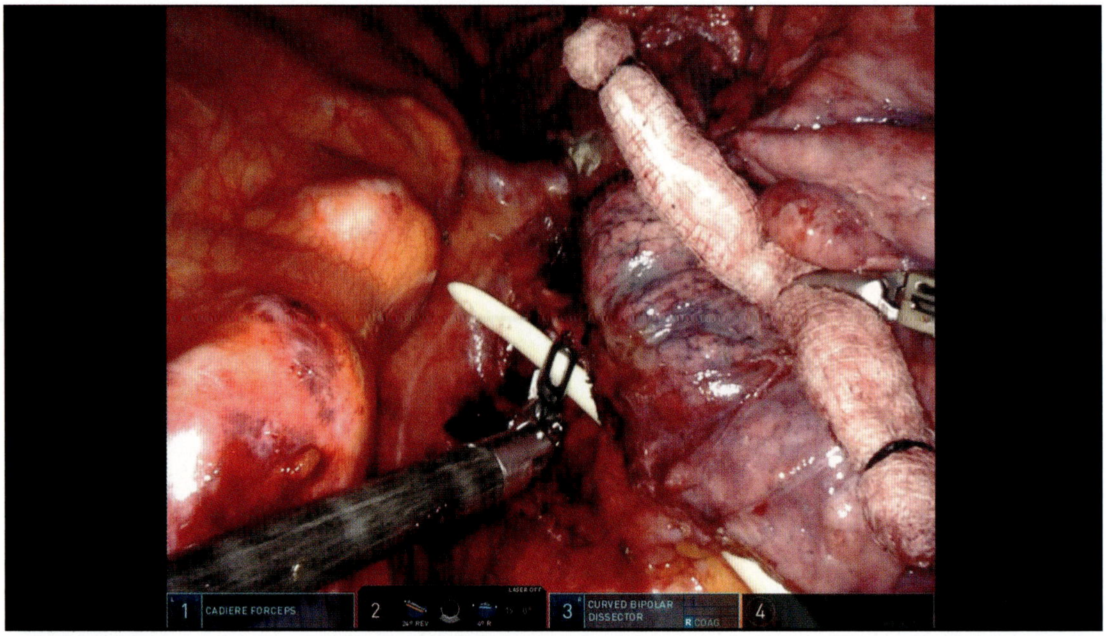

FIGURE 7.4 ▌ Isolation of the right inferior pulmonary vein using a blunt-end vessel loop.

- The lung is positioned posteriorly and the branch points of the middle and superior pulmonary veins are identified.
- Dissection of the fissure begins at the anterior hilum between the right middle and right upper lobes (Figure 7.5).

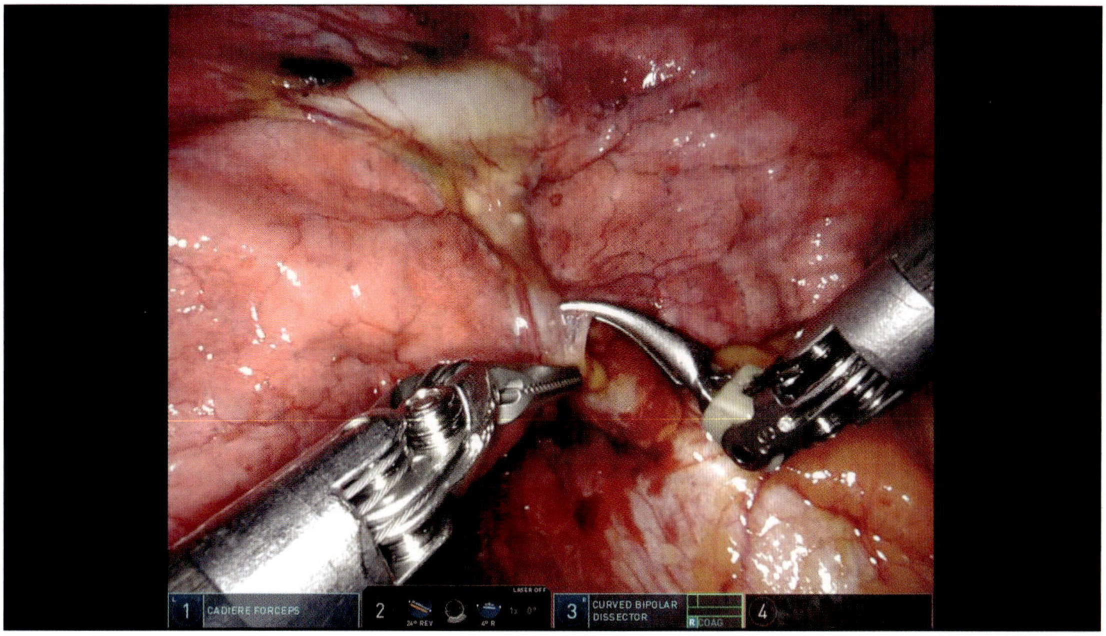

FIGURE 7.5 ▮ Dissection of the anterior oblique fissure over the inferior pulmonary vein between the right middle lobe (screen right) and right lower lobe (screen left).

- The ongoing right lower lobe artery is dissected out until the right middle lobe and superior segmental arterial branches are visualized (Figure 7.6).

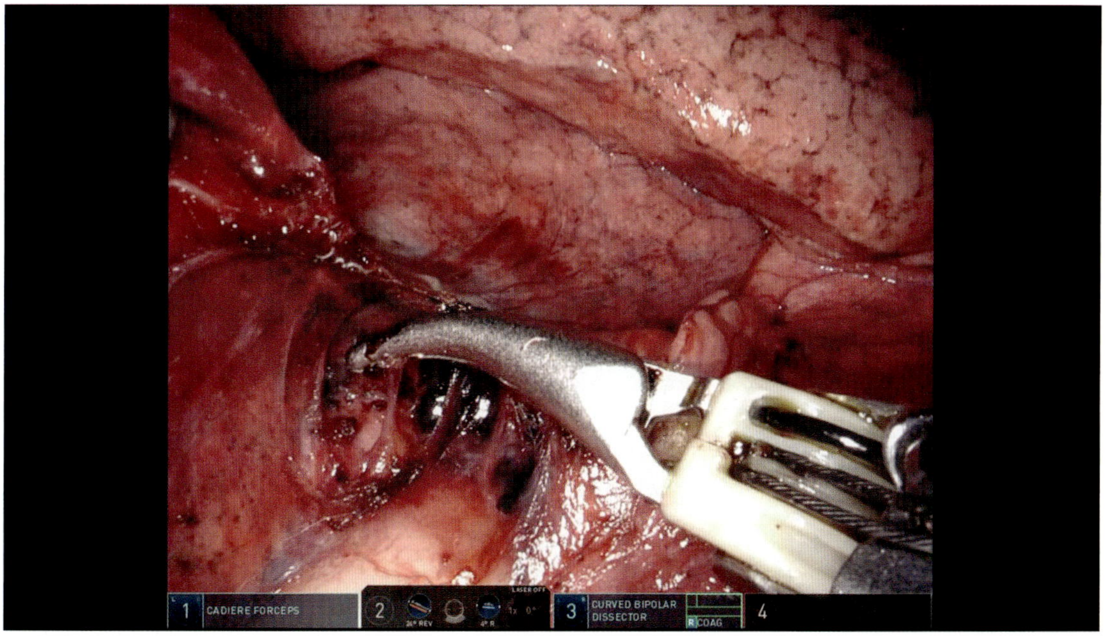

FIGURE 7.6 ▮ Development of the areolar plane just above the right inferior pulmonary artery (foreground). The superior segmental artery is seen just below the tip of the bipolar. Level 12 lymph nodes reside near the branch point of the artery.

- For incomplete fissures, development of an anterior-to-posterior areolar tunnel from the pulmonary artery at the triple-point to the posterior hilum at lymph node station 11R allows for visualization of all arterial branches and safe passage of the stapling device (Figure 7.7).

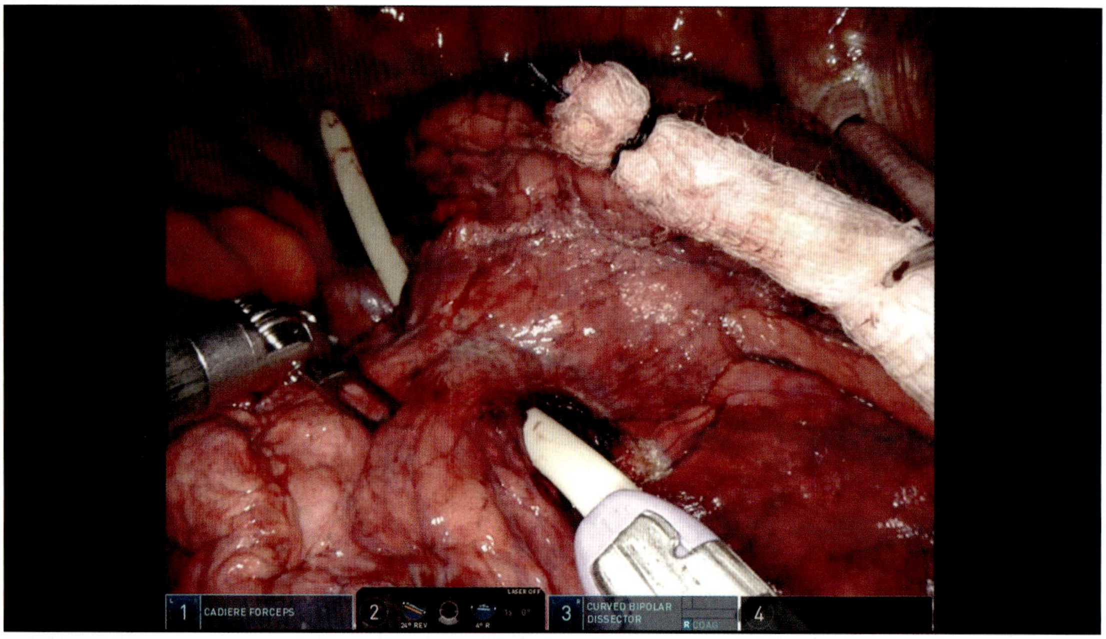

FIGURE 7.7 ▌ Division of the posterior oblique fissure. Placement of a blunt-end vessel loop over the pulmonary arteries and through the tunnel made between the ongoing right inferior pulmonary artery anteriorly, and station 11 posteriorly. The robotic vessel loop is attached to the curved tip of the stapler to allow safe passage around the parenchymal bridge at the fissure.

- If the fissure is complete, the pleura over the pulmonary artery is incised and its branches are exposed and identified.
- The superior segmental artery and right basilar artery are then encircled with a vessel loop and transected using an endovascular stapler (Figure 7.8).

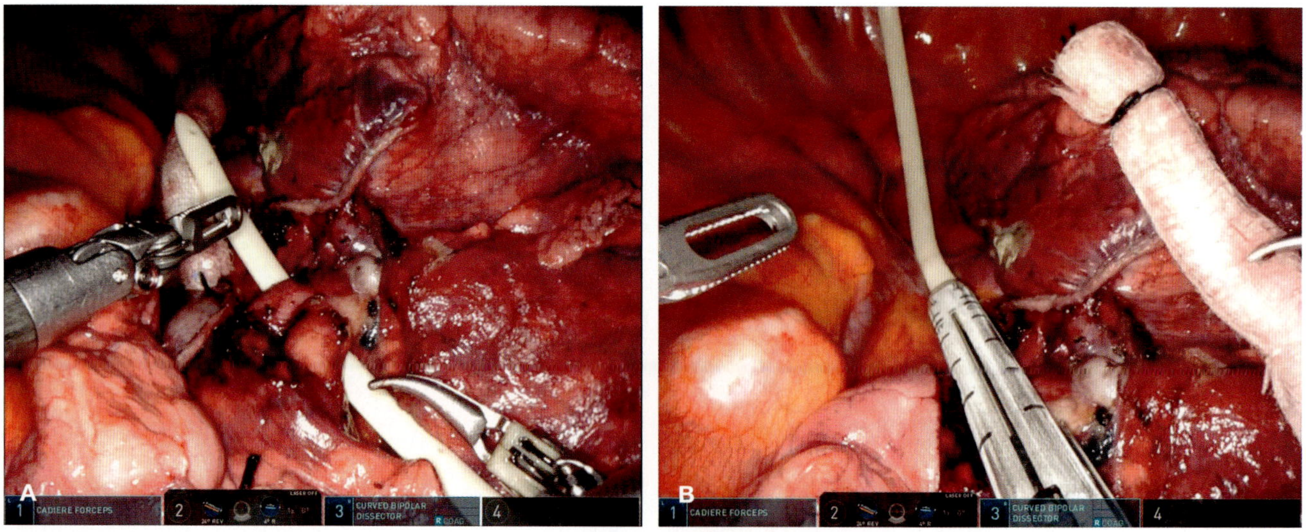

FIGURE 7.8 ▌ Isolation and division of the right lower lobe arteries. **A.** The right superior segmental artery and right basilar artery are encircled with the vessel loop. **B.** The stapler is closed across the right lower lobe arteries and preservation of the right middle lobe artery is ensured (seen here clear of the stapler jaws).

TIPS

The right lower lobe artery is transected only when the safety of the right middle lobe artery is ensured.

- After arterial control, the isolated inferior pulmonary vein is transected in the same fashion (Figure 7.9).

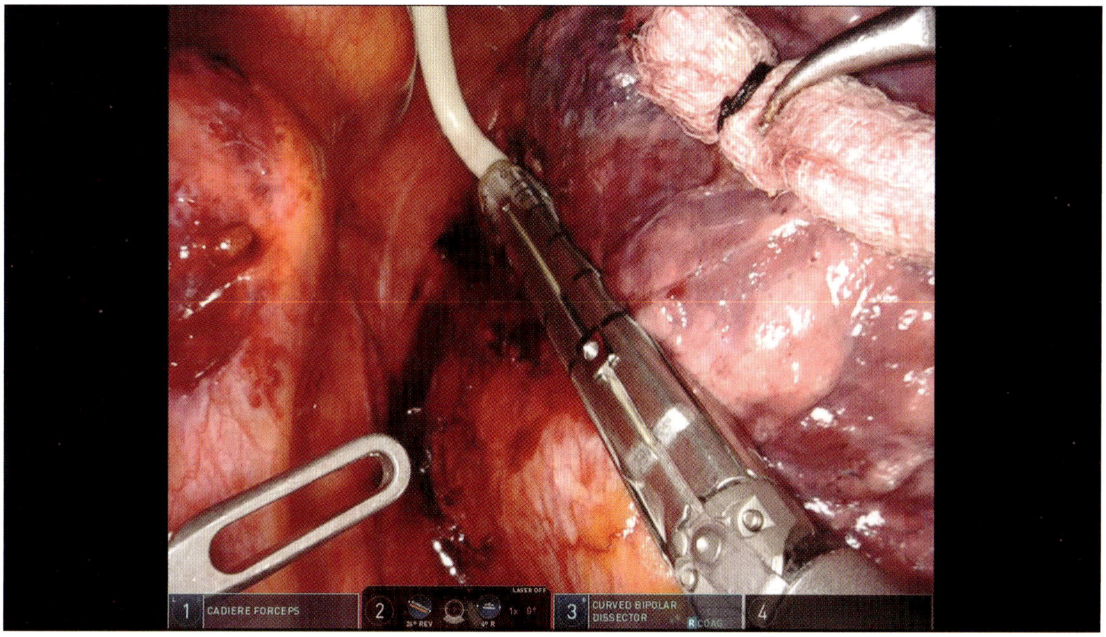

FIGURE 7.9 ▮ Division of the inferior pulmonary vein. Prior to firing the stapler, the right middle lobe vein is identified and preserved.

- Any remaining parenchymal attachments to the middle or upper lobes are then divided with a linear stapler.
- The lower lobe is retracted skyward and the peribronchial tissue is bluntly swept into the specimen. At this point, the right middle lobe bronchus is identified and the right lower lobe bronchus is isolated (Figure 7.10A).

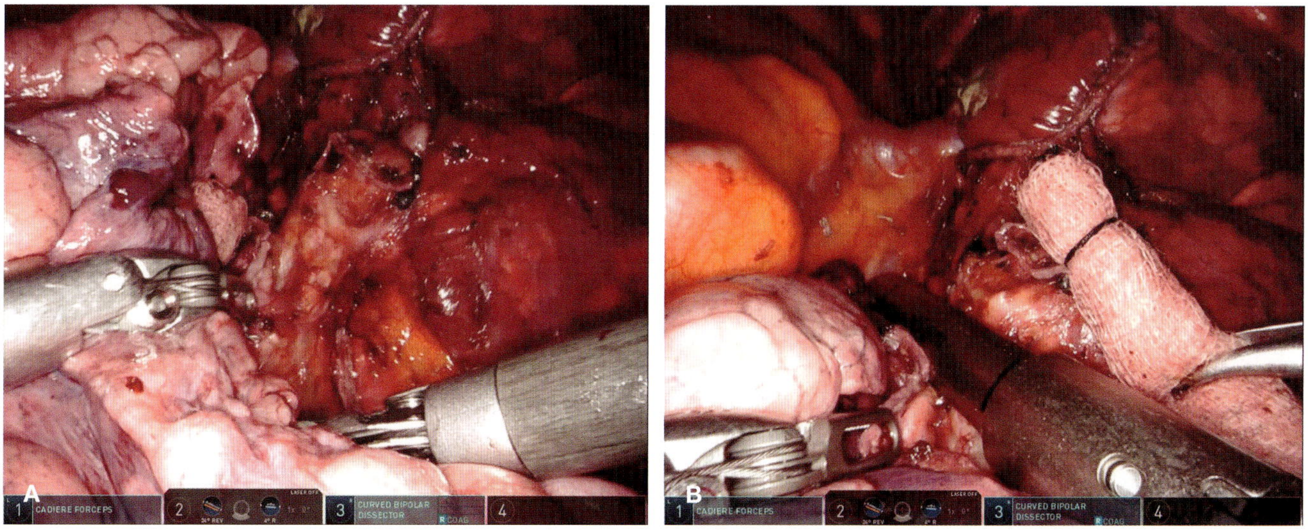

FIGURE 7.10 ▮ **A.** Skeletonization of the right lower lobe bronchus. **B.** Placement of the stapler across the right lower lobe bronchus while ensuring preservation of the right middle lobe bronchus (visualized above and to the right of the staple jaws).

- The stapler is closed around the bronchus and ventilation to the right middle lobe is assessed with either a test-breath or pediatric bronchoscope visualization.
- The bronchus is stapled across and the specimen is removed (Figure 7.10B).
- The mediastinal lymph node dissection, assessment of hemostasis, intercostal nerve blocks, chest tube placement, and chest closure continue as described in the following section (VATS).

TIPS

Prior to closure, the insufflation is turned off, lung ventilation is confirmed, and the robot is undocked.

Video-Assisted Thoracoscopic Surgery

Port Site Placement

- Three ports are routinely utilized in VATS lobectomy (Figure 7.11).
  - The camera port is typically placed through the 8th or 9th interspace at the mid-axillary line.
  - A 3 to 4 cm working incision is made at the level of the superior pulmonary vein at the anterior axillary line (typically the 4th interspace).
  - The utility port is placed through the 7th or 8th interspace at the posterior axillary line off the tip of the scapula.

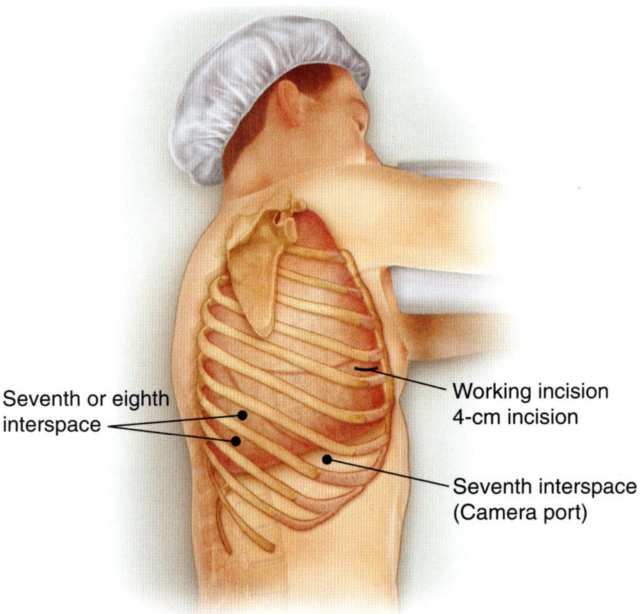

FIGURE 7.11 ▮ Illustration of standard port site placements for video-assisted thoracoscopic surgery pulmonary procedures. (From Weyan MJ. Right lower lobe: VATS. In: Mathisen DJ, Morse C, eds. *Master Techniques in Surgery: Thoracic Surgery—Lung Resections, Bronchoplasty*. Wolters Kluwer; 2015:143-152. Figure 14.2A.)

TIPS

Camera port placement is performed first and thoracoscopy is used to ensure optimal placement of the working incision and utility port.

Intrathoracic Assessment

- Upon placement of the camera within the chest, the pleura, diaphragm, and chest wall are inspected for evidence of metastatic disease, and any suspicious lesions or effusions are sampled for immediate pathologic or cytologic evaluation, respectively.
- Using an angled-ring clamp though the accessory port to provide countertraction, the lung is digitally palpated through the working incision to identify the lesion.

TIPS

Pleural adhesions encountered during inspection are lysed via sharp dissection or electrocautery.

Isolation and Division of the Pulmonary Vein

- The inferior pulmonary ligament is put under tension by providing gentle upward traction on the right lower lobe using a ring clamp.
- Using either thoracoscopic DeBakey forceps or a pediatric suction device, the inferior pulmonary ligament is splayed out and divided by electrocautery up to the inferior pulmonary vein.

TIPS

Level 9 lymph nodes within the inferior pulmonary ligament, if present, reside adjacent to the vein.

- The inferior pulmonary vein is then exposed by blunt dissection using a pediatric suction device or a "peanut" against countertraction provided by thoracoscopic forceps.

TIPS

The vein can be safely manipulated if held carefully and broadly. The artery should never be grasped.

- The inferior pulmonary vein is then encircled using a large blunt right-angled clamp and isolated using a vessel loop.
- Prior to dividing this vein, it is imperative to identify the middle lobe vein as it can drain into the inferior pulmonary vein, and must be spared.
- Through the working incision, a curved-tip endovascular stapler is visualized being placed around the inferior pulmonary vein and the vessel loop is removed.
- The stapler is then closed and the vein is transected.

TIPS

For any staple fire, if the angles are suboptimal, the stapler can be placed though one of the other two ports and the camera moved accordingly.

Isolation and Division of the Pulmonary Arteries

- Complete fissure
  - If the major fissure is complete or near-complete and the pulmonary artery is identified at the base of the fissure, the pleura over the right lower lobe pulmonary artery can be incised and the artery carefully isolated by gentle blunt dissection.

  - The middle lobe and superior segmental arteries are then identified.
  - The superior segmental artery and common arterial trunk to the right lower lobe are isolated through careful blunt dissection, encircled with a vessel loop either individually or together, and are transected using a curved-tip endovascular stapler introduced through the working incision.
- Incomplete fissure
  - The presence of a grossly incomplete fissure may require division of the right lower lobe bronchus prior and isolation of the artery from an inferior approach.
  - In the inferior approach to the artery, the endovascular stapler is again introduced through the working incision.

Isolation and Division of the Right Upper Lobe Bronchus

- If the pulmonary artery has been transected, the right lower lobe can be lifted away from the hilum to elevate and expose the bronchus.
- To dissect the bronchus, the peribronchial fat and lymphatic tissue should be bluntly swept up into the specimen.
- Exercise caution when bluntly dissecting behind the bronchus, where the lower lobe pulmonary artery is prone to injury.

TIPS

Always remember that the pulmonary artery lies directly behind the bronchus.

- An endoscopic GIA stapler with a purple staple cartridge (45 mm) is placed the working incision and around the bronchus while care is taken not to encroach onto the right middle lobe bronchus which runs from left to right.
- Once the right lower lobe bronchus is isolated, the stapler can be closed and patency of the right middle lobe bronchus is verified either by anesthesia giving a right-sided test breath or by direct visualization using a pediatric bronchoscope.
- The stapler is then fired and the bronchus is transected.

Division of the Fissure and Removal of the Specimen

- The remaining major fissure is then transected using tissue-appropriate endoscopic GIA staplers through the working incision.
- The right lower lobe is then placed into an endoscopic retrieval bag and removed through the working incision.

TIPS

For bulky tumors, the working incision can be extended by dividing the pleura and intercostal muscles alone. Occasionally, the skin incision may also need to be extended.

Mediastinal Lymph Node Assessment

- Principles of mediastinal lymph node dissection are discussed in detail in Chapter 13, Principles of Mediastinal Lymph Node Dissection of this textbook.
- For right lower lobectomy, mediastinal lymph node dissection at stations 2R/4R, 7, 8, and 9 aid in accurate staging and postoperative management.
- To minimize bleeding and risk of chyle leak during nodal sampling, we dissect just off the nodal capsule using electrocautery while picking up directly on the node or nodal packet with endoscopic forceps (Figure 7.12).
- Should bleeding incur, a combination of direct compression, hemostatic gauze, and localized electrocautery while keeping nearby structures (eg, nerves, bronchus, esophagus) in mind, is almost always sufficient.

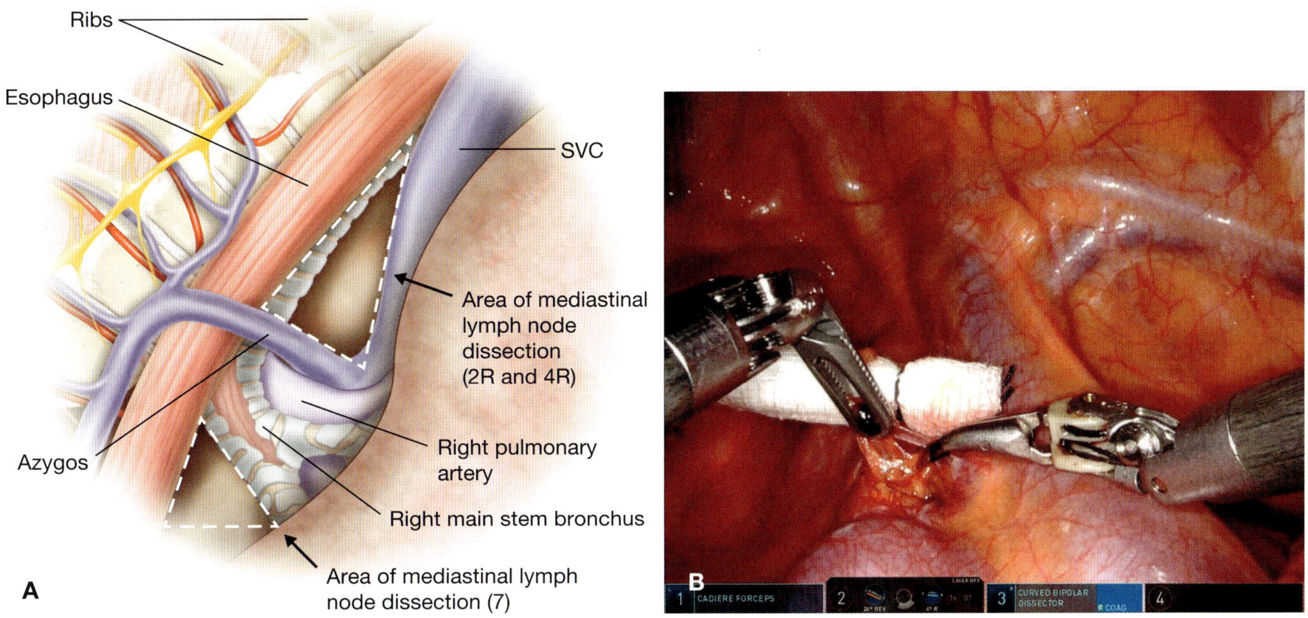

FIGURE 7.12 ▮ Mediastinal lymph node dissection during right-sided robotic lobectomy. **A.** A schematic showing the relevant nodal stations for dissection right-sided lobectomy. **B.** Robotic dissection of station 4R triangulated between the superior vena cava (anterior), azygous vein (inferior), and trachea (posteriorly). (**A.** From Wei B, Cerfolio RJ. Robotic approach to lobectomy. In: Mathisen DJ, Morse C, eds. *Master Techniques in Surgery: Thoracic Surgery—Lung Resections, Bronchoplasty*. Wolters Kluwer; 2015:209-222. Figure 20.6.)

Closing

- Intercostal nerve block
  - Using a mediastinoscopy needle though the working incision, 0.25% Marcaine with epinephrine is injected adjacent to the intercostal nerve bundles just under the endothoracic fascia while avoiding the neurovascular bundles (Figure 7.13).

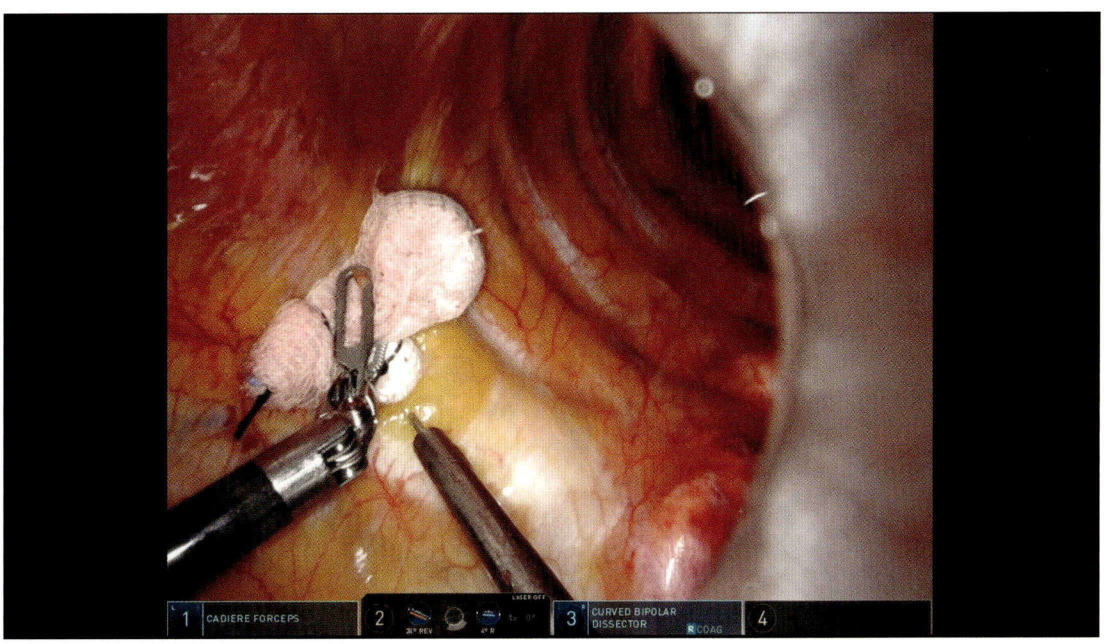

FIGURE 7.13 ▮ Intercostal nerve block. By occluding the intercostal space above the site of injection, local anesthetic is directed longitudinally along multiple rib spaces superiorly and inferiorly.

TIPS

Proper instillation of the local anesthetic is confirmed by the creation of an expanding weal along the course of the intercostal space. Always withdraw on needle before injection to confirm absence of blood (ie, vascular access).

- We aim to perform nerve blocks from one space above the working incision to one space below the camera port.

Thoracostomy Tube Placement

- Typically, a 24F chest tube is placed through the camera port and positioned along the posterior hilum up until it lies just off the apex.

TIPS

At the skin, the chest tubes can either be tunneled or the incision around the tube closed primary to prevent air leak.

- The tube is then secured to the skin with a 0-silk stitch and placed to a chest drainage system at −20 cm H_2O, until the patient arrives in the recovery area where the tube is placed on water seal.

Port Site Closure

- Each port is examined using the thoracoscope and hemostasis is ensured using electrocautery.
- The working incision is closed using a 0 Vicryl running stitch on the muscle, a 2-0 Vicryl running stitch on the superficial fascia, and a 4-0 Vicryl or Monocryl running subcuticular stitch on the skin.
- The camera port and utility ports are closed in two layers—the superficial fascia and skin.
- Sterile adhesive strips are applied over the incision and topped with occlusive sterile dry dressings.

Thoracotomy

Incision Placement

- The posterolateral thoracotomy incision is a gentle S-shaped incision following the course of the 5th rib as it extends from the anterior axillary line to the level of T4 or higher between the scapula and spine (Figure 7.14).
- The incision has two slight curves—at the inferior and superior angles of the scapula.
- The subcutaneous tissue is divided along the entire incision using electrocautery until the investing fascia of the latissimus dorsi muscle is encountered. This muscle can either be divided or fully mobilized and retracted posteriorly (muscle-sparing thoracotomy).
- The serratus anterior is then separated parallel to its muscle fibers along the 5th rib and the thoracic fascia is exposed.
- To confirm thoracotomy positioning at the 5th interspace, the ribs are counted manually using a hand-held scapular retractor to elevate the scapula while passing a free hand under the scapula to develop a plane superiorly until the 1st rib is identified.
- The periosteum is then incised over the length of the 5th rib using electrocautery and reflected superiorly off of the rib with a periosteal elevator.
- The fate of the lower rib is ultimately decided based on the operative circumstances; however, to ensure adequate rib spreading while maintaining structure integrity of the chest we typically use a rib cutter and Kocher forceps to remove the most posterior 2 cm of the rib.

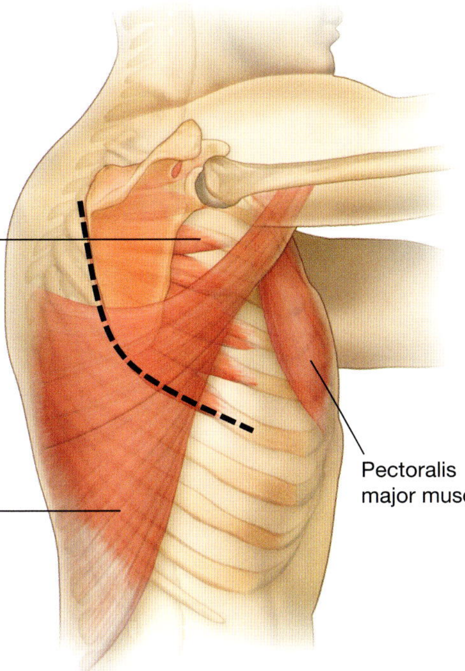

FIGURE 7.14 | Posterolateral thoracotomy: An incision is made 1 to 2 cm below the scapular tip and continued anteriorly along the direction of the rib and posteriorly between the scapula and the spine. The latissimus dorsi is either divided or preserved and the serratus muscle is retracted anteriorly. (From Raz DJ. Techniques/Complications of Thoracotomy; **A.** From Wei B, Cerfolio RJ. Robotic approach to lobectomy. In: Mathisen DJ, Morse C, eds. *Master Techniques in Surgery: Thoracic Surgery—Lung Resections, Bronchoplasty*. Wolters Kluwer; 2015:85-93. Figure 8.1.)

TIPS

To get around the inferior rib without injuring the neurovascular bundle, keep the tip of the periosteal elevator right on the rib by directing it up and under the rib. The bundle is then pried away using a gentle rocking motion.

- The pleura over the superior border of the rib is incised using electrocautery along the extent of the incision.
- For a planned intercostal muscle flap, the intercostal muscle, neurovascular bundle, and pleura are separated from the inferior border of the 5th rib, the muscle is divided, and the ongoing intercostal vessels are suture ligated at the anterior chest wall (Figure 7.15).
- A rib spreader is placed incorporating the inferior rib, the superior rib, and the tip of the scapula and opened to expose the pleural space.

TIPS

If more separation of the ribs is needed for better exposure, the parietal pleura can be incised further anteriorly and posteriorly to provide laxity.

Intrathoracic Assessment

- Upon entry into the chest, the pleura, diaphragm, and chest wall are inspected for evidence of metastatic disease, and any suspicious lesions or effusions are sampled for immediate pathologic or cytologic evaluation, respectively.
- Pleural adhesions, if present, are lysed by sharp dissection.
- The location of the tumor is then confirmed and resectability is assessed.

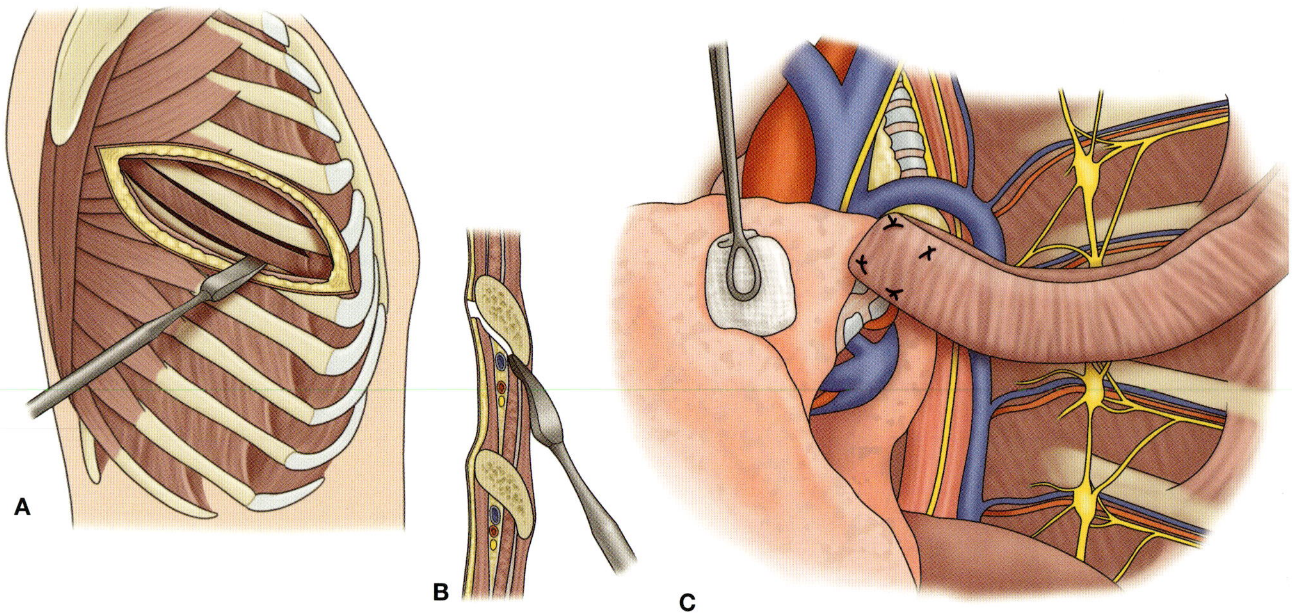

FIGURE 7.15 ▌ Intercostal muscle flap buttressing of the bronchial stump during open lobectomy. **A** and **B.** The intercostal muscle flap is harvested directly on the rib as described in the text to avoid injury to the neurovascular pedicle. **C.** The intercostal muscle flap is left attached to the origin of its vascular supply, placed into the chest after removal of the surgical specimen, and sutured to the bronchial stump to reduce the risk of bronchopleural fistula formation.

Hilar Dissection and Inferior Pulmonary Vein Isolation

- The lung is retracted posteriorly using a sponge stick to expose the hilum and the mediastinal pleural over the pulmonary artery and vein is sharply incised and gently brushed aside by blunt dissection with a "peanut" or pediatric suction device.

TIPS

When exposing the pulmonary veins, make sure to localize the right middle lobe vein branch.

- Hilar lymphadenectomy (station 10) will aid in defining vascular branch points.
- The inferior pulmonary ligament is then exposed on tension and divided using electrocautery by retracting the right lower lobe superiorly. The station 9 lymph node within the ligament, if present, is resected as described above.
- The inferior pulmonary vein is isolated by blunt dissection, encircled using a blunt right angle and snared using a vessel loop.

TIPS

Wait to divide the vein until after the arterial supply is transected to prevent lobar venous congestion and increased parenchymal bleeding.

- The lung is then retracted anteriorly and the posterior hilum is exposed by sharply incising the mediastinal pleura overlying the artery and vein posteriorly.
- Once the posterior hilum is exposed, access to the paraesophageal (station 8) and subcarinal (station 7) lymph nodes allows for lymphadenectomy.

TIPS

When working on the posterior hilum, beware of electrocautery near the esophagus and vagus nerve.

Isolation and Division of the Right Lower Lobe Arteries

Anatomic Variations of the Pulmonary Artery

- A clear understanding of the pulmonary arterial anatomy is critical for performing safe lung resections.
- In 77.8% of cases, there is a single superior segmental artery. However, there are two branches in 20.7% of cases and three in about 1.5% of cases.
- The majority of superior segmental arteries branch from the main pulmonary artery, though in 6.7% of cases it arises from the posterior basal segmental artery and travels though the superior segment of the lower lobe.

TIPS

Keep in mind that in 14% of cases the posterior ascending branch to the right upper lobe arises from the superior segmental artery of the lower lobe rather than the main trunk.

Division of the Right Lower Lobe Arteries and the Inferior Pulmonary Vein

- The visceral pleura is incised where the major and minor fissure meet and the lung parenchyma is dissected using blunt dissection and electrocautery along the course of the pulmonary artery.

TIPS

An endoscopic stapling device can also be used if a tunneled plane between the artery and parenchyma is well developed.

- Station 11 lymph nodes reside within the crotches of vascular branch points in this location and their resection optimizes arterial exposure.
- Both the basilar and superior segmental arteries are identified, encircled by standard methods, and divided using a curved-tip endovascular stapler.
- The anterior fissure is then divided from below the takeoff of the right middle lobe artery to the inferior border of the right middle lobe vein using an endo GI stapling device.
- If posterior fissure remains, it is divided with a linear stapler from just above the superior segmental artery stump to the posterior hilum.
- The inferior pulmonary vein is now divided using an endovascular stapling device.

Approach to the Right Lower Lobe Bronchus

Isolation and Division of the Bronchus

- The lung is retracted away from the hilum and both the right lower lobe bronchus and right middle lobe bronchus are identified. This is facilitated by brushing the peribronchial tissue up into the specimen along the bronchus and performing lymphadenectomy at stations 11 and 12.
- The right lower lobe bronchus is isolated circumferentially to its origin by blunt dissection and an endoscopic GIA stapler is placed flush with the takeoff of the lower bronchus without narrowing the right middle lobe bronchus.
- The stapler is closed and a test-breath is administered to ensure collapse of the right lower lobe and ventilation of the right middle lobe. Airway patency can also be directly visualized using a pediatric bronchoscope.
- The right lower lobe specimen can then be removed and sent for pathological assessment.

Bronchial Stump Coverage

- As patients treated with neoadjuvant chemo- or radiotherapy are at risk for developing bronchopleural fistula, we routinely reinforce their bronchial stumps with a pedicled intercostal muscle flap.

TIPS

Pedicled flaps using pericardial fat, pleura, diaphragm, or latissimus dorsi muscle can also be used to buttress the bronchial stump.

- The flap, made during thoracotomy, is lowered into the chest and its orientation is confirmed so that there is no twisting of the muscle and the pleural side is opposed to the bronchial staple line.
- Typically, four vertical mattress stitches are placed from the muscle to the wall of the bronchus—one adjacent to each corner of the staple line and one at the halfway point along each side of the staple line (Figure 7.15).

TIPS

When sewing the pedicled flap bronchus, start with the staple line corner nearest to the origin of the flap to allow exposure for subsequent stitches.

Mediastinal Lymph Node Assessment

- Lymphadenectomy at stations 2 and 4R are performed as discussed previously.
- Additional sampling at previously dissected stations (7, 8, 9, 10, and 11) can also be performed at this point.

Closing

Bronchial Stump Testing

- The pleural space is bathed in warm saline and the right lung is gently reinflated to assess for leakage of air.
- Should a staple line defect be identified, the area is oversewn with 4-0 or 5-0 PDS and the air leak test is repeated.

Thoracostomy Tube Placement

- With open thoracotomy, two chest tubes are typically placed—one anteriorly for air leak control and one posteriorly for fluid drainage.
- The first, a 19-French round Blake drain, is tunneled though a new incision one or two rib spaces below the thoracotomy at the anterior axillary line and positioned along the diaphragm and posterior hilum up to just below the apex.
- The second, a 24-French argyle chest tube, is tunneled though a third skin incision just adjacent to the Blake drain and positioned along the anterior chest up to the apex.
- Both tubes are secured to the skin with a 0-silk stitch, placed to a chest drainage system at −20 cm H_2O and managed postoperatively.

Thoracotomy Closure

- The chest is irrigated with warm normal saline and the surgical field is evaluated for bleeding.
- Once hemostasis is achieved, the fifth and sixth ribs are reapproximated with two or three broad figure-of-eight stitches using nonabsorbable pericostal sutures (number one or two Ethibond).

TIPS

During chest closure, the intercostal bundle is avoided by entering and exiting the chest at the superior border of each rib.

- The serratus anterior muscle and latissimus, if divided, is reapproximated using a running stitch (0-Vicryl).

TIPS

The latissimus dorsi muscle is typically closed in two layers.

- The superficial fascia and skin are closed with running stitches using 2-0 Vicryl and 4-0 Monocryl sutures, respectively.
- The incision is covered with adhesive strips and a sterile dry occlusive dressing.

Postoperative Care

- Effective analgesia is paramount in promoting effective pulmonary toilet and early ambulation to prevent respiratory compromise secondary to pneumonia and venous thromboembolism, respectively.
- We typically use patient-controlled analgesia until the patient is tolerating a regular diet, at which point they are transitioned to multimodal oral pain medication (eg, acetaminophen, ibuprofen, gabapentin, topical lidocaine patches).
- Every patient should be educated on the proper use of their incentive spirometer.
- Depending on surgeon preference, argyle chest tubes are placed on H_2O seal in the OR or to −20 cm H_2O of suction until the patient reaches the recovery unit, at which point they are placed to water seal. A postoperative chest radiograph is obtained.
- Blake drains are kept until the volume of drainage is <200 to 300 mL/d and the character has become thin and serous.

TIPS

Argyle chest tubes have low resistance and are useful for detecting air leaks. Blake drains are fluid draining tubes of higher resistance and can be kept on suction or H_2O seal until removal pending surgeon preference and CXR findings.

- After uncomplicated lobectomy, we routinely begin a clear liquid diet once recovered from anesthesia and advance to a regular diet on the first postoperative day.
- Maintenance IV fluids are administered until the patient is able to self-hydrate (usually postoperative day 1).
- If an indwelling urinary catheter was placed preoperatively, we will remove it the morning after surgery provided the patient has mobilized.
- Postoperative DVT prophylaxis is essential to preventing venous thromboembolic events in this susceptible patient population. We typically begin daily LMWH (Lovenox) or subcutaneous heparin TID on the first postoperative day.

PEARLS AND PITFALLS

- The main steps of right lower lobectomy are similar across modalities.
- A large part of the lymph node dissection is done in parallel to the lobectomy, as removal of key nodal stations will reveal critical anatomy.
- To avoid lobar congestion and increased bleeding risk, the arterial supply to the right lower lobe should be transected prior to the vein.
- Always keep in mind the anatomic variations of the superior segmental artery.
- Always identify and preserve the right middle lobe vein branch prior to transection of the inferior pulmonary vein. Visually confirm presence of a superior pulmonary vein.
- When preparing to divide the right lower lobe bronchus, define the right middle lobe bronchus and take care not to narrow it at its takeoff.

Suggested Readings

1. Schmid RA, Kocher GJ. Right lower lobe: open. In: Mathisen DJ, Morse CM, Fischer JE, eds. *Master Techniques in Surgery: Lung Resections, Bronchoplasty*. Wolters Kluwer; 2015:135.
2. Wei B, Cerfolio RJ. Robotic approach to lobectomy. In: Mathisen DJ, Morse CM, Fischer JE, eds. *Master Techniques in Surgery: Thoracic Surgery—Lung Resections, Bronchoplasty*. Wolters Kluwer; 2015:209.
3. Weyant MJ. Right lower lobe: VATS. In: Mathisen DJ, Morse CM, Fischer JE, eds. *Master Techniques in Surgery: Thoracic Surgery—Lung Resections, Bronchoplasty*. Wolters Kluwer; 2015:143.

Chapter 8

Left Upper Lobectomy: Robotic-Assisted Surgery/ Video-Assisted Surgery/ Thoracotomy

JUSTIN D. BLASBERG

Perioperative Considerations

- The left upper lobe represents 50% of the left lung by volume and over 20% of the total lung capacity in most patients.
- Resection of the left upper lobe, either open or minimally invasive, is a common and reproducible operation for both benign and malignant etiologies.
- Patient selection is a critically important consideration prior to left upper lobectomy, and should include cardiac risk stratification, assessment of a patient's performance status, a discussion of the risks and benefits of surgery and alternatives relative to the stage of disease (in the setting of cancer), and pulmonary function tests to define expectations for postoperative pulmonary reserve.
- Left upper lobectomy, particularly for lung cancer, can be the most technically challenging lobar resection given the anatomic variability of the pulmonary artery (PA) branches.

TIPS

- *Preoperative thin-cut chest imaging with IV contrast and 3D reconstruction can help significantly with preoperative planning and the identification of pulmonary artery branches.*
- *Complete hilar and mediastinal lymphadenectomy should be performed first to allow for exposure and circumferential mobilization of all vascular and airway structures.*
- *A "flyover" technique using the robotic/VATS stapler should be considered prior to division of vascular or airway structures so that the angle of the stapler and comfort with the trajectory can be achieved.*
- *Preoperative discussion between the surgeon and anesthesiologist about the particulars of surgery, airway concerns, preferences for isolation, and peripheral access to ensure optimal patient outcomes is important.*

Instruments and Equipment

Robotic-Assisted Thoracic Surgery

- S retractors
- 30° robotic 3-dimensional camera (0° can also be used)
- 2 × 8-mm robotic ports and 2 × 12-mm robotic ports with reducers (allow for exchange of robotic instruments and larger stapling devices while maintaining insufflation)

- 12-mm AirSeal port for the assistant (a 12-mm trocar can also be used with CO_2 insufflation if AirSeal is not available)
- Preferred robotic instruments:
  - Maryland bipolar (alternative: long bipolar)
  - Double fenestrated grasper (alternative: tip-up grasper)
  - Cadiere grasper (alternative: fenestrated bipolar)
  - Robotic vessel sealer
  - Robotic scissors
- Beside instruments:
  - 5-mm Snowden grasper
  - Laparoscopic suction irrigator
  - Endocatch bag (preferably a large bag that fits through the assistant 12-mm port)
- Ancillary tools:
  - Vessel loop cut to 12 to 14 cm
  - 10-French Rob-Nel red rubber catheter cut to 12 cm or prepackaged endoleader

Video-Assisted Thoracic Surgery

- 30°, 5- or 10-mm video thoracoscope
- 5-mm Maryland-tip LigaSure of laparoscopic length
- 12-mm Thoracoport (US Surgical) trocar with nonconductive sleeve ×2
- Alexis wound protector (Applied Medical)
- Endoscopic Kittners
- Endo GIA stapler, curved- and straight-tip 45-cm stapler with vascular and thick tissue loads
- Foerster/long lung graspers
- Thoracoscopic tonsil clamp
- Thoracoscopic right angle clamp
- Long-tip monopolar cautery with protected tip
- Vessel loop cut to 20 cm

Open

- Finochietto rib spreader and Balfour retractor
- 5-mm Maryland-tip LigaSure
- Long-tip monopolar cautery with protected tip
- Vessel loop cut to 20 cm
- Endoscopic Kittners
- Right-angled clamp (blunt tip)
- Lung graspers (Forrester clamps)/Duval clamps
- Endo GIA stapler, curved- and straight-tip 45-cm stapler with vascular and thick tissue loads
- 12-mm Thoracoport for stapling access inferior/anterior to the incision

Anesthesia

- All patients at our institution, regardless of approach, are managed within an Enhanced Recovery After Surgery (ERAS) protocol to ensure optimal outcomes.
- Preoperative 8 oz carbohydrate load 2 hours prior to surgery
- Oral acetaminophen and gabapentin 30 minutes prior to intubation
- Chlorhexidine gluconate mouthwash (15 mL of solution in mouth for 30 seconds and then spit) for pneumonia prevention
- First-generation cephalosporins within 30 minutes of incision
- Subcutaneous heparin 5000U intramuscularly
- Thromboembolic stockings/sequential compression devices
- Arterial line and Foley catheter are routinely placed.
- Double-lumen endotracheal tube is placed with bronchoscopic assistance and is the preferred technique for lung isolation.
- Alternate technique for lung isolation: single-lumen endotracheal tube with a bronchial blocker (however, suctioning through a bronchial blocker is inferior to a double-lumen endotracheal tube and may lead to technical challenges associated with inadequate lung deflation)

Positioning

- Right lateral decubitus position with the left side up
- Axillary roll (towel or gel) is placed just inferior to the axilla in a transverse direction (this is better referred to as a "subaxillary" roll).
- The bed is flexed at the patient's hip to allow for flattening of the chest wall such that the anterior superior iliac supine is parallel to the chest wall.
- The bed is rotated or the patient position adjusted so the posterior axillary line represents the highest point of the chest (Figure 8.1).

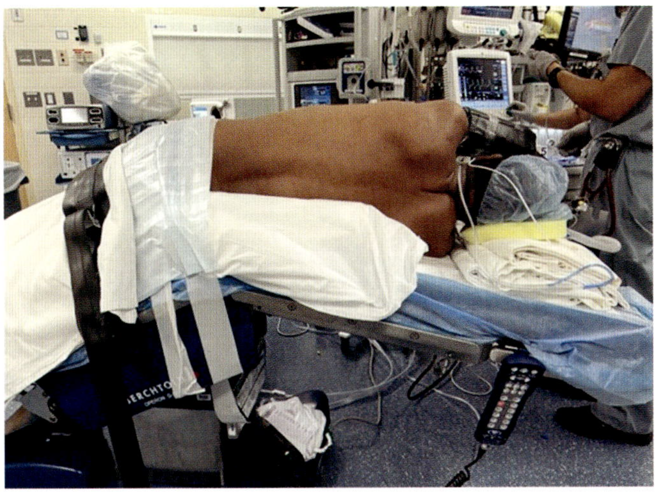

FIGURE 8.1 | The bed is flexed, and the patient positioned such that the anterior superior iliac spine and the chest wall are flat and parallel to the ground.

- Patients are secured in place with rolled blankets placed longitudinally on either side and tied together under the patient with a stockinette.
  - Alternatively, a deflatable bean bag can be placed under the patient.
- Silk tape is used to secure the patient to the bed at the level of the anterior superior iliac spine.
- The lower extremities are separated with pillows and the bottom leg flexed slightly.
- The left arm is padded at pressure points and placed in an Allen arm rest at 90 degrees of shoulder and elbow flexion at a height where the arm rests in a neutral position (avoid shoulder abduction beyond 90°).
- Pillows can be used between the arms if an Allen arm rest is not available.
- The left arm is available to anesthesia in the event where additional access is required.

Robotic Positioning

- DaVinci Xi can be placed on either side of the table based on space constraints of the operating room.
- If the operating space will accommodate, we aim to bring the boom toward the table from the patient's right for a left upper lobectomy, which allows the assistant to stand on the left side of the bed.
- The boom is brought in as cephalad as possible and 90° to the bed to allow for maximum flexibility of the arms.
- This positioning also allows for thoracotomy incision if required during conversion.

Technique

Robot-Assisted

- Robotic lobectomy is performed using a 4-arm technique, with a fifth port for the bedside assistant.
- Ports are positioned in the same interspace or within two adjacent interspaces.
- The initial 8-mm port is placed into the eighth intercostal space (ICS) posterior axillary line, entering the chest with knife and then cautery dissection with the assistance of S retractors to enter the left pleural space.

- Other techniques for entry include tonsil spreading into the pleural space or the use of an Optiview trocar for entry (a video-assisted 5-mm camera is needed as the Intuitive 8-mm camera does not fit inside the robotic port with the trocar in place).
- Do not make this port too large: (1) insufflation can escape and lead to subcutaneous emphysema and (2) telescoping of the port when undocked can lead to inadvertent injuries.
- With the first port placed, insufflate to a pressure of 8 mm Hg and a flow of 5 L/min.
- Intercostal injections with either 0.5% Marcaine or a Marcaine/Exparel mix (1:1) to all interspaces where ports are planned as well as one above and below
- Additional ports:
  - Eighth ICS infrascapular position (12 mm) (can be used for stapling)
  - Eighth ICS paraspinous position (8 mm)—aligns with the superior segment of the left lower lobe—externally located 2-3 cm anterior to the spine
  - Seventh or Eighth ICS anterior axillary line one interspace above the camera port for left-handed stapling
  - Assist port placed in the ninth ICS half the distance between the camera and infrascapular ports (Figure 8.2)

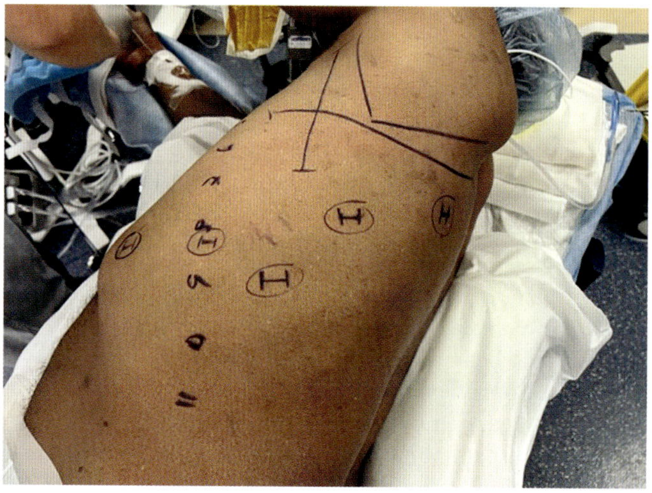

FIGURE 8.2 | Robotic ports are placed in the seventh, eighth, and ninth intercostal spaces for left upper lobectomy. We recommend marking out both a posterolateral and vertical muscle-sparing thoracotomy incision in case they are needed during the case.

  - Alternative assist port location: anterior and inferior ninth ICS between the camera and anterior axillary ports
- Target to the pulmonary hilum, dock the remaining robotic arms, and insert instruments under direct vision.
- Proceed with maneuvers that are best exposed and most safely performed rather than a standard order of the operation that might not be technically feasible in every patient.
- Division of the superior pulmonary vein early in the procedure often leads to lung congestion and a significantly more challenging experience manipulating the lung.
- Perform complete hilar and mediastinal lymphadenectomy prior to dividing vascular or airway structures.
- During robotic lobectomy, there is no tactile feedback and learning visual cues are necessary to avoid inadvertent injury.
- Instead of grabbing the lung directly, retraction with a cigar helps reduce parenchymal tearing.
- The most posterior arm is loaded with a double fenestrated grasper to facilitate left lower lobe retraction in a cephalad direction.
- The inferior pulmonary ligament is divided and level 8 and 9 lymph nodes are harvested (Figure 8.3).
- The lung is retracted anteriorly and the posterior hilum is opened, allowing dissection of the subcarinal space/level 7 lymph nodes in the space between the inferior pulmonary vein and the left lower lobe bronchus.
- If the lung is not deflated and with inadequate retraction, this maneuver can be very challenging, thus limiting level 7 harvesting.

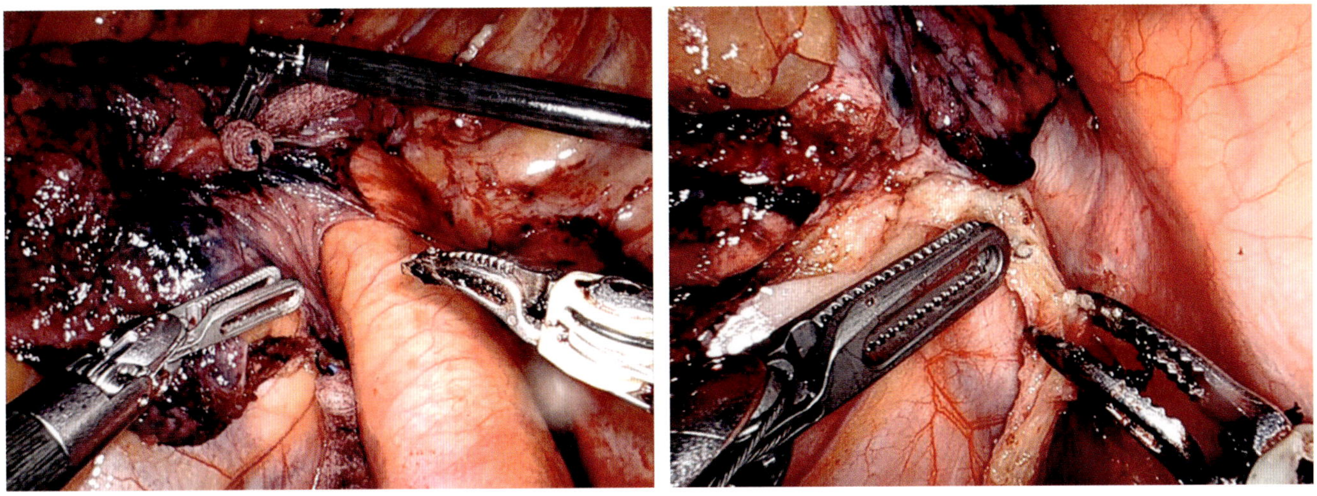

FIGURE 8.3 ▌ The inferior pulmonary ligament is divided to the level of the inferior pulmonary vein with Maryland bipolar and cigar retraction. Level 8 and 9 lymph nodes are harvested.

- Level 11 lymph nodes are harvested off the posterior aspect of the ongoing PA at the level of the fissure and the remainder of the posterior hilum is opened with bipolar energy.
- Level 10 lymph nodes can also be harvested from this position.
- The use of bipolar energy with either a Maryland or long bipolar instrument is a significant advantage over monopolar energy given the lack of thermal spread.
- From this position, the posterior ascending PA branch is identified and the inferior aspect of the vessel dissected out (Figure 8.4).

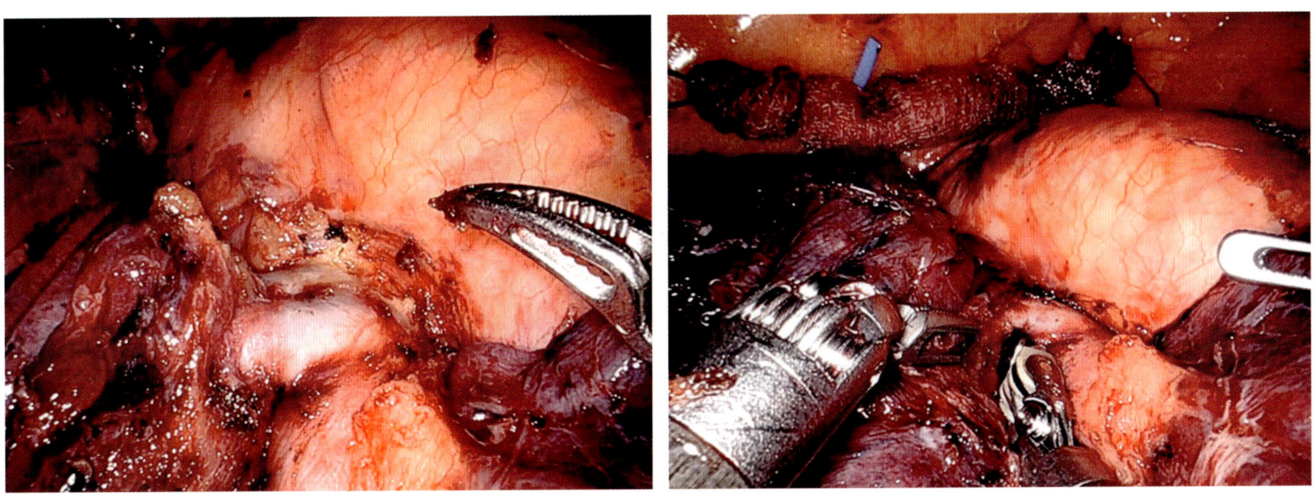

FIGURE 8.4 ▌ With the posterior hilum and pulmonary artery (PA) exposed, the posterior ascending PA branch can be mobilized prior to division of the truncus PA branch, allowing safe passage of a stapler.

- It is critically important to be directly on the PA as it enters the fissure, which allows for separation of the parenchyma from the PA to facilitate staple division of the posterior fissure.
- The lung is retracted in a caudal direction with the most posterior arm and the superior aspect of the pulmonary hilum is dissected out as well as level 5 and 6 lymph nodes.
- Care must be taken to preserve both the left recurrent laryngeal nerve and the ongoing vagus nerve (Figure 8.5).
- The posterior aspect of the truncus branch of the PA can also be dissected out from this location, which is helpful prior to anterior dissection, facilitating stapling of the truncus.
- Attention then turns to the major fissure where the ongoing PA is identified and dissected out.
- Level 11 lymph nodes are harvested, which separates the PA from the surrounding parenchyma.
- Both anterior and posterior aspects of the major fissure can be developed using blunt dissection and small spreading with the Cadiere grasper to separate the PA and its branches from surrounding

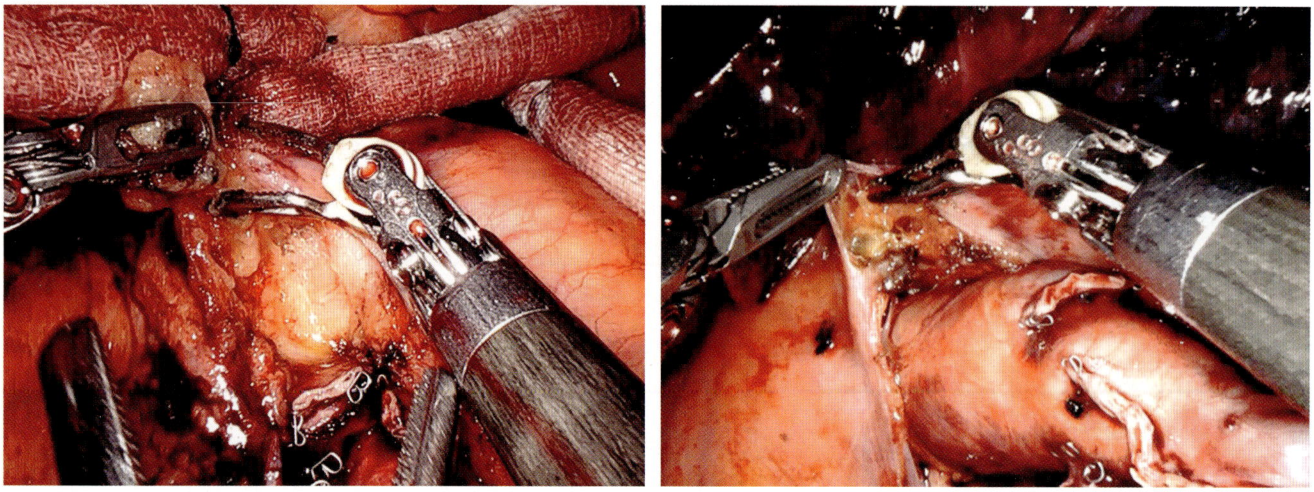

FIGURE 8.5 ■ Dissection of level 5 lymph nodes from the AP window (with attention paid to avoid injury to the recurrent laryngeal nerve and ongoing vagus nerve). (Image taken after completion of lobectomy to better illustrate anatomy.)

parenchyma. Staying directly on the PA is the safest place to develop the fissure and avoids inadvertent injury to both vascular branches and lung parenchyma (Figure 8.6).

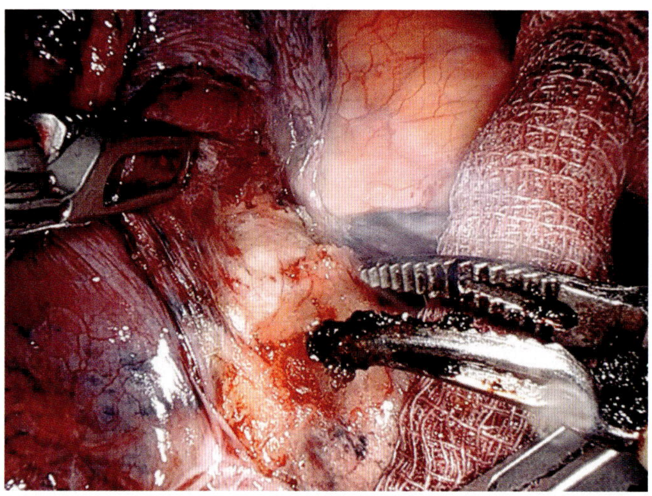

FIGURE 8.6 ■ Dissection directly on the pulmonary artery within the major fissure and complete resection of adjacent lymph nodes facilitates division of the fissure.

- The lung is retracted posteriorly and the bifurcation of the upper and lower lobe bronchus is developed.
- Level 10 lymph nodes are harvested to expose this bifurcation and develop the anterior aspect of the major fissure.
- The underside of the ongoing PA will come into view with resection of this lymph node and care should be taken to avoid injury.
- A long instrument can be passed from either anterior to posterior or posterior to anterior to confirm that the anterior fissure is mobilized (Figure 8.7).
- A 30-mm or 45-mm thick tissue stapler is used to complete the anterior and posterior fissures; use of a vessel loop or endoleader is encouraged if the angle of staple firing is challenging (Figures 8.8 and 8.9).
- With the fissures complete, access to the lingular PA branch is significantly improved.
- After circumferential mobilization and resection of any remaining lymph nodes, the lingular PA can be divided with a curved-tip vascular load 30-mm stapler, usually with the left hand (Figure 8.10).
- The left upper lobe bronchus is exposed by retracting the lung posteriorly.
- The superior pulmonary vein is exposed with bipolar energy and circumferentially mobilized.
  - It is easiest and safest to free up the posterior aspect of the vein with blunt dissection and gentle spreading with a Cadiere forceps or a Maryland dissector (Figure 8.11).

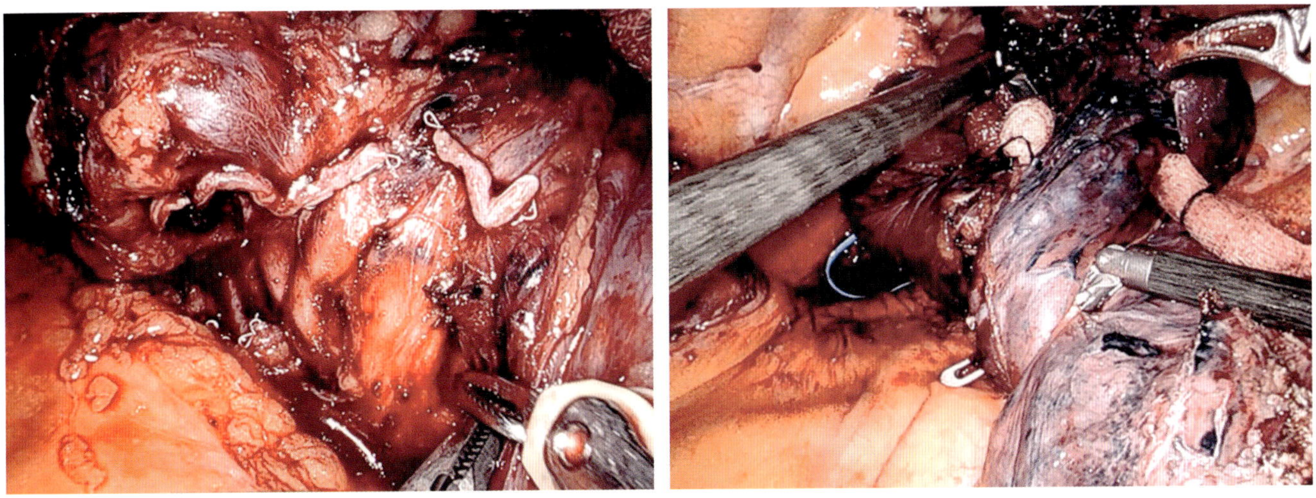

FIGURE 8.7 ▮ Dissection of hilar lymph nodes at the junction of left upper lobe and left lower lobe bronchus helps facilitate identification on the ongoing pulmonary artery (PA) and division of the anterior aspect of the fissure. An instrument can be passed along the anticipated trajectory of the stapler with the PA in view to confirm that this dissection is adequate.

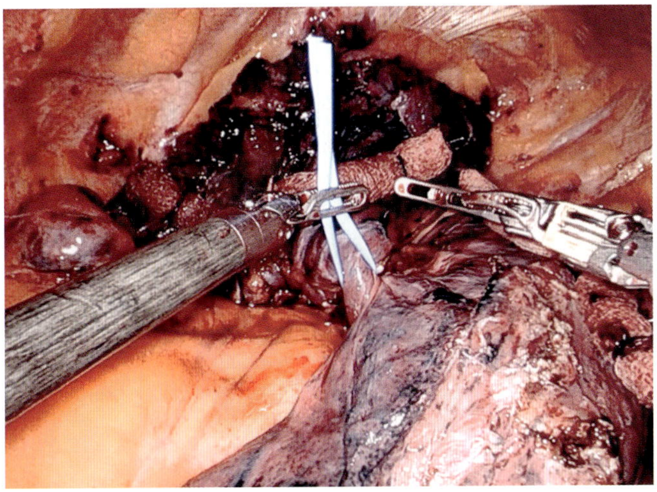

FIGURE 8.8 ▮ The anterior fissure is elevated away from the lingular and ongoing pulmonary artery (PA) with a vessel loop to facilitate staple firing, usually in an anterior-to-posterior direction with the left hand. A curved-tip stapler is preferred to facilitate safe passage in the vicinity of the lingular PA.

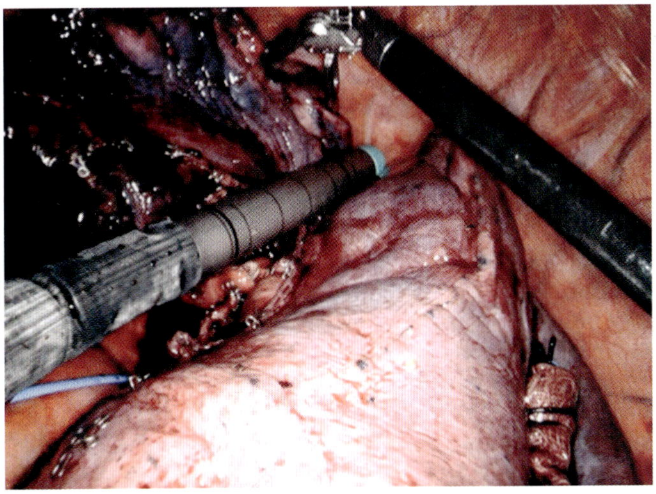

FIGURE 8.9 ▮ The remainder of the posterior fissure can be divided from anterior to posterior.

- The bronchus is directly posterior to the vein. Passing an instrument or stapler behind the vein should be performed with caution as the rigid left upper lobe bronchus could result in back wall injury of the vein.
- A vessel loop cut to 12 cm can be passed behind the vein (Figure 8.12).
- Occasionally, the lingular and superior pulmonary veins are divided separately.

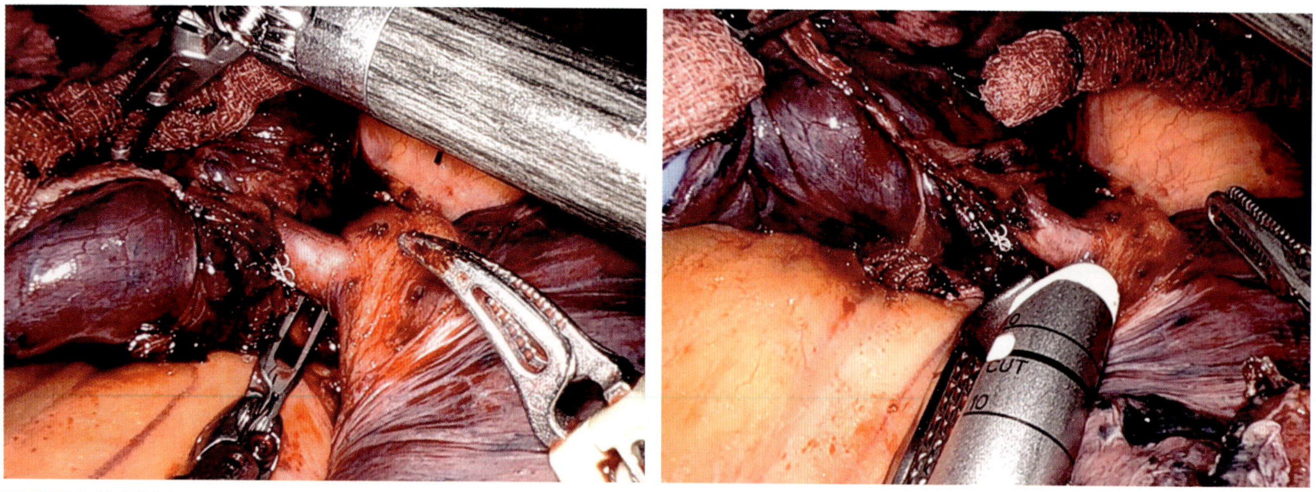

FIGURE 8.10 ▮ Division of the anterior and posterior fissure allows for circumferential mobilization of the lingular pulmonary artery branch.

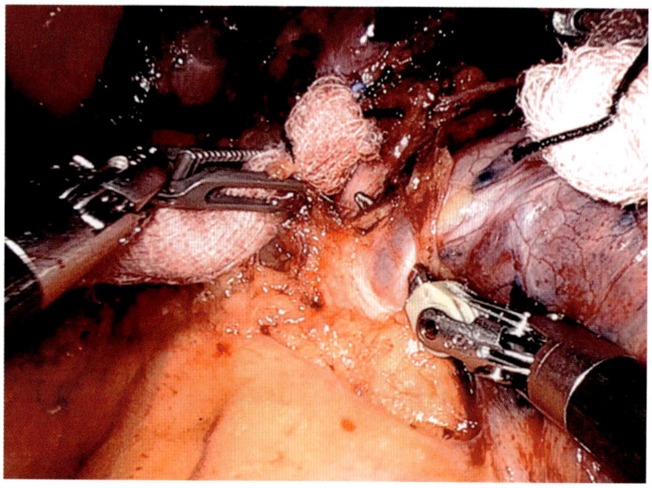

FIGURE 8.11 ▮ Lingular vein circumferentially mobilized using a two-handed approach; cigar in the left hand functions as an endoscopic Kittner to bluntly dissect adjacent soft tissue.

- A "flyover" technique is recommended to optimize safety.
  - The stapler is oriented at the necessary angle and passed directly above the vein to ensure this trajectory is achievable.
- With the superior pulmonary vein divided, the anterior aspect of the truncus branch of the PA and ongoing PA are in view.
- Additional level 11 lymph nodes are dissected off this bifurcation, facilitating anterior exposure of the truncus branch of the PA.
- We routinely flip the lung anteriorly to inspect the posterior aspect of the truncus PA to avoid inadvertent injury to adjacent vascular branches.
- Placement of a vessel loop confirms isolation of the truncus PA branch and is helpful to expose this structure (Figure 8.13).
- A similar "flyover" technique is recommended prior to division of the truncus PA branch.
- Posterior PA branches should be identified and divided prior to division of the left upper lobe airway.
- In circumstances where the stapler is too large or the space around a small vessel is too tight, consider clipping the PA branch (small metal or medium-sized plastic clip) and/or use of the vessel sealer as an alternative, particularly for vessels <7 mm (Figure 8.14).
- The lung is retracted anteriorly and posterior ascending PA branches that were previously identified are ligated and divided.
  - Retraction is facilitated with the posterior right hand retracting the lung anteriorly, allowing for the use of the other two hands to divide the PA.
  - A Cadiere in the left hand is useful or additional retraction of the lung in the immediate proximity of the PA branch.

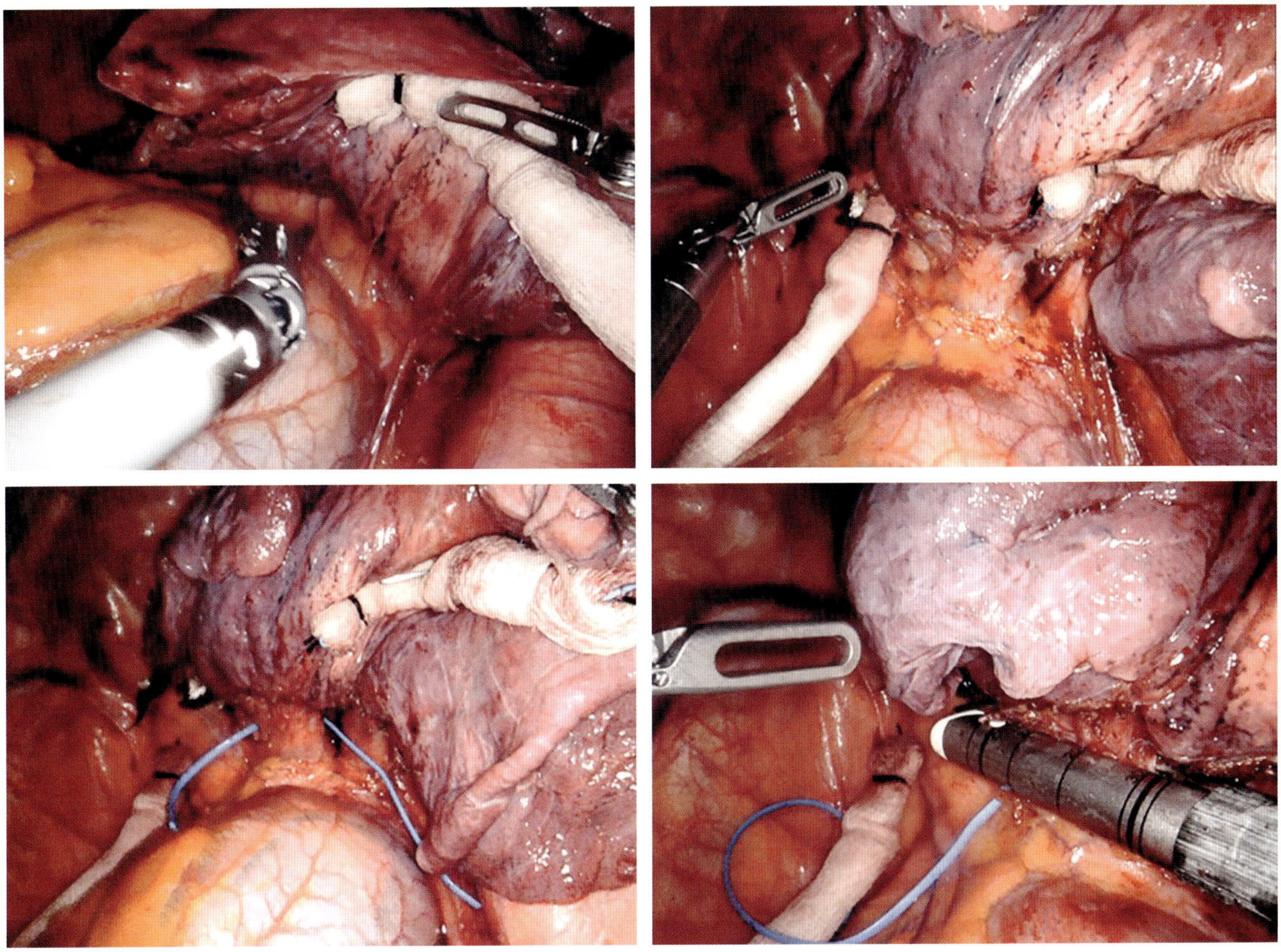

FIGURE 8.12 | A cigar grasped in the left robotic instrument is used to brush away soft tissue as the right-handed Cadiere grasper bluntly dissects behind the vein. Stapling of the vein is performed with a 30-mm curved-tip vascular load in the right hand.

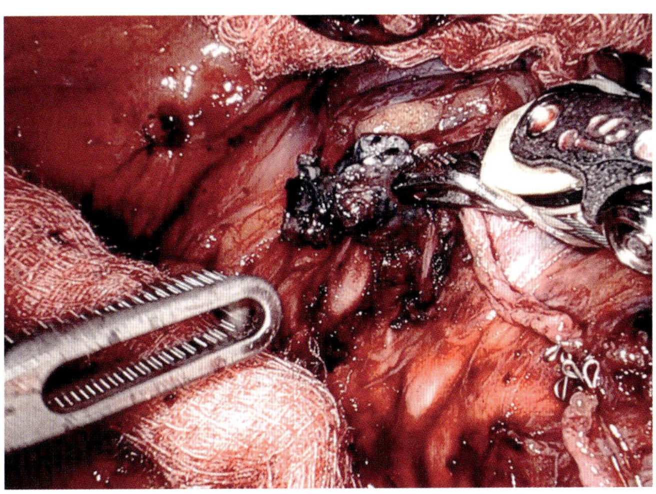

FIGURE 8.13 | Resection of the level 11 lymph node at the junction of the truncus branch of the pulmonary artery (PA) and the ongoing PA helps to expose the anterior aspect of the truncus, facilitating division.

- Anterior and lateral (toward 10 o'clock) retraction will open the space between the lung and the PA, allowing for passage of the stapler with the right hand (Figure 8.15).
- The use of a vessel loop may help with exposure to facilitate stapling.
- Any remaining lymph nodes adjacent to the left upper lobe bronchus are dissected out with bipolar energy.
- A cigar is used as a Kittner to sweep all remaining soft tissue toward the specimen.

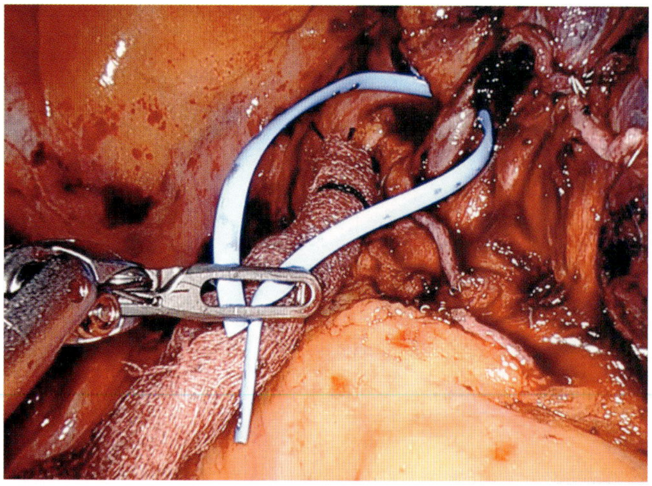

FIGURE 8.14 | The truncus pulmonary artery (PA) branch is circumferentially mobilized, divided with a curved-tip vascular load 30-mm stapler, and approached using the right hand. A vessel loop around the vessel helps with small adjustments to minimize tension on the PA.

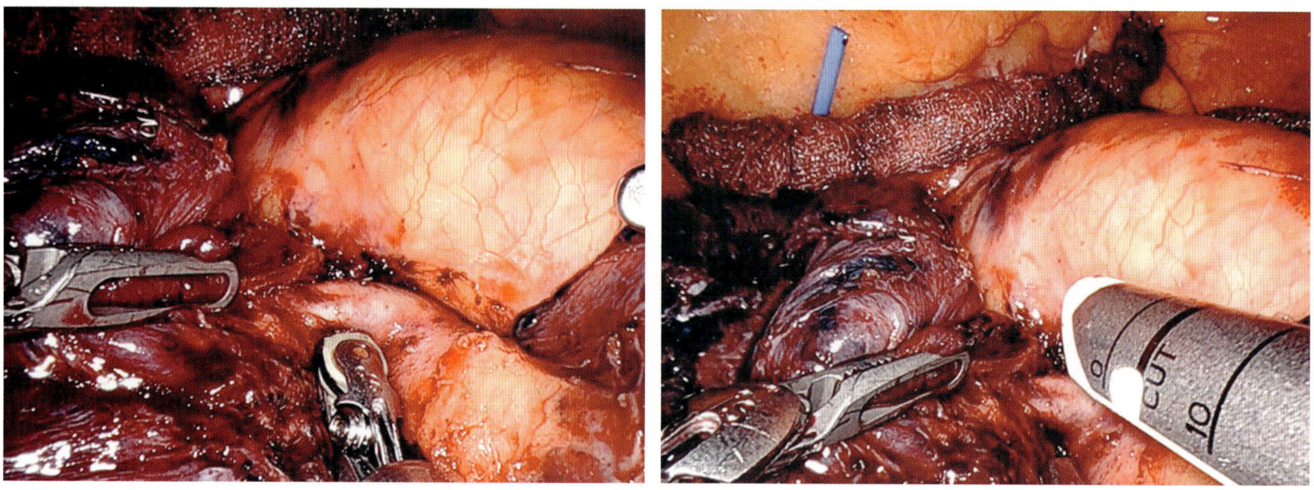

FIGURE 8.15 | Mobilization and division of the posterior ascending pulmonary artery branch is best accomplished with a stapler in the right hand.

- A vessel loop can be placed around the bronchus for retraction.
- Either a 30-mm curved-tip stapler or 45-mm straight stapler with a thick tissue load can be used to divide the airway and free the specimen (Figure 8.16).
- The specimen is placed in an endocatch bag and removed via the assistant port or anterior incision, which often requires enlargement to approximately 2 to 2.5 cm for removal.

Top-Down Modification

- This technique is used for cases where there is concern that dissecting into the fissure will lead to a significant postoperative air leak.
- This technique is similar regardless of minimally invasive or open approach.
- Much of the operation is as described above including the hilar and circumferential mobilization and division of all associated vascular structures.
- Thorough posterior hilar dissection to identify any aberrant PA branches is helpful with the lung retracted anteriorly, and the "top-down" division of hilar vessels is almost exclusively from the anterior hilum.
- The lymph node packet from the bifurcation of the left upper and lower lobe airway is resected as described above, with identification of the ongoing PA within the fissure, which is dissected away from the overlying parenchyma.
- A 45-mm stapler from the left hand can be used to divide the anterior aspect of the major fissure by parking the stapler at the bifurcation of the airway with the stapler tip above the PA.

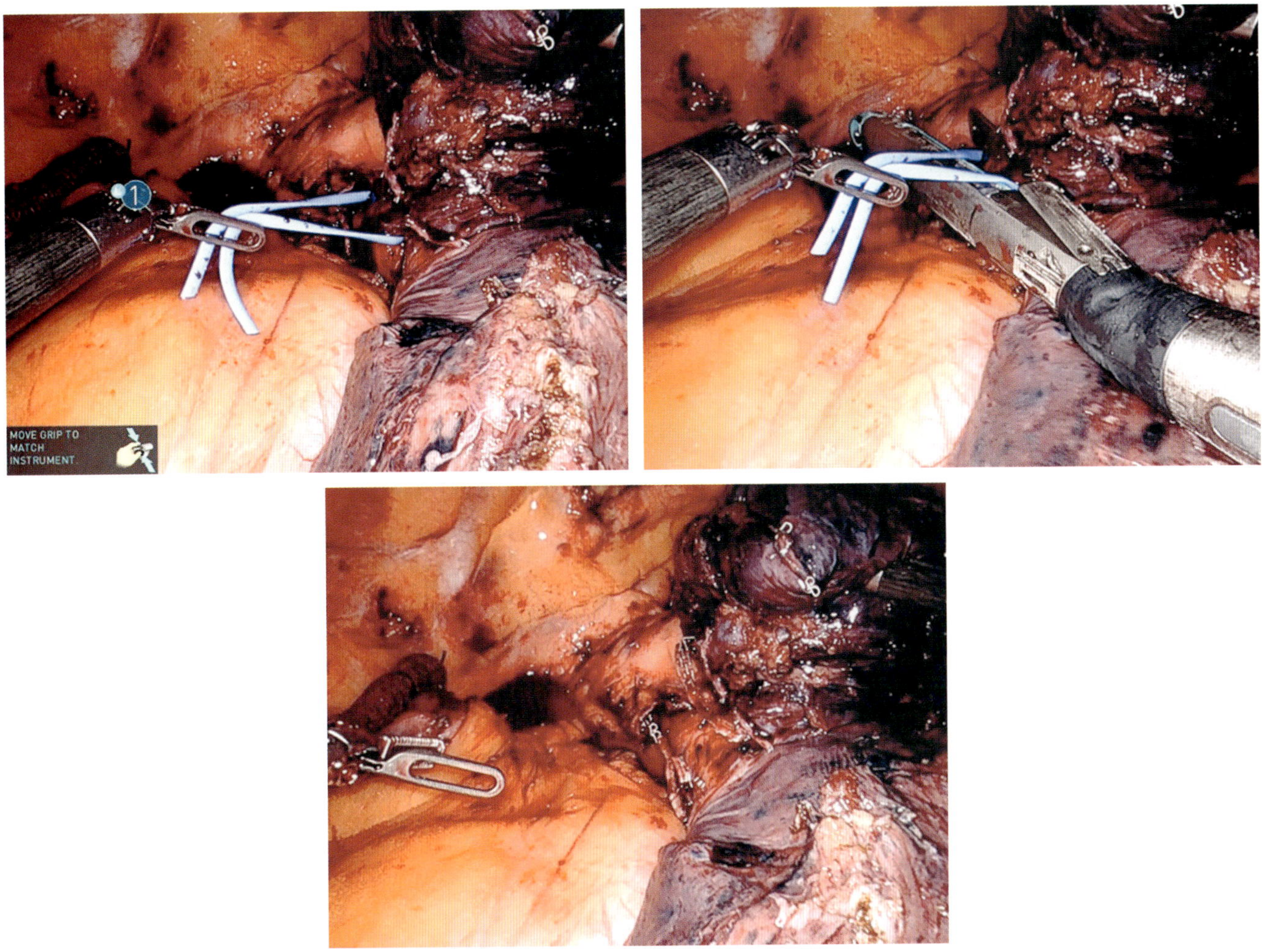

FIGURE 8.16 ▌ Circumferential mobilization of the left upper lobe bronchus helps free any loose attachments between the airway and pulmonary artery. A vessel loop can be used for gentle anterior retraction of the airway using the left hand while stapling with the right hand.

- Fissure division to the level of the airway helps create space for stapling hilar structures (Figures 8.17 and 8.18).
- The lung is retracted posteriorly and the left upper lobe bronchus is mobilized (Figure 8.19).
- The right-handed instrument can be exchanged for a curved-tip 30-mm stapler for division of the left upper lobe bronchus.

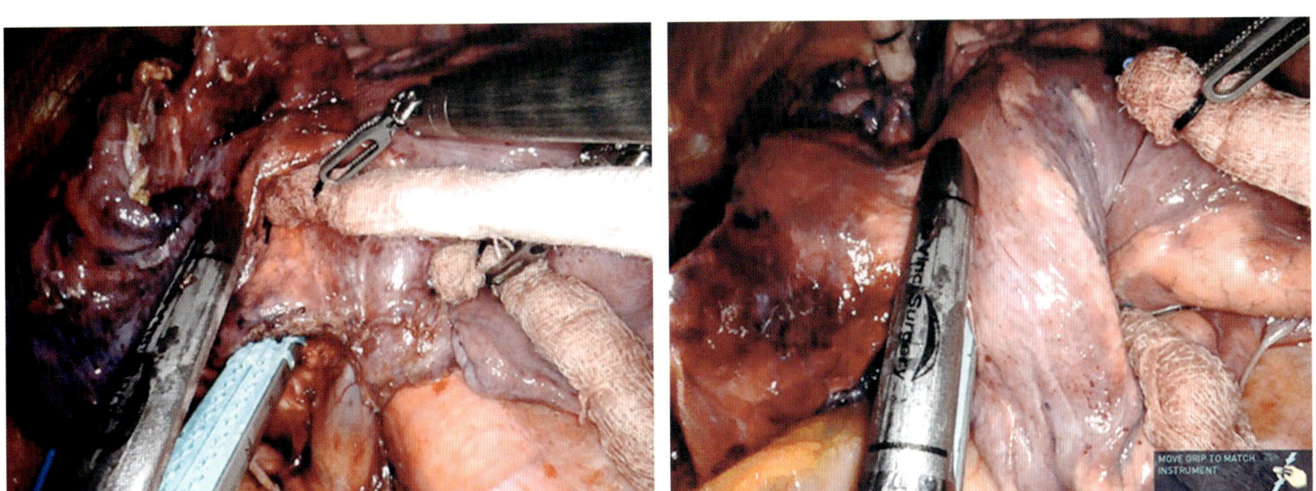

FIGURE 8.17 ▌ With the bifurcation of the airway dissected out, a thick tissue stapler is parked at that junction and the anterior aspect of the major fissure is divided.

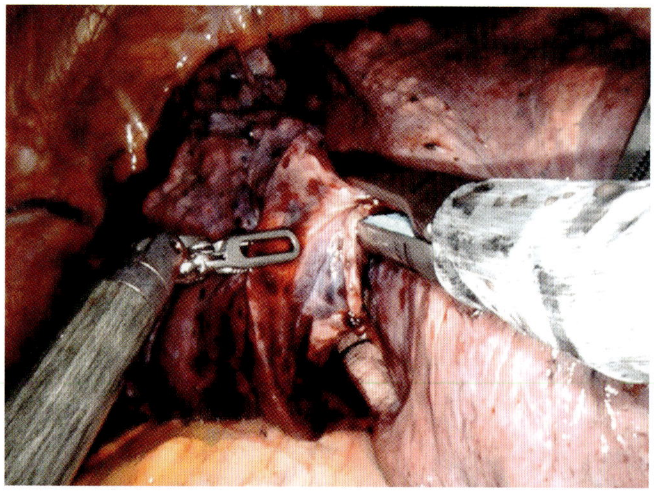

FIGURE 8.18 ▌ With the pulmonary artery in view and dissected away from the fissure, anterior-to-posterior stapling further divides the fissure and exposes the left upper lobe bronchus.

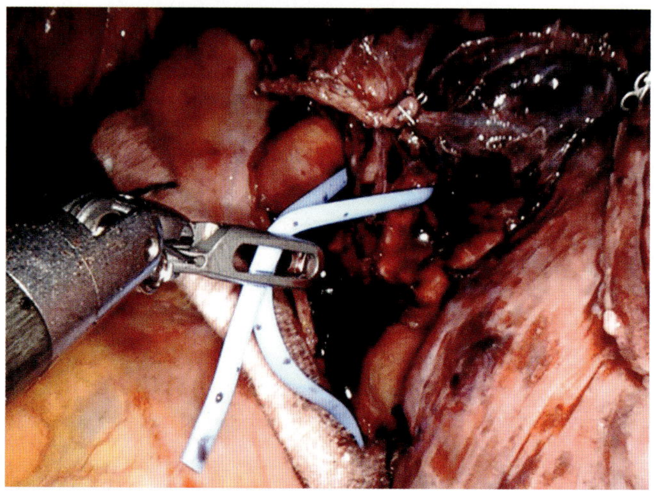

FIGURE 8.19 ▌ Mobilization of the left upper lobe bronchus is performed prior to completion of the major fissure. Use of a vessel loop should be considered given the possibility of aberrant pulmonary artery branches behind the airway.

- The lung is retracted posteriorly and laterally using the posterior right hand to expose the lingular PA branch for division.
- In the right hand, a curved-tip 30-mm stapler vascular load is used to divide the lingular PA.
- In the event the angle or vessel trajectory is not appropriate for stapling, consideration for clipping and division with a vessel sealer may be a safer option (Figure 8.20).

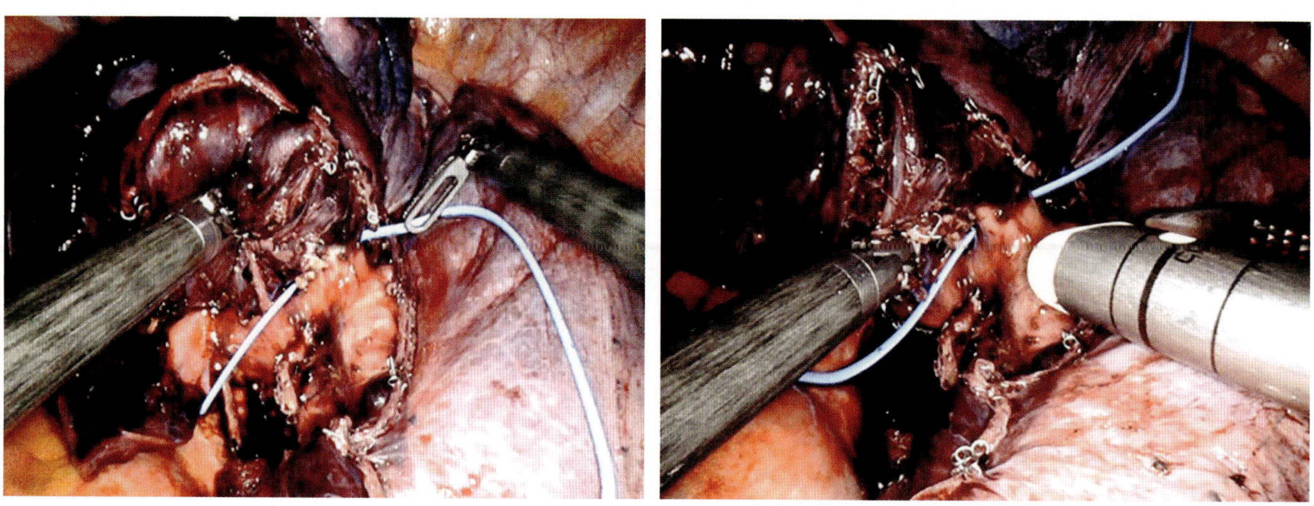

FIGURE 8.20 ▌ With the left upper lobe retracted away from the hilum, the lingular pulmonary artery branch is exposed, dissected out, and divided either with a stapler or clips/energy.

- With just the major fissure remaining, the lung is grasped and retracted toward the lateral chest wall and a 45-mm straight stapler is used to complete the fissure anterior to posterior usually from the left hand.
- When placing the stapler down the line of the fissure, the ongoing PA should always be kept in view to avoid inadvertent injury.
- Additionally, the descending aorta should also be kept in view and the tip of the stapler kept on top of this vessel to avoid injury.

Video-Assisted Thoracic Surgery

- Positioning and setup of a video-assisted thoracic surgery (VATS) lobectomy is similar to that previously described for robotic-assisted thoracic surgery (RATS) lobectomy.
- Flexion of the bed is important to prevent restriction of instruments that might contact the ipsilateral hip, particularly from the anterior incision.
- Entry into the left pleural space begins in the seventh ICS posterior axillary line where a 12-mm Thoracoport is placed.
- Intercostal injections with either 0.5% Marcaine or a Marcaine/Exparel mix (1:1) to all interspaces where ports are planned as well as one above and below
- Additional ports:
  - Fourth ICS anterior axillary line—4-cm incision and an extra-small Alexis wound protector is placed
  - Sixth ICS mid-axillary line—12-mm Thoracoport for both camera viewing and stapling
  - Fifth ICS paraspinous—12-mm Thoracoport just posterior to the tip of the scapula
- 5-mm ports and camera can be used instead of 12 mm; however, we routinely exchange the camera for stapler, and therefore, a 12-mm port in the seventh ICS is often needed.
- VATS lobectomy is performed with thoracoscopic lung graspers (Foerster clamps) to provide lung retraction and exposure.
- A 30° thoracoscope helps to visualize critical structures by providing adjustable viewing angles.
- The critical aspects of VATS lobectomy are similar to the description of robotic left upper lobectomy, including the importance of complete lymphadenectomy.
- The lung is retracted to facilitate resection of inferior pulmonary ligament (level 9) lymph nodes, the subcarinal space (level 7), as well as AP window (level 5) and prevascular space (level 6).
- This dissection is best accomplished with a LigaSure energy or monopolar cautery device.
- The curved Maryland-tip LigaSure is particularly useful as both a dissector and for hemostasis.
- Circumferential hilar dissection is performed typically from the front to back via the utility incision while retracting from the posterior port, then switching the instruments for the posterior dissection.
- Endoscopic Kittners are used to assist with circumferential vascular dissection, followed by passage of either a thoracoscopic right angle via the access incision or a thoracoscopic tonsil clamp via the camera port to elongate and isolate each structure.
- A top-down approach allows for safe division of bronchial and vascular structures with division of the major fissure last, reducing the risk of postoperative air leak.
- From the camera port, the superior pulmonary vein, followed by the truncus branch of the PA can be ligated and divided using a curved tip vascular load/stapler.
- Similar to RATS, a vessel loop can be used for gentle retraction away from the hilum to help isolate and facilitate stapler division.
- The lung is then retracted anteriorly and posterior branches are dissected out.
- Ligation and division is accomplished with a curved-tip vascular load/stapler also inserted via the camera port.
- Lymph nodes adjacent to the bronchus are resected and remaining soft tissue adjacent to the bronchus is swept toward the specimen.
- After removal of any suction device inside of the airway, a thick tissue load/stapler is placed via the camera port and around the airway, facilitated by posterior retraction of the lung via the posterior Thoracoport.
- With the left upper lobe bronchus divided, the lingular PA branch is identified with posterior retraction of the lung, circumferentially mobilized, and divided with a curved tip vascular load/stapler placed via the camera port.
- The ongoing PA is now in view, and with thick tissue loads/stapler, sequential firings from the camera port from anterior to posterior allow for safe completion of the fissure.

- Depending on the patient habitus and anatomy, fissure division may also be accomplished via the utility incision.
- Once divided, the specimen is placed in an endocatch bag and removed via the utility incision.
- A single 24-French chest tube is placed via the camera port in a posterior and apical position and secured with a heavy braided suture.

Open

- Elective open left upper lobectomy can be performed through a variety of incisions and with both muscle-dividing or muscle-sparing techniques.
- To facilitate recovery, a complete muscle-sparing thoracotomy can and should be performed as the exposure is similar to thoracotomy with muscle division.
- A muscle-sparing thoracotomy can be performed either with a 15-cm vertical incision from the axilla in the posterior axillary line just anterior to the latissimus muscle or in a transverse direction similar to a traditional thoracotomy incision, without division of the latissimus (Figure 8.2).
  - Advantages of the muscle-sparing approach include the ease of muscle mobilization, including the latissimus muscle, which is mobilized from anterior to posterior, as well as the serratus from a caudal to cranial direction.
  - Often lower serratus attachments require separation/division from the chest wall to adequately expose the fourth ICS.
  - Generous latissimus mobilization posteriorly allows for less chest wall spreading under tension as well as access to the posterior aspect of the ICS.
- Entry into the left pleural space via the fourth ICS using cautery as far anterior as possible without injuring the left internal mammary artery and posteriorly to the erector spinae muscles without dividing them
- Shingling the fifth rib is preferred with preservation of the neurovascular bundle.
  - This technique reduces postoperative pain and is preferable to rib fracturing that can occur with vigorous chest wall spreading.
- A Finochietto rib spreader is used to open the pleural space, as well as a Balfour retractor placed at 90° to improve exposure.
- In most cases, stapling is best facilitated by making a 12-mm incision in the eighth ICS anterior axillary line and inserting a Thoracoport, similar to the stapling access during VATS lobectomy.
- Special considerations:
  - During urgent conversion of RATS/VATS lobectomy, we do not recommend a muscle-sparing approach as this technique takes significantly more time.
  - As part of the timeout for a minimally invasive lung resection, we draw an emergency thoracotomy incision in the event access to the chest is needed (Figure 8.2).
  - Our preferred technique for urgent conversion is for the assistant to hold pressure on the site of bleeding using a cigar held in place with a 5-mm Snowden grasper while the circulator or surgeon removes the instruments, undocks the system, and moves it out of the way, so that the thoracotomy incision can be accessed.
  - In these cases, muscle division of the latissimus is preferred and may also be necessary for the serratus based on the emergent need for access to the pleural space.
  - Communication with both the anesthesia and scrub teams is critical to reduce blood loss and facilitate safe conversation.
  - Simulation of these scenarios is very helpful for the team to develop proficiency, and a discussion of critical points of conversion during timeout or prior to a case is a very useful exercise.
- The steps of open left upper lobectomy are similar to what has been outlined in the minimally invasive discussion.
- Lung retraction is typically accomplished with ring clamps or Duval clamps.
- Dissection of the inferior pulmonary ligament can be performed with monopolar cautery or a Maryland-tip LigaSure energy device.
- Circumferential mobilization of vascular structures is accomplished with a right angle that has a blunt tip.
- A Kittner, similar to the minimally invasive technique, is used in the opposite hand to clear off adjacent soft tissue when the right-angled instrument is passed behind structures of interest.
- Vessel loops are used when needed to allow for safe passage of a stapler.
- A curved-tip Endo GIA stapler is preferred in a similar fashion to minimally invasive resection, allowing for isolation of a target structure while reducing the risk that the lower jaw of the stapler inadvertently injuries an adjacent structure.

- Complete hilar and mediastinal lymphadenectomy allows for:
  - Identification of relevant vascular and airway structures to the left upper lobe
  - Elongation of vessels to facilitate division
  - Reduced risk of inadvertent injury during the passage of a stapler
- After completion of lobectomy and mediastinal lymph node dissection, irrigation of the left pleural space and pressure testing of the left upper lobe stump to 30 mm Hg is performed to ensure no air leak.
- If there is parenchymal leaking from the left lower lobe, an adjunct sealing agent can be considered or pledgeted repair with Vicryl.
- A 24-French chest tube is placed via the stapling port in a posterior and apical position, secured with a heavy braided suture.
- The thoracotomy is closed with #2 Vicryl placed in figure-of-eight fashion ×4 around adjacent rib spaces, with careful attention paid to not injure the neurovascular bundle under the rib immediately inferior to the interspace being closed.
- The lung is recruited with a low pressure but sustained Valsalva maneuver and the pericostal sutures are tied down.
- In a muscle-sparing thoracotomy, the serratus is reapproximated to its surrounding soft tissue with running 0 Vicryl, the latissimus to surrounding soft tissue with running 0 Vicryl suture, and the remainder of the incision closed in layers.
- For a latissimus-dividing approach, we routinely close this muscle in two layers with running 0 Vicryl, the deep layer catching the posterior fascia and half of the muscle, and the anterior layer the other half of the muscle body and the anterior fascia.

Preoperative, Intraoperative, and Postoperative Care

- Open and minimally invasive lobectomy patients are managed according to an ERAS protocol.

Preoperatively

- Patients are administered Tylenol 1000 mg PO and celecoxib 200 mg PO unless contraindicated.
- Finger-stick glucose is obtained to document normoglycemia (glucose of 140-180) with insulin provided if appropriate.
- Preanesthetic antiemetic medications are considered based on preoperative risk.
- IV antibiotics are administrated within 60 minutes of the surgical incision (cefazolin IV or vancomycin IV if a penicillin allergy is documented) and chlorhexidine mouthwash in the holding area for pneumonia prevention.
- Weight-dosed thromboembolic prophylaxis with subcutaneous heparin or low-molecular-weight Lovenox

Intraoperatively

- Aim for a net zero fluid balance for all patients
- Normothermia with a goal core temperature of >36°C using forced air warming blankets, heated IV fluids, and an upper body warming blanket
- Patients are assessed using the Apfel score and treated with at least two antiemetics if appropriate (ex. ondansetron, Decadron, or scopolamine patch).
- A lung protection strategy is recommended, which includes reduced tidal volumes and induction with propofol combined with short-acting opioids only if opioids are needed.
- Regional anesthesia is utilized in all patients including either intercostal blocks with Marcaine 0.5% or Exparel or with implantable catheters (On-Q pain pump).
- Patients receive IV Tylenol prior to emergence.

Postoperatively

- Postoperative pain control includes Tylenol 975 mg q6h, Toradol 15 mg IV q6h × 5 days if Celebrex is not used, otherwise Celebrex dosed 12 hours postoperatively or Zofran IV PRN, with the addition of scopolamine/Compazine/Dramamine or Decadron PRN.
- IV fluid is discontinued on POD #0 and patients are started on regular diet sitting in a chair starting POD #0.

- Finger-stick glucose is checked every 24 hours and corrected to maintain normoglycemia (glucose 140-180).
- DVT prophylaxis includes Lovenox 40 mg subcutaneous until discharge and chest tubes are removed when drainage <350 mL/24 hours.
- Patients are assisted with early ambulation including at least three walks per day.
- Atrial fibrillation prophylaxis with diltiazem is utilized if the patient is not on a home beta-blocker and continued after discharge if postoperative atrial fibrillation develops.

PEARLS AND PITFALLS

- Complete mediastinal lymphadenectomy is the key to a successful lung resection for both open and minimally invasive resection.
- Dissection directly onto the PA to separate it from surrounding tissue is the safest method to prevent injury.
- The use of rolled sponges/"cigars'" to provide lung retraction and a dry field is helpful to reduce retraction injuries—it is almost never necessary to directly grab the left lower lobe.
- Careful attention is required to recognize visual cues, particularly when placing an instrument or stapler underneath a structure—if the instrument appears to pull that structure with it, insufficient posterior dissection has been achieved.
- A "flyover" technique helps to fine-tune the angle of entry of a stapler under a vascular structure particularly in circumstances where there is no tactile feedback.

Suggested Readings

1. Batchelor TJP, Rasburn NJ, Abdelnour-Berchtold E, et al. Guidelines for enhanced recovery after lung surgery: recommendations of the Enhanced Recovery After Surgery (ERAS®) Society and the European Society of Thoracic Surgeons (ESTS). *Eur J Cardio Thorac Surg*. 2019;55(1):91-115.
2. Gan TJ, Belani KG, Bergese S, et al. Fourth consensus guidelines for the management of postoperative nausea and vomiting. *Anesth Analg*. 2020;131(2):411-448.
3. Geraci TC, Ng T. When is it safe to operate for lung cancer? Selection of fiscally responsible cardiopulmonary function tests for limited resection (wedge resection and segmentectomy), standard lobectomy, Sleeve lobectomy, and pneumonectomy. *Thorac Surg Clin*. 2021;31(3):255-263.
4. Haro GJ, Sheu B, Marcus SG, et al. Perioperative lung resection outcomes after implementation of a multidisciplinary, evidence-based thoracic ERAS program. *Ann Surg*. 2021;274(6):e1008-e1013.
5. Hennington MH, Ulicny KS Jr, Detterbeck FC. Vertical muscle-sparing thoracotomy. *Ann Thorac Surg*. 1994;57(3):759-761.
6. Rogers LJ, Bleetman D, Messenger DE, et al. The impact of Enhanced Recovery After Surgery (ERAS) protocol compliance on morbidity from resection for primary lung cancer. *J Thorac Cardiovasc Surg*. 2018;155(4):1843-1852.
7. Uzzaman MM, Robb JD, Mhandu PCE, et al. A meta-analysis comparing muscle-sparing and posterolateral thoracotomy. *Ann Thorac Surg*. 2014;97(3):1093-1102.

Chapter 9

Left Lower Lobectomy

SAMUEL S. KIM
J. MARK ERFE

Perioperative Considerations

- Consider preoperative bronchoscopy to characterize the airway in terms of pathologic findings (eg, tracheomalacia, endobronchial tumor, ulceration), to clean out secretions, and to confirm proper endotracheal tube positioning.
- Widely opening the mediastinal pleura and complete mobilization of hilar structures help identify the lower lobe pulmonary artery (PA), vein, and bronchus.
- The order of dissection and transection of lower lobe vessels is subject to surgeon preference, operative approach, tumor location, and anatomic considerations. Classically, the fissure is opened, and the lower lobe basilar and superior segmental PAs are divided first, followed by the inferior pulmonary vein and the lower lobe bronchus. Some surgeons believe in dividing the inferior pulmonary vein first to prevent the dissemination of malignant cells during lung manipulation with the trade-off that the lower lobe lung parenchyma can become engorged when venous drainage is disrupted.
- Avoid fissure dissection in the lung with incomplete fissure to prevent postoperative air leaks. The lobectomy can be accomplished using the "fissureless" technique by stapling and dividing the lower lobe vein first, followed by the lower lobe bronchus, lower lobe PA branches, and then the interlobar fissure.

Instruments and Equipment

- Double-lumen endotracheal tube or bronchial blocker.
- Video-assisted thoracoscopic surgery (VATS)—a small wound protector, 5-mm camera, and one 5-mm retraction port.
- Robot—4 robotic ports (two 8 and 12 each).
- CO_2 insufflation and smoke evacuator for VATS and robotic-assisted surgery (RAS).
- Stapler.

Positioning

- Right lateral decubitus positioning.
- The anterior-superior iliac crest should be positioned at the level of the break in the bed so flexing can open the intercostal spaces (ICSs).
- The right arm is extended out on an armrest, and the left arm is slightly flexed and suspended using an arm extension device.

Technique

- Incision and port placement for thoracotomy, VATS, and RAS.
- For an open approach, the posterolateral thoracotomy is made on the fifth ICS. The posterior aspect of the rib is typically shingled to allow for a more generous exposure.
- For VATS, the 4 cm minithoracotomy is made over the midclavicular line just over the hilum (fourth to fifth ICS), and additional camera ports and retraction ports are placed.

- For RAS, the 8-mm camera port is placed over the anterior axillary line over the eighth ICS. An additional 12-mm stapling port is placed along the same ICS.
- The traditional four robotic ports for the basic lobectomy setup are 2 × 8 mm and 2 × 12 mm. The majority of stapling is done anteriorly. Additionally, a fifth port (12 mm) is used for CO_2 insufflation and assistance (Figure 9.1A).

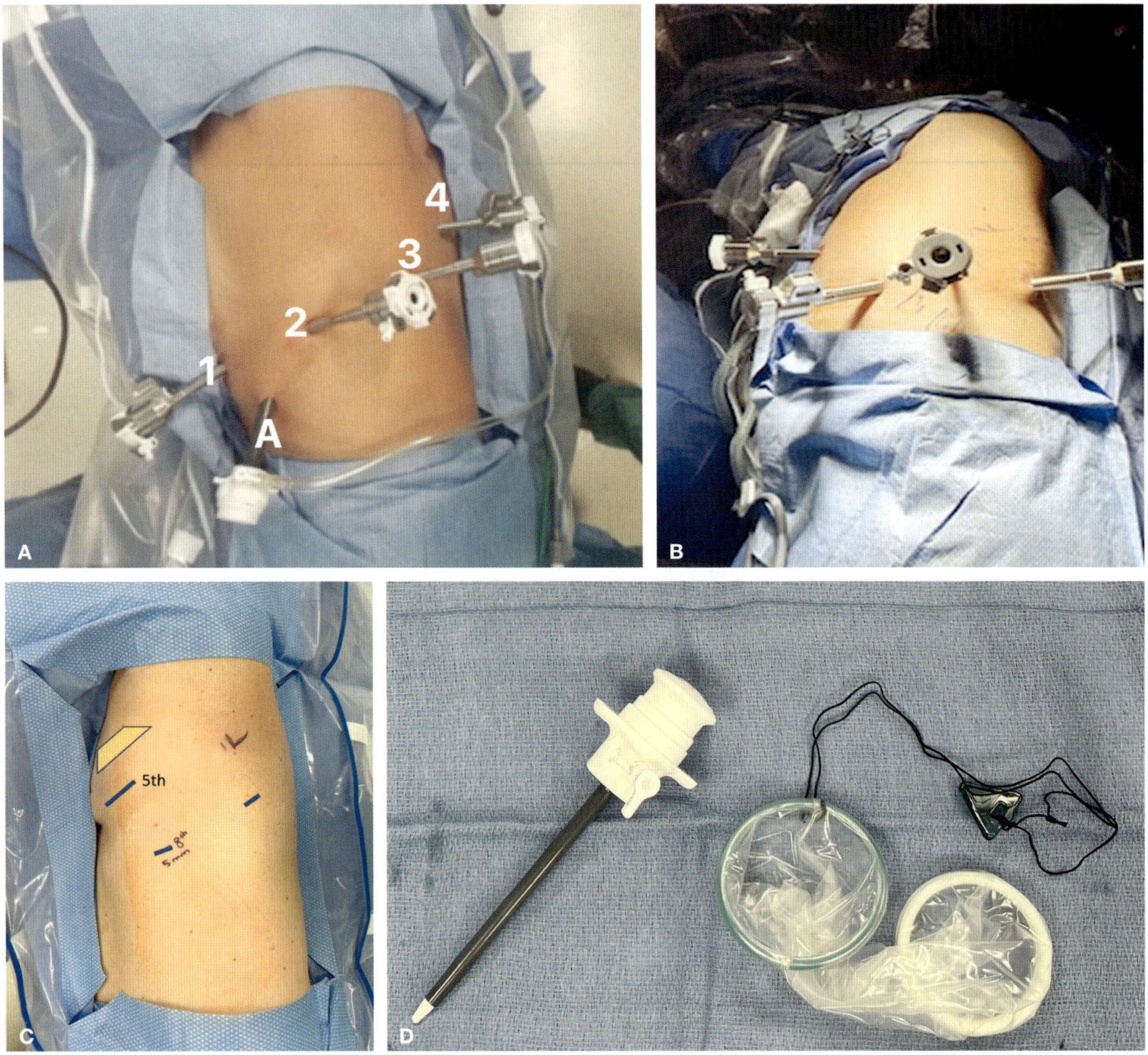

FIGURE 9.1 ❙ A and B. Four robotic ports and an insufflation port are used for left lower lobectomy. **C and D.** Port placement for video-assisted thoracoscopic surgery lower lobectomy and instruments.

- Alternative port placement can be considered, such as moving the most posterior 8-mm retraction port anteriorly to avoid significant pain and neuralgia related to the posterior port (Figure 9.1B).
- Robotic arm 2 is used for the camera port (8 mm), which is inserted in the ninth ICS posterior-axillary line. If the computed tomography of the chest demonstrates a higher diaphragm, a higher port placement can be considered.
- Robotic arm 1 inserted a hand's breadth (6 cm) ventrally and anteriorly from the camera port near the anterior axillary line.
- Robotic arm 3 (12 mm) is placed about one hand's breadth (6 cm) posterior toward the spine and caudal to the scapula. This port can be moved lower (1-2 rib spaces) to ensure a straight stapling angle.

- Robotic arm 4 (8 mm) is placed about 1 to 2 rib spaces cranially from arm 3 and 2 cm from the spine. This port can be associated with significant postoperative pain and neuralgia. Alternatively, it can be moved anteriorly over the fifth to sixth ICS along the submammary line.
- The assistant's hand port (12 mm) is placed caudal to robot arms 1 and 2 in a triangulated setup. An assistant port can be avoided for experienced surgeons (Figure 9.1B).
- A camera port is placed in the eighth ICS in the anterior axillary line (Figure 9.1C).
- A 5 cm utility incision is made over the fifth ICS or just over the hilum to perform the majority of dissections. A wound protector can be placed over the incision, making the operation easier (Figure 9.1D).
- A retraction port is placed posteriorly 3 to 4 cm below the scapula, which can also be used to staple hilar structures.

Resection

Important to note is that the dissection for a VATS or open approach follows similar principals as described in the section that follows:

1. First, dissect the inferior pulmonary ligament (IPL) up to the inferior pulmonary vein (Figure 9.2). Remove the level 9 node (Figure 9.3).

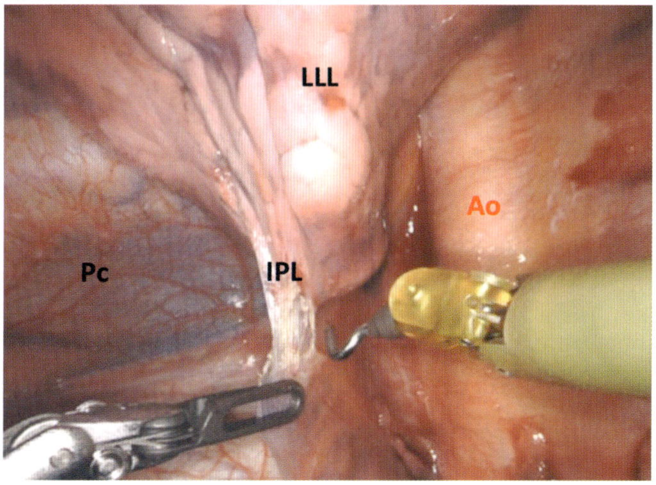

FIGURE 9.2 | Cauterization of the inferior pulmonary ligament. Ao, aorta; IPL, inferior pulmonary ligament; LLL, left lower lobe; Pc, pericardium.

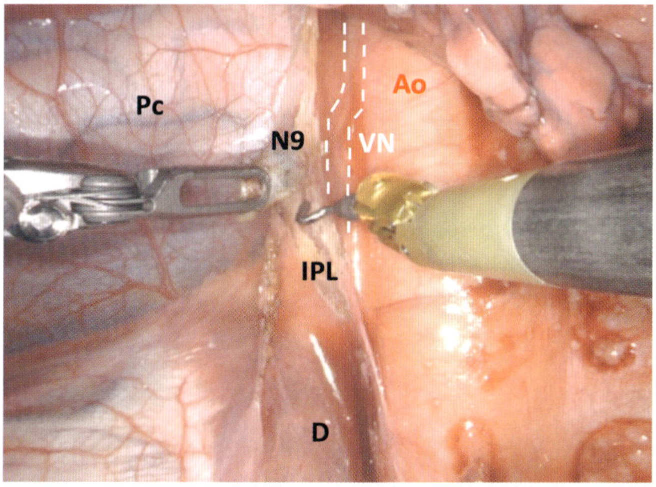

FIGURE 9.3 | Removal of node 9. Ao, aorta; D, diaphragm; IPL, inferior pulmonary ligament; LLL, left lower lobe; Pc, pericardium; VN, vagus nerve.

2. Retract the lower lobe anteriorly and expose the posterior aspect of the left lower lobe. Open the posterior mediastinal pleura (Figure 9.4).

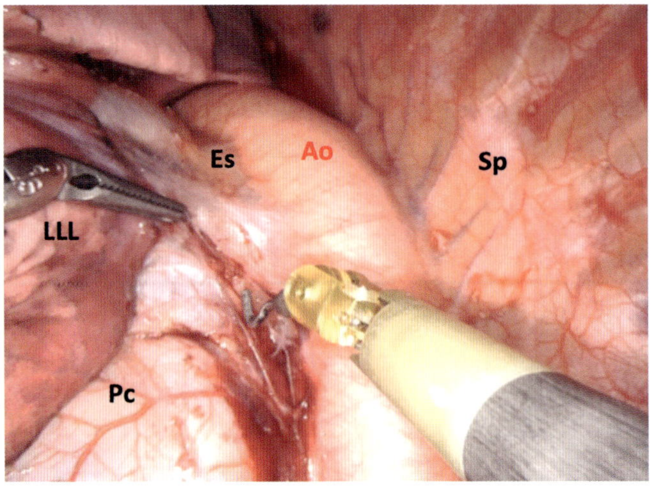

FIGURE 9.4 ▌ Opening the posterior mediastinal pleura posterior to left lower lobe, lateral to the esophagus, anterior to descending aorta. Ao, aorta; Es, esophagus; LLL, left lower lobe; Pc, pericardium; Sp, spine.

TIPS

- *In some patients, enlarged arterial branches along IPL may retract and bleed postoperatively. Careful dissection and complete hemostasis should be achieved.*
- *Identify and avoid the vagus nerve, which courses laterally along the esophagus. Damage can cause gastroparesis postoperatively.*

3. Anterior retraction of the lung opens up the posterior hilum. The posterior mediastinal pleura is incised, exposing the inferior pulmonary vein, the left main bronchus, and the main PA (Figure 9.5). Hilar dissection continues superiorly above the main PA. The level 10 lymph node (LN) on top of the main PA is removed, exposing the avascular plane along the PA. The lung is retracted superiorly. Superior and inferior pulmonary veins should be identified, and the LN between them should be removed (Figure 9.6). The inferior pulmonary vein is isolated and divided (Figures 9.7 and 9.8).

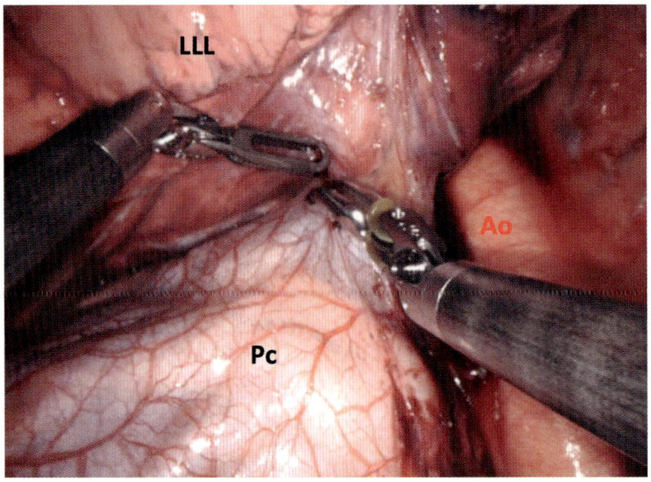

FIGURE 9.5 ▌ The mediastinal pleura is opened, exposing the anterior aspect of the lower lobe vein. Ao, aorta; LLL, left lower lobe; Pc, pericardium.

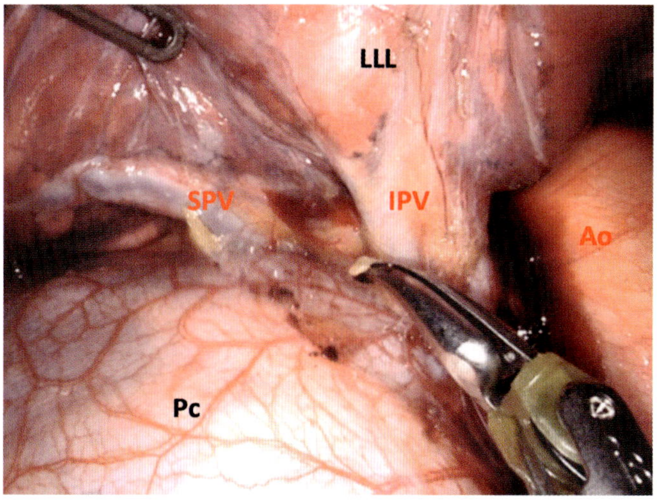

FIGURE 9.6 | Cephalad retraction of lower lobe and separation of superior pulmonary vein (SPV) and inferior pulmonary vein (IPV). Removal of the lymph node between SPV and IPV creates a dissection plane around IPV. Ao, aorta; LLL, left lower lobe; Pc, pericardium.

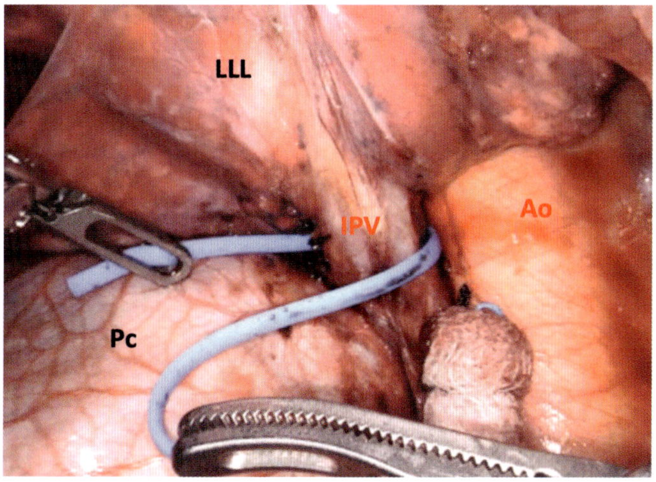

FIGURE 9.7 | Isolation of inferior pulmonary vein with vessel loop. Ao, aorta; IPV, inferior pulmonary vein; LLL, left lower lobe; Pc, pericardium.

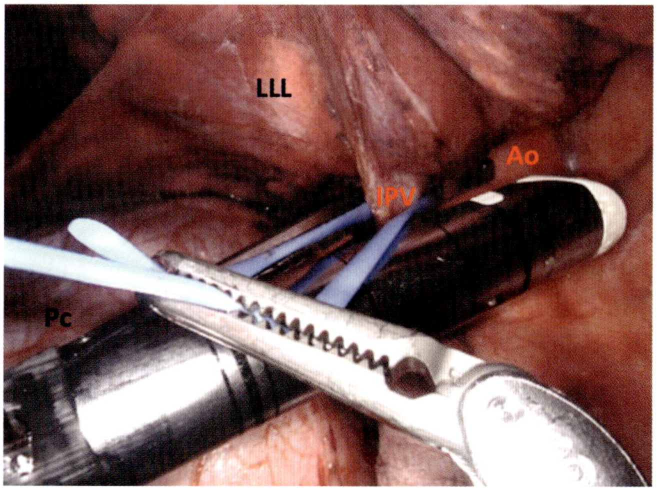

FIGURE 9.8 | Stapling across inferior pulmonary vein. Ao, aorta; IPV, inferior pulmonary vein; LLL, left lower lobe; Pc, pericardium.

4. Resect the node between the lower lobe bronchus and PA posteriorly and then retract the lung cephalad (Figure 9.9). Dissect out and identify the bifurcation between upper and lower lobe bronchus and remove the interlobar node (Figure 9.10). Dissect around the lower lobe bronchus. Place a vessel loop for retraction and division of the left lower lobe bronchus.

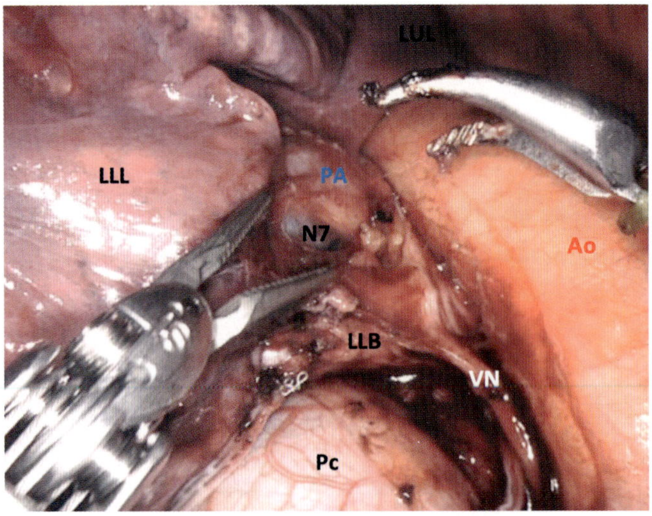

FIGURE 9.9 ▍ Anterior lower lobe retraction and removal of the node between the main pulmonary artery and lower lobe bronchus. Ao, aorta; LLB, lower lobe bronchus; LLL, left lower lobe; N7, node 7; PA, main pulmonary artery; Pc, pericardium; VN, vagus nerve.

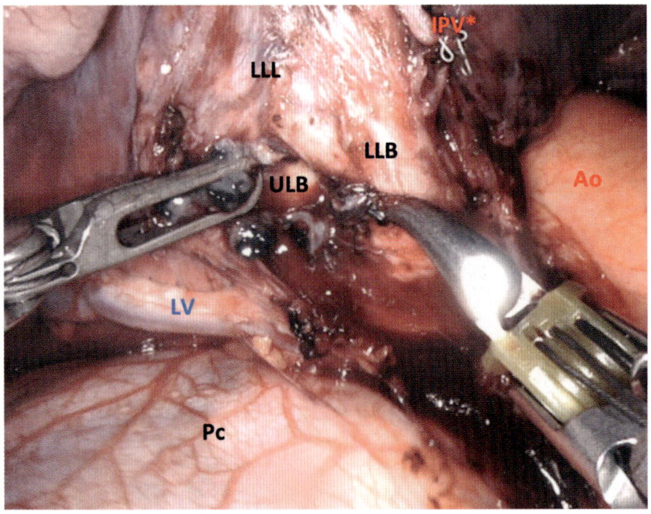

FIGURE 9.10 ▍ Lower lobe is retracted cephalad, and node 11 between upper and lower lobes is removed. Ao, aorta; IPV*, inferior pulmonary vein stump; LLB, left lower bronchus; LLL, left lower lobe; LV, lingular vein; Pc, pericardium; ULB, upper lobe bronchus.

PEARLS AND PITFALLS

- Removing the LN between the PA and the lower lobe bronchus improves the speed and safety of subsequent dissection around the lower lobe bronchus.
- Remember that the left lower lobe PA is deep to the interlobar node and is at risk of injury.
- Avoid capsular disruption when removing the LN. This will minimize bleeding.

5. Dissect around and divide the lower bronchus (Figures 9.11 and 9.12).

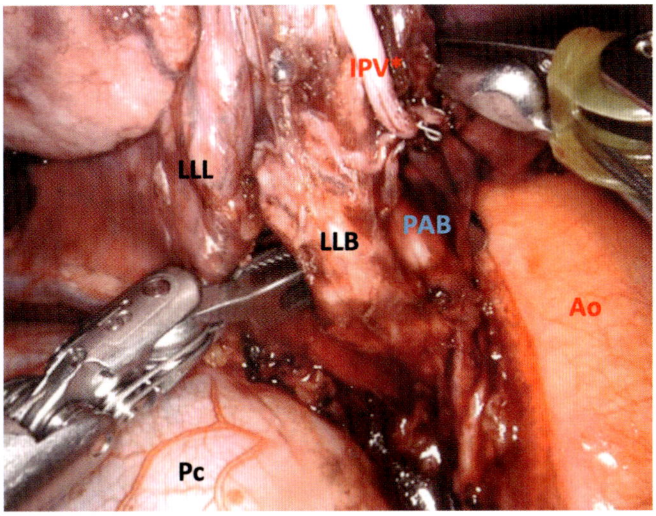

FIGURE 9.11 ❙ Bluntly dissect around lower lobe bronchus. Ao, aorta; IPV*, inferior pulmonary vein stump; LLB, lower lobe bronchus; LLL, left lower lobe; PAB, basilar pulmonary artery; Pc, pericardium.

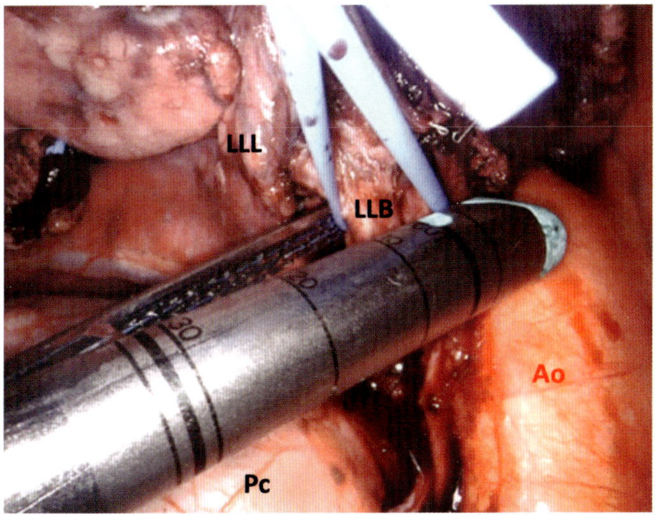

FIGURE 9.12 ❙ Passage of vessel loop behind lower lobe bronchus and stapling. Ao, aorta; LLB, left lower bronchus; LLL, left lower lobe; Pc, pericardium.

PEARLS AND PITFALLS

- Hug the lower lobe bronchus while dissecting around it. The space created by removing the LN between the PA and the bronchus in step 4 should aid in getting around the lower lobe bronchus and avoid inadvertent injury to the main PA.
- Make sure to identify the bifurcation between the upper and lower lobe bronchi before dividing the lower lobe bronchus.

6. Grasp the bronchial stump and gently retract cephalad, exposing the lower lobe PA (Figure 9.13). Divide in sequential order the left lower lobe pulmonary arterial branches (basilar and superior segments) (Figures 9.14 and 9.15).

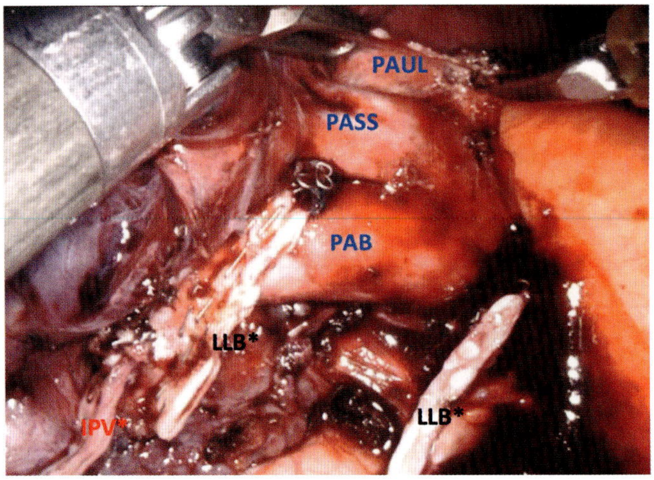

FIGURE 9.13 ▮ Anterior retraction of lower lobe exposes pulmonary artery branches deep to lower lobe bronchial stump. Dissection here shows multiple arterial branches. IPV*, inferior pulmonary vein stump; LLB*, lower lobe bronchial stump; PAB, basilar pulmonary artery; PAUL, upper lobe pulmonary artery; PASS, superior segment pulmonary artery.

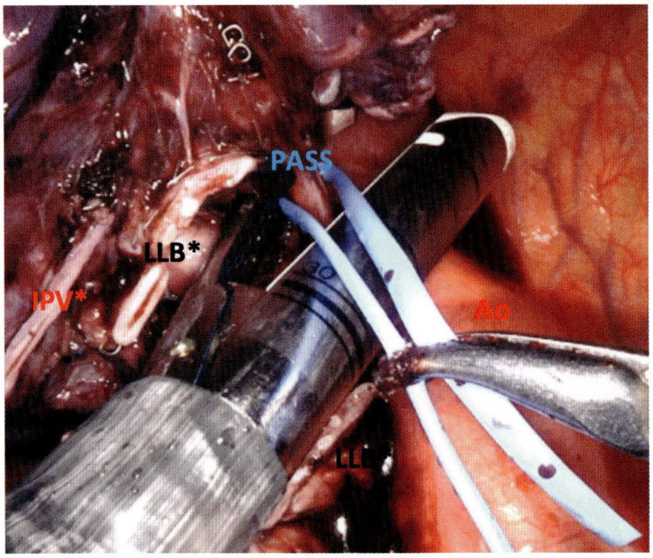

FIGURE 9.14 ▮ Vessel loop isolation and stapling of superior segment artery. Ao, aorta; IPV*, inferior pulmonary vein stump; LLB*, lower lobe bronchial stump; PASS, superior segment pulmonary artery.

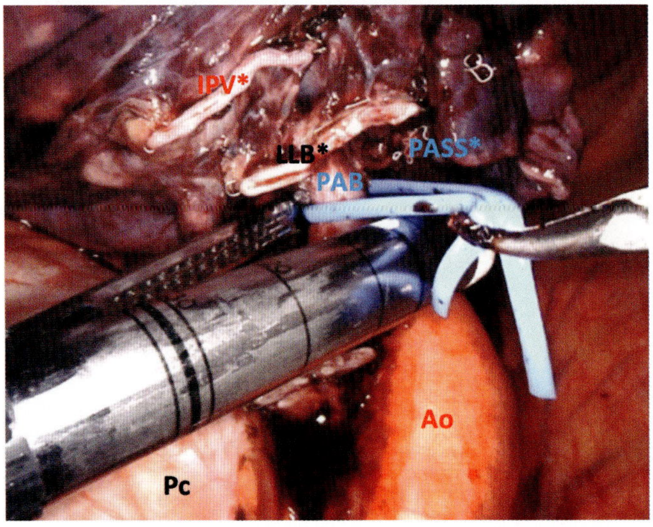

FIGURE 9.15 ▮ Vessel loop ligation and division of basilar artery. Ao, aorta; IPV*, inferior pulmonary vein stump; LLB*, lower lobe bronchial stump; PAB, basilar pulmonary artery; PASS, superior segment pulmonary artery; Pc, pericardium.

7. Divide the fissure (Figure 9.16). Complete the mediastinal LN dissection (Figures 9.17 and 9.18).
8. Removal of lower lobe specimen through the appropriate access incision.

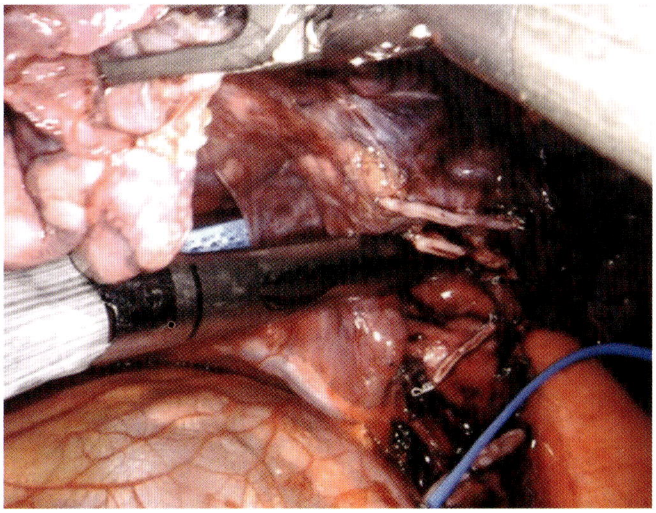

FIGURE 9.16 | Gently retract the lung and slide stapler beneath the divided pulmonary artery to separate the fissure.

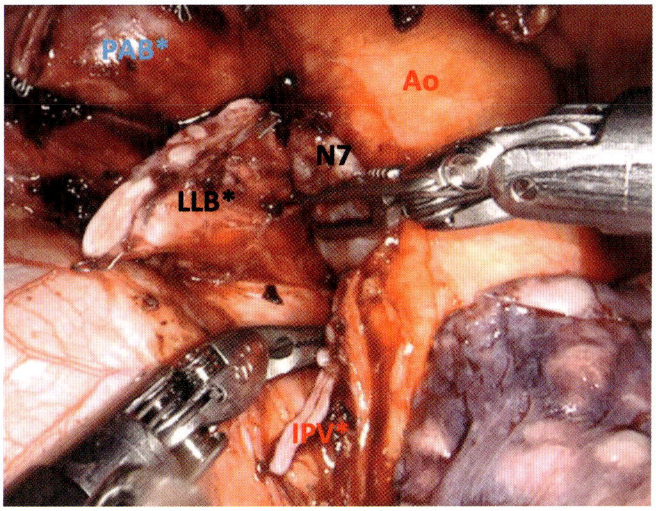

FIGURE 9.17 | Deeper node 7 dissection after greater retraction of lower lobe. Ao, aorta; IPV*, inferior pulmonary vein stump; LLB*, lower lobe bronchial stump; N8, node 8; PAB*, basilar artery stump.

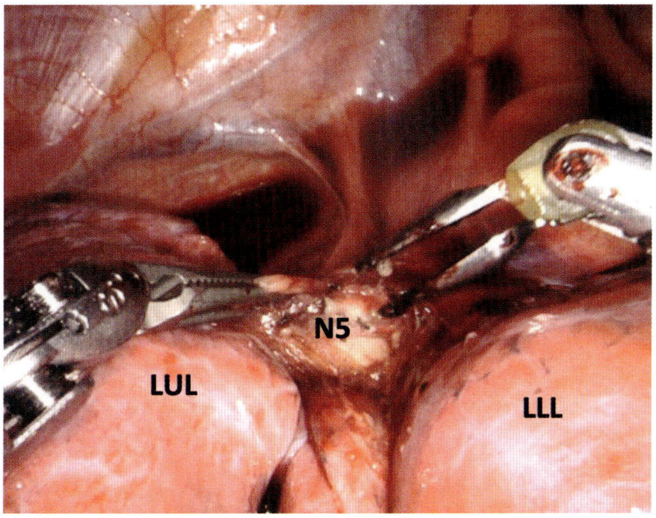

FIGURE 9.18 | Posterior retraction of lung and dissection of node 5 near aortic arch. LLL, left lower lobe; LUL, left upper lobe; N5, node 5.

Postoperative Care

- Postresection, intraoperative nerve blockade with local anesthetic is useful for immediate postoperative pain control.
- A chest tube (24 French) is left for drainage.
- Chest tubes are usually removed if there is no air leak and output is low (<300 mL/d).

Suggested Readings

1. Fell SC, DeCamp MM, Feins RH. Technical aspects of lobectomy. In: Locicero J III, Feins RH, Colson YL, Rocco G, eds. *Shields' General Thoracic Surgery*. 8th ed. Wolters Kluwer; 2019:388-411.
2. Grenda T, Lin J. Lobectomy: robotic. In: Hawn MT, Mulholland MW, eds. *Operative Techniques in Thoracic and Esophageal Surgery*. Wolters Kluwer; 2015:48-60.
3. Hanna JM, Onaitis MW, D'Amico TA. Lung cancer: minimally invasive approaches. In: Sellke FW, del Nido PJ, Swanson SJ, eds. *Sabiston & Spencer: Surgery of the Chest*. 9th ed. Elsevier; 2016:318-326.
4. Wei B, Cerfolio RJ. Robotic approach to lobectomy. In: Mathisen DJ, Morse CR, eds. *Thoracic Surgery: Lung Resections, Bronchoplasty*. Wolters Kluwer; 2015:209-222.

Chapter 10

Pneumonectomy: Robotic/Video-Assisted Thoracic Surgery/Thoracotomy

ROBERT E. MERRITT

Perioperative Considerations

- Pneumonectomy is defined as a resection of the whole lung. The operation is typically performed for centrally located lung tumors involving the hilar structures, such as the main bronchus, pulmonary artery, or the pulmonary veins. The operation can also be performed with a thoracotomy or with a minimally invasive approach, such as video-assisted thoracic surgery (VATS) or robotic-assisted surgery.
- The key technical steps are the same regardless of whether the surgeon utilizes a thoracotomy or a minimally invasive technique to perform a pneumonectomy.
- A standard cardiopulmonary evaluation should include pulmonary function testing, nuclear medicine split lung perfusion study, and an echocardiogram prior to pneumonectomy.
- Pulmonary function tests should be obtained to measure the forced expiratory volume in 1 second (FEV_1) and diffusion capacity. Patients with a history of chronic obstructive pulmonary disease will have diminished values for FEV_1 and diffusing capacity of lung for carbon monoxide (DLCO); therefore, they will be at increased risk for perioperative respiratory complications. A postoperative predicted FEV_1 of less than 1 L is predictive of postoperative pulmonary complications.
- A transthoracic echocardiogram should be obtained to assess the left ventricular ejection fraction and left ventricular wall motion. A treadmill cardiac stress test should be obtained when the echocardiogram findings are abnormal. In addition, a right ventricular systolic pressure greater than 35 mm Hg could indicate significant pulmonary hypertension, and a right cardiac catheterization should be obtained to measure the pulmonary artery pressure. Pulmonary hypertension is a relative contraindication for pneumonectomy.
- Patients with marginal pulmonary function (FEV_1 and/or DLCO < 60% predicted) should undergo a cardiopulmonary exercise testing to measure the VO_2 maximum value (>20 mL/kg/min).

Anesthesia and Patient Positioning

- Patients can be intubated with a double-lumen endotracheal tube for single-lung isolation. A right-sided double-lumen tube is preferable for left pneumonectomy and a left-sided double-lumen tube for right pneumonectomy. Endobronchial blockers should be avoided in cases involving pneumonectomy. The endobronchial blocker would need to be removed prior to stapling the bronchus. In cases in which the bronchial stump is opened and sutured, ventilation will not be optimal unless the single-lumen tube is advanced into the contralateral main bronchus.
- Optimal single-lung ventilation during pneumonectomy is critical to maintain adequate oxygenation and ventilation.
- A thoracic epidural catheter with continuous infusion of a local anesthetic and an opioid is recommended for patients who undergo open thoracotomy to optimize postoperative pain management and pulmonary toilet.
- Close monitoring of tidal volumes and airway pressures is recommended to avoid barotrauma to the contralateral lung during pneumonectomy.

- Perioperative antibiotics should be given within 30 minutes of the first incision. Compression boots are placed on the lower extremities and subcutaneous unfractionated heparin is given to minimize the risk of postoperative deep venous thrombosis (DVT).
- An arterial line is recommended for continuous blood pressure monitoring during pneumonectomy. A central line is optional and can facilitate assiduous intraoperative fluid management to avoid intravascular volume overload, which can lead to pulmonary edema.
- Patients are positioned in the lateral decubitus position with a padded bean bag or rolls.
- Joints should be in neutral position and bony protuberances should be well padded to avoid pressure-induced soft-tissue injuries and pressure ulcers.
- The arms should be secured on padded arm boards. Care should be taken to prevent tension on the brachial plexus.

Instruments and Equipment

Open Thoracotomy

- Finochietto retractor
- Balfour retractor
- Standard open thoracotomy tray
- Linear endomechanical stapler
- Assortment of vascular clamps
- 5-mm LigaSure vessel sealer
- Double-armed Prolene suture
- Pneumonectomy balanced drainage system

Video-Assisted Thoracic Surgery

- Three 12-mm thoracoscopic ports
- 10-mm, 30° thoracoscope
- Linear endomechanical stapler
- 5-mm LigaSure vessel sealer
- 5-mm laparoscopic atraumatic graspers
- 5-mm laparoscopic suction catheter
- Pneumonectomy balanced drainage system

Robotic-Assisted Surgery

- Three 8-mm robotic ports
- 12-mm robotic port
- 12-mm air seal port
- 8-mm, 30° robotic thoracoscope
- Robotic 45-mm stapler
- Tip-up fenestrated grasper
- Cadiere grasper
- Long bipolar grasper
- Pneumonectomy balanced drainage system

Technique

- The open right and left pneumonectomy are performed through a posterior lateral thoracotomy (Figure 10.1). The latissimus dorsi and serratus anterior muscles are divided and the thoracic cavity is entered in the fifth intercostal space.
  - An intercostal muscle flap can be harvested at the time of thoracotomy.

TIPS

An intercostal muscle flap can be harvested at the time of thoracotomy.

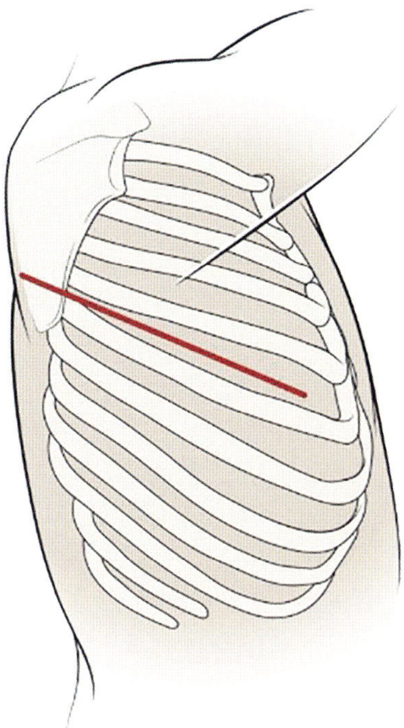

FIGURE 10.1 ▮ Standard posterior lateral thoracotomy for exposure for open pneumonectomy. (Reproduced with the permission of The Ohio State University.)

- For the VATS technique, a 12-mm port is placed in the eighth intercostal space anteriorly and in the seventh intercostal space posteriorly. A 3- to 4-cm access incision is placed in the fifth intercostal space anteriorly (Figure 10.2).

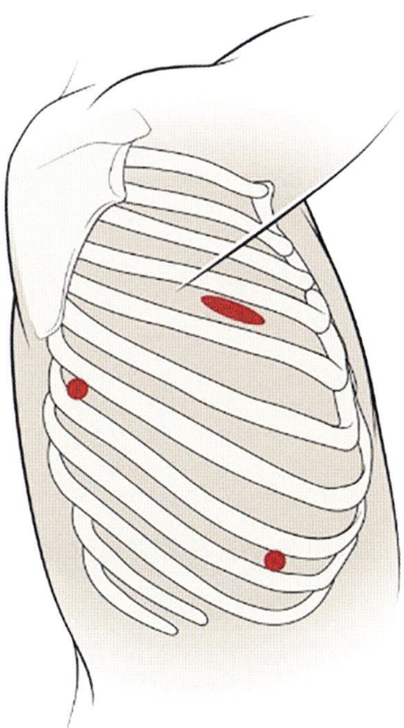

FIGURE 10.2 ▮ Port incision location for the video-assisted thoracic surgery approach for pneumonectomy. (Reproduced with the permission of The Ohio State University.)

- For the robotic technique, three 8-mm ports and one 12-mm port are placed in the eighth intercostal space. A 12-mm air seal port is placed in the 10th intercostal space and carbon dioxide insufflation is initiated with a pressure of 5 mm Hg (Figure 10.3).
- The pulmonary veins are usually dissected initially (Figure 10.4). The inferior pulmonary ligament is incised to expose the inferior pulmonary vein. The superior vein is then dissected from the

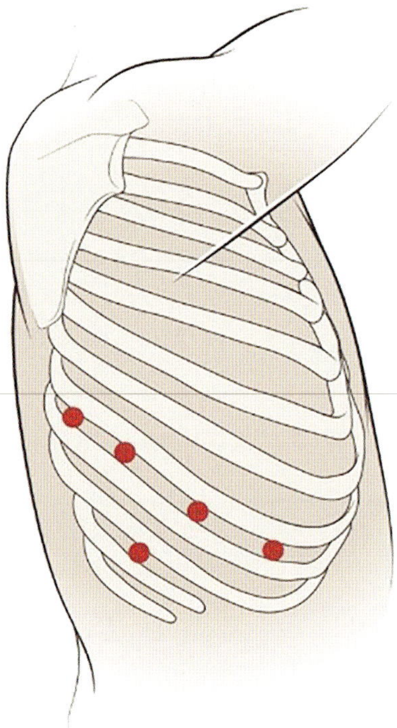

FIGURE 10.3 ▮ Port incision location for the robotic-assisted approach for pneumonectomy. (Reproduced with the permission of The Ohio State University.)

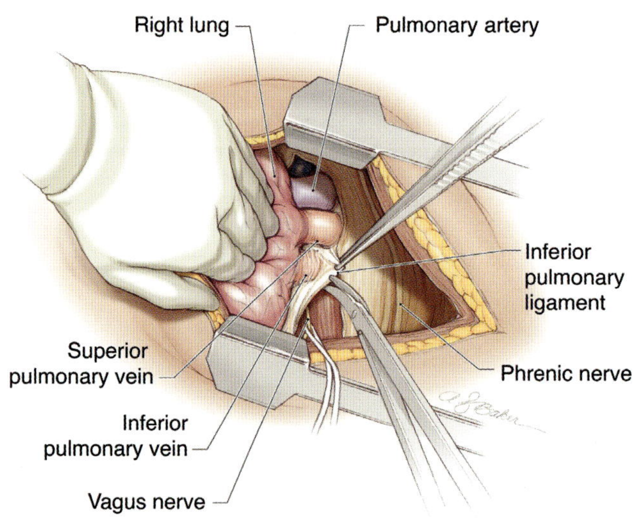

FIGURE 10.4 ▮ Dissection of the right pulmonary veins in the hilum. (Reproduced with the permission of The Ohio State University.)

pulmonary artery and bronchus. The pulmonary veins can be divided with a linear endomechanical stapler with vascular reloads (Figure 10.5).

- The right main pulmonary artery can be identified as it courses underneath the superior vena cava. The right main pulmonary can be dissected from the right main bronchus with a large right angle clamp or dissected with blunt finger dissection (Figure 10.6). Care must be taken to not injure the right main pulmonary artery when passing a clamp or a stapler.
- The left main pulmonary artery can be identified as it courses underneath the aortic arch. The truncus anterior branch is typically located proximally. The left main pulmonary artery should be dissected from the left main stem bronchus with blunt finger dissection or with a right angle clamp (Figure 10.7).
- The left and right main pulmonary arteries can be divided with a linear endomechanical stapler with vascular reloads (Figure 10.8).

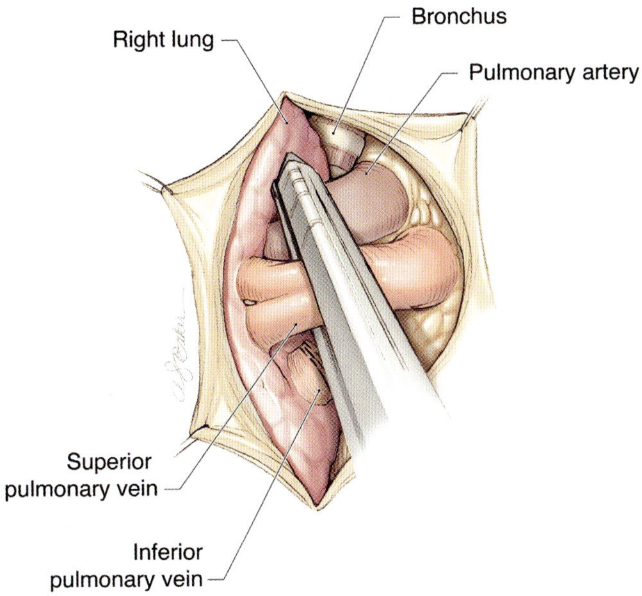

FIGURE 10.5 | Division of the right superior pulmonary vein with a linear endomechanical stapler. (Reproduced with the permission of The Ohio State University.)

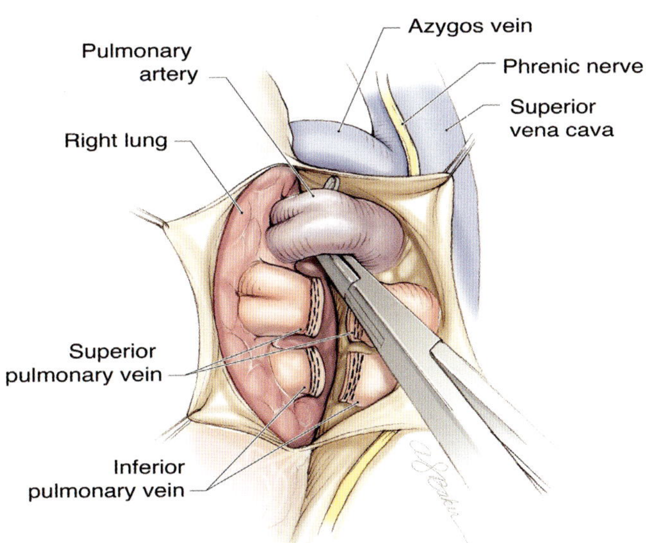

FIGURE 10.6 | Dissection of the right main pulmonary artery in the right hilum as it courses underneath the superior vena cava. (Reproduced with the permission of The Ohio State University.)

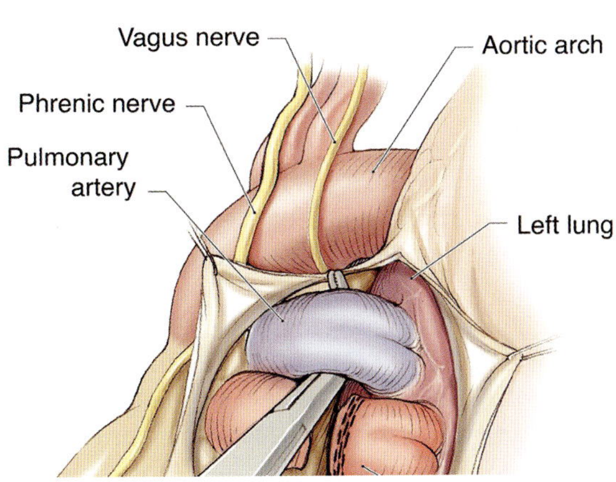

FIGURE 10.7 | Dissection of the left main pulmonary artery in the left hilum as it courses underneath the descending thoracic aorta. (Reproduced with the permission of The Ohio State University.)

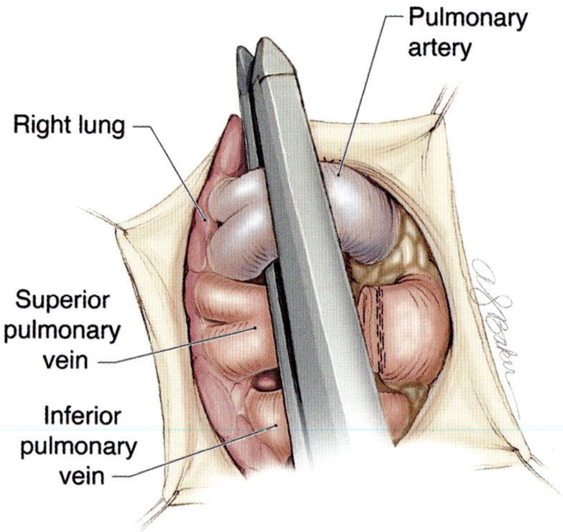

FIGURE 10.8 | Division of the right main pulmonary artery with a linear endomechanical stapler. (Reproduced with the permission of The Ohio State University.)

- The bronchus is typically the last structure to be divided during pneumonectomy. The right main stem bronchus can be divided with a linear endomechanical stapler at the bifurcation at the main carina (Figure 10.9).

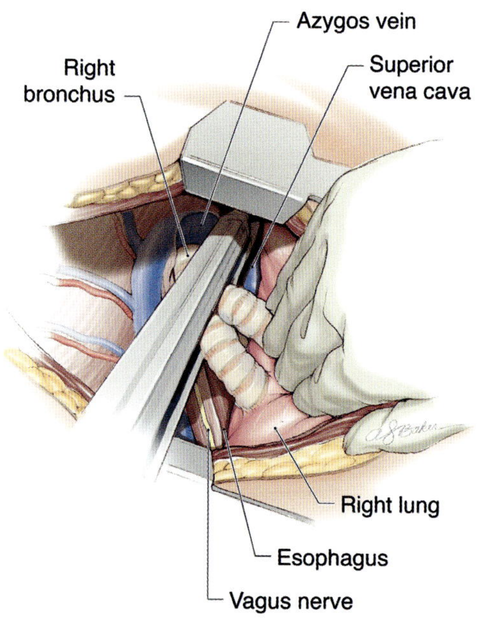

FIGURE 10.9 | Division of the right main stem bronchus with an endomechanical stapler. (Reproduced with the permission of The Ohio State University.)

- The left main stem bronchus courses underneath the descending thoracic aorta. The bronchus should be divided as close to the carina as possible with the stapler.
- The bronchial stump is typically covered with a vascularized pedicle such as an intercostal muscle (Figure 10.10) or a serratus anterior muscle. The vascularized pedicle should be sutured to the bronchial stump to ensure adequate coverage of the staple line or the suture line. Even for minimally invasive pneumonectomy, the bronchial stump should still be covered with a vascularized pedicle.
- A systematic lymph node dissection or sampling should be performed during pneumonectomy. For right pneumonectomy, levels 4R, 7, 8, 9R, 10R, and 11R should be sampled/dissected. For left pneumonectomy, levels 5, 6, 7, 9L, 10L, and 11L should be sampled/dissected.
- A "test clamp" of the main pulmonary artery is not necessary prior to division.

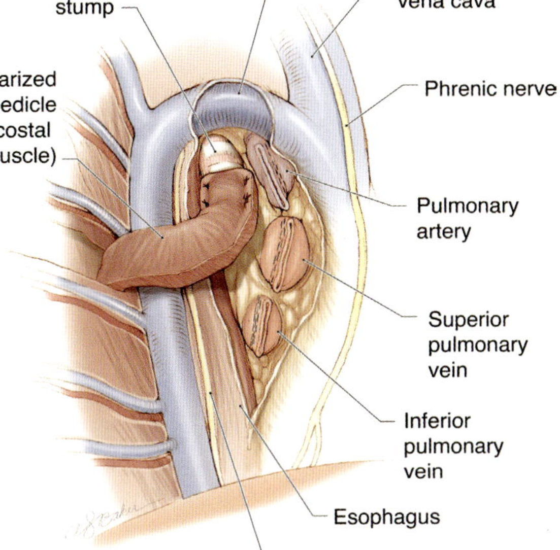

FIGURE 10.10 ▮ Coverage of the right main stem bronchial stump with an intercostal muscle flap. (Reproduced with the permission of The Ohio State University.)

Postoperative Care

- The administration of intravenous fluid should be very conservative after pneumonectomy to minimize the risk of pulmonary edema and respiratory failure.
- Patients should be extubated in the operating room if possible. A chest radiograph should be obtained in the recovery room or intensive care unit.
- A chest tube should be placed in the postpneumonectomy cavity for at least 24 hours to assess for bleeding.
  - The chest tube should **not** be placed on suction, which will result in significant mediastinal shifting and hypotension and potential mortality.

TIPS

*The chest tube should **not** be placed on suction, which will result in significant mediastinal shifting and hypotension and potential mortality.*

- An early postoperative arterial blood gas should be obtained to assess for hypoxia and hypercarbia.
- Patients should be mobilized from the bed early with frequent ambulation.
- Routinely administered subcutaneous heparin should be ordered in the postoperative period to mitigate the risk of DVT and pulmonary embolism.
- Aggressive pulmonary toilet with incentive spirometry, coughing, and deep breathing is essential to avoid postoperative pneumonia.
- Chest tubes should be removed as early as possible and balanced Pleur-evacs are preferred to minimize mediastinal shifting.
- An epidural catheter should be placed for postoperative pain management. Epidural infusion of local anesthetic minimizes postthoracotomy pain and allows patients to participate in pulmonary toilet exercises.
- Fiberoptic bronchoscopy is recommended for evaluation of suspected early bronchopleural fistula.
- Pulmonary edema, pneumonia, pulmonary embolism, and aspiration pneumonitis can cause devastating complications after pneumonectomy and should be avoided at all costs.

PEARLS AND PITFALLS

- The pericardium can be incised to gain access to the proximal pulmonary artery for intrapericardial division when there is proximal tumor encasement of the main pulmonary artery.
- Pericardial defects should be closed primarily or with a synthetic or biologic patch to prevent herniation of the heart and subsequent cardiac torsion and cardiac arrest.
- The bronchial stump should be as short as possible to minimize the risk of dehiscence and bronchopleural fistula.
- The bronchial closure can be performed with primary sutured technique or with endomechanical staplers.
- The bronchial stump should be covered with a vascularized pedicle, such as intercostal muscle, a pericardial fat pad, or the serratus anterior muscle.
- A complete lymph node dissection should be performed during pneumonectomy. Removing the hilar lymph nodes can make the dissection of the pulmonary artery and bronchus easier.
- In some cases, the tumor may encase the proximal pulmonary vein, which will need to be divided at the junction of the vein and the left atrium. A thicker stapler reload should be used in this situation. In addition, consideration should be given to reenforcing the staple line with interrupted Prolene sutures with pledgets to minimize the risk of suture line dehiscence and hemorrhage.

Suggested Readings

1. Alvarez JM, Tan J, Kejriwal N, et al. Idiopathic postpneumonectomy pulmonary edema: hyperinflation of the remaining lung is a potential etiologic factor, but the condition can be averted by balanced pleural drainage. *J Thorac Cardiovasc Surg*. 2007;133(6):1439-1447.
2. Craig SR, Walker WS. Initial experience of video assisted thoracoscopic pneumonectomy. *Thorax*. 1995;50(4):392-395.
3. Graham EA, Singer JJ. Landmark article Oct 28, 1933. Successful removal of an entire lung for carcinoma of the bronchus. By Evarts A. Graham and J. J. Singer. *JAMA*. 1984;251(2):257-260.
4. Groth SS, Burt BM, Sugarbaker DJ. Management of complications after pneumonectomy. *Thorac Surg Clin*. 2015;25(3):335-348.
5. Henon MW, Kumar A, Devisetty H, et al. Mininally invasive do not compromise outcomes for pneumonectomy: a comparison using the national cancer databse. *J Thorac Oncol*. 2019;14(1):107-114.
6. Louie BE. Robotic pneumonectomy. *Thorac Surg Clin*. 2014;24(2):169-175.

Chapter 11

Sleeve Resection/ Bronchoplasty via Minimally Invasive/Thoracotomy

CHRISTINA L. COSTANTINO
HUGH G. AUCHINCLOSS

Overview

- Neoplasms involving the central airways require more complex planning for resection and reconstruction.
- Bronchoplasty involves resection of a central airway tumor with preservation of the lung parenchyma either by primary reconstruction or sleeve reconstruction.
- Sleeve lobectomy refers to an anatomic lung resection taken en bloc with a circumferential segment of the mainstem bronchus.
- Low-grade bronchial malignancies, including carcinoid, mucoepidermoid, and adenoid cystic cancers, as well as primary non-small cell lung cancer represent the bulk of these lesions.
- Right upper lobes are the most common sleeve lobectomies performed.
- Technique for airway anastomoses includes a running suture for minimally invasive techniques and standard interrupted suture for open procedures.
- Wristed movement of robotic instruments improves upon the technical challenges with minimally invasive sleeve lobectomies.
- Surveillance bronchoscopy can be performed on postoperative day 5 or 6 to ensure anastomotic healing prior to discharge to home.
- Adjuvant treatment, including radiation, may be started at 6 to 8 weeks from surgery following bronchoscopy to ensure healing.

Perioperative Considerations

- Patients should undergo a preop bronchoscopy and chest computed tomography (CT) with contrast (Figure 11.1).
- Patients should undergo staging including mediastinal evaluation, including positron emission tomography CT, endobronchial ultrasonography or mediastinoscopy, and brain magnetic resonance imaging.
- Perioperative evaluation with bronchoscopy in the operating room should be used to fully assess the extent of endobronchial involvement and determine the resectability of airway. This is typically performed by the surgeon performing the procedure either at the time of the procedure or in a separate setting.
- If there is evidence of bronchial obstruction and postobstructive pneumonia, we recommend consideration of endobronchial debulking and antibiotic administration prior to surgical resection.
- Anticoagulation including coumadin, Xarelto, Eliquis, and Plavix is held preoperatively. Patients who require bridging may transition with therapeutic Lovenox with the last injection being the night prior to surgery.

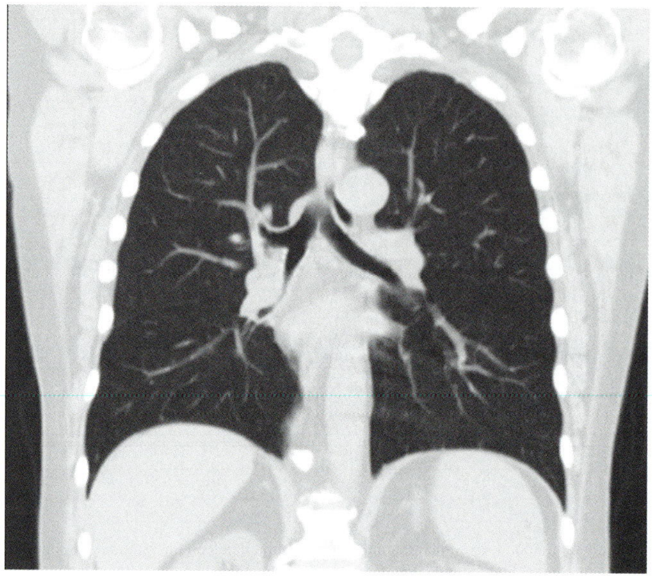

FIGURE 11.1 ▮ Computed tomography scan of the endobronchial lesion requiring right middle and right lower sleeve resection.

Anesthesia and Patient Positioning

- Induction of general anesthesia and placement of a double-lumen endotracheal tube in supine position. For a left-sided sleeve resection, consider the placement of a right-sided double lumen endotracheal tube.
- Turn the patient to a lateral decubitus position (side of resection up) with bed flexed to maximize the aperture of intercostal spaces.

Instruments and Equipment

Open Technique via Posterolateral Thoracotomy

- Finochietto retractor, Balfour retractor
- 4-0 Vicryl RB1 (70 cm), coat with mineral oil
- Long needle driver
- Linear EndoGIA stapler

Minimally Invasive Robotic Technique

- Standard 8-mm 3-Trocar technique
- 1 to 12 mm Trocar
- Suction and air seal insufflation (pressure set at 8)
- Cadiere forceps, Maryland bipolar forceps (coagulation energy 3), tip-up fenestrated grasper, monopolar curved scissors, and large needle driver
- SureForm stapler curved tip (white and blue loads)
- 3-0 Vicryl suture
- 3-0 V-Loc suture × 2

Technique

Open Technique via Posterolateral Thoracotomy

Dissection and Resection of the Airway

- Dissection for a sleeve lobectomy begins with the requisite mobilization of the hilar structures, identifying and dividing the pulmonary artery and veins.
- If fissures are incomplete, these should be divided with linear staplers to assist in complete mobilization of the lobe.
- The bronchus should be identified and followed proximally to its origin. Level 11 and 12 lymph nodes should be completely excised to better expose the airway.
    - Careful attention should be paid to avoid devascularizing the airway.

- Transection of the airway can be undertaken under bronchoscopic guidance.
  - Insert a 25G needle into the airway to define where best to begin incising the airway. The airway is then transected sharply proximally and distally.
  - Start conservatively, so as not to take more airway than is needed. Sending an additional margin of airway is preferable to confirm it is negative for the disease on frozen section.

Open Anastomotic Techniques for Reconstruction

- Two 3-0 Vicryl traction sutures are placed at each cartilaginous membranous margin on both bronchial stumps.
- 4-0 Vicryl interrupted sutures (mineral oil) are then placed in series, beginning with the cartilaginous wall.
- Traction sutures are typically tied to bring the airway together, followed by interrupted sutures placed on the anterior wall, followed by the posterior wall interrupted sutures.
  - A 3-0 PDS may alternatively be used in a running fashion on the membranous wall, followed by interrupted 4-0 Vicryl sutures to the anterior cartilaginous wall.
- A well-vascularized pedicle (pericardial fat or intercostal muscle) can be used to buttress the anastomosis, tied down with silk sutures. If intercostal muscle is used, it is important not to circumferentially wrap the bronchus for fear of airway stricture with any calcification of the periosteum. A buttress is also placed between the airway and pulmonary artery to prevent fistula.

Minimally Invasive Robotic Technique

Port Placement (Figure 11.2)

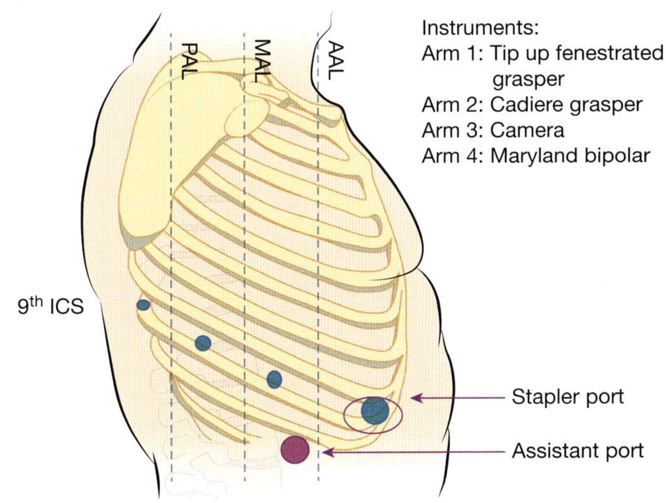

FIGURE 11.2 ▮ Robotic port placement. (Reprinted by Permission of SAGE Publications from Onwugbufor MT, Predina JD, Osho AA, Schumacher LY. 10 commandments of robotic lobectomy. *Innovations*. 2021;16(2):123-126.)

- 8-mm port placed at eighth intercostal space (camera port)
- Insufflate chest to 8 cm H_2O
- Additional ports placed under thoracoscopic visualization
- 8-mm port just lateral to paraspinal ligament at the tip of the lower lobe superior segment, 8 mm port in posterior axillary line in the ninth intercostal space, 12 mm port placed just posterior to costal margin in anterior chest, and 12 mm AirSeal port placed just above the diaphragm for the bedside assistant

Dissection and Division of Airway (Video 11.1)

- Dissection for a sleeve lobectomy begins with the requisite mobilization of the hilar structures, identifying and dividing the pulmonary artery and veins.

- If fissures are incomplete, these should be divided with linear staplers to assist in complete mobilization of the lobe.
- The bronchus should be identified and followed proximally to its origin. Level 11 and 12 lymph nodes should be completely excised to better expose the airway.
  - Careful attention should be paid toward not devascularizing the airway.
- Transection of the airway proximally and distally is done sharply using monopolar curved scissors (Figure 11.3).

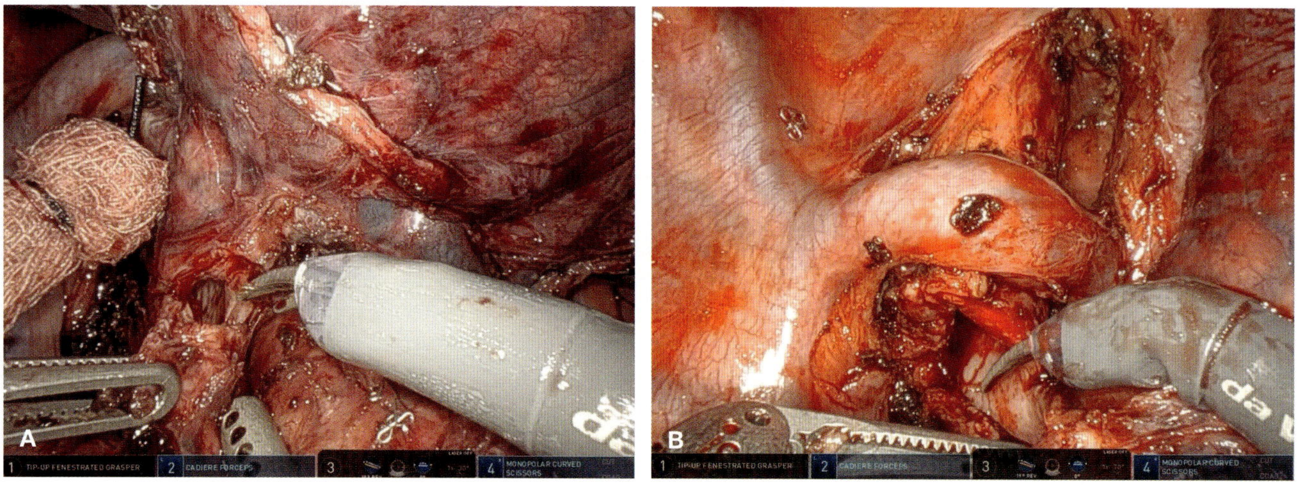

FIGURE 11.3 ▮ Sharp division of the airway in a right upper lobe sleeve lobectomy. **A.** Division of the bronchus intermedius and **B.** right mainstem.

  - This should be done under bronchoscopic guidance.
  - Start conservatively, so as not to take more airway than is needed. Sending an additional margin of airway is preferable to confirm it is negative for disease on frozen section.

Anastomotic Techniques for Reconstruction (Figure 11.4)

- Placement of 3-0 Vicryl traction suture at the medial cartilaginous-membranous junction, tied to bring the two bronchial stumps together (Figure 11.4A).
- A 3-0 V-lock suture is used to begin with the membranous wall to create a running anastomosis. This first portion of the anastomosis is run from one membranous cartilaginous junction on the medial aspect to the lateral aspect (Figure 11.4B).
- A second 3-0 V lock suture beginning at the medial membranous cartilaginous junction is used to run the anterior wall to join our previous suture (Figure 11.4C).
- The two sutures were then tied together to complete a circumferential bronchial anastomosis (Figure 11.4D).
- A well-vascularized pedicle (pericardial fat or intercostal muscle) can be used to buttress the anastomosis, tied down with silk sutures.

TIPS

- *Careful attention must be paid to reduce any amount of tension across the anastomosis. Traction sutures, preservation of airway length and blood supply, and release maneuvers will aid in reducing the risk of anastomotic complications.*
- *Well-vascularized pedicles (pericardial fat and intercostal muscle) should be mobilized and placed to buttress the airway and vascular stumps.*

Postoperative Care

- Pain management to improve pulmonary toilet and secretion mobilization.
- Diet: clear liquid diet for postoperative day 0 to 1, followed by resumption of the normal diet.

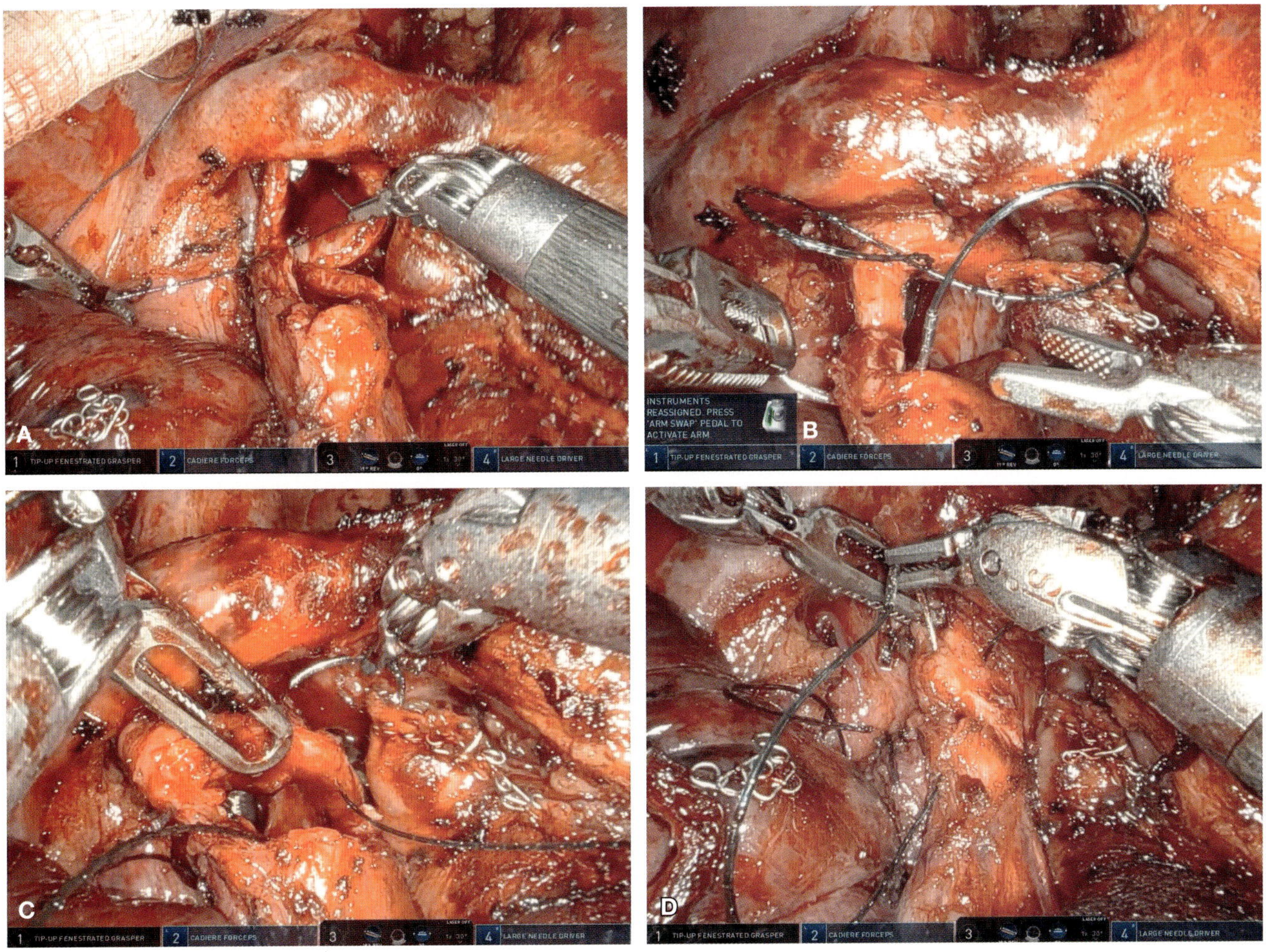

FIGURE 11.4 | Robotic airway anastomosis. **A.** 3-0 Vicryl stay suture, medial, cartilaginous-membranous junction. **B.** Running of V-loc suture, membranous wall, medial to lateral. **C.** Running of V-loc suture, cartilaginous wall, medial to lateral. **D.** Two V-loc sutures tied together to complete a circumferential bronchial anastomosis.

- Medications:
  - AFib prophylaxis—low-dose beta blockade
  - Around the clock saline nebulizers, which can be supplemented with Mucomyst or DuoNeb depending on the secretion burden
- Surveillance bronchoscopy at postoperative day 5 or 6 in the operating room
  - Laryngeal mask airway
  - Flexible bronchoscopy to evaluate vocal cord movement, followed by topical lidocaine to vocal cords
  - Evaluation of integrity of airway anastomosis, therapeutic suctioning of secretions
  - Nothing by mouth for 2 hours following topical lidocaine to vocal cords

Complications

- Retained secretions: encourage excellent pulmonary toilet, mobilization of secretions, may require bronchoscopy if the patient is unable to mobilize secretions.
- Anastomotic complications: early inpatient surveillance bronchoscopy at postoperative day 5 to 6 can identify any early signs of impaired anastomotic healing.
  - Treatment with hyperbaric oxygen, antibiotics, or ongoing observation may be sufficient for conservative management.
  - If impending dehiscence is identified, surgical intervention is required, often necessitating a completion pneumonectomy with buttressing of the stump to prevent fistula formation.
  - Anastomotic strictures may be observed expectantly unless becomes clinically symptomatic (postobstructive pneumonia and shortness of breath).

PEARLS AND PITFALLS

- Intraoperative assessment of bronchial margin is essential to assess for negative margin at the proposed anastomosis.
- Careful spacing of sutures will help accommodate any size discrepancy; however, there may require some degree of intussusception based on the size of the airways.
  - Depth of airway bites are typically ~3 mm in depth and 2 to 4 mm apart.
- Placement of knots outside the airway is preferable.
- Reconstruction must avoid any anastomotic tension on the airway anastomosis, and we recommend buttressing with a well-vascularized tissue such as pericardial fat or intercostal muscle.
  - Hilar release maneuver may assist in releasing airway tension.
- An air leak test is performed to test the bronchial anastomosis, and any required repair is made at that time.
- At the conclusion of the case, the double-lumen endotracheal tube is replaced with a laryngeal mask airway and the anastomosis is evaluated under bronchoscopic guidance.

Suggested Readings

1. Ashiku S, DeCamp MM. Parenchymal-sparing procedures in lung cancer: sleeve resection of the lung for proximal lesions. *Oper Tech Thorac Cardiovasc Surg*. 2006;11(4):295-309.
2. Cerfolio RJ. Robotic sleeve lobectomy: technical details and early results. *J Thorac Dis*. 2016;8(suppl 2):S223-S226.
3. Costantino CL, Wright CD. Extended pulmonary resection by sleeve lobectomy and carinal pneumonectomy: selection and technique. *Thorac Surg Clin*. 2021;31(3):273-281.
4. Mathisen DJ, Morse CR. *Masters Techniques in Thoracic Surgery: Lung Resections, Bronchoplasty*. Wolters Kluwer Health; 2014.
5. Merritt RE, Mathisen DJ, Wain JC, et al. Long-term results of sleeve lobectomy in the management of non-small cell lung carcinoma and low-grade neoplasms. *Ann Thorac Surg*. 2009;88(5):1574-1582. discussion 1581-1582.
6. Qiu T, Zhao Y, Xuan Y, et al. Robotic sleeve lobectomy for centrally located non-small cell lung cancer: a propensity score-weighted comparison with thoracoscopic and open surgery. *J Thorac Cardiovasc Surg*. 2020;160(3):838-846.e2.

Chapter 12

Anterior and Posterior Approach to Superior Sulcus Tumors

K. ROBERT SHEN

Perioperative Considerations

- Lung cancers that occur in the apex of the chest and invade any of the apical chest wall structures including the most superior ribs, the lower nerve roots of the brachial plexus, the sympathetic chain, or the subclavian blood vessels are classified as superior sulcus tumors, or Pancoast tumors (Figures 12.1-12.3).
- These tumors are categorized into anterior, middle, and posterior compartment tumors depending on the location of the chest wall involvement in relation to the insertions of the anterior and middle scalene muscles on the first rib.
- Patients frequently present with shoulder pain and pain radiating down the arm on the affected side as a manifestation of brachial plexus involvement following the distribution of the ulnar nerve. Invasion of the stellate ganglion causes Horner syndrome (ipsilateral ptosis, miosis, and anhydrosis).
- In patients with a potentially resectable, nonmetastatic superior sulcus tumor (and good performance status), it is recommended that preoperative concurrent chemoradiotherapy be administered before resection.
- In patients who undergo resection of a superior sulcus tumor, it is recommended that every effort be made to achieve a complete resection.
- It is recommended that resection of a superior sulcus tumor consists of a lobectomy (instead of a nonanatomic wedge resection or segmental resection) as well as the involved chest wall structures.
- In patients with either completely or incompletely resected super sulcus tumors, postoperative radiotherapy is not recommended because of lack of evidence supporting a survival benefit.

Preoperative Evaluation

- In patients with a superior sulcus tumor, a tissue diagnosis should be obtained before treatment is initiated.
- Patients with superior sulcus tumors who are being considered for curative surgical resection should have an MRI of the thoracic inlet and brachial plexus to rule out tumor invasion of unresectable vascular structures or the extradural space. They should also undergo invasive mediastinal staging (endobronchial ultrasound/mediastinoscopy), brain MRI, and PET/CT scan.
- Involvement of mediastinal lymph nodes, extrathoracic metastases, pleural metastases, and spinal canal involvement as well as invasion of the brachial plexus above the T1 nerve root (C8, C7) are contraindications to surgical resection.
- Vertebral body involvement is not a contraindication to surgical treatment if a complete resection can be achieved. Similarly, invasion of subclavian blood vessels is not a contraindication as long as a complete resection of the involved vessels can be achieved and revascularization can be done.

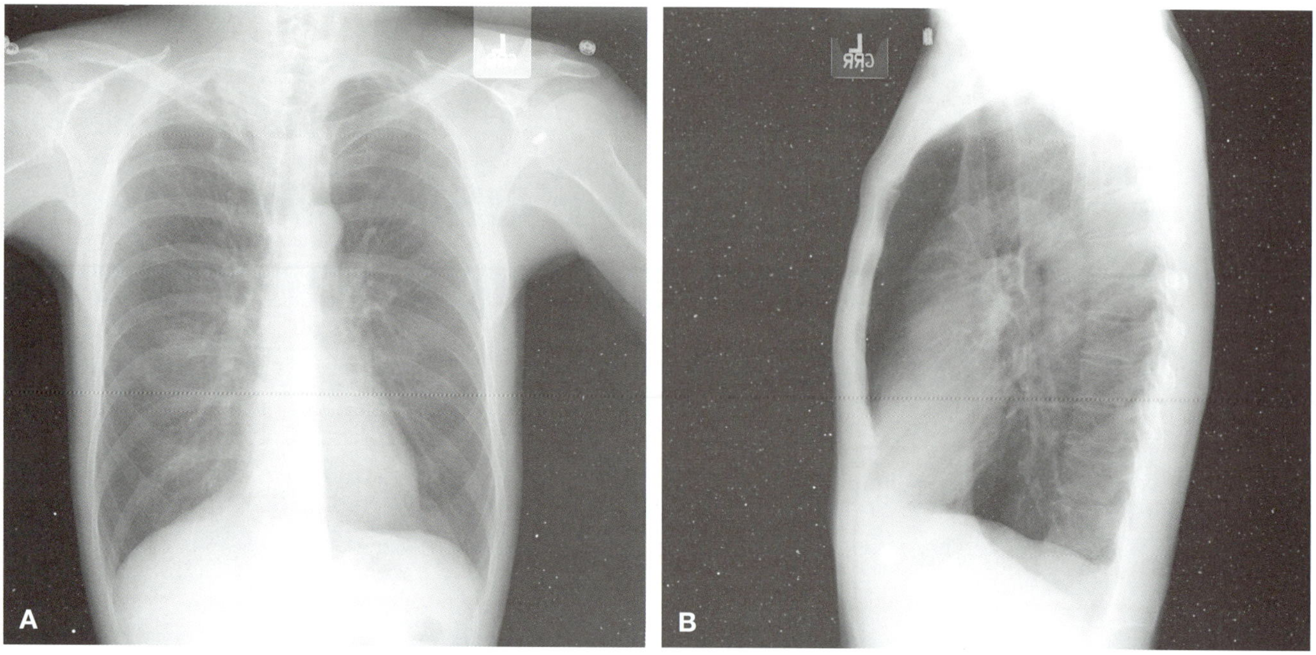

FIGURE 12.1 ▌ A and B. PA and lateral CXR from 63-year-old man with a 40 pack-year smoking history who developed pain in his right shoulder and back. Radiograph demonstrates a 3 cm opacity in the apex of the right chest posteriorly.

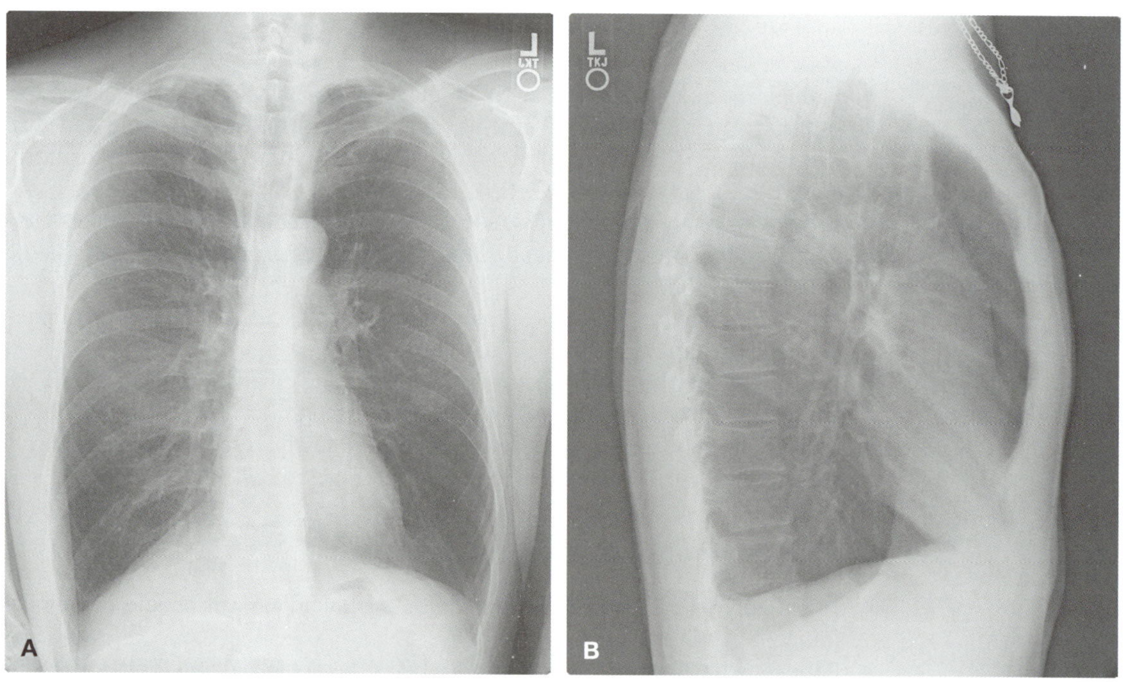

FIGURE 12.2 ▌ A and B. PA and lateral CXR 1 year prior.

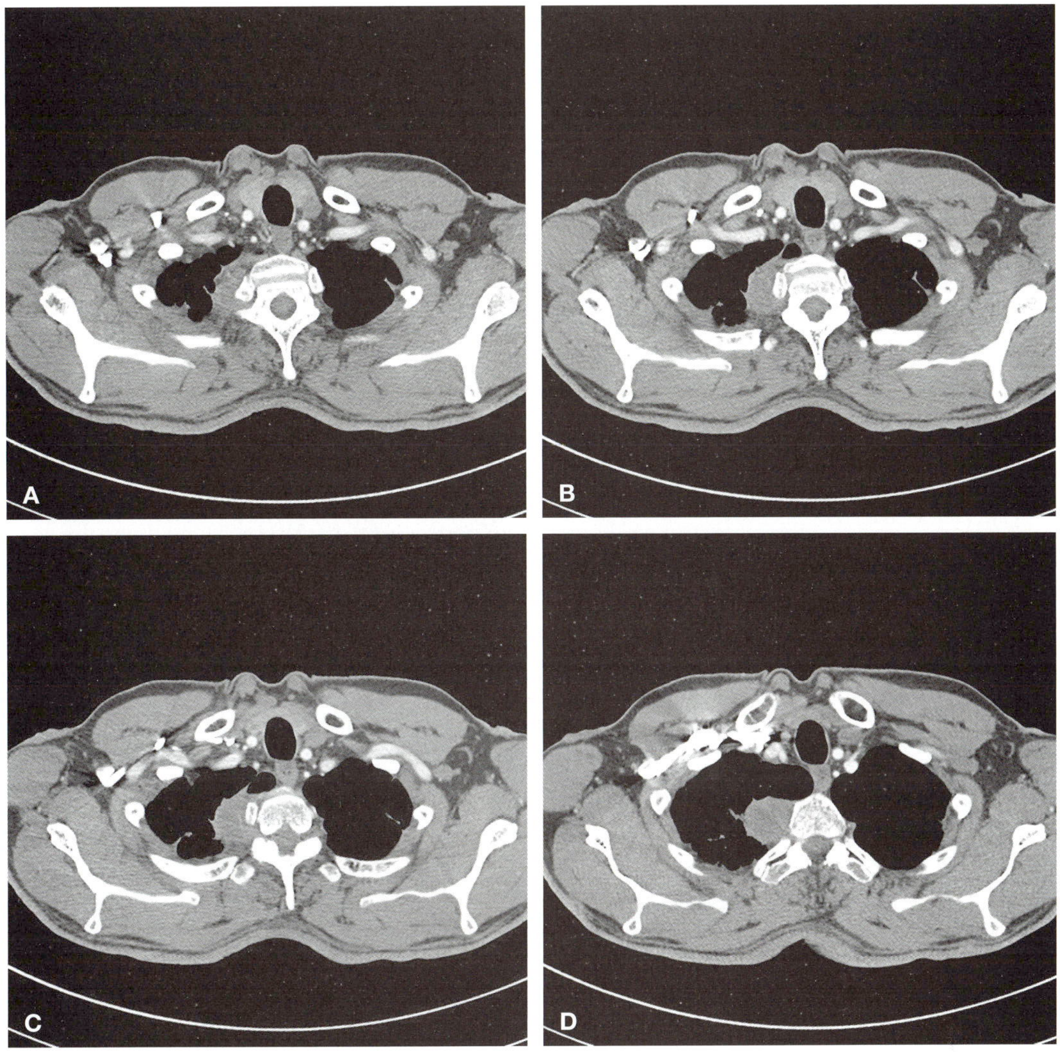

FIGURE 12.3 ▌ A-D. Chest CT scan with representative sections demonstrating 3 × 3.5 cm posterior mass abutting the T1 and T2 vertebral bodies and encasing the proximal first rib.

TIPS

- *The posterolateral thoracotomy approach has certain advantages over the anterior transcervical approach. It is preferred for posterior tumors, particularly those that invade the vertebral bodies and/or the brachial plexus. If unanticipated invasion of the subclavian artery is found at the time of operative exploration, this approach can still be utilized if proximal and distal control of the artery can be obtained, complete resection of the involved artery performed, and revascularization done with a polytetrafluoroethylene graft, bovine pericardial patch, or primary end-to-end anastomosis. If invasion into the subclavian vessels is identified or highly suspected on preoperative evaluation, the anterior approach is strongly recommended as the preferred surgical approach.*

Technique

Posterior Approach

Anesthesia and Patient Positioning

- General anesthesia with double-lumen endotracheal tube
- Thoracic epidural catheter, Foley catheter, arterial line
- Lateral decubitus position with the arm on the involved side sterilely prepped and draped to allow repositioning of the arm during the case
- Skin prep should be to the midline of the back and high up to the base of the neck.

Initial Exploration

- Limited posterolateral thoracotomy incision with entry into the chest between the two ribs nearest but uninvolved with the tumor, usually the fourth or fifth intercostal space.
- Pleural space, lung, chest wall, and mediastinum are inspected for evidence of metastatic disease, tumor resectability, and the extent of resection required to incorporate all of the disease, or any findings that would preclude complete resection.
- Once resectability is confirmed, the thoracotomy incision is extended superiorly and toward the midline to the base of the neck.

Anterior Chest Wall Resection

- Latissimus dorsi muscle is divided, and anterior serratus anterior muscle is spared and reflected anteriorly.
- The rhomboid, trapezius, and posterior serratus muscles are divided with cautery, which allows the posterior aspect of the scapula to be elevated.
- The Finochietto chest retractor is placed with one arm under the posterior aspect of the scapula and the other arm on the cephalad portion of the fifth rib. This allows the scapula to be lifted anteriorly off the ribs (Figure 12.4).

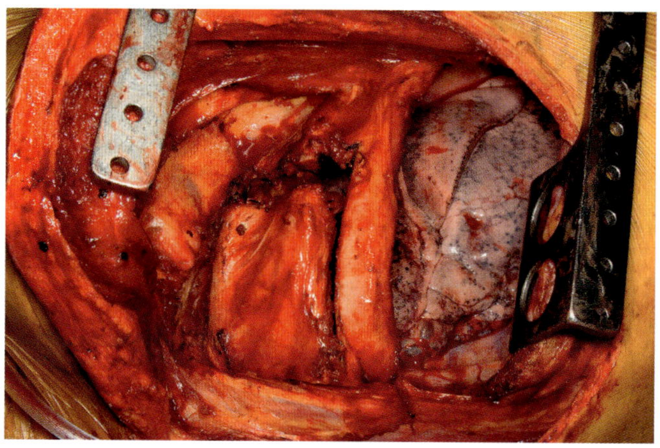

FIGURE 12.4 ▌ Posterior approach. Finochietto chest retractor has one arm under the scapula and one arm on the fifth rib. Ribs 2 and 3 have been divided anteriorly.

- Anterosuperior attachments of the serratus anterior muscle are divided from the first and second ribs, which exposes the middle and posterior scalene muscle attachments to the first and second ribs.
- Middle and posterior scalene muscle attachments to the first rib are divided with cautery, which exposes the subclavian artery and brachial plexus.
- The tumor is palpated with a hand inside the chest to identify the extent of rib involvement. The ribs to be resected are marked with cautery to delineate the extent of resection.
- A 3- to 4-cm margin of normal rib and intercostal muscle around the tumor is optimal.
- Usually the first three ribs are resected en bloc with the tumor but larger tumors may require additional ribs resected depending on the extent of tumor involvement.
- The chest wall resection is initiated with anterior division of the lowest rib to be resected. The periosteum on the rib is scored with cautery and a subperiosteal plane is developed with a periosteal elevator over a 1- to 2-cm distance. A 1- to 2-cm piece of the anterior portion of the rib to be resected is removed. This allows the section of the chest wall to be resected to fall inward as each successive piece of rib is removed. Removal of a segment of rib also facilitates exposure to the neurovascular bundle associated with each rib, which will need to be successively individually ligated and divided as the rib resection proceeds cephalad.
- Once the second and third ribs have been divided anteriorly and pushed into the chest cavity, the first rib is exposed. The subclavian artery is retracted superiorly and a subperiosteal plane is circumferentially developed around the first rib. A right angle clamp is passed around the first rib and a Gigli saw is used to cut the first rib.

TIPS

- *If the tumor is bulky and the portion of the chest wall resection with attached tumor is obscuring exposure to the hilar structures once the anterior ribs have been divided and the ribs/tumor have been pushed within the chest cavity, it is sometimes helpful to divide the lung parenchyma with a stapler to facilitate the lobectomy by allowing the tumor with attached ribs to be reflected anteriorly and the remaining portion of the lung parenchyma to fall away, providing a better view of the hilar structures.*

Lobectomy

- A standard en bloc upper lobectomy with a mediastinal lymph node dissection is performed.

Posterior Chest Wall Resection

- The paraspinal muscles are elevated from the spine to expose the transverse processes of the ribs that are to be resected.
- In order to disarticulate the rib from the transverse process, the costotransverse ligament is divided with cautery.
- Pushing inward on the portion of the chest wall that had been freed anteriorly allows the costotransverse junction to separate slightly to allow an osteotome to be inserted into the synovial cavity.
- The osteotome is used to lever the rib tubercle, neck, and head of the rib away from the transverse process and vertebral body. This leverage exposes the neurovascular bundle, which can then be individually ligated (Figure 12.5).

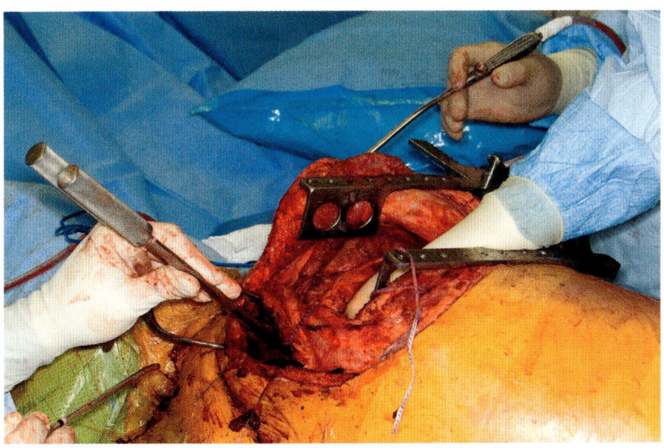

FIGURE 12.5 ▌ Hemilaminectomy of T1-T4 has been performed and photo illustrates spine surgeon working posteriorly and thoracic surgeon working anteriorly to perform vertebral osteotomy of T1-T3.

- In most cases, the T1 nerve room must be sacrificed to ensure a negative margin.
- If the T1 nerve root is sacrificed proximally, the distal root is divided just proximal to its junction with the C8 nerve root and entry into the brachial plexus proper.
- Effort should be made to avoid division of the C8 nerve root because of its importance in supplying a wide distribution of branches to the ulnar and median nerves as well as dorsal motor nerves of the arm and shoulder.
- The specimen is brought out en block through the chest wall defect (Figure 12.6).

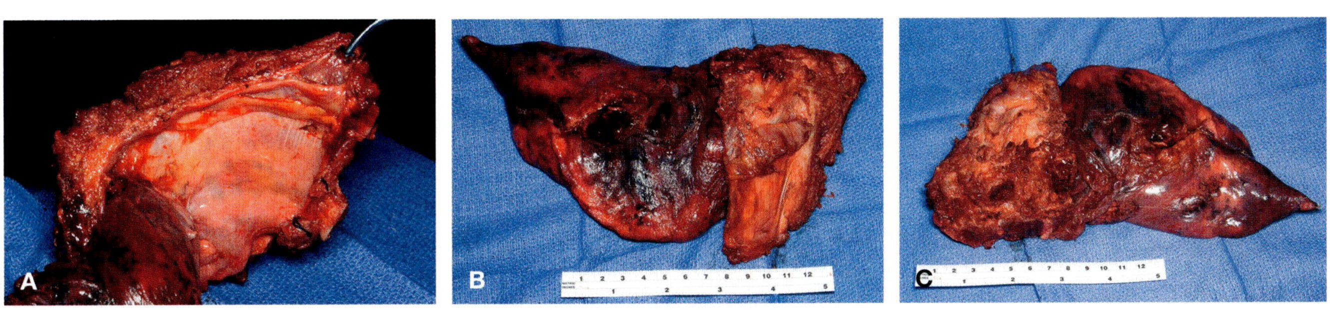

FIGURE 12.6 ▌ **A-C.** Resected specimen. En bloc resection of tumor encompassing right first, second, and third ribs with right upper lobe of lung and portions of right T1-T3 vertebral bodies. Patient had posterior spinal fusion (C7-T4) using right posterior iliac crest autograft.

- If more than three ribs have been resected, reconstruction of the chest wall defect with a prosthetic mesh such as 2-mm Gor-Tex is recommended to avoid entrapment of the tip of the scapula. Otherwise, the scapula will adequately cover the chest wall defect.

PEARLS AND PITFALLS

- Potential complications related to injury to the neurovascular bundles or nerve roots during disarticulation of the rib from the transverse process include tension pneumocephalus, cerebrospinal fluid leak, or a progressive hematoma causing spinal compression.
- Placement of a hemoclip or ligature near the exit of the neurovascular bundle from the intervertebral foramen is recommended.

Anterior Approach

- Superior sulcus tumors arising anteriorly in the apex of the chest were long considered unresectable because of early invasion of the vascular structures that were difficult to address through the conventional posterolateral Paulson-Shaw approach.
- These tumors became resectable when Dartevelle and colleagues developed an anterior transclavicular approach (1981, 1993).
- In the years since Dartevelle popularized the cervicothoracic transclavicular approach, several different surgical approaches to anterior superior sulcus tumors have been proposed: the Masaoka anterior trans-sternal approach performed through a proximal median sternotomy combined with extension into the anterior fourth intercostal space, Bains and colleagues described a hemiclamshell approach in 1994 and 1998, Grunenwald and Spaggiari proposed the transmanubrial approach in 1997.
- There is no consensus on the ideal anterior approach.

TIPS

- *The transmanubrial approach provides excellent access for anterior tumors involving the subclavian vessels with safe resection of neurovascular outlet structures involved by apical chest tumors and has the advantage of avoiding the functional and cosmetic consequences of clavicle resection required by the cervicothoracic transclavicular approach.*

Anterior Transmanubrial Approach

Anesthesia and Patient Positioning

- General anesthesia with double-lumen endotracheal tube
- Thoracic epidural catheter, Foley catheter, arterial line
- Skin should be prepped from high neck to the knees in the event autologous vein needs to be harvested.
- Supine position with the arm on the involved side sterilely prepped and draped to allow repositioning of the arm during the case. Arms abducted 90°.
- Shoulder roll placed under the shoulder to allow full extension of the neck and anterior elevation of surgical side of the chest
- Head extended and turned away from surgical side

Initial exploration

- L-shaped skin incision in made vertically from the angle of the manubrium on the anterior border of the sternocleidomastoid muscle (SCM) down to the manubrium (Figure 12.7). The incision is then gently curved horizontally three finger widths below the clavicle along the third rib toward the axilla.

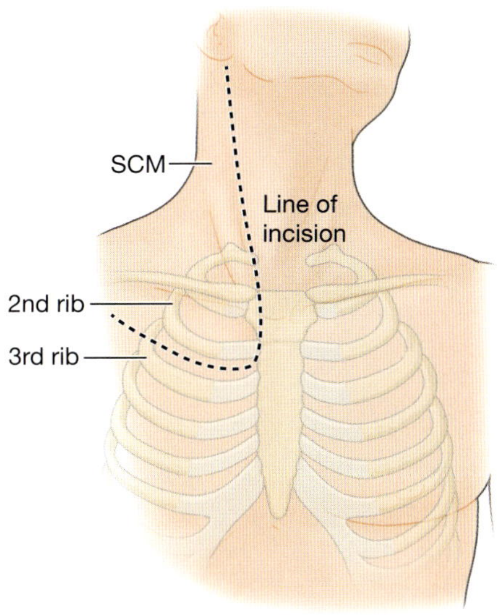

FIGURE 12.7 | Patient positioned in supine position with shoulder roll placed behind the shoulder to elevate the operative side. Skin incision extends vertically along the sternocleidomastoid muscle (SCM) down toward the manubrium and then gently curves horizontally parallel to the third rib toward the axilla.

- Clavicle and its muscular insertions are not divided.
- Pectoralis major muscle is spared and the pectoralis muscle fibers are split in the direction of their fibers detaching the pectoralis muscle and attachments of the SCM to the sternum and clavicle are divided with electrocautery (Figure 12.8).

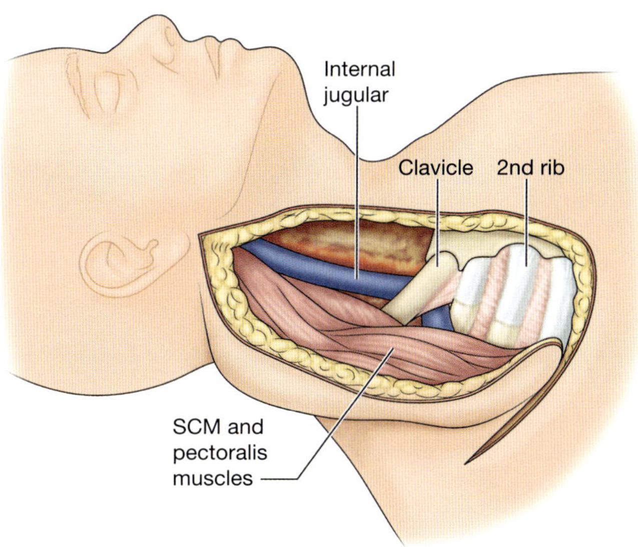

FIGURE 12.8 | The sternocleidomastoid muscle (SCM) and pectoralis major muscles have been dissected off the manubrium, clavicle, and chest wall. This provides exposure to the strap muscles, internal jugular vein, and anterolateral chest wall. The muscle and skin are folded laterally together as a myocutaneous flap.

- SCM is freed along its anterior part from cervical tissue up to the internal jugular vein exposing the sternal manubrium.
- The manubrium is divided through an L-shaped incision, resecting the sternoclavicular articulation but preserving the sternoclavicular joint (Figure 12.9).
- The intercostal muscle on the inferior side of the clavicle is divided with cautery, which allows access to the first rib at the junction with the first costal cartilage. The first rib is divided on the sternal side with a Gigli saw. This allows exposure to the costoclavicular ligament, which is divided and allows the clavicle to be rotated out laterally. The first rib is then divided distally after dividing the subclavius muscle (Figure 12.10).
- Starting at the internal jugular vein and moving laterally toward the confluence of the internal jugular vein and the subclavian vein, the subclavian vein is carefully dissected from the subclavius muscle (Figure 12.11).

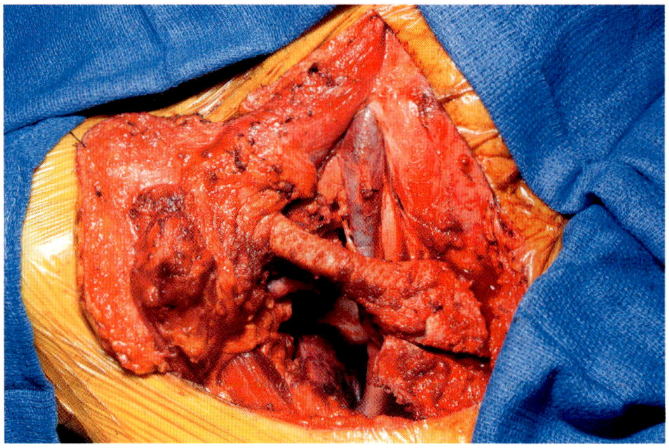

FIGURE 12.9 ▮ Removal of the proximal clavicle or rotation of the proximal portion of the clavicle using the transmanubrial approach provides excellent exposure of the first rib and subclavian vessels.

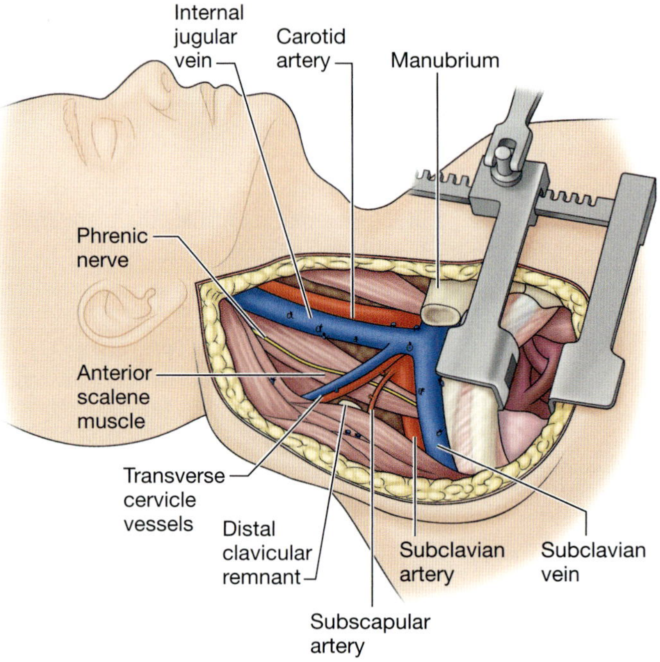

FIGURE 12.10 ▮ The manubrium is divided through an L-shaped incision, resecting the sternoclavicular articulation but preserving the sternoclavicular joint.

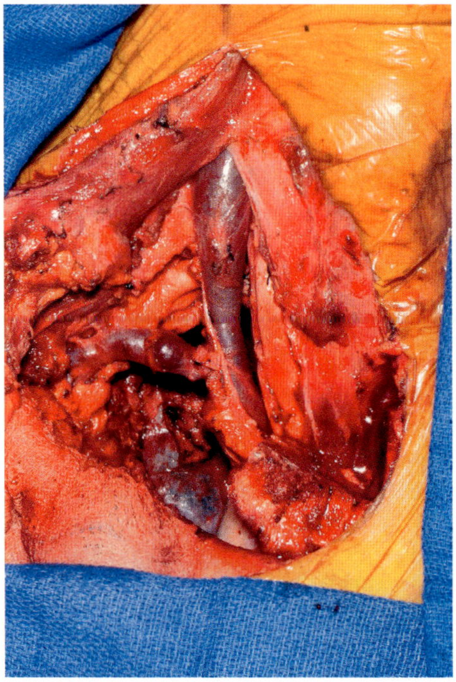

FIGURE 12.11 ▮ Transmanubrial approach demonstrating excellent exposure to confluence of internal jugular vein and subclavian vein after the clavicle has been divided from manubrium and rotated laterally.

- Venous branches of the subclavian vein can be divided to expose the main axis and expose the phrenic nerve and anterior scalene muscle.
- If the subclavian vein is invaded by tumor it is resected. Reconstruction of the subclavian vein is not required.
- The phrenic nerve is rotated medially and preserved unless involved by tumor.
- The anterior scalene muscle is divided above the level of the tumor. This exposes the subclavian artery.
- The subclavian artery is fully mobilized and the various small branches are divided to provide adequate mobility (Figure 12.12).

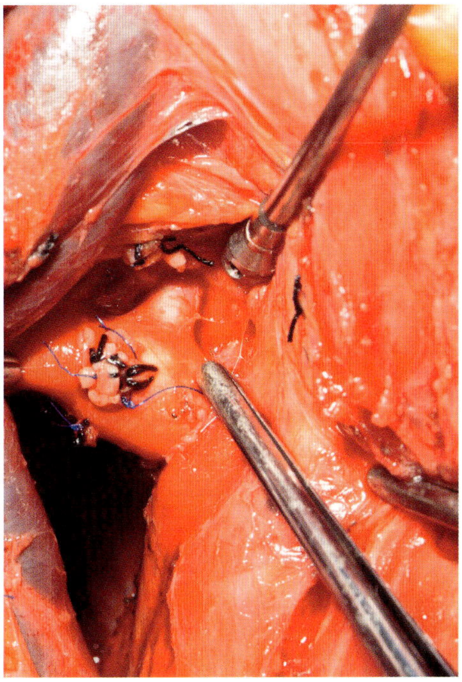

FIGURE 12.12 ▌ Confluence of right subclavian artery and internal carotid artery. The thyrocervical branch and internal mammary artery branches have been ligated.

- If the artery is invaded by tumor, it is resected and reconstructed using a 6- or 8-mm synthetic graft.
- Once the apical portion of the tumor is completely freed from the anterior cervicothoracic structures, the upper lobectomy and mediastinal lymph node dissection is performed through an anterolateral muscle-sparing thoracotomy (Figure 12.13).

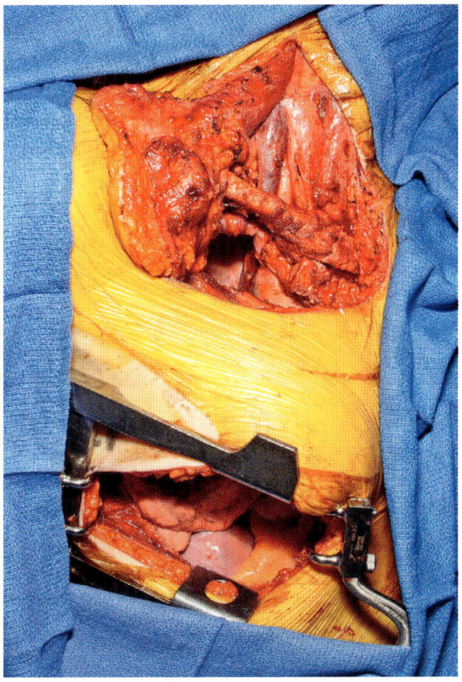

FIGURE 12.13 ▌ Once the apical portion of the tumor is completely freed from the anterior cervicothoracic structures, the upper lobectomy and mediastinal lymph node dissection is performed through an anterolateral muscle-sparing thoracotomy.

- Once the lobectomy is completed, the clavicle is reattached to the manubrium with several interrupted steel sternal wires (Figure 12.14).

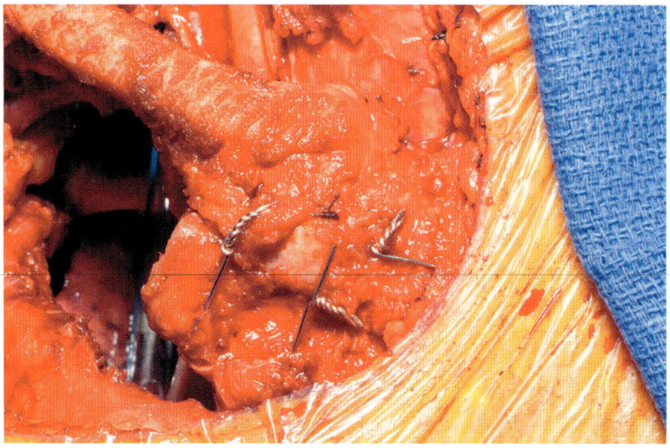

FIGURE 12.14 ▮ The clavicle is reattached to the manubrium with several interrupted steel sternal wires.

TIPS

- *For patients where the tumor is suspected of invasion into the subclavian arteries and who might require resection of the subclavian arteries and/or vertebral arteries, a cerebral angiogram is recommended.*
- *A 10-minute test balloon occlusion of the vertebral artery can provide useful information about collateral flow from the contralateral vertebral artery.*

Suggested Readings

1. Bains MS, Ginsberg RJ, Jones WG, et al. The clamshell incision: an improved approach to bilateral pulmonary and mediastinal tumors. *Ann Thorac Surg*. 1994;58:30-32.
2. Dartevelle PG, Chapelier AR, Macchiarini P, et al. Anterior transcervical-thoracic approach for radical resection of lung tumors invading the thoracic inlet. *J Thorac Cardiovasc Surg*. 1993;105(6):1025-1034.
3. Dartevelle PG, Levasseur P, Rojas-Miranda A, et al. Combined cervical and thoracic approach to the removal of tumours responsible for the Pancoast and Tobias syndrome. *Nouv Presse Med*. 1981;10:1051-1054.
4. Grunenwald D, Spaggiari L. Transmanubrial osteomuscular sparing approach for apical chest tumors. *Ann Thorac Surg*. 1997;63(2):563-566.
5. Korst RJ, Burt ME. Cervicothoracic tumors: results of resection by the "hemiclamshell" approach. *J Thorac Cardiovasc Surg*. 1998;115(2):286-295.
6. Masaoka A, Ito Y, Yasumitsu T. Anterior approach for tumor of the superior sulcus. *J Thorac Cardiovasc Surg*. 1979;78(3):413-415.
7. Rusch VW, Giroux DJ, Kraut MJ, et al. Induction chemoradiation and surgical resection for superior sulcus non-small cell lung carcinomas: long-term results of Southwest Oncology Group Trial 9416 (Intergroup Trial 0160). *J Clin Oncol*. 2007;25(3):313-318.

Chapter 13

Principles of Mediastinal Lymph Node Dissection

MICHAEL LANUTI

Perioperative Considerations

- Mediastinal staging prior to lung resection should be considered when there are anatomically enlarged or fluorodeoxyglucose-avid mediastinal lymph nodes and/or the target lung nodule ≥3 cm in the periphery, or the lung nodule is centrally located.
- Mediastinal lymph node dissection is primarily associated with pulmonary resection for lung cancer at the time of surgery and can be lobe specific, but it is encouraged to perform a standard lymph node dissection for right-sided tumors (lymph node stations 2, 4, 7, and 9R) or for left-sided tumors (5, 6, 7, 9L). This can be done with minimally invasive technique (video-assisted thoracic surgery [VATS], robotic-assisted thoracic surgery [RATS]) or an open technique (thoracotomy).

TIPS

Mediastinal lymph node dissection can also be considered for patients undergoing pulmonary metastasectomy for extrathoracic neoplasm, but its role is controversial and believed to be prognostic and not therapeutic.

Anesthesia and Patient Positioning

- General anesthesia with endotracheal intubation and paralysis is the standard; however, there are published series that report tubeless pulmonary resection with spontaneous breathing.
- The patient is placed in a modified lateral decubitus position with patient's xiphoid placed at the level of flexion of the operating room table. The table should be flexed to open the rib spaces and lower the ipsilateral hip.
- Reverse Trendelenburg can be used to level the chest in the horizontal plane.

Instruments and Equipment

- 5- to 10-mm, 30° thoracoscope
- 5- to 10-mm thoracoscopic port, additional ports can be used at other utility sites
- Energy device (cautery, harmonic scalpel or LigaSure, Maryland bipolar)
- Wound protector (optional)
- VATS or RATS instruments (lung grasper, dissecting tools, robotic cadiere forceps, curved scissors, 5- to 10-mm endopeanut)

Technique

Port Placement

- If the procedure is performed minimally invasively, then port placement differs for VATS versus RATS as seen in Figure 13.1A and B below. Port sizes range from 8 to 12 mm. Improper placement of ports can make lymph node dissection more difficult.

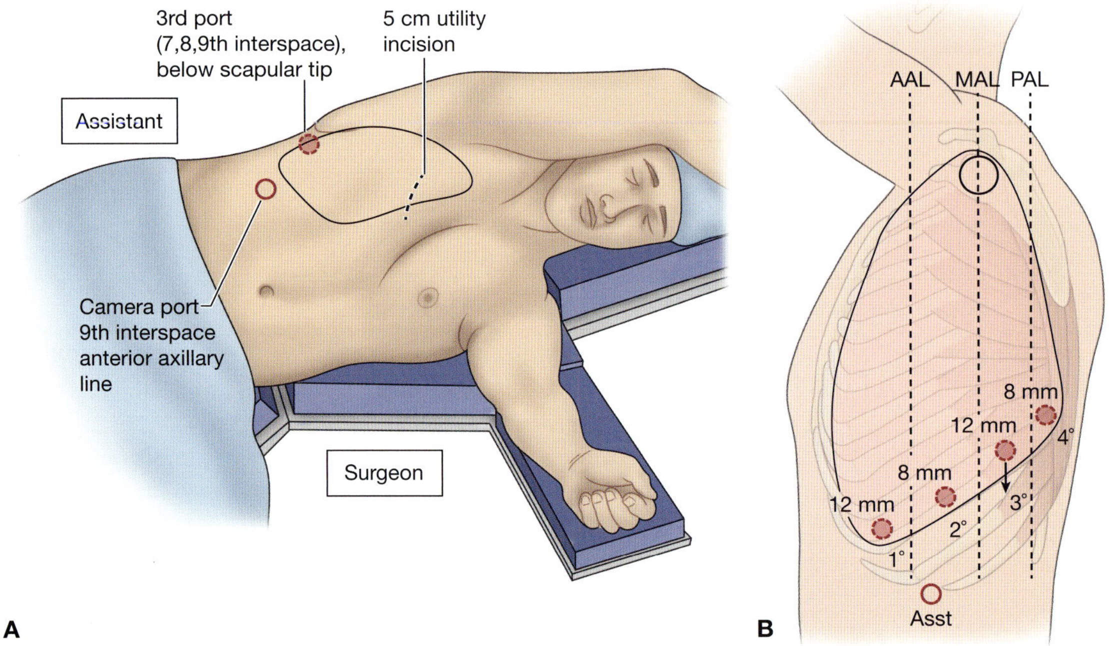

FIGURE 13.1 ▮ **A.** Ideal port placement for video-assisted thoracic surgery pulmonary resection and lymph node dissection. **B.** Standard port placement for robotic-assisted pulmonary resection and lymph node dissection. AAL, anterior axillary line; MAL, mid-axillary line; PAL, posterior axillary line.

Nodal Stations

- Familiarize oneself with accessible nodal stations and appropriate labels to assure complete and accurate nodal staging at the time of pulmonary resection (Figure 13.2).

Right Paratracheal Lymph Node Dissection (2R and 4R)

- The lymph node dissection in the right paratracheal region can include both stations 3A and 3P. The superior border of the dissection is the apex of the right hemithorax, whereas the inferior border is the azygos vein. The lateral border is the trachea and vagus nerve, and medial border is superior vena cava and phrenic nerve (Figure 13.3).

Left Paratracheal Lymph Node Dissection

- The left paratracheal lymph nodes (2L and 4L) cannot be easily dissected from a left-sided approach either with a thoracotomy or minimally invasive approach. The 4L lymph node station can be accessed under the aorta while reflecting the pulmonary artery down and medially. The ligamentum arteriosum is often divided to improve visualization (Figure 13.4A and B).

Aortopulmonary Lymph Nodes (Level 5/6 Lymph Nodes)

- AP window lymph nodes are also termed “prevascular lymph nodes” (Figure 13.5A-C).
- Level 5 is located below the aortic arch close and just above the level of the left pulmonary artery.
- Level 6 is located above the aortic arch and is often not visualized during pulmonary resections.

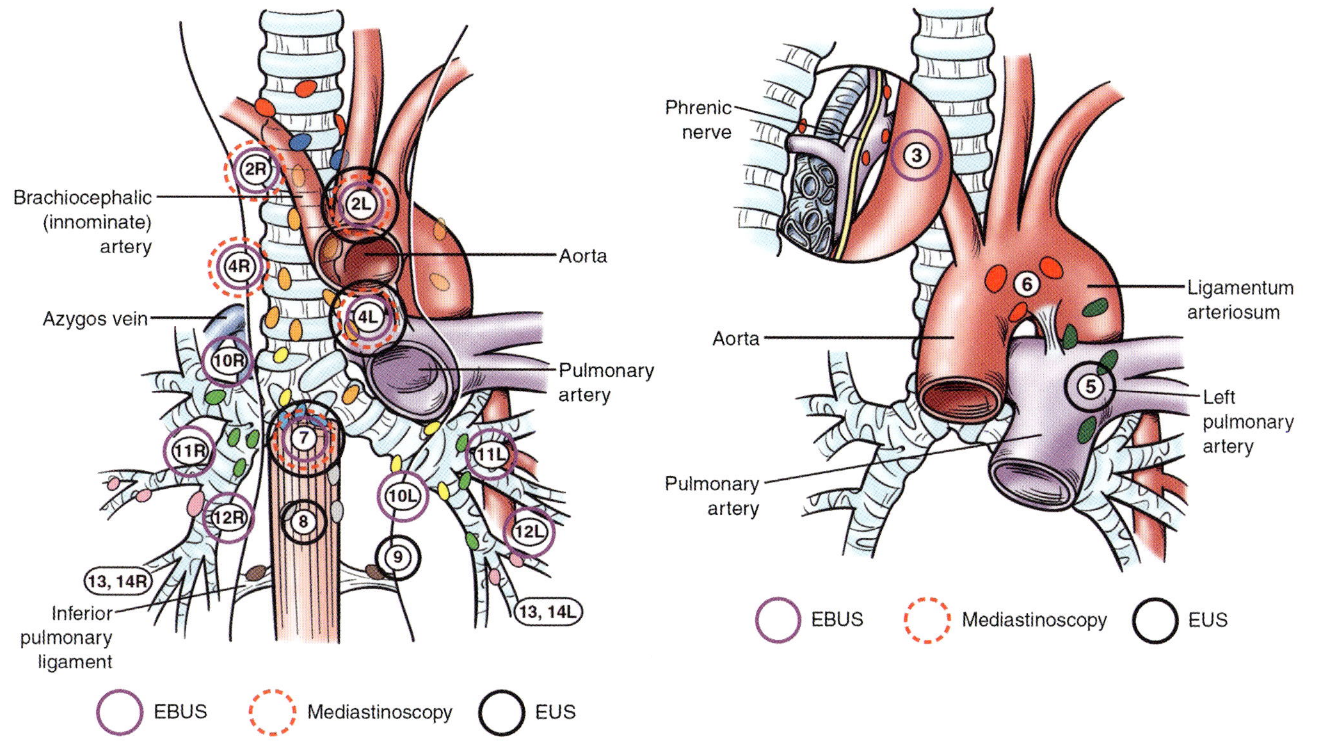

FIGURE 13.2 | Map depiction of thoracic lymph node stations according to accessibility by common staging modalities endobronchial ultrasound (EBUS), cervical mediastinoscopy, esophageal ultrasound (EUS), mediastinotomy, and video-assisted thoracic surgery (VATS). (Reprinted from Mountain CF, Dresler CM. Regional lymph node classification for lung cancer staging. *Chest*. 1997;111:1718-1723c, with permission from Elsevier.)

Subcarinal Lymph Node Dissection (Level 7)

TIPS

Some surgeons prefer to perform mediastinal lymph node dissection prior to a planned pulmonary resection to rule out the presence of occult node-positive disease or to facilitate the subsequent dissection.

- The subcarinal lymph node can be reached from the right (Figure 13.6A-D) or left side (Figure 13.7A-C). Accessing this lymph node station from the left side is more challenging when using a minimally invasive technique.
- If this lymph node station is accessed via a thoracotomy, dissection and hemostasis can be easily achieved. Since the subcarinal lymph node station is often more vascular and associated with bronchial arteries, dissection in this area is more commonly associated with bleeding.

Inferior Pulmonary Vein Lymph Node Dissection (9R and 9L)

- The inferior pulmonary ligament is divided on the right (Figure 13.8A-C) or left (Figure 13.9A-C) to achieve lymph node dissection in this region. Level 8 lymph nodes are typically more inferior and adjacent to the esophagus.

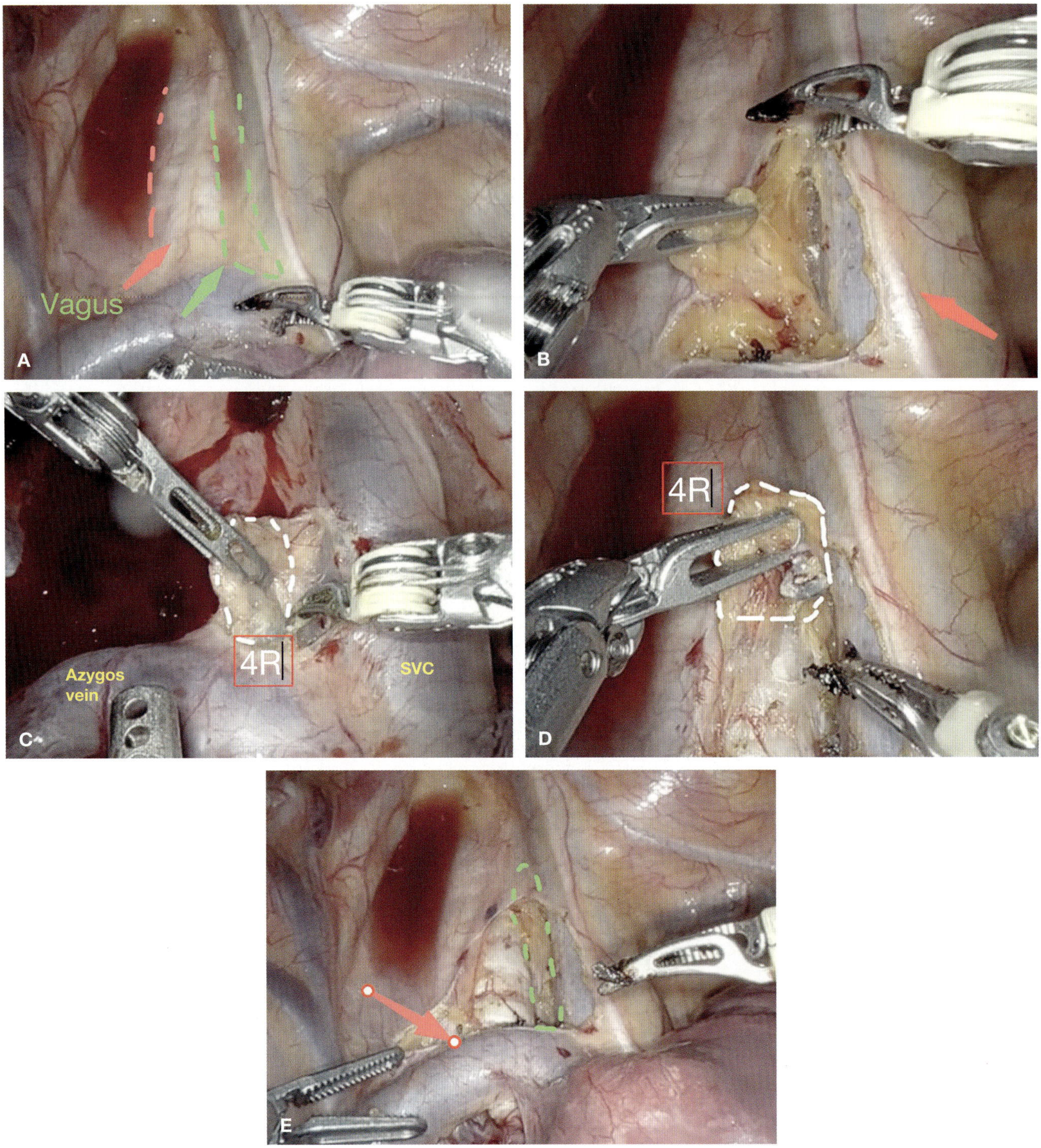

FIGURE 13.3 ▮ A. Borders of the right paratracheal lymph node dissection (green dotted line and green arrow). The lateral border is the trachea (red dotted line, lateral border of the trachea; red arrow marks the vagus nerve). The inferior border is azygos vein and medial border is superior vena cava (SVC). **B.** Parietal pleura is incised over the right paratracheal region and lymph nodes are dissected. The phrenic nerve over the SVC (red arrow).**C** and **D.** 4R lymph nodes are dissected free. White dotted line depicts the 4R lymph node. **E.** Completely dissected right paratracheal lymph node basin. Red arrow depicts azygos vein, green dotted line is border of 4R lymph node basin.

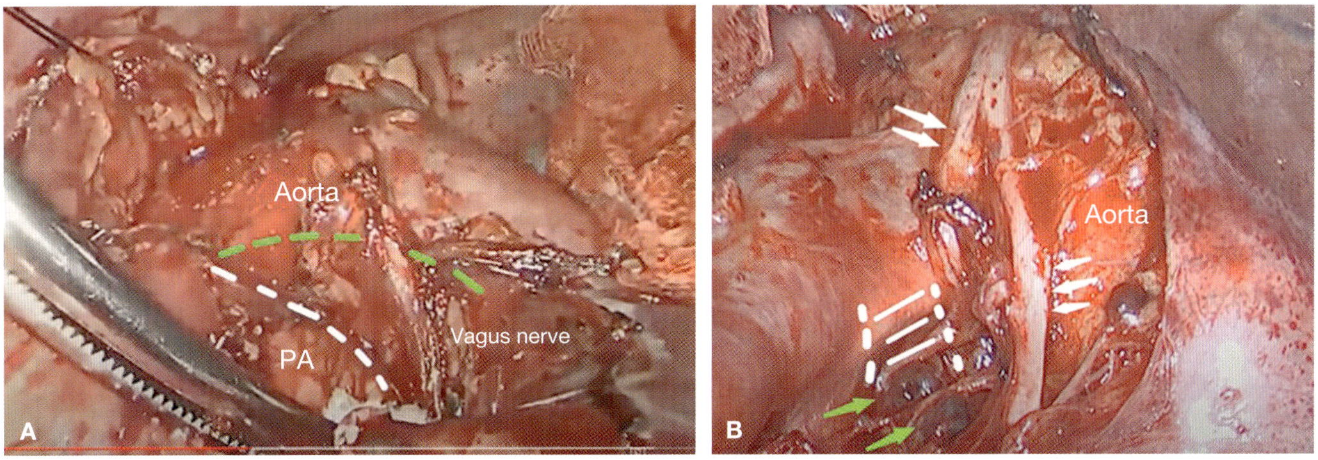

FIGURE 13.4 ▮ A. Left-sided view where the segmental pulmonary artery (PA) branches to left upper lobe have been divided. The left PA is reflected inferomedial, (white dotted line superior border of PA) to work under the aortic arch depicted by green dotted line. **B.** Dissection under the aortic arch where left recurrent laryngeal nerve (double white arrow) and vagus nerve (triple white arrow) can be seen. The 4L lymph nodes (green arrows) are just on top of the trachea (white ladder).

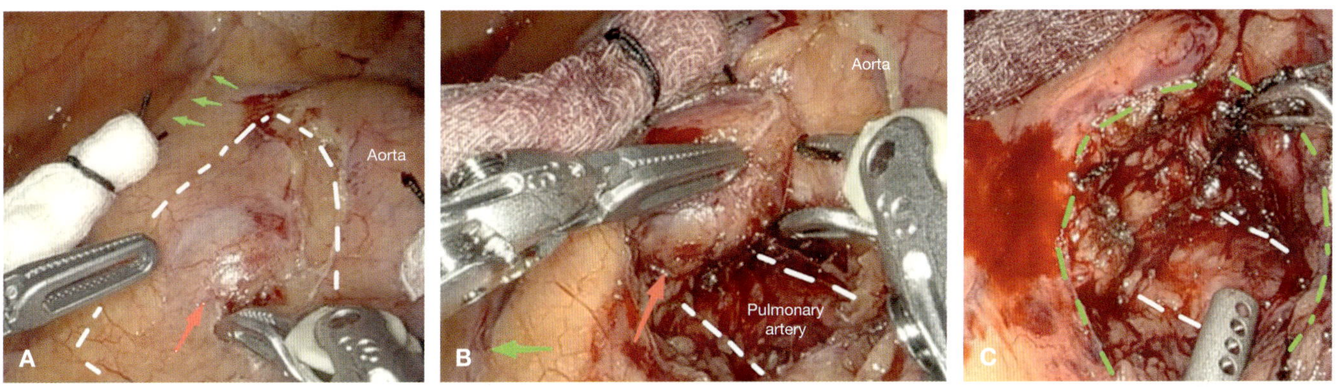

FIGURE 13.5 ▮ A. The border of dissection after the parietal pleura is incised (white dotted line) includes aortic arch superiorly and laterally and superior vena cava medially. The left phrenic nerve is also medial to the bed of dissection (green arrows). The enlarged level 5 lymph is bulging in the mid field (red arrow). **B.** The left main pulmonary artery (white dotted line) is at the floor of the dissection where the aorta is the roof. The enlarged level 5 lymph node (red arrow) can be very vascular. Phrenic nerve (green arrow) is medial in the field and can be easily injured during this dissection. **C.** The bed of the resected level 5 lymph node is demonstrated (bordered by green dotted lines). The left PA is at the floor of the dissection (white dotted lines).

Postoperative Care

- Patients undergoing mediastinal lymph node dissection will often have a chest tube in place postoperatively as part of management of bleeding and air leak.
- Achieving hemostasis after lymph node dissection is critical since this can often be a reason for postoperative bleeding and return to the operating room for exploration.
- High chest tube output that is not blood should invoke the possibility of chyle leak where the patient can be challenged with fat-containing diet to look for turbid or milky effluent. The chest tube effluent can be tested for either triglycerides or chylomicrons.

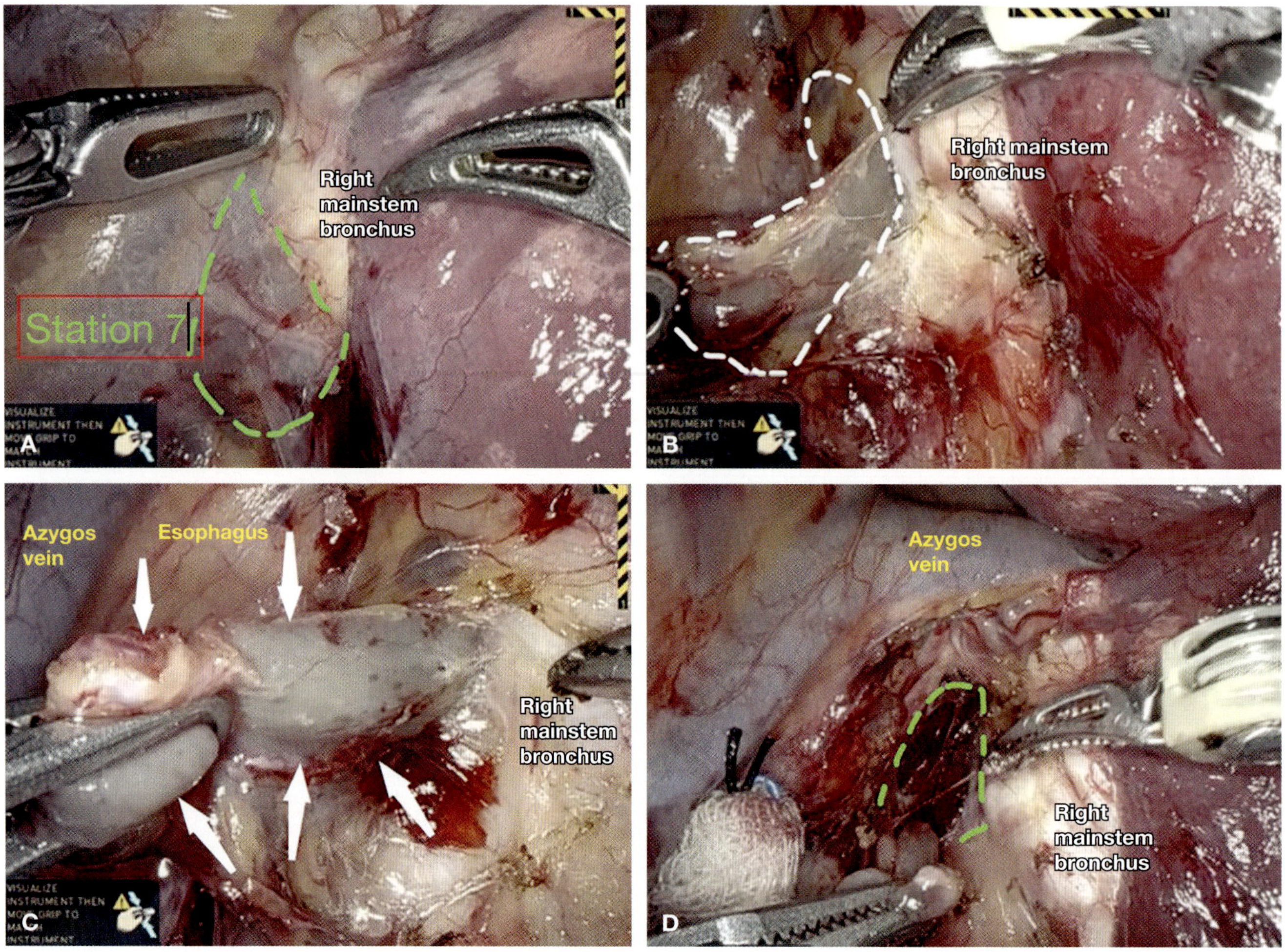

FIGURE 13.6 ‖ A. Subcarinal lymph node dissection from the RIGHT. The pleura over the subcarinal lymph node station (level 7) is incised. The borders of surgical dissection (green dotted line) include the right mainstem bronchus superiorly and medially, thoracic spine laterally, and esophagus along the floor. **B.** Parietal pleura is opened, and the level 7 lymph node packet (white dotted line) is visualized and mobilized with an energy device, cautery, or blunt dissection. **C.** Lymph node (highlighted in white arrows) extraction. **D.** Level 7 lymph node dissection bed (green dotted line) as seen from a right-sided approach.

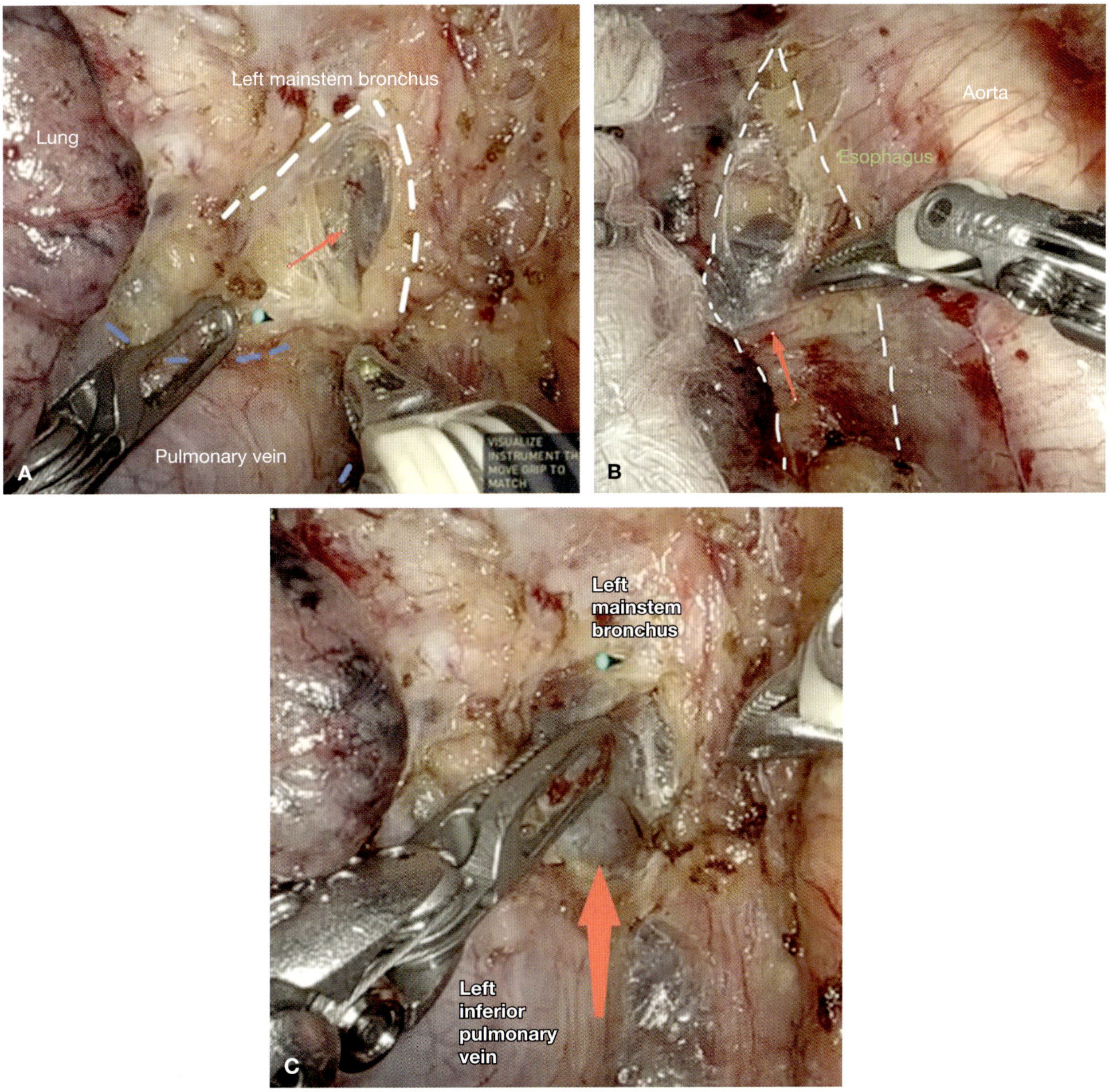

FIGURE 13.7 | **A** and **B. Subcarinal lymph node dissection from the LEFT.** The subcarinal space via the left is bordered by the left mainstem bronchus superiorly, the esophagus and aorta laterally, and the left inferior pulmonary vein inferiorly. The white dotted line depicts border of level 7 lymph node dissection. The red arrow marks level 7 lymph node. **C.** Subcarinal lymph node (red arrow) as seen with deeper dissection. Esophagus is lateral along with the vagus nerve.

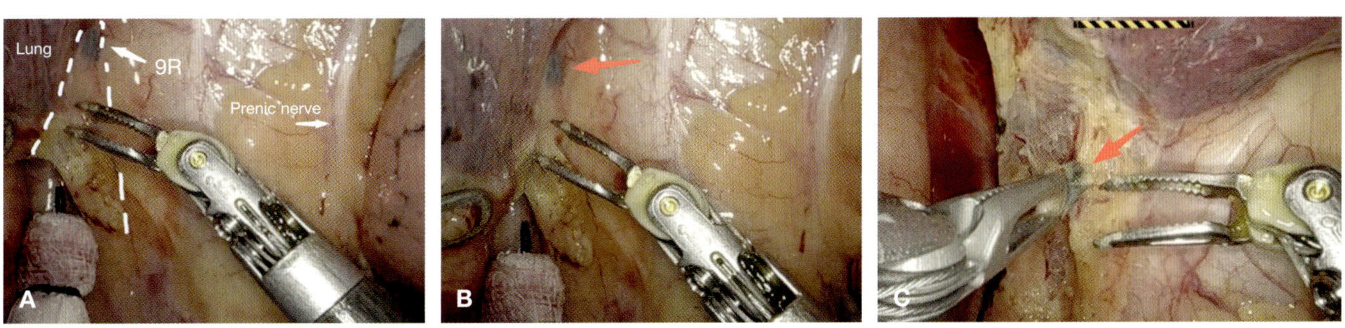

FIGURE 13.8 | **A.** Right inferior pulmonary ligament is highlighted in white dotted line with 9R lymph node (white arrow) at the apex. **B** and **C.** Right inferior pulmonary ligament is divided with energy device for hemostasis. Red arrow depicts level 9R lymph node. *Avoid injury to the lung since this is a source of air leak.*

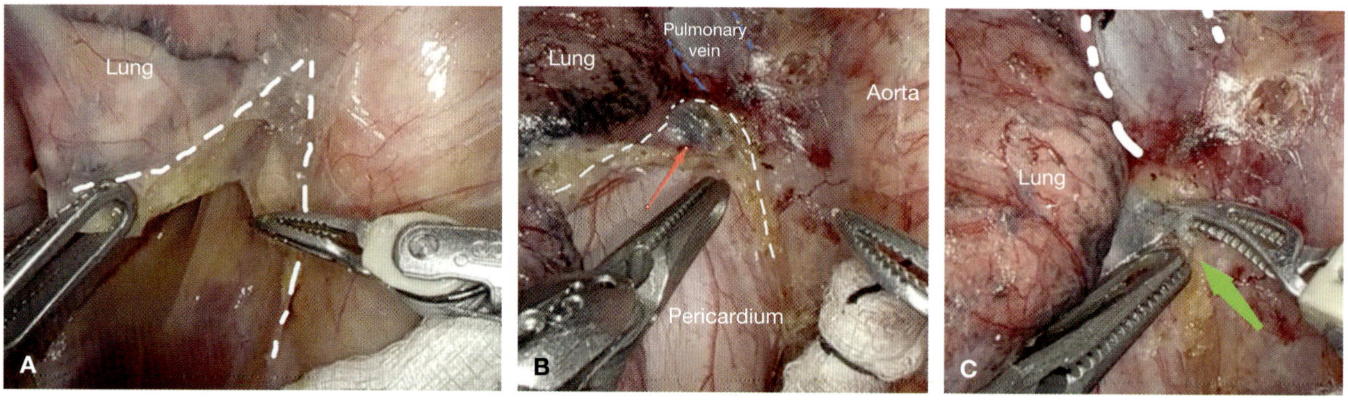

FIGURE 13.9 ▮ A. The left inferior pulmonary ligament (marked by white dotted line) is divided with cautery or energy device toward the left inferior pulmonary vein. **B.** The left inferior pulmonary vein is at the superior border of the dissection (dotted white lines) and the 9L lymph node is visualized (arrow). **C.** Magnified view of left inferior pulmonary vein (white dotted lines) and the 9L lymph node is visualized (arrow).

PEARLS AND PITFALLS

- Lymph nodes are adjacent to bronchovascular structures, so dissecting on the lymph node is the safest strategy to avoid bleeding or injury to a bronchus.
- The paratracheal and aortopulmonary lymph nodes are in close proximity to nerves (phrenic, vagus). In particular, the AP window (level 5) lymph node region is also in close proximity to the left recurrent laryngeal nerve where the nerve can be directly injured.
- Hemostasis with lymph node dissection improves with energy devices that minimize thermal transmission to surrounding structures or with precision cautery or hemoclips.
- Lymph nodes should be labeled by a numbered station to avoid ambiguity when interpreting final pathology.
- Becoming familiar with lymph node regions and nomenclature is paramount when submitting specimens from the operating room (Figure 13.2).
- If lymph node dissections are performed with blunt technique, there is a higher risk of chyle leak postoperatively.

Suggested Readings

1. Detterbeck FC, Lewis SZ, Diekemper R, Addrizzo-Harris D, Alberts WM. Executive summary: diagnosis and management of lung cancer, 3rd ed—American College of Chest Physicians evidence-based clinical practice guidelines. *Chest*. 2013;143(5 suppl):7S-37S.
2. Kiss G. Technical issues and patient safety in non-intubated thoracic anesthesia. *Thorac Surg Clin*. 2020;30(1):1-13.
3. Mountain CF, Dresler CM. Regional lymph node classification for lung cancer staging. *Chest*. 1997;111(6):1718-1723c.

Chapter 14

Lung Decortication: Open Thoracotomy and Video-Assisted Thoracoscopic Surgery

ELIZA D. HOMPE
CHRISTOPHER R. MORSE
PHILICIA MOONSAMY

Background

- Lung decortication is the surgical management for an empyema. Decortication can be the first-line approach or performed after more conservative options have failed, such as tube thoracostomy and intrapleural fibrinolysis.
- The goals of a decortication operation are: (1) to completely drain the infected pleural space and (2) to fully reexpand the lung.
- The choice of minimally invasive approach or open thoracotomy depends on the stage of the empyema, patient factors, and surgeon experience. For a stage II (fibrinopurulent phase) empyema, a minimally invasive procedure (video-assisted thoracoscopic surgery [VATS]) can be efficacious. For a stage III (chronic organizing phase) empyema, open thoracotomy is often necessary to remove the pleural rind, completely reexpand the lung, and evacuate the empyema.

Perioperative Considerations

Anesthesia and Positioning

- Decortication is performed under general anesthesia. Single-lung ventilation is facilitated by either a double-lumen endotracheal tube or a bronchial blocker.
- Access is established with two large-bore IVs and an arterial line is placed for continuous blood pressure monitoring if the patient has specific comorbidities (coronary artery disease, heart failure, etc.). There is a potential for significant blood loss with removal of pleural rind from the raw lung surface. The patient should therefore have an active type and screen and appropriate vascular access.
- After general anesthesia is administered and a double-lumen endotracheal tube placed, the patient is positioned supine with the xiphoid process at the level of the break in the operating room table. The patient is then repositioned in the standard lateral decubitus position with the affected side up.
- Our preference is to use blanket rolls on either side of the patient, but a bean bag positioner can also be used. The operating room table is flexed and the patient is secured to the operating room table. All pressure points are padded.
- Once the positioning of the double-lumen endotracheal tube is confirmed with bronchoscopy, the patient is placed on single-lung ventilation with isolation of the affected lung.

Instruments and Equipment

- Open
    - Standard thoracotomy instrument tray
    - Cobb elevator (Figure 14.1)

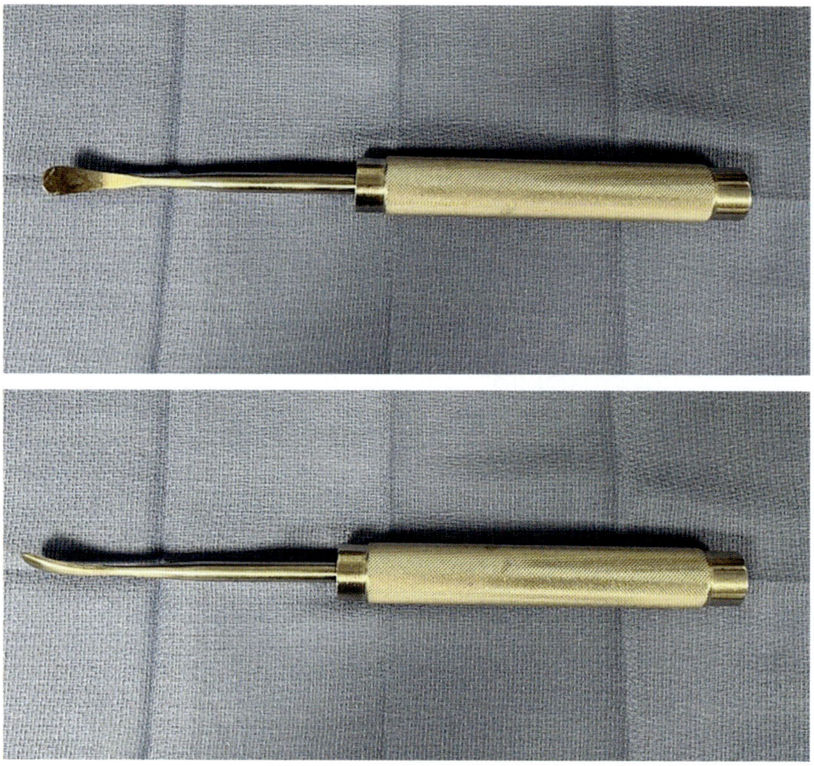

FIGURE 14.1 ▮ Cobb elevator for lung decortication.

-
    - Peanut dissector or endoscopic Kittner
- VATS
    - 10-mm, 30° thoracoscope
    - Ring forceps and curved ring forceps
    - Endoscopic Kittner
    - A standard thoracotomy instrument tray should be readily available in the event of the need for conversion to an open operation.

TIPS

- *Even in experienced hands, the conversion rate from VATS to open thoracotomy for decortication has been cited at 10% to 15%. The most important predictor for conversion thoracotomy is the chronicity or time interval between onset of symptoms and surgery, with >2 weeks significantly increasing the likelihood of conversion.*

Technique

Open

- The incision is planned based on the location and size of the empyema on preoperative imaging. In the operating room, a needle thoracentesis can be performed directly over the anticipated location of a dependent fluid pocket and trapped lung (the eighth intercostal space in Figure 14.2). Once fluid is successfully aspirated, a thoracotomy incision can be made at that rib level.

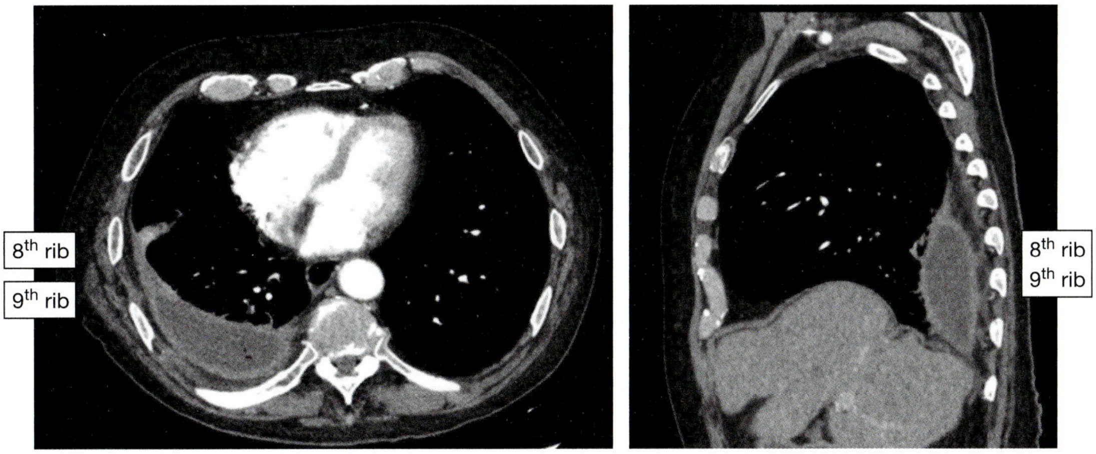

FIGURE 14.2 | Preoperative imaging of an empyema (chest CT, axial and sagittal views) for incisional planning.

- For an anticipated complete lung decortication, a standard posterolateral thoracotomy incision is made one to two fingerbreadths below the tip of the scapula and curving around the scapular border.
- The subcutaneous tissues and latissimus dorsi muscle are divided with electrocautery. The serratus anterior muscle is preserved and freed from the chest wall.
- A scapular retractor is used to elevate the scapula and count the ribs in the subscapular space, identifying the sixth rib and the fifth intercostal space immediately superior to it.
- The periosteum is scored along the entire extent of the rib and then removed from its rib bed using a periosteal elevator. Often, there is rib crowding (Figure 14.3), which may necessitate resection of a rib (usually fifth) to gain adequate exposure.

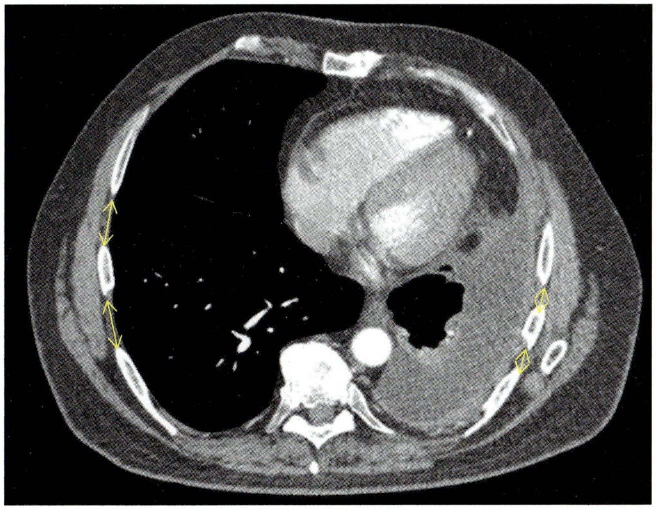

FIGURE 14.3 | Rib crowding on chest CT (axial view).

- The intercostal muscles are divided with electrocautery and the pleural space is entered. Blunt dissection with a finger or sponge stick may need to be carried out superiorly and inferiorly for a few centimeters to facilitate insertion of the rib-spreading (Finochietto) retractor.
- It is very important to correctly identify the appropriate layers at this point. If there is a thick pleural rind, it should be incised sharply with a scalpel until the lung is visualized. Then, the correct dissection plane between the lung surface and the pleural rind is identified and developed. This can be facilitated by inflating the lung with low tidal volumes to better visualize the anatomic planes. This helps to avoid injuries to the lung parenchyma and resultant postoperative air leaks.
- We favor performing most of the decortication bluntly with a Cobb elevator.
- The entire lung is meticulously separated from the pleural rind, taking care to minimize injuries to the lung parenchyma. Once a segment of pleural rind has been mobilized away from the lung,

it is divided with scissors and removed. The lung is mobilized inferiorly until it is freed from the diaphragm and superiorly all the way to the apex. Anteriorly, the extent of decortication is limited by the mediastinum and care should be taken not to damage the critical structures. Specifically, avoid decortication close to the phrenic nerve, internal mammary artery, and the subclavian vessels.
- Pleural fluid should be sent for aerobic and anaerobic cultures. Pleural rind should be sent for both microbiology and pathology.
- Once a complete decortication is performed, the lung is ventilated to ensure that it expands fully. Any areas of incomplete expansion will require additional decortication.
- Multiple, large-bore chest tubes are placed to widely drain the chest as air leaks are anticipated. At our institution, we routinely place anterior and posterior 28-French tubes and may sometimes place an additional third tube to ensure adequate drainage. The thoracotomy incision is closed in layers.

Video-Assisted

- We prefer to use three ports for a thoracoscopic decortication, when possible.
    - A camera port in the seventh intercostal space in the mid-axillary line. It is important not to place this port too inferior as there can be volume loss and contraction from a chronic empyema. Placement of this port may also be guided by needle thoracentesis, as described above.
    - A posterior port in the seventh or eighth intercostal space
    - A 3- to 4-cm working port in the fourth intercostal space anteriorly
- The chest is entered in the seventh intercostal space in the mid-axillary line and the thoracoscope is introduced. A Yankauer or metal tip suction catheter is introduced to drain any effusion and break up loculations to create a working space as well as space for additional port placement.
- The pleural space is debrided and any fibrinous material removed using a ring forceps. Adhesiolysis is performed. The lung is then decorticated from the apex to the diaphragm using the technique described previously with an endoscopic Kittner or the metal tip suction catheter.
- An intercostal nerve block is performed for local analgesia using Marcaine 0.25% with epinephrine.
- At the conclusion of the procedure, the lung is reexpanded under direct visualization and multiple, large-bore chest tubes are placed for drainage. The VATS incisions are closed in layers.

TIPS

Benefits of a minimally invasive approach include decreased hospital length of stay, lower postoperative pain, and reduced postoperative morbidity. However, the VATS approach should be abandoned if it compromises the goal of complete decortication and reexpansion of the lung.

Postoperative Care

- The patient is extubated in the operating room and transferred to the postoperative care unit, followed by the inpatient floor.
- For pain control, we favor a thoracic epidural catheter or patient-controlled analgesia in the immediate postoperative period, followed by a multimodal oral regimen.
- The chest tubes will remain in until all air leaks resolve. This may take several days depending on the extent of parenchymal tears created during the decortication. The decision to place the chest tubes to suction or water seal is a balance between ensuring lung inflation and not perpetuating the air leaks and preventing them from sealing off. The patient will undergo daily chest x-rays.
- Aggressive pulmonary toilet and early mobilization is encouraged.
- Duration and choice of antibiotics is informed by intraoperative cultures.

PEARLS AND PITFALLS

- In a chronic empyema, volume loss can cause the interspaces between ribs to narrow on the affected side relative to the contralateral hemithorax, creating the appearance of rib crowding on axial imaging (Figure 14.3).
- It is important to review a patient's preoperative axial imaging carefully to determine if there is rib crowding. This finding may lead the surgeon to start with an open thoracotomy and plan for complete resection of a rib to gain adequate exposure for decortication.
- It is sometimes difficult to enter the correct plane between the visceral and parietal pleura due to dense adhesions. In these cases, it may be easier to enter the extrapleural plane and perform a pleurectomy to complete the decortication. It is important to avoid injury to the phrenic nerve, internal mammary artery, subclavian artery, and sympathetic chain during pleurectomy since these structures can become obscured and adherent to the pleura due to the chronic infection.
- Inflating the affected lung with low tidal volumes helps to identify the correct dissection plane when removing the pleural rind.

Suggested Readings

1. Chambers A, Routledge T, Dunning J, Scarci M. Is video-assisted thoracoscopic surgical decortication superior to open surgery in the management of adults with primary empyema? *Interact Cardiovasc Thorac Surg*. 2010;11(2):171-177.
2. Lardinois D, Gock M, Pezzetta E, et al. Delayed referral and gram-negative organisms increase the conversion thoracotomy rate in patients undergoing video-assisted thoracoscopic surgery for empyema. *Ann Thorac Surg*. 2005;79(6):1851-1856.
3. Shen KR, Bribriesco A, Crabtree T, et al. The American Association for Thoracic Surgery consensus guidelines for the management of empyema. *J Thorac Cardiovasc Surg*. 2017;153(6):e129-e146.
4. Tong BC, Hanna J, Toloza EM, et al. Outcomes of video-assisted thoracoscopic decortication. *Ann Thorac Surg*. 2010;89(1):220-225.
5. Towe CW, Carr SR, Donahue JM, et al. Morbidity and 30-day mortality after decortication for parapneumonic empyema and pleural effusion among patients in the Society of Thoracic Surgeons' General Thoracic Surgery Database. *J Thorac Cardiovasc Surg*. 2019;157(3):1288-1297.e4.

Chapter 15

Tracheal Resection and Reconstruction/Postintubation Tracheal Stenosis

SARAH A. BROWNLEE
DOUGLAS J. MATHISEN

History

- Prior prolonged intubation
- Prior tracheostomy
- Symptoms—dyspnea, stridor, and cough

Airway Management on Presentation (Acute)

- Sit upright
- O_2, Heliox
- Steroids to reduce edema and inflammation
- Chest computed tomography (CT) scan if stable airway

TIPS

- *Avoid attempts at intubation or flexible endoscopy in emergency ward for fear of losing airway.*
- *Avoid emergency cricothyroidotomy as it may be at the level of stenosis or above stenosis and may be unable to pass tracheostomy tube.*

Perioperative Considerations

- Resolve all medical issues before resection and reconstruction.
- Obtain contrast CT scan of neck and chest to evaluate stenosis (Figure 15.1A and B).
- Wean steroids if previously started. Delay surgery for 1 week for every week of steroid use. May have to dilate to maintain airway during this interval.

Contraindications to Tracheal Surgery

- Chronic high-dose steroids
- Ventilator-dependent
- Prior high-dose radiation (some exceptions)
- Severe comorbidities (consider T-tube or tracheostomy as alternative to repair)

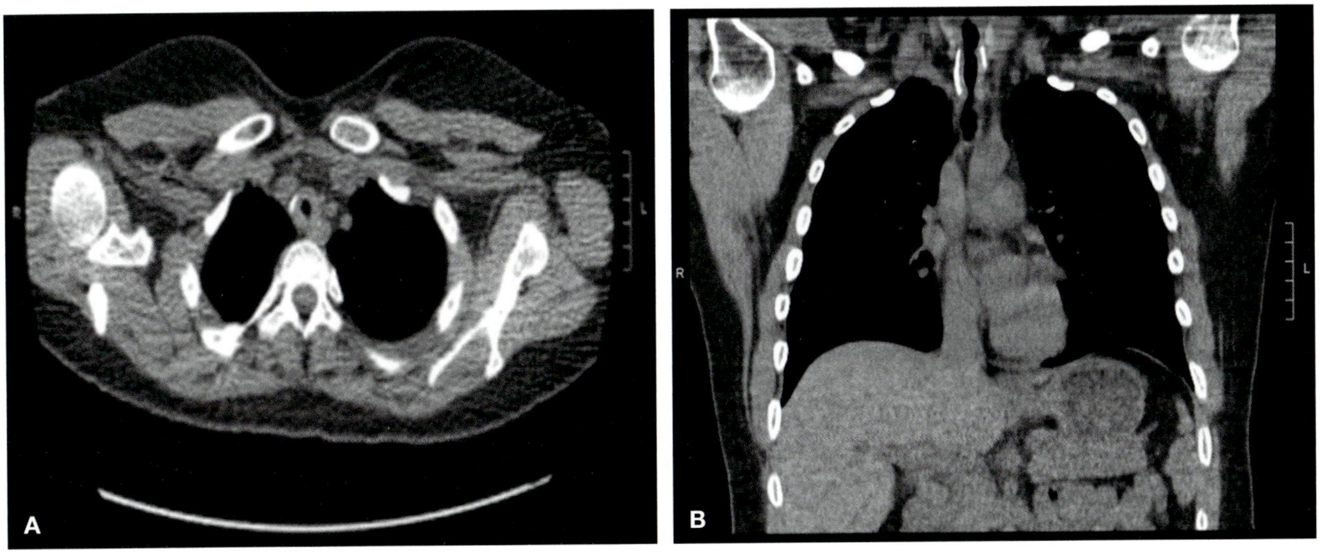

FIGURE 15.1 | Axial **(A)** and coronal **(B)** chest computed tomography demonstrating tracheal stenosis.

- Extensive length of stenosis
- Active pneumonia or tracheobronchitis (must clear first)

TIPS

- *Stents are contraindicated for benign inflammatory conditions as may (a) extend injury, (b) become incorporated in stenosis if stent uncovered, and (c) tracheobronchitis may be exacerbated with increased inflammation.*

Positioning

- Supine
- Gently extend neck using blankets or inflatable thyroid bag, don't overextend (Figure 15.2)

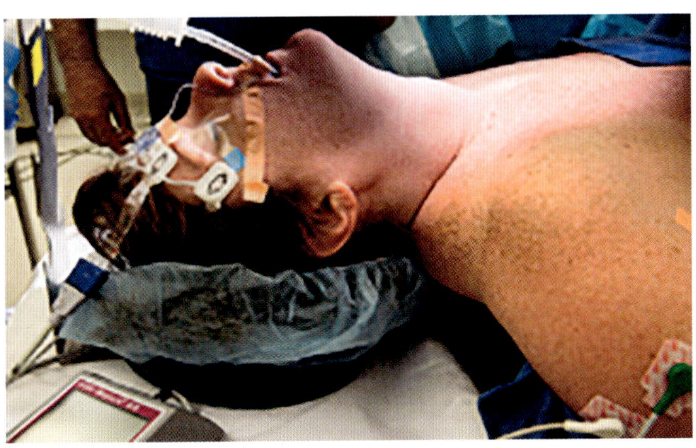

FIGURE 15.2 | Don't overextend the neck because of the risk of spinal cord ischemia. Use thyroid bag or blankets to achieve desired position.

- Raise back of bed 15°
- Prep widely in case partial sternotomy is required

Surgical Technique

- Start with careful flexible and rigid bronchoscopic evaluation and gentle dilation to provide an airway during the operation (Figure 15.3A-C).

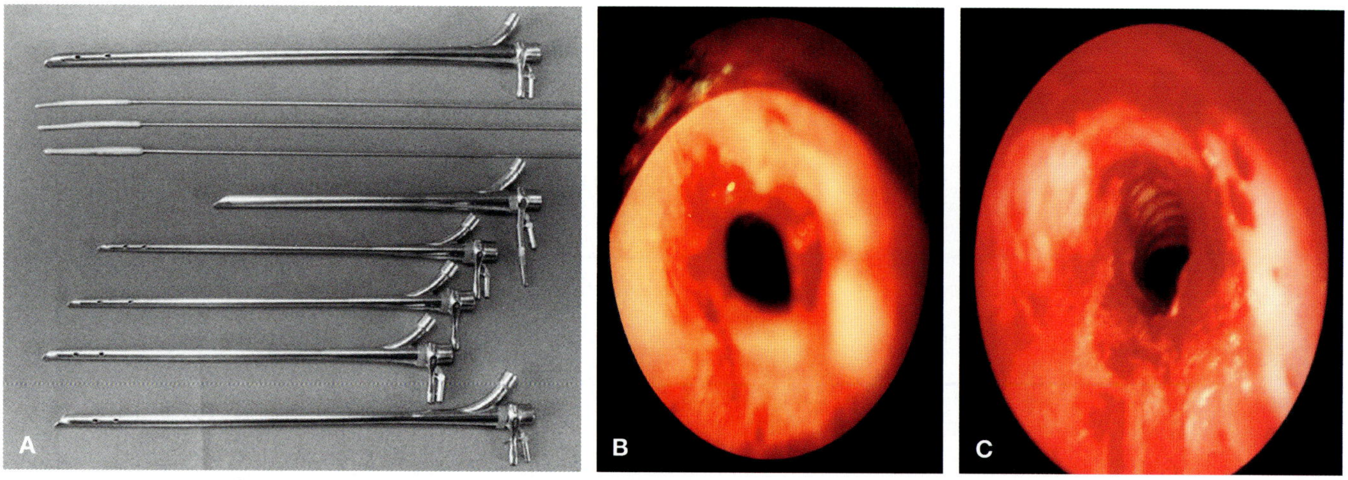

FIGURE 15.3 ▮ **A.** Rigid dilators and assortment of pediatric to adult bronchoscopes. **B.** Tight postintubation tracheal stenosis. **C.** Successful dilation with graduated rigid bronchoscopes to adult #8 bronchoscope. (From Mathiesen DJ. Rigid/flexible bronchoscopy. In: Mathiesen DJ, Morse CR, eds. *Master Techniques in Surgery: Thoracic Surgery—Lung Resections, Bronchoplasty*. Wolters Kluwer; 2015:1-6. Figure 1.4.)

- Once airway adequately dilated, a small endotracheal tube can be inserted either through a laryngeal mask airway or over a bronchoscope (Figure 15.4A and B).

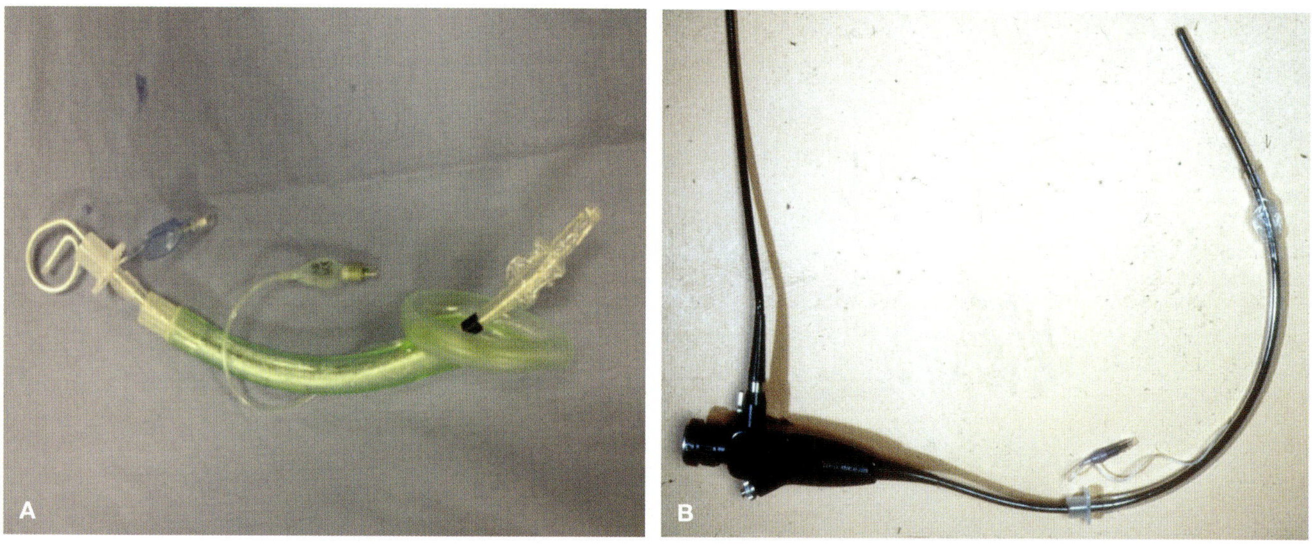

FIGURE 15.4 ▮ **A.** Endotracheal tube through laryngeal mask airway (LMA). **B.** 5.5 endotracheal tube over adult flexible bronchoscope. (From Mathiesen DJ. Rigid/flexible bronchoscopy. In: Mathiesen DJ, Morse CR, eds. *Master Techniques in Surgery: Thoracic Surgery—Lung Resections, Bronchoplasty*. Wolters Kluwer; 2015:1-6. Figure 1.3.)

- Incision—low cervical collar (most common) (Figure 15.5), partial sternotomy versus full sternotomy (rare) (Figure 15.6A and B).

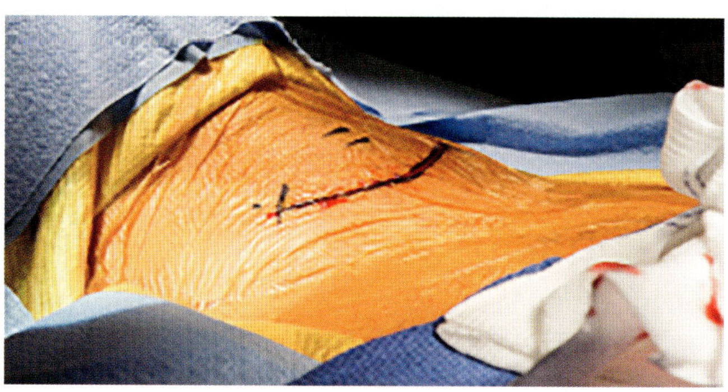

FIGURE 15.5 ▮ Two short horizontal lines are marking location of cricoid cartilage. Skin incision centered a little higher for proximal resection as in this case—finger breadth above suprasternal notch for lower resection.

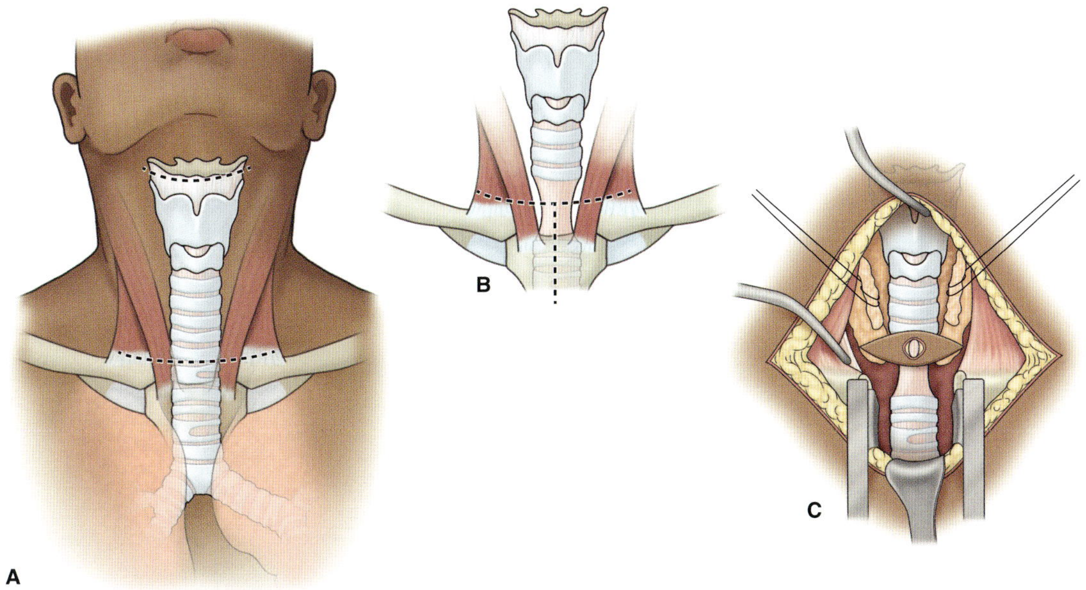

FIGURE 15.6 | **A.** Incisions for repair of postintubation tracheal lesions. Collar incision is basic. For low lesions, the upper sternal incision (manubrium) is added. Laryngeal release is performed through a short incision overlying the hyoid bone (upper dotted line). **B and C.** Exposure of trachea from partial upper sternotomy—pediatric sternal retractor is used. (From Auchincloss H, Mathisen DJ. Tracheoesophageal fistula. In: Mathisen DJ, Morse CR, eds. *Master Techniques in Surgery: Thoracic Surgery—Transplantation, Tracheal Resections, Mediastinal Tumors, Extended Thoracic Resections*. Wolters Kluwer; 2015:361-367. Figure 38.2.)

- Mobilize airway.
  - Divide thyroid isthmus (Figure 15.7).
  - Perform bronchoscopy to localize stenosis, use needle through trachea to mark proximal and distal ends of stenosis, and mark with sutures (Figure 15.8).
  - Careful dissection on the wall of trachea inside the thyroid gland—don't electively visualize recurrent laryngeal nerves as you may injure them (Figure 15.9).
  - Initial airway incision through a damaged portion of the airway (Figure 15.10A-C). Care should be taken not to devascularize airway or injure esophagus (adherent posteriorly). Resection of the trachea proceeds from this point (Figure 15.11A and B).
  - Traction sutures: 2-0 Vicryl are placed both proximally and distally usually around a ring in the midlateral airway (Figure 15.12A and B). These control the airway and allow testing for whether

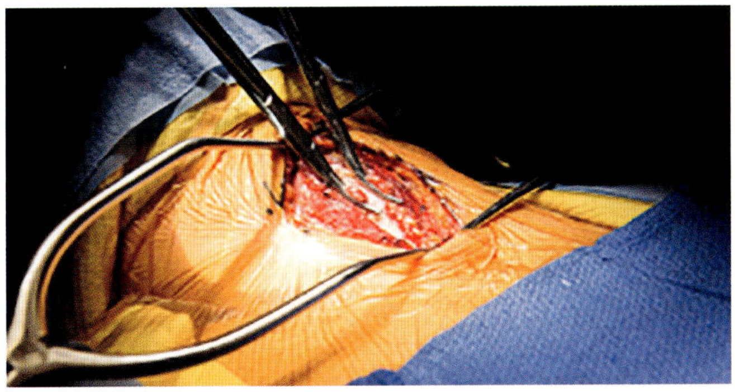

FIGURE 15.7 | Divided thyroid isthmus.

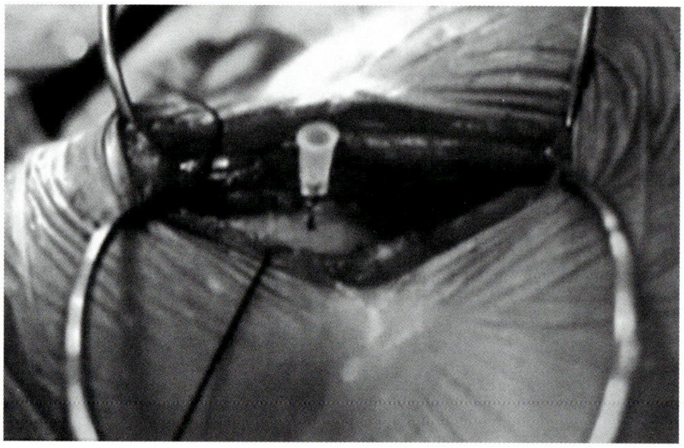

FIGURE 15.8 ▮ Light from bronchoscope. Needle to identify proximal and distal stenosis inserted through trachea. Proximal and distal extent masked with suture.

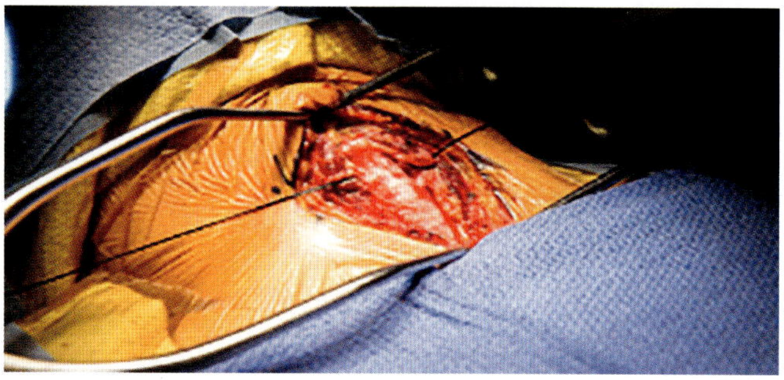

FIGURE 15.9 ▮ Thyroid isthmus divided. Sutures on divided ends of thyroid isthmus. Dissection close to wall of trachea inside retracted thyroid gland. Dissection can be circumferential at the level of stenosis. Recurrent laryngeal nerves allowed to fall away—never attempt to identify as may injure.

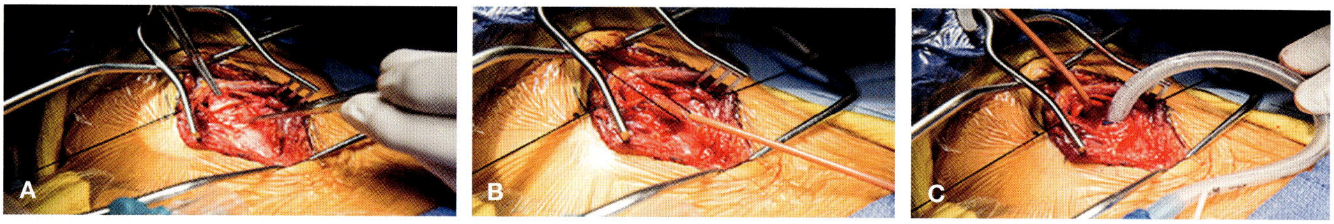

FIGURE 15.10 ▮ A. The trachea is opened conservatively through stenosis. **B.** Red rubber catheter secured to oral secured to oral endotracheal tube and pulled back proximally out of field. **C.** Flexible armored endotracheal tube (Tovell) in distal airway for crossfield ventilation. Sterile connecting tubing passed off the anesthesia staff to maintain ventilation.

the airway can be approximated with acceptable tension. If concern exists regarding excessive tension, it is best to perform a suprahyoid laryngeal release (Figure 15.13A-C).

TIPS

- *Better to do suprahyoid release during mobilization of trachea if indicated, before trying to tie the anastomotic sutures and finding excessive tension.*

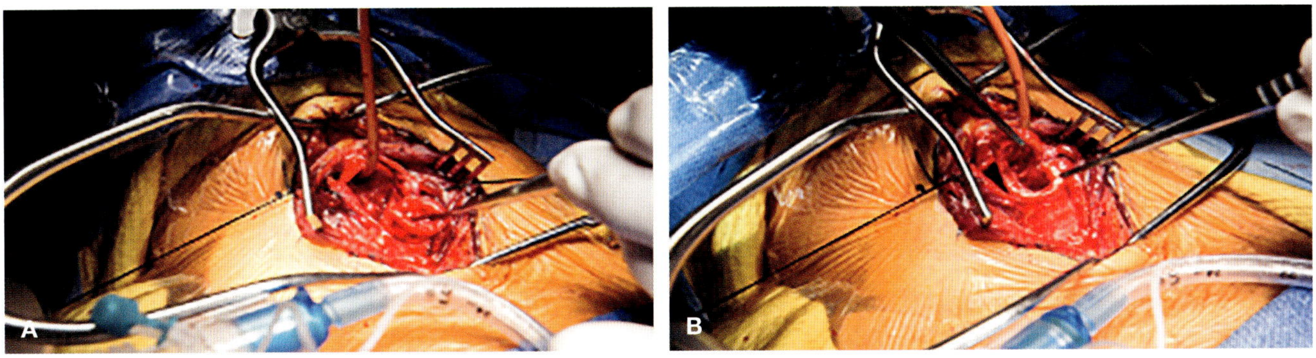

FIGURE 15.11 ▌ . Damaged tracheal segment mobilized **(A)**. The damaged segment is resected. Traction sutures are used to approximate proximal and distal tracheal ends to assess tension. It is desirable to get to normal mucosa and healthy nonmalacic tracheal rings. 2-0 Vicryl stay sutures are placed in midlateral position of proximal and distal airways around the tracheal ring **(B)**.

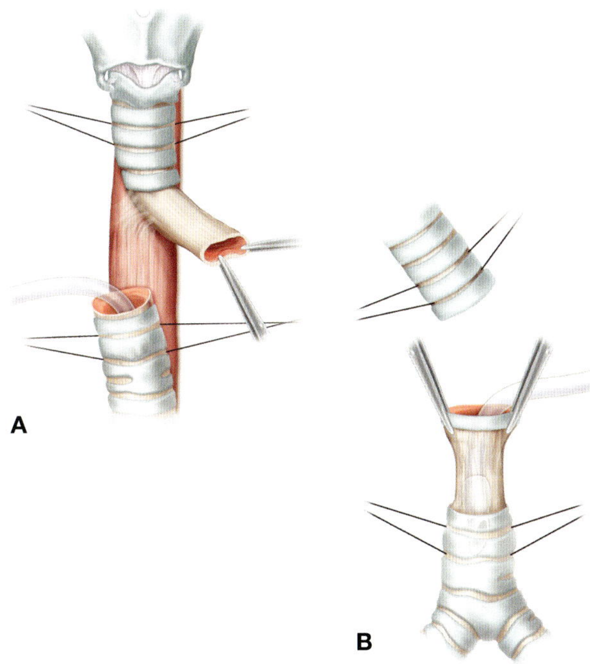

FIGURE 15.12 ▌ A. Traction sutures are placed at a midlateral position. **B.** Proximally and distally full thickness around a ring. (From Muniappan A. Tracheal resection. In: Mathisen DJ, Morse CR, eds. *Master Techniques in Surgery: Thoracic Surgery—Transplantation, Tracheal Resections, Mediastinal Tumors, Extended Thoracic Resections*. Wolters Kluwer; 2015:327-334. Figure 35.5.)

Anastomotic Techniques

- 4-0 Vicryl sutures
- Sutures by convention are placed so that the knots are on the outside of the airway, 3 to 4 mm in depth, with 3 to 4 mm between each suture (Figure 15.14).
- See Tables 15.1 and 15.2.

Tracheal Anastomosis

- The anastomosis starts with a 4-0 Vicryl suture placed in the posterior midline membranous wall with the resulting knots on the outside (Figure 15.15A-D).
- Subsequent sutures are placed in front of the previously placed suture.
- Organizing anastomotic sutures by clipping to drapes. The sutures are not tied until they are all placed. Instead, each suture is placed, snapped, and clipped to the drapes in order.
- Once all sutures are placed, the bag beneath the shoulders is deflated and the neck is flexed.
- With the neck flexed, the traction sutures are tied on either side, which is facilitated by pulling the anterior anastomotic sutures in opposite directions to help approximate the two ends of the airway.
- The anterior sutures are tied first.

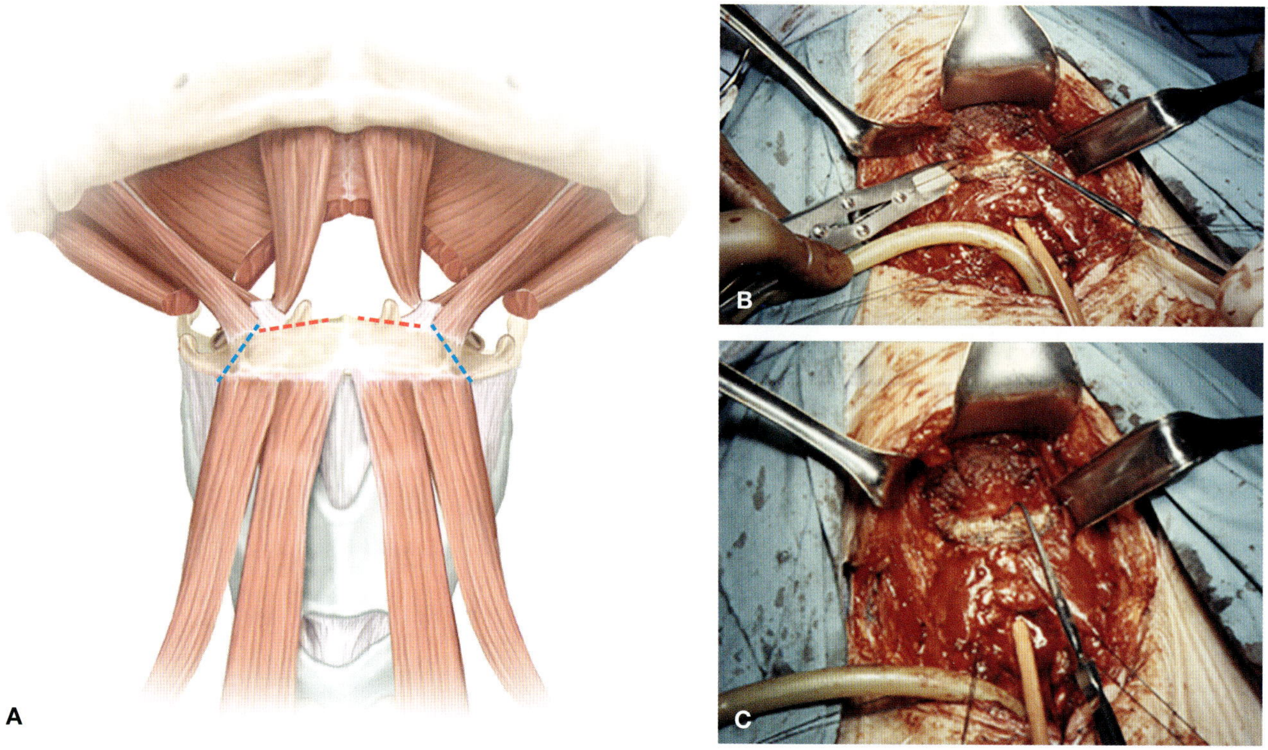

FIGURE 15.13 | A. Muscles attaching to hyoid are divided. Hyoid bone is divided as shown by the dotted line. **B.** Muscles attaching to the superior aspect of hyoid are divided. **C.** Hook pulls down on hyoid after dividing giving 1 to 2 cm of relaxation. (From Nasir BS, Liberman M. Release maneuvers: suprahyoid laryngeal release. In: Mathisen DJ, Morse CR, eds. *Master Techniques in Surgery: Thoracic Surgery—Transplantation, Tracheal Resections, Mediastinal Tumors, Extended Thoracic Resections*. Wolters Kluwer; 2015:303-307. Figure 31.3.)

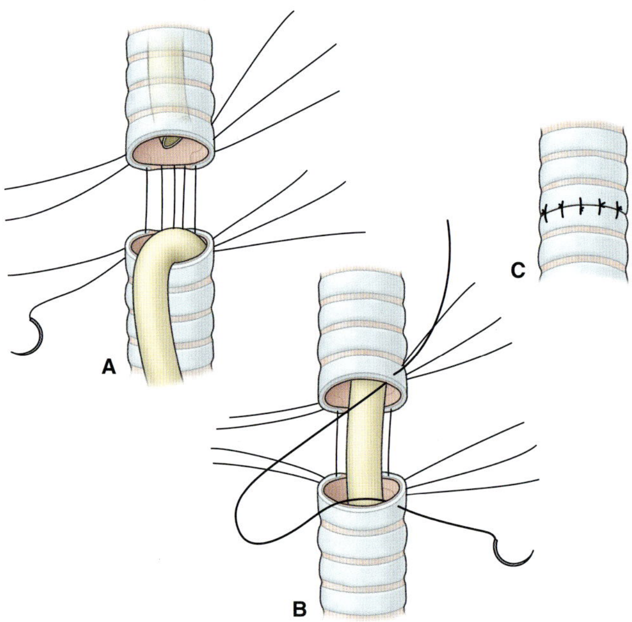

FIGURE 15.14 | A and B. Anastomotic open technique allowing precise placement of sutures 3 to 4 mm apart and around ring preferably. Sutures are placed so knots are on the outside first suture placed posteriorly (6 o'clock) each suture placed in front of previous suture and clipped to drapes cephalad to caudad.

TABLE 15.1 | Risk Factors for Anastomotic Complications

Risk Factors	Odds Ratio
• Diabetes	3.32
• Reoperation	3.03
• <17 y	2.26
• Resection >4 cm	2.01
• Preoperative tracheostomy	1.79

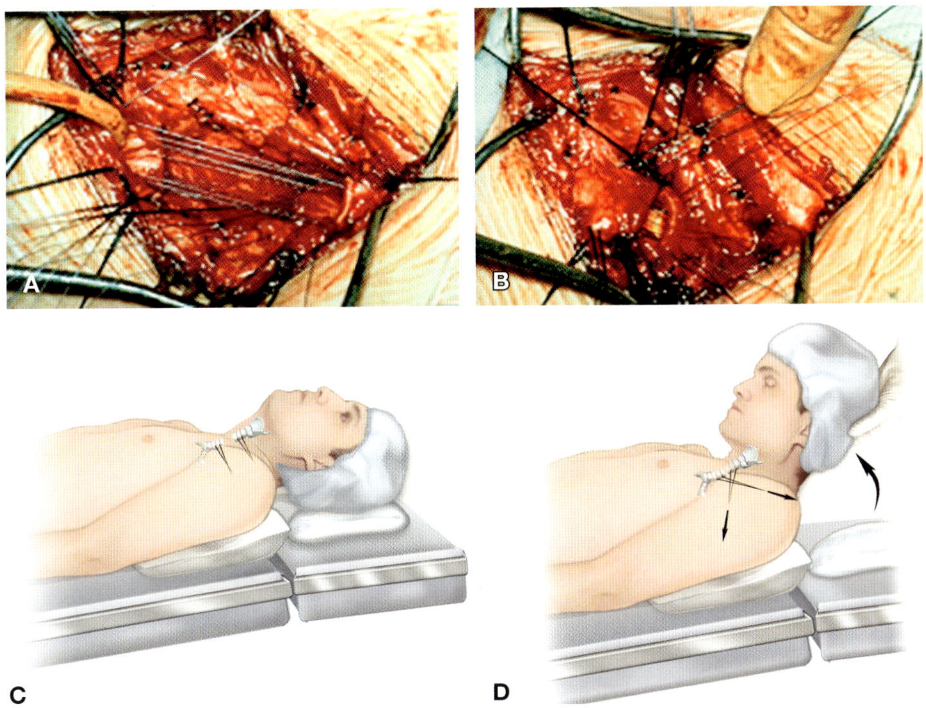

FIGURE 15.15 ▌ A. First suture by convention placed in 6 o'clock position. Knots will be on the outside. Each subsequent suture is placed so that it is placed "inside" the previous suture and clipped in a cranial to caudal fashion to the drapes. This system allows the sutures to be kept untangled. **B.** Traction sutures are pulled together and tied. All sutures are placed circumferentially. Anastomotic sutures are clipped to the drapes from cephalad to caudad. Each suture is placed "inside" the previous suture and when all placed, tied in reverse order. Traction sutures are drawn together and tied reducing tension on the anastomotic sutures. Anastomotic sutures are tied in reverse order of placement starting with anterior sutures. **C and D.** The neck is flexed to reduce tension as anastomotic sutures are tied. (From Muniappan A. Tracheal resection. In: Mathisen DJ, Morse CR, eds. *Master Techniques in Surgery: Thoracic Surgery—Transplantation, Tracheal Resections, Mediastinal Tumors, Extended Thoracic Resections*. Wolters Kluwer; 2015:327-334. Figure 35.8.)

TABLE 15.2 ▌ Results—Repair of Postintubation Tracheal Stenosis 1993-2017

	N	Good/Satisfactory %	Failure %	*P*
Postintubation tracheal stenosis	301	95.6	3.3	—
Laryngotracheal	91	84.5	15.4	.005
Reoperation	43	91	9	.075
Complications	131	80	19	<.001
Calcified airway	70	87	12	.059
Steroids at surgery	34	91	9	.458
Length ≥5 cm	12	89	8.5	.554

- The posterolateral sutures on either side are tied by retracting the traction suture away from the side being tied, giving exposure to the individual sutures. The back row is tied somewhat blindly.

TIPS

- *Don't overflex the neck as this can potentially cause spinal cord ischemia and result in paralysis.*

Anastomotic Integrity Check

- When all anastomotic sutures have been tied, the anastomosis is checked for air tightness by deflating the balloon and insufflating to pressures between 20 and 40 cm water through the endotracheal tube (Figure 15.16).
- Any air leak that is identified must be repaired even if it requires taking down the anastomosis.

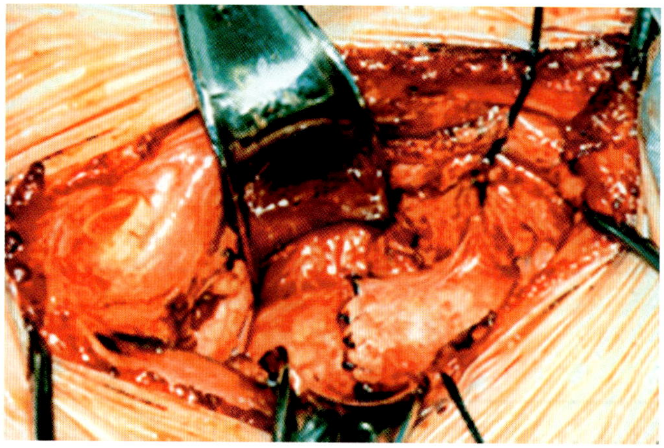

FIGURE 15.16 ▮ All anastomotic sutures have been tied. The endotracheal balloon is deflated, and a large breath is given (30-40 cm of water pressure) listening for air around the tube. The mouth and nose are occluded, a large breath to 20, 30, and 40 cm of air given with the anastomosis submerged in saline to check for air leak.

Closure

- The anastomosis is covered by mobilization of the strap muscles.
- Dead space is eliminated, and the wound is irrigated with antibiotic solution because of the potential contamination from an open airway.
- A #10 Jackson-Pratt drain is placed.
- If concern exists about the integrity of reconstruction, place small tracheostomy tube two rings below anastomosis as described earlier and buttress with strap muscle.
- After skin closure, a heavy #2 Vicryl suture is placed as a "Guardian stitch" from the submental crease to the presternal skin to remind the patient to maintain the neck flexion (Figure 15.17).

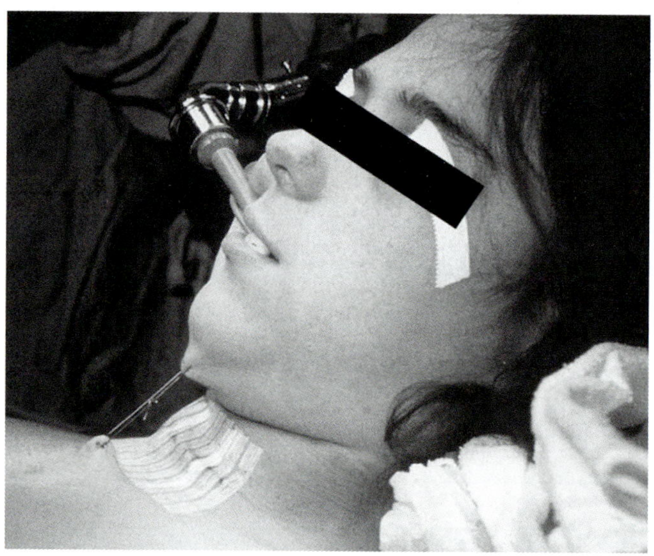

FIGURE 15.17 ▮ Guardian stitch. After the neck is closed and prior to extubation, a heavy No. 2 suture is placed to remind the patient to maintain neck flexion. The stitch is passed from the submental crease to the presternal skin. (From Muniappan A. Tracheal resection. In: Mathisen DJ, Morse CR, eds. *Master Techniques in Surgery: Thoracic Surgery—Transplantation, Tracheal Resections, Mediastinal Tumors, Extended Thoracic Resections*. Wolters Kluwer; 2015:327-334. Figure 35.12.)

- If stridulous at extubation, reintubate with 5 or 5.5 tube over flexible bronchoscope. Treat edema and return to operating room for controlled trial extubation at 48 hours. (If fails, small tracheostomy tube may need to be placed.)

TIPS

- *A few extra sutures buttressed by strap muscle usually suffice for anterior leaks. Posterior leaks may require opening anterior anastomosis and placing sutures under direct vision leaving knots inside.*
- *Mobilizing the strap muscles to cover the anastomosis serves as a buttress, may provide some ingrowth of blood vessels, separates the anastomosis from the subcutaneous tissues in case of a superficial wound infection, and also serves to separate the anastomosis from the innominate artery, thereby avoiding the risk of tracheoinnominate artery fistula.*
- *Mild neck flexion is maintained throughout to avoid tension.*

Postoperative Care

- Keep neck flexed with blankets or pillows for 6 to 7 days.
- Voice rest 6 to 7 days to minimize vocal cord edema.
- Humidified O_2.
- Nothing by mouth except meds 6 to 7 days (to avoid aspiration secondary to vocal cord dysfunction and incomplete closure of epiglottis).
- Avoid narcotics because of nausea and provide antiemetics around the clock to avoid nausea/vomiting.
- Check airflow every day at the bedside. The patient should blow in and out against your hand.

TIPS

- *At the bedside, assess the ability to move air in and out easily. Restriction on inhaling suggests edema or vocal cord issue.*

- Cut chin stitch at 6 to 7 days.
- Repeat bronchoscopy typically performed at postoperative day 7 (Figure 15.18).
- See Table 15.3.

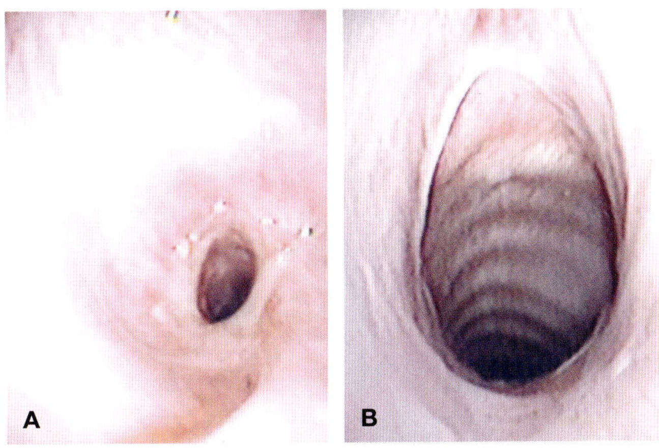

FIGURE 15.18 | A. Preoperative bronchoscopy of tight stenosis. **B.** Postoperative photo is 6 weeks postop.

TABLE 15.3 | Influence of Prior Treatments on Outcomes

	N	Good/Satisfactory %	Failure %	Death %	*P*
No prior treatment	31	97	3	3	—
Tracheostomies (preop)	275	91	8	0.8	.041
Removed	152	96	4	—	N.S.
Present at surgery	123	86	13	0.8	.002
Postoperative protecting	27	74	26	—	<.001
Postoperative after surgery	24	38	54	—	<.001
T-tubes	61	90	10	0	.034
Stents	44	90	10	0	.038
Laser/dilations	82/202	96	4	0.5	.2
Tracheal operations	43	91	9		.075

PEARLS AND PITFALLS

- Prior prolonged intubation
- Prior tracheostomy
- Symptoms—dyspnea, stridor, and cough
- Sit upright
- O_2, Heliox
- Steroids to reduce edema and inflammation
- Chest CT scan if stable airway

Suggested Readings

1. Axtell A, Mathisen DJ. *Management of tracheal stenosis*. In: *Cameron: Current Surgical Therapy 12/e*. Elsevier; 2017:882-887.
2. Chitilian HV, Bao X, Mathisen DJ, Alfille PH. *Anesthesia for airway surgery*. In: *Thorac Surg Clinics*. Elsevier; 2018:249-255.
3. Mathisen DJ. Tracheal resection and reconstruction: how I teach it. *Ann Thorac Surg*. 2017;103(4):1043-1048.
4. Stock C, Gukasyan N, Muniappan A, Wright C, Mathisen D. Hyperbaric oxygen therapy for the treatment of anastomotic complications after tracheal resection and reconstruction. *J Thorac Cardiovasc Surg*. 2014;147(3):1030-1035.
5. Tapias LF, Wright CD, Lanuti M, et al. Hyperbaric oxygen therapy in the prevention and management of tracheal and oesophageal anastomotic complications. *Eur J Cardiothorac Surg*. 2020;57(6):1203-1209.
6. Wright CD, Li S, Geller AD, et al. Postintubation tracheal stenosis: management and results 1993 to 2017. *Ann Thorac Surg*. 2019;108(5):1471-1477.

Chapter 16
Tracheostomy

CHINMAY HARIDAS
HUGH G. AUCHINCLOSS
CHI-FU JEFFREY YANG

Perioperative Considerations

- Know the anatomic locations of the thyrohyoid membrane, hyoid bone, sternomastoid muscle, cricothyroid membrane, thyroid gland, thyroid cartilage, and cricoid cartilage.
- Select an appropriate tracheostomy tube, and factors such as diameter, presence or absence of an inner cannula, length, whether the tube is cuffed or cuffless, and the presence or absence of a fenestration should be considered.
- The thyroid isthmus lying across the second to fourth tracheal rings may be encountered while performing a tracheostomy. An isthmectomy may be performed in such a case.

Indications

- Tracheostomy may be needed in the event of upper airway obstruction to provide a safe airway. Causes of upper airway obstruction include tumors of the larynx, tongue, pharynx, or upper trachea; bilateral vocal fold paralysis as a complication of thyroidectomy; and craniofacial abnormalities.
- Tracheostomy is also often needed in the setting of prolonged mechanical ventilation.

Contraindications

- Cervical spine injury, evidence of infection at the insertion site, uncontrolled coagulopathy, and complex anatomy (eg, morbid obesity, short neck, limited neck movement)

Patient Positioning (Figure 16.1)

- Place the patient in supine position.
- Extend the neck (if possible) by placing a shoulder roll underneath the patient's scapulae.
- Stabilize the head on a head ring or use a pillow/towel.

TIPS

- *Tracheotomy is an incision in the trachea, while tracheostomy refers to making a semipermanent or permanent opening/stoma.*
- *Be careful not to overextend the neck because this can lead to a tracheostomy placed too low (toward the carina) and too close to the innominate artery. This can be especially true when performing a tracheostomy on children.*

Instruments and Equipment

- Medications: For sedation, pain control, and inducing paralysis
- Flexible video bronchoscope
- Silicone lubricant
- Saline
- Surgical lubricant

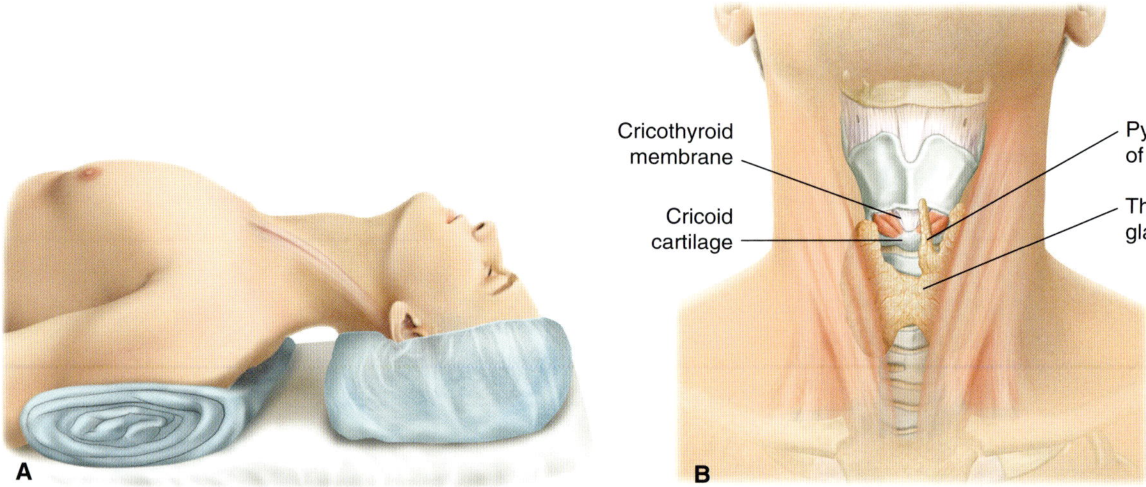

FIGURE 16.1 ▮ A and B: Patient positioning and relevant anatomy. (From Goldberg AJ, Pathak AS. Procedures. In: Britt LD, Peitzman A, Barie P, Jurkovich G, eds. *Acute Care Surgery*. Wolters Kluwer; 2013:808-815. Figure 64.1.)

- Dissecting instruments
- Tracheostomy tube and collar
- For performing percutaneous tracheostomy: A kit that includes a number 15 surgical scalpel blade, an introducer needle, dilators, a protective sheath, a tracheal loading trocar, and a small slip-tip syringe.
- Tracheostomies can be performed with either an open or percutaneous technique. Studies have found no significant clinical differences between the two approaches.

Technique

Open Surgical Tracheostomy

Mark the incision site and inject it with a local anesthetic.

Identify the entry site by palpating the essential anatomical landmarks: the thyroid cartilage, cricoid cartilage, and the sternal notch (Figure 16.2).

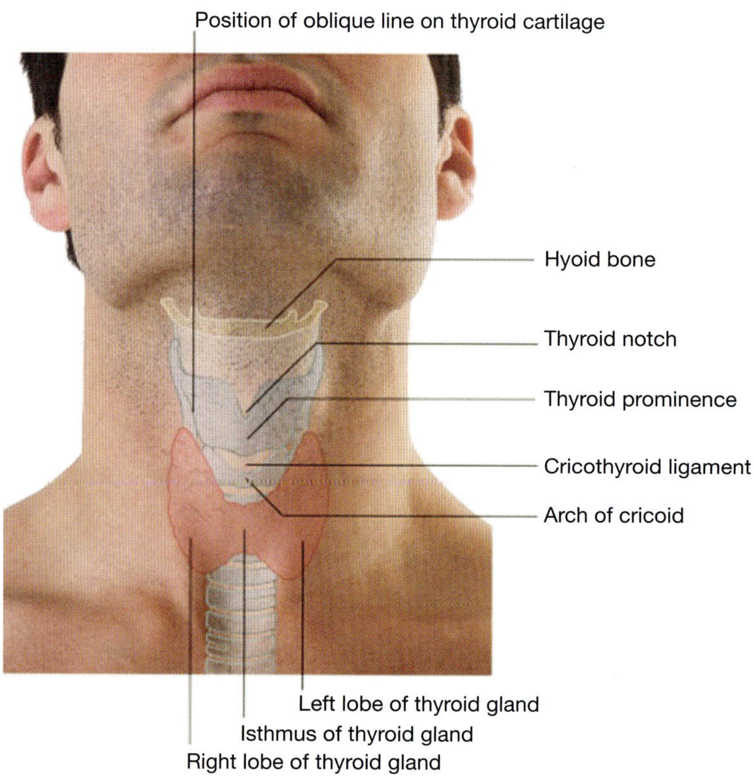

FIGURE 16.2 ▮ Identification of anatomical landmarks. (Reprinted from Lee B. Chapter 68: Transtracheal block. In: Gray AT, ed. *Atlas of Ultrasound-Guided Regional Anesthesia*. 3rd ed. Elsevier; 2019:353-356, with permission from Elsevier.)

The skin incision can be made vertically or in a transverse fashion (Figure 16.3). A transverse incision, which we commonly use, should be made approximately two fingerbreadths above the sternal notch. If choosing to make a vertical incision, make this incision 2 to 3 cm in the midline of the neck, from the cricoid cartilage to just above the sternal notch.

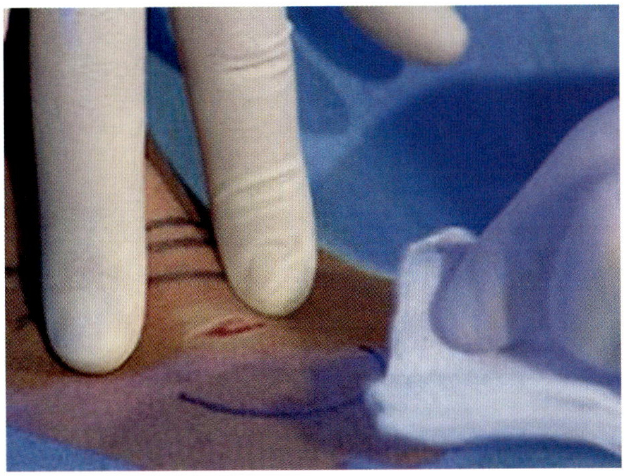

FIGURE 16.3 ▌ Skin incision. (From Koscielny S. Methods of surgical tracheotomy/tracheostomy. In: Klemm E, Nowak A, eds. *Tracheotomy and Airway*. Cham: Springer; 2020.)

- Once the skin has been incised, continue incising through the platysma muscle. Once this is done, identify the strap muscles. Retract the strap muscles laterally; retraction of the sternohyoid and sternothyroid muscle can expose the cricoid cartilage and the thyroid gland. Dissect and divide the thyroid isthmus if necessary.
  - The anterior tracheal wall can now be identified. Use large retractors to ensure adequate exposure and clear off the soft tissues overlying the trachea (Figure 16.4).

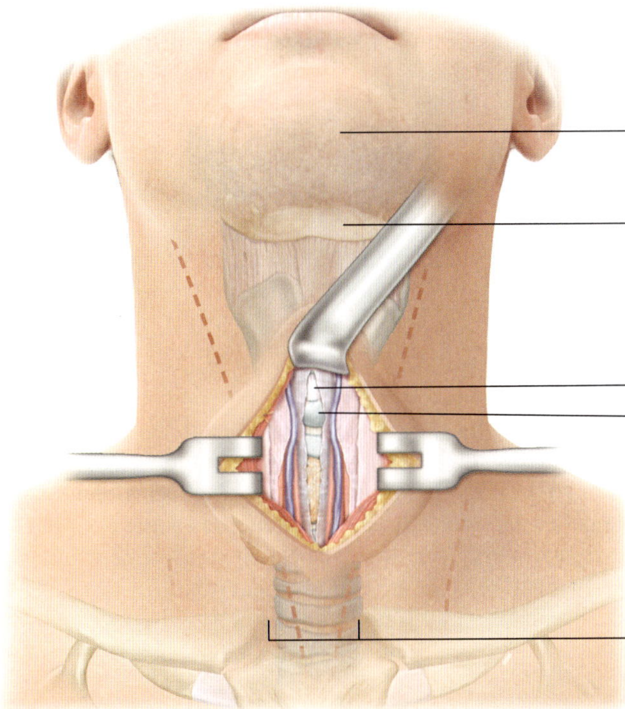

FIGURE 16.4 ▌ Dissection to the trachea. (From Goldberg AJ, Pathak AS. Procedures. In: Britt LD, Peitzman A, Barie P, Jurkovich G, eds. *Acute Care Surgery*. Wolters Kluwer; 2013:808-815. Figure 64.2.)

- Place a cricoid hook beneath the cricoid cartilage to provide upward traction on the larynx and trachea. The second and the third thyroid cartilages can now be visualized. Ask the anesthesiologist to hold ventilation and let the cuff down on the endotracheal tube. To open the trachea, divide the membrane between the second and third rings horizontally and then cut the corresponding rings through the midline. Then make an incision between the corresponding tracheal rings (divide a ring) and place the tracheostomy tube (Figure 16.5).

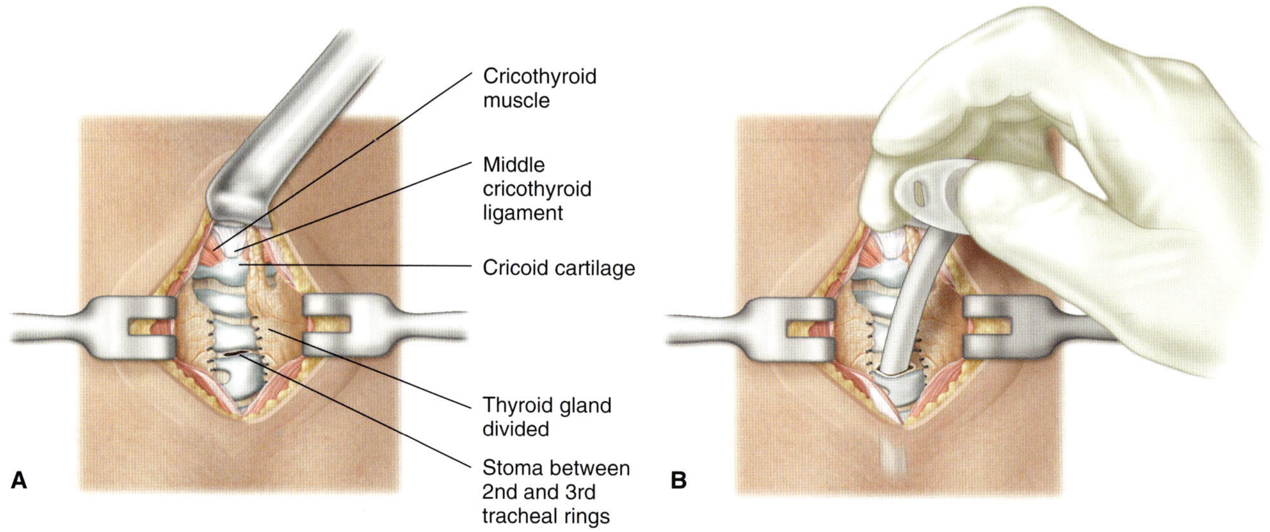

FIGURE 16.5 ▮ A and B. Exposure of the trachea and insertion of the tracheostomy tube. (From Goldberg AJ, Pathak AS. Procedures. In: Britt LD, Peitzman A, Barie P, Jurkovich G, eds. *Acute Care Surgery*. Wolters Kluwer; 2013:808-815. Figure 64.3.)

- Have the anesthesia team begin to withdraw the tube and stop when the tip is immediately above the tracheotomy. The tracheostomy tube is inserted at a 90-degree angle and then gently rotated in place.
- Inflate the tracheostomy cuff and confirm its correct placement by direct visualization and by evaluating the end-tidal CO_2, oxygen saturation, ease of ventilation, breath sounds in both lungs, and chest rise.

TIPS

If you cannot easily advance the tracheostomy tube, pull the tracheostomy tube back, advance the endotracheal tube back into the airway past the tracheotomy, inflate the cuff, and reestablish the airway.

- After the tracheostomy tube is in place and confirmed, remove the cricoid hook from the tracheotomy and secure the tracheostomy tube with sutures and ties or Velcro tapes. Every attempt should be made to stop bleeding around the trachea under direct visualization. However, there are times when the patient has coagulopathy and there is some low-level oozing around the trachea. In this case, the tracheostomy can be packed with surgical or a hemostatic dressing. Apply the tracheostomy dressing and remove the endotracheal tube.
- Perform a bronchoscopy through the tracheostomy tube and evaluate the positioning of the tube. Suction out any blood or secretions from the trachea, bilateral mainstem, and segmental bronchi.

TIPS

Although we suture the tracheostomy tube to the skin, one needs to be careful and watch out for skin ulceration. If sutures are used, do make sure to cut the sutures on ~postoperative day 7. Make sure to tape the obturator to the patient's chest before leaving the room.

Percutaneous Tracheostomy

The neck should be carefully palpated, and the thyroid cartilage, cricoid cartilage, and the sternal notch should be identified.

- Make a 2- to 3-cm vertical incision approximately 2 cm below the cricoid cartilage and clear the pretracheal tissue with blunt dissection. The incision can also be made transversely, two finger-breadths above the sternal notch.

TIPS

- *For patients with coagulopathy concerns, tie a purse-string suture surrounding the tracheostomy incision for additional hemostatic control.*
- *If an ultrasound is used for guidance, the "blinking frog" sign can be referenced to avoid damage to pretracheal vasculature.*
- *Ultrasound guidance may be considered during percutaneous dilatational tracheostomy to identify and avoid the vasculature in the pretracheal or paratracheal regions, thus minimizing the risk of bleeding. In Figure 16.6A, the trachea with inferior thyroid veins resembles the head of a frog with its eyes open. Application of pressure makes the vessels disappear, which resembles the closing of the eyes (Figure 16.6B). This is called the "blinking frog sign."*
- *Advance a bronchoscope via a swivel adaptor down the oral endotracheal tube until you see the trachea. The bronchoscopy can be performed by either the anesthesia team or the surgeon's assistant.*
- *The surgeon should then palpate the trachea and insert an introducer needle at the level of the second tracheal ring under direct bronchoscopic visualization.*
- *To visualize this needle, the anesthesia team will need to deflate the endotracheal tube cuff and slowly withdraw the endotracheal tube proximally enough so that the bronchoscope can visualize the finder needle (Figure 16.7).*

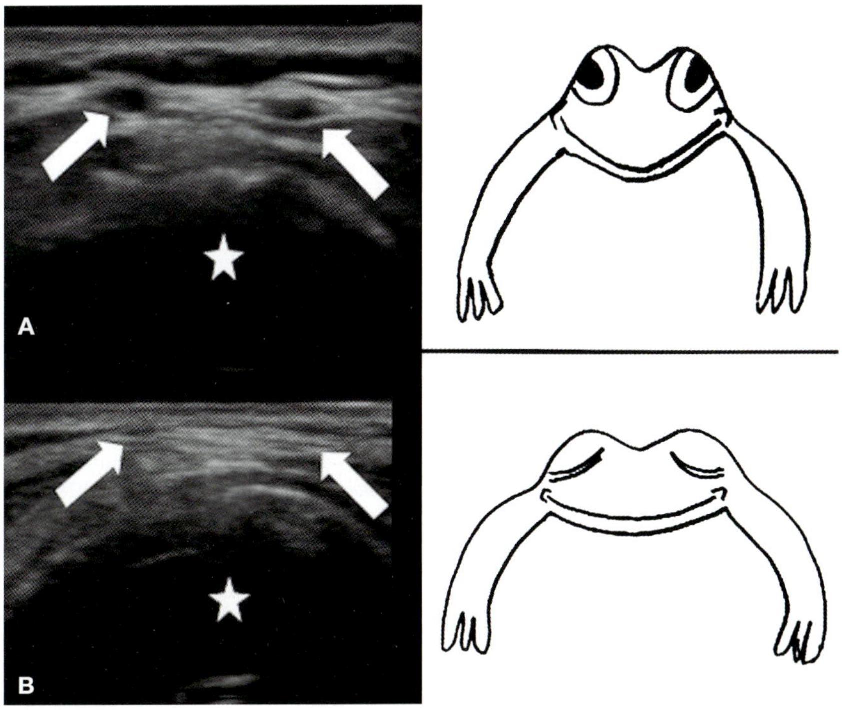

FIGURE 16.6 | The 'blinking frog' ultrasound sign establishes the presence of pretracheal vasculature. In the ultrasound images, the white star marks the trachea. The white arrows show the presence of two pretracheal vessels **(A)** which are compressible **(B)**. (From Tuinman PR, van Westerloo D, Slot S, Touw HRW. The 'blinking frog' ultrasound sign establishes the presence of pretracheal vasculature. *Intensive Care Med*. 2019;45(2):261-262. Figure 1.)

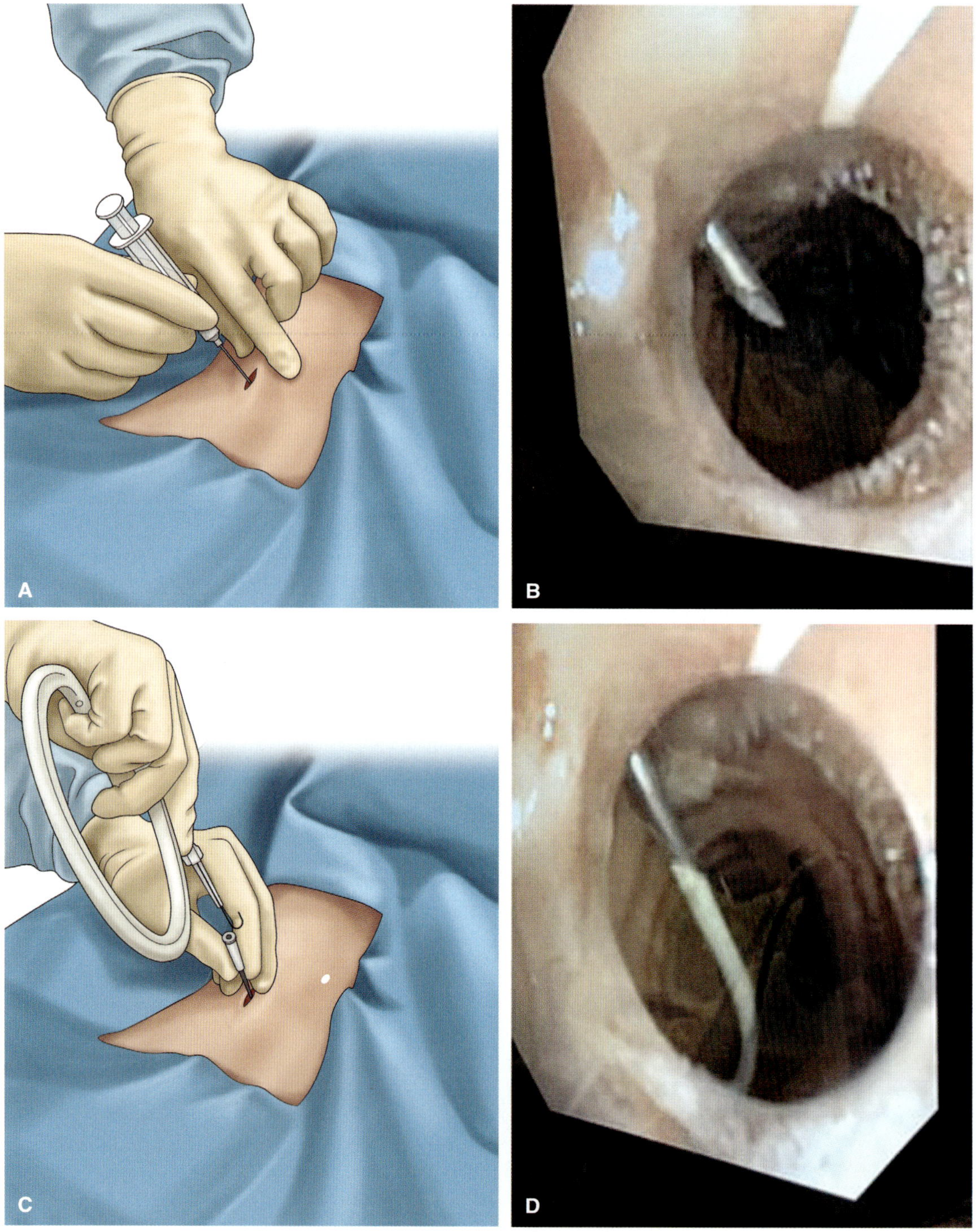

FIGURE 16.7 ▮ A. Insertion of an introducer needle with **(B)** endoscopic view. **C.** Insertion of a guidewire with **(D)** endoscopic view. (**B and D.** Reprinted from Lerner AD, Yarmus L. Percutaneous dilational tracheostomy. *Clin Chest Med*. 2018;39(1):211-222, with permission from Elsevier.)

TIPS

- *Transillumination may also be used to facilitate the positioning of the tube. In order to ensure control of the airway, the bronchoscope is kept within the oral endotracheal tube at all times.*
- *The needle bevel should face downward while being introduced into the tracheal wall to insert the guidewire into the distal trachea.*
- *Special care should be taken to avoid damaging the balloon on the oral endotracheal tube when inserting the finder needle.*

- Insert the guidewire through the needle. It can be seen as advancing distally down the trachea, toward the carina on the bronchoscope.
  - Remove the needle and advance the first small tracheal dilator to dilate the tract. Progressively larger dilators are then used to dilate the tract further (Figure 16.8).
  - Keeping the wire and the protective sheath in place, remove the progressive dilator and insert the tracheostomy tube, with the curve directed toward the patient's head, directly into the trachea over the wire. As the tube is advanced into the patient's trachea, rotate the tube 180° to its standard orientation, which will prevent the creation of a pretracheal plane (Figure 16.9).

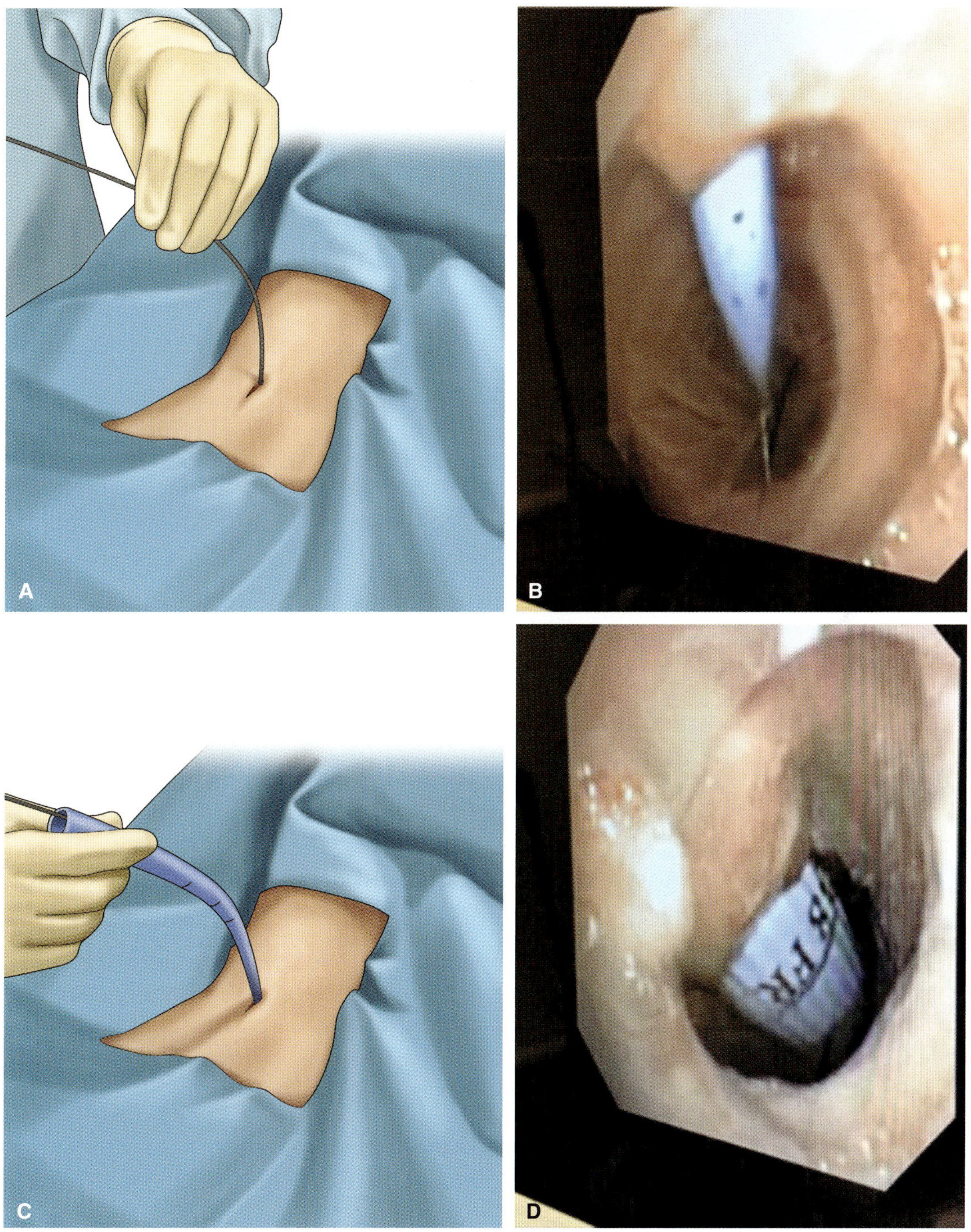

FIGURE 16.8 ▌ A. Insertion of a 14 French dilator over wire and **(B)** endoscopic view. **C.** Insertion of dilator and **(D)** endoscopic view. (**B and D.** Reprinted from Lerner AD, Yarmus L. Percutaneous dilational tracheostomy. *Clin Chest Med*. 2018;39(1):211-222, with permission from Elsevier.)

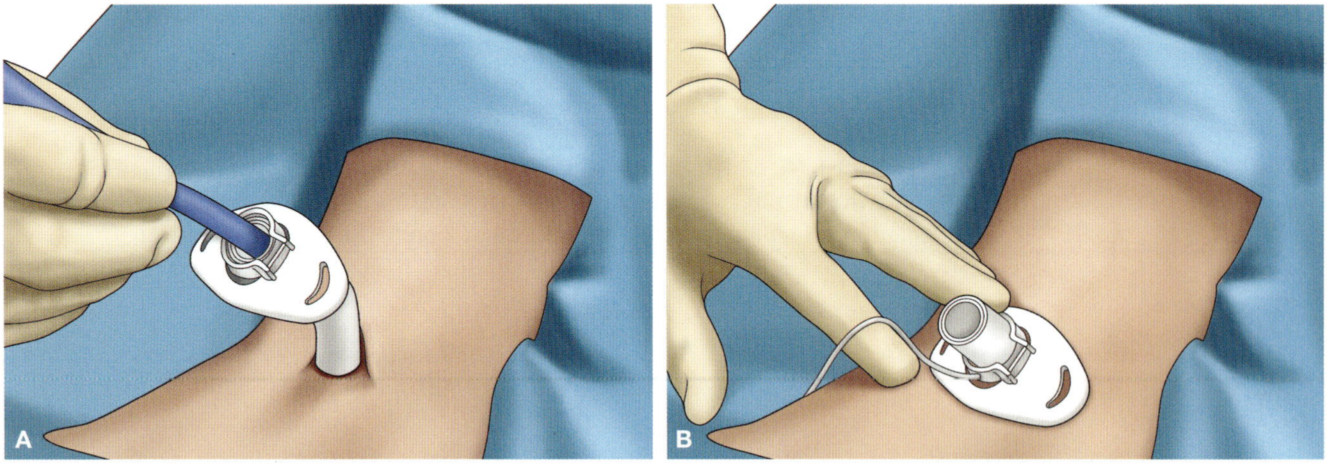

FIGURE 16.9 ▌ **A.** Insertion of tracheostomy tube over the introducer. **B.** Tracheostomy tube in the final position. (From Lerner AD, Yarmus L. Percutaneous dilational tracheostomy. *Clin Chest Med*. 2018;39(1):211-222.)

- The protective sheath and wire can be removed now. Inflate the tracheostomy cuff at low pressure, and resume ventilation.
- The presence of end-tidal carbon dioxide confirms placement in the airway. Evaluate for bilateral breath sounds and chest rise as well. Also, pay attention to the oxygen saturation, which should be stable.
- Once satisfactory placement of the tracheostomy tube is confirmed, remove the oral endotracheal tube, and secure the tracheostomy tube with a tracheostomy collar. Closing the skin incision around the tracheostomy with a suture is optional.

Complications

Immediate Complications (Perioperative Period)

- Hemorrhage, severe if blood vessels are damaged
- Tube occlusion, tube misplacement
- Pneumothorax
- Surgical emphysema
- Loss of the upper airway

Delayed Complications (Postoperative Period <7 days)

- Tube blockage with secretions or blood
- Tube displacement
- Stomal infection
- Infection of the bronchial tree
- Development of tracheoinnominate fistula
- Formation of a tracheo-oesophageal fistula

Late Complications (Late Postoperative Period >7 days)

- Granulation tissue formation
- Tracheal dilation, stenosis, tracheomalacia
- Pneumonia
- Dysphagia
  - Development of tracheoinnominate fistula
  - Development of a tracheo-oesophageal fistula

PEARLS AND PITFALLS

Use of Tracheostomy During the COVID-19 Pandemic

- Patients may undergo either open tracheostomy or percutaneous dilatational tracheostomy. Techniques that minimize aerosolization should be utilized.
- The use of personal protective equipment is recommended to minimize the risk of any infection during the procedure.
- While performing percutaneous tracheostomy, a complete neuromuscular paralysis helps minimize the cough reflex and involves a period of apnea when the ventilatory circuit is considered open.
- A novel percutaneous tracheostomy technique has been described to reduce the risk of aerosolization, thus minimizing the risk of infection for healthcare workers.

Suggested Readings

1. Angel L, Kon ZN, Chang SH, et al. Novel percutaneous tracheostomy for critically ill patients with COVID-19. *Ann Thorac Surg*. 2020;110(3), 1006-1011.
2. Bacchetta MD, Girardi LN, Southard EJ, et al. Comparison of open versus bedside percutaneous dilatational Tracheostomy in the cardiothoracic surgical patient: outcomes and financial analysis. *Ann Thorac Surg*. 2005.79(6), 1879-1885,
3. Cheung NH, Napolitano LM. Tracheostomy: epidemiology, indications, timing, technique, and outcomes. *Respir Care*. 2014;59(6):895-919. discussion 6-9.
4. Freeman BD. Tracheostomy update: when and how. *Crit Care Clin*. 2017;33(2):311-322.
5. Hashimoto DA, Axtell AL, Auchincloss HG. Percutaneous tracheostomy. *N Engl J Med*. 2020;383(20):e112.
6. Kidane B, Pierre AF. From open to bedside percutaneous tracheostomy. *Thorac Surg Clin*. 2018;28(3):263-276.
7. McGrath BA, Brenner MJ, Warrillow SJ, et al. Tracheostomy in the COVID-19 era: global and multidisciplinary guidance. *Lancet Respir Med*. 2020;8(7):717-725.
8. Mecham JC, Thomas OJ, Pirgousis P, Janus JR. Utility of tracheostomy in patients with COVID-19 and other special considerations. *Laryngoscope*. 2020;130(11):2546-2549.
9. Okonkwo I, Cochrane L, Fernandez E. Perioperative management of a child with a tracheostomy. *BJA Educ*. 2020;20(1):18-25.

Chapter 17

Postpneumonectomy Bronchopleural Fistula

JAMES T. NAWALANIEC
DOUGLAS J. MATHISEN

Perioperative Considerations

- Bronchopleural fistula (BPF) is best avoided by identifying high-risk patients and using precise, atraumatic technique during the index operation (Table 17.1).

TABLE 17.1 | Risk factors and operative considerations for BPF.

Risk Factors for BPF	Operative Considerations to Prevent BPF
• Right pneumonectomy	• Avoid devascularizing the bronchial stump
• Completion pneumonectomy	• Avoid excessive nodal dissection
• Postoperative positive pressure ventilation	• Ensure a short bronchial stump remains
• Preexisting infection (ie, TB)	• Avoid excessive tension on bronchial closure
• Prior irradiation	• Consider prophylactic coverage of high-risk stumps with a pedicled tissue flap
• Malnutrition	• We prefer sutured bronchial closure, although staples are acceptable
• Steroids	

BPF, bronchopleural fistula; TB, tuberculosis

- The incidence of BPF after lung resection is about 3% to 6% (range 9%-14% in the literature).
- Patients with a postoperative BPF usually present with a productive cough and a new or enlarging air-fluid level on chest radiograph (Figure 17.1).
  - Patients with a suspected BPF require several diagnostic studies to guide treatment. Chest computed tomography with intravenous contrast is the best test to define the location of the BPF relative to the hilar structures, most importantly the pulmonary artery (Figure 17.2).
  - Flexible bronchoscopy is used to visualize the fistula location on the bronchial stump (Figure 17.3).

TIPS

If the fistula is not readily apparent, the surgeon may gently probe with flexible closed biopsy forceps, keeping in mind that the pulmonary artery can be very close.

  - Thoracoscopy may be helpful if bronchoscopy is equivocal. Locate pleural space with needle aspiration, then insert the thoracoscope. Insufflate through endotracheal tube to 30 to 40 cm of pressure to identify the presence of air bubbles.
  - Bronchogram and V/Q scan are rarely used.

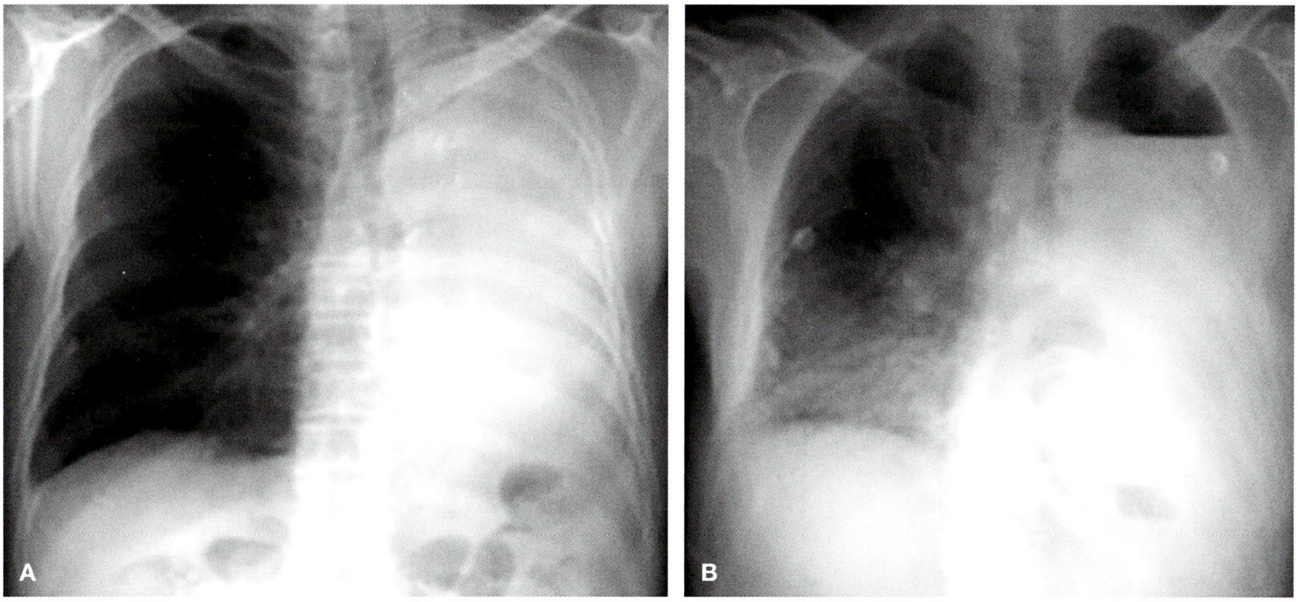

FIGURE 17.1 ▌ New air-fluid level seen postpneumonectomy. Chest x-ray at discharge shows the pleural space is filled with fluid (**A**). Chest x-ray 3.5 weeks later demonstrates a new air-fluid level (**B**).

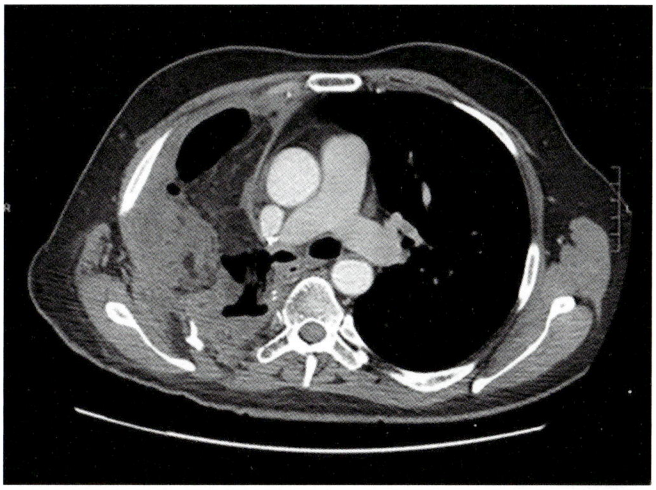

FIGURE 17.2 ▌ CT scan with contrast demonstrating right mainstem bronchopleural fistula (BPF). Notice proximity of right main pulmonary artery stump to the right main bronchus and BPF.

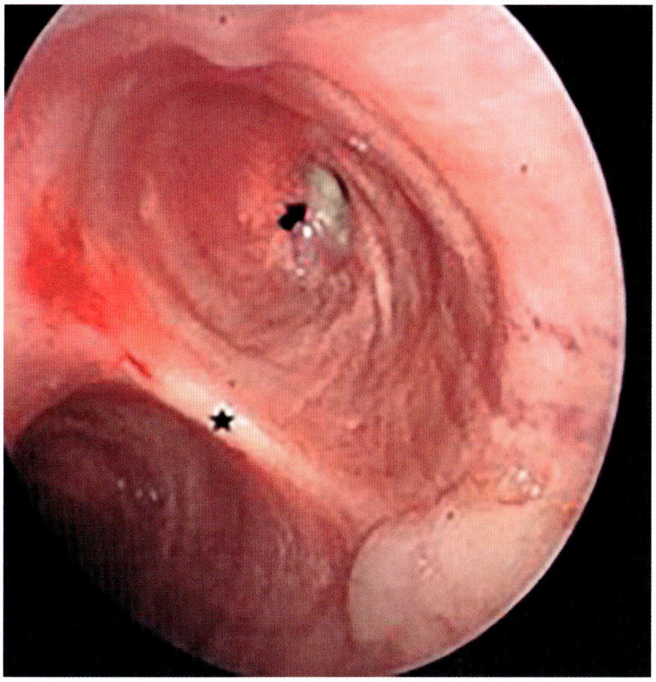

FIGURE 17.3 ▌ Bronchopleural fistula (BPF) seen in the right main bronchus. Note the long bronchial stump, which increases the risk of developing a BPF.

Management

- The specific management for BPF depends on the timing of presentation relative to the index operation. However, the same three basic principles apply: (1) control the infection with drainage of the chest, (2) identify, excise, and repair the BPF, and (3) obliterate the residual pleural space.

Acute BPF—0 to 7 Days Postoperative (Implies Technical Failure)

- Immediate management:
  - Sit upright or operated side down to avoid aspiration and contamination of the opposite lung.
  - Administer broad-spectrum antibiotics.
  - Place a chest tube in a dependent position in the pleural cavity (Figure 17.4).

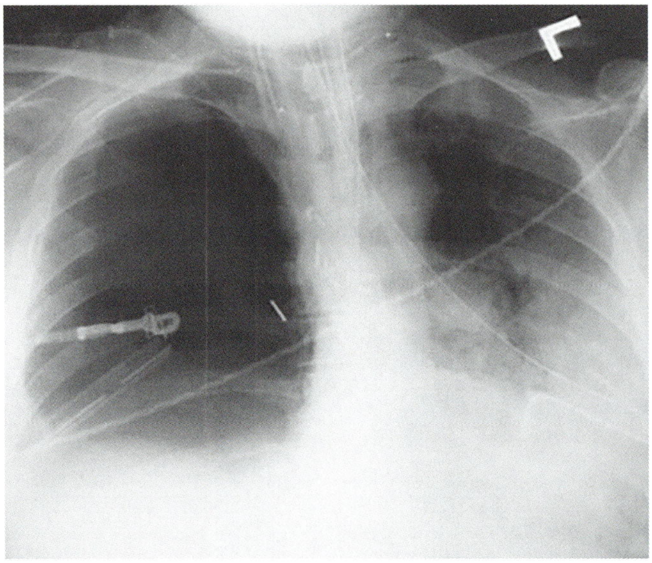

FIGURE 17.4 Chest x-ray showing complete drainage of fluid by a large dependent empyema drainage tube.

  - Definitive management
    - In early BPF, immediate reoperation is indicated. The healthy lung must be protected with either a long single-lumen endotracheal tube or double-lumen tube to prevent contamination and pneumonia.

Intermediate BPF—7 to 14 Days Postoperative (Pleural Fluid Cultures Are Positive But There Is No Frank Pus)

- Initial management is similar to acute BPF. Immediately begin antibiotics and place a large, dependent chest tube in the pleural space.
- If conditions permit (not grossly contaminated and minimal surgical inflammation), operative intervention is indicated to close and buttress the fistula as one would with an acute BPF. However, given the longer contamination of the pleural cavity with the possibility of developing infection, open drainage of the pleural space is preferred.
- In cases of gross contamination or significant inflammation, the BPF is managed with window thoracostomy, delayed repair, and obliteration of the pleural space with vascularized tissue flaps. This is similar to management for a late BPF (see next section).

LATE BPF—More Than 14 Days Postoperative (Established Infection With Pus Is Present in the Pleural Space)

- As with early and intermediate BPF, the first step in management is controlling the infection with chest tube drainage and antibiotics. Convert to open window thoracostomy drainage early (Figure 17.5).
  - For a window thoracostomy, it is important to make a generous window to allow for contraction of the wound. A U-shaped, inferiorly based skin flap is sewn carefully to the edges of the wound, which helps maintain a window and decrease contraction.

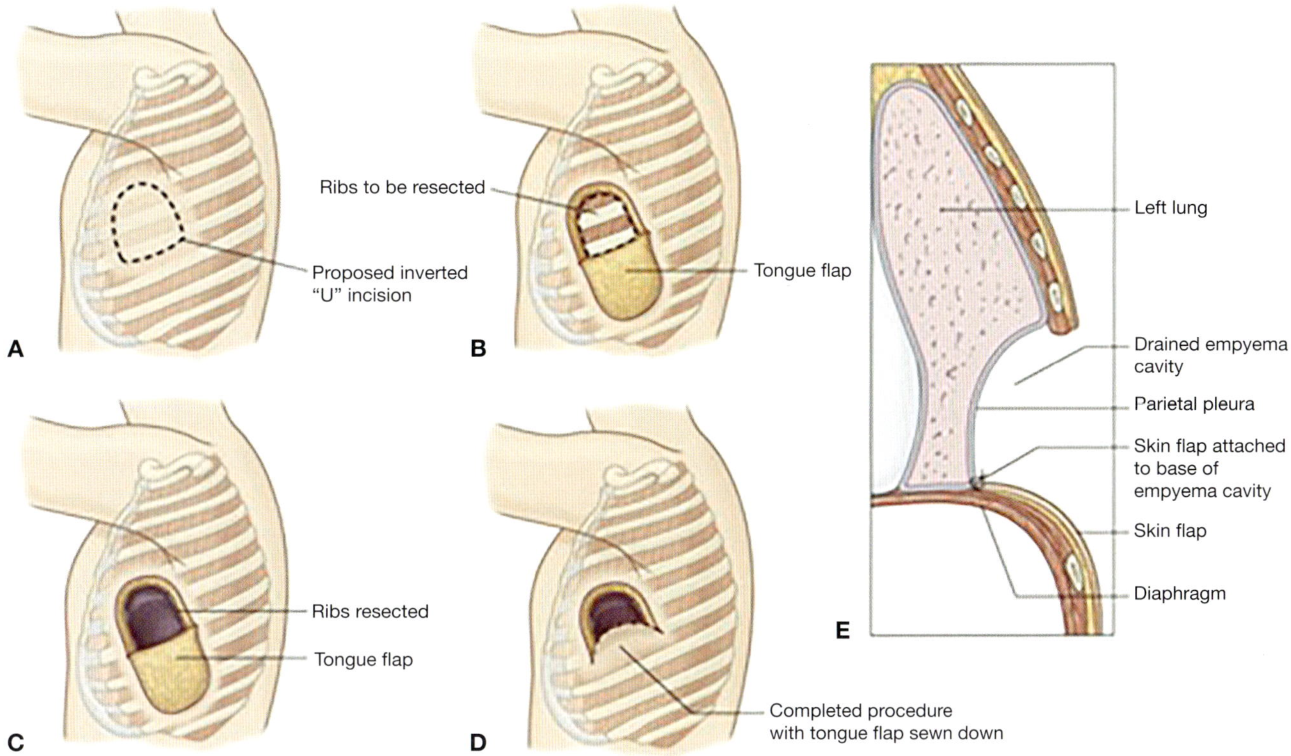

FIGURE 17.5 ▮ A-E. Open window thoracostomy—Eloesser flap and Clagett procedure. (From Albomoz CR, Kerrigan CL, Vidal EDC, et al. Evidence-based medicine and health services research in plastic surgery. In: Song DH, Neligan PC, eds. *Plastic Surgery: Volume 4—Lower Extremity, Trunk, and Burns*. 4th ed. Elsevier; 2018:115-134. Figure 10.20.)

Principles of Definitive Management

- Define the anatomy of the BPF using bronchoscopy and CT with IV contrast as discussed.
- Wide open drainage of the pleural space. Pack space (tightly if large air leak) and change dressings frequently as needed or at least twice daily.
- Irrigation and intravenous antibiotics are determined by culture data (10 days is sufficient). The key to success is mechanical debridement of the space.
- Must be extremely clean before repair (usually weeks later) is considered.

Technique

Acute BPF

- Perform a wide thoracotomy.
- Send pleural fluid for Gram stain and culture.
- Debride the bronchus and fistula, and primarily close the defect with interrupted 3-0 or 4-0 Vicryl absorbable sutures.
- Buttress the bronchial repair with intercostal or serratus muscle, or omentum. Pericardial fat is not recommended.

TIPS

If dealing with a short mainstem stump, one may have to pull the endotracheal tube back to manually oppose bronchus and membranous wall of the trachea. Intermittent apnea is used to place sutures. Reinsert tube or cover bronchus with finger during periods of ventilation.

- Wash out the pleural space with copious amounts of saline and antibiotic solution.
- Management of the residual pleural space.

- Fill with empiric antibiotics if clean and Gram stain is negative.
- Angiocatheter is left in the chest to irrigate with antibiotics postoperatively (Figure 17.6). Culture effluent every 2 days and adjust antibiotics accordingly if cultures are positive.
- Remove catheter after 5 to 7 days if cultures are negative. Fill with appropriate antibiotic solution (antibiotic concentration to equal desired serum concentration) prior to removal.
- If cultures are positive, may have to convert to open drainage (see below).

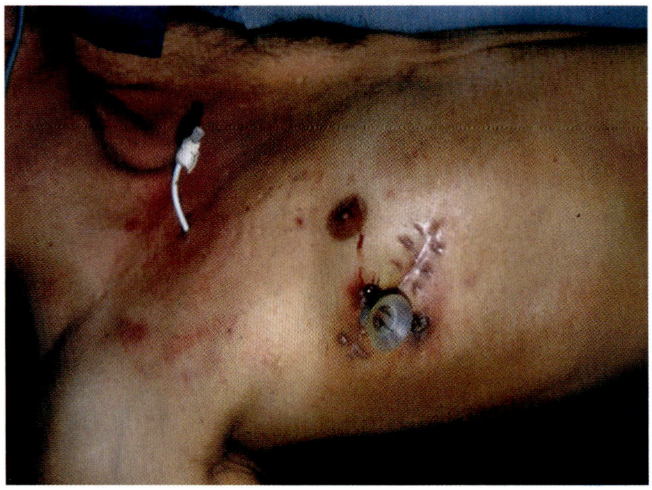

FIGURE 17.6 ▮ Delayed closure of residual cavity with catheter placement for antibiotic irrigation and drainage through empyema tube.

TIPS

If the bronchial stump cannot be closed without tension, sew a pedicled muscle flap to the bronchial opening carefully as if doing an anastomosis. Must leave a chest tube or open window thoracostomy until certain the BPF is closed.

Late BPF—Transthoracic Approach

- It is important to again emphasize the utility of a preoperative CT chest with IV contrast to understand the location of the BPF relative to the pulmonary artery to avoid inadvertent injury during the case.
- Begin the dissection by very carefully peeling the inflammatory tissue and scarring away from the site of the BPF (Figure 17.7). The tissue usually comes off layer by layer, like peeling an onion.

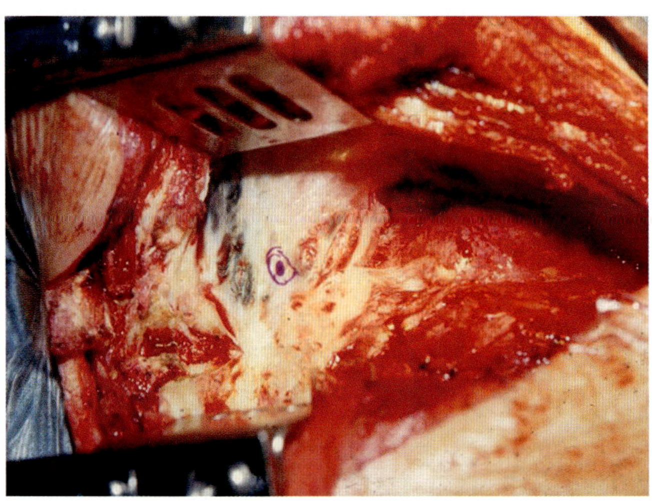

FIGURE 17.7 ▮ Small fistulous opening circled by marker. Thick scar is evident.

- Eventually, under the thick rind of scar, soft, healthy mediastinal tissue will be exposed (Figure 17.8).

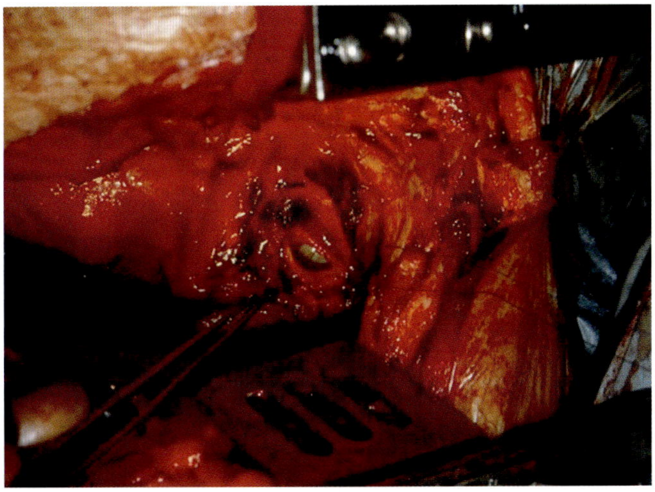

FIGURE 17.8 ▌ The thick scar has been cleared to expose soft mediastinal tissue and the bronchus. The bronchopleural fistula and distal bronchial stump have been amputated, leaving healthy bronchus. The endotracheal balloon of the long single-lumen tube is seen in the bronchial lumen.

- At this point, the origin of the fistula at the bronchus must be adequately exposed to evaluate the anatomy of the fistula and assess options for repair. The fistulous tract to the bronchus is excised (Figure 17.9).

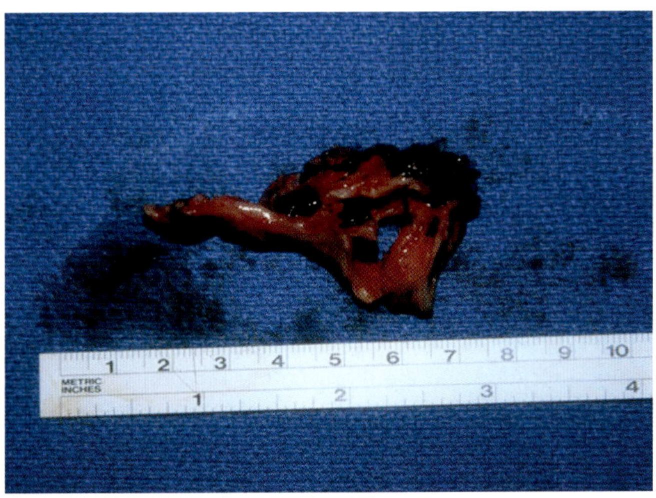

FIGURE 17.9 ▌ Long fistulous tract excised.

- If enough bronchus exists to reamputate the bronchus, this should be done. If not, freshen the bronchial stump to prepare it for closure.
- The bronchial stump is closed with interrupted 3-0 or 4-0 Vicryl sutures (Figure 17.10).

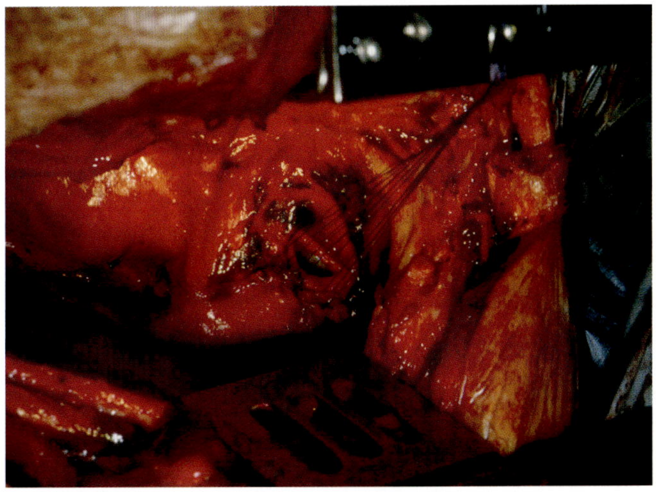

FIGURE 17.10 ▌ Interrupted absorbable sutures are used to close the bronchus.

- Buttress the bronchial closure with vascularized tissue (our preference is with an omental flap, see Figure 17.11).

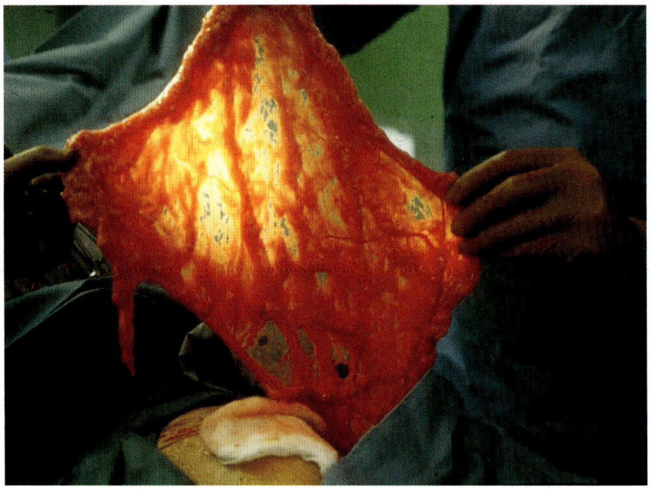

FIGURE 17.11 ▮ Omentum mobilized on a right gastroepiploic artery.

- A detailed description of an omental flap harvest is beyond the scope of this chapter, but in general, the blood supply to the omentum is ligated except for the right gastroepiploic artery and vein, which serves as the vascular pedicle. The freed omentum is then passed through a substernal tunnel, and then sewn to the bronchial closure (Figures 17.12-17.15).
- Obliterate any remaining pleural space with vascularized tissue flaps (Figure 17.16).
- Muscle buttress options:
  - Latissimus
  - Serratus (Figure 17.17)
  - Pectoralis major
  - Free flap with microvascular anastomosis
- Once the pleural space has been completely filled, a chest tube is placed and the thoracotomy incision is closed (Figure 17.18).
- If there is not enough tissue to completely fill the pleural space, any remaining space may instead be filled with antibiotic solution and the thoracotomy incision closed in multiple layers to avoid leakage of fluid (Clagett procedure).
  - Note, if there is concern for residual infection in the remaining pleural space that cannot be obliterated with a tissue flap, the wound may be left open for regular antibiotic-soaked dressing changes on the floor until there is satisfactory clearance of all remaining infection. Once the residual space is clean, then the antibiotic solution may be instilled and the wound closed.

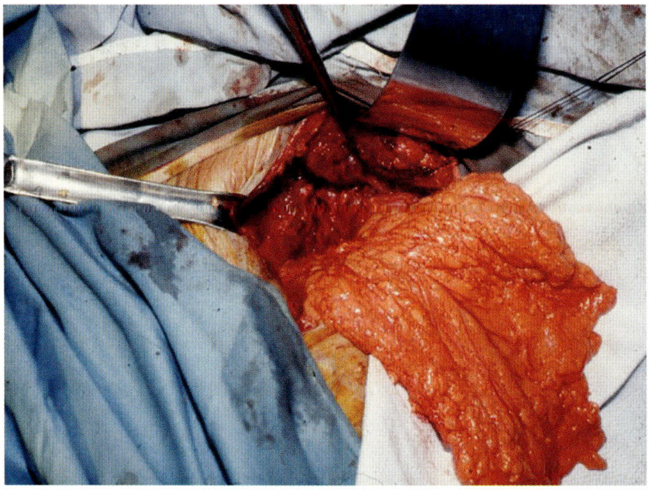

FIGURE 17.12 ▮ The omentum is brought substernally and an opening is created in thick scar above the pericardium. The opening must be generous so as not to compromise the blood supply of the omentum.

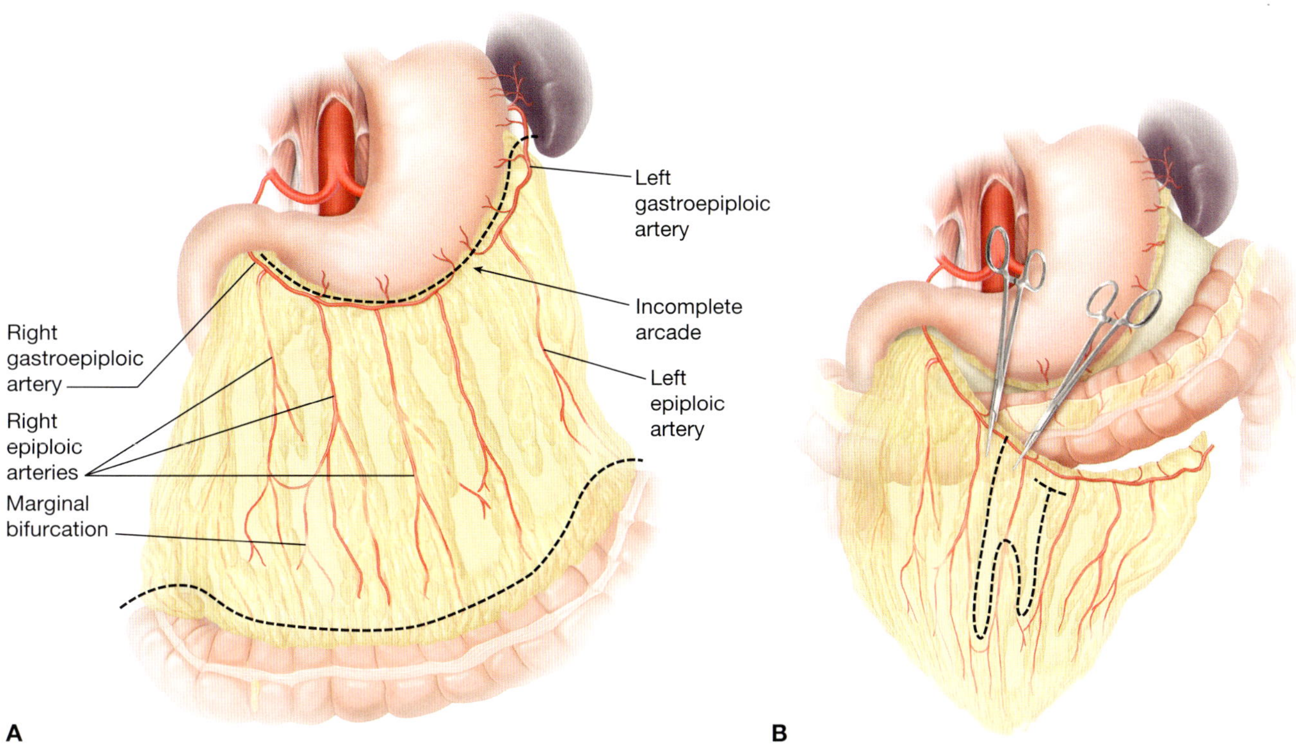

FIGURE 17.13 | A. Anatomy of the omentum. The dashed lines represent the line of division of the omentum from the stomach and from the transverse colon. Note that great care should be taken to identify and preserve the right gastroepiploic artery, the primary blood supply for this flap when rotated to the chest. **B.** If further lengthening of the flap is needed, the arcade can be divided at one or more points to produce a longer pedicle. If this is necessary, vascular clamps are first placed at the sites of potential transection and the distal omentum is examined for viability before vascular division. (From Burt BM, Shrager JS. Omental flap In: Mathisen DJ, Morse C, eds. *Master Techniques in Surgery: Thoracic Surgery—Lung Resections, Bronchoplasty*. Wolters Kluwer; 2015:495-501. Figure 51.1.)

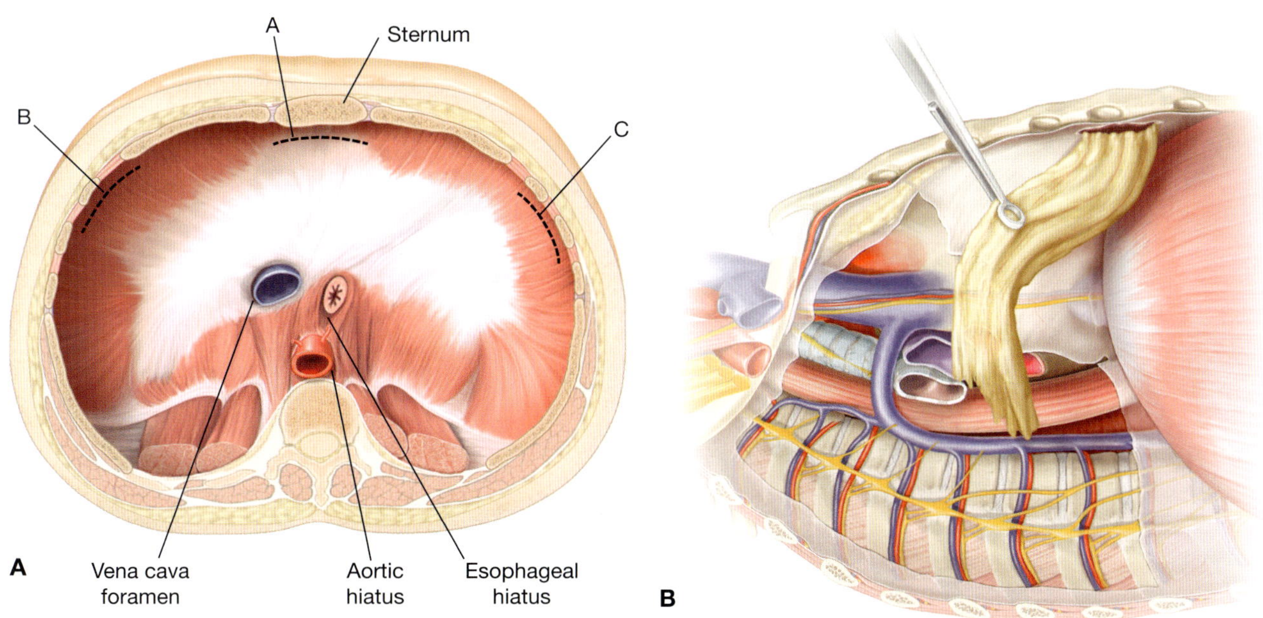

FIGURE 17.14 | A. Dashed lines labeled A, B, and C indicate possible diaphragmatic apertures for transposition of the omentum. The opening for substernal transfer is shown in the retrosternal position **(A)**, and the lateral incisions indicate the region for anterolateral passage into the hemithorax. **B.** Following placement in a retrosternal pocket during the abdominal portion of this procedure, the mediastinal pleura is divided inferiorly and the omentum is retrieved. (From Burt BM, Shrager JS. Omental flap. In: Mathisen DJ, Morse C, eds. *Master Techniques in Surgery: Thoracic Surgery—Lung Resections, Bronchoplasty*. Wolters Kluwer; 2015:495-501. Figure 51.2.)

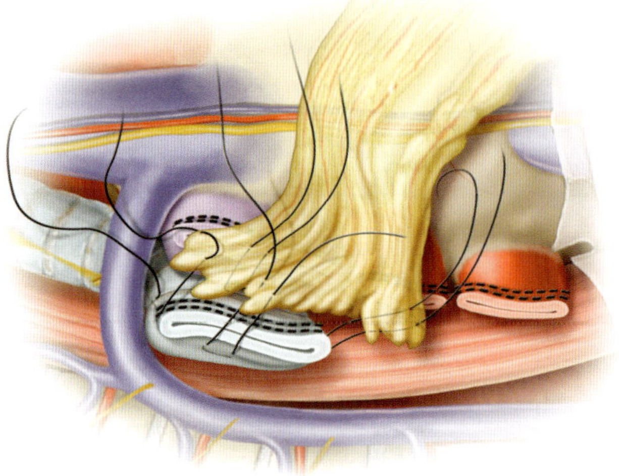

FIGURE 17.15 ▌ Buttress of a pedicled omental flap to the bronchial stump following pneumonectomy. This diagram shows four sutures (more can be used) that are placed to secure the omentum over the stump prior to tying them down. The sutures are all placed before any are tied. They are taken as partial-thickness, horizontal mattress bites through the omentum and then to the bronchus, 3 to 4 mm proximal to the line of closure. (From Burt BM, Shrager JS. Omental flap. In: Mathisen DJ, Morse C, eds. *Master Techniques in Surgery: Thoracic Surgery—Lung Resections, Bronchoplasty*. Wolters Kluwer; 2015:495-501. Figure 51.3.)

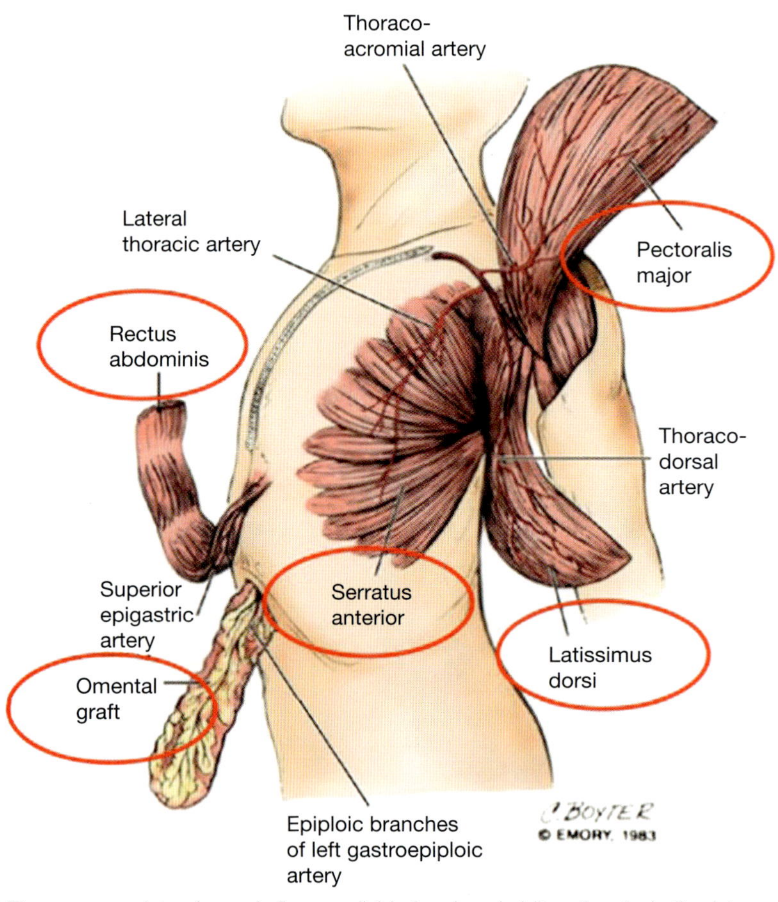

FIGURE 17.16 ▌ There are a variety of muscle flaps available for pleural obliteration, including intercostal, latissimus, serratus, pectoralis, and rectus muscles. The omentum is also an option if not used for the bronchial closure buttress. (From Chapter 98. In: Patterson GA, Pearson FG, eds. *Pearson's Thoracic & Esophageal Surgery*. 3rd ed. Elsevier; 2008. Figure 98.7.)

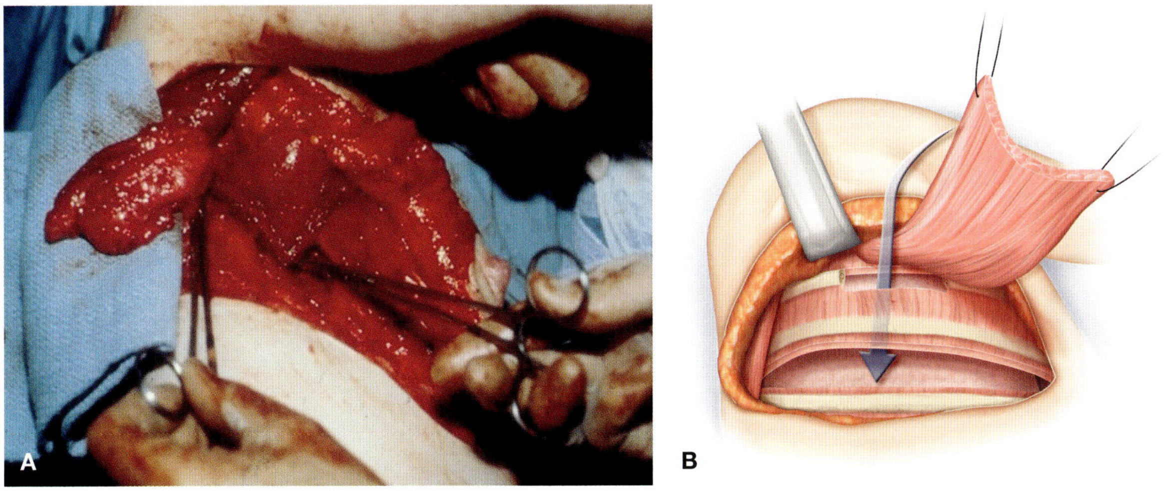

FIGURE 17.17 | Mobilization of chest wall muscle (ie, serratus, pectoralis, or latissimus muscles) to fill the residual cavity (left, **A**). Illustration of serratus mobilization and transposition into the thoracic cavity after removing a segment of the ipsilateral third rib (right, **B**). (B from Nichols FC. Transthoracic repair bronchopleural fistula. In: Mathisen DJ, Morse C, eds. *Master Techniques in Surgery: Thoracic Surgery—Lung Resections, Bronchoplasty*. Wolters Kluwer; 2015:477-484. Figure 49.3.)

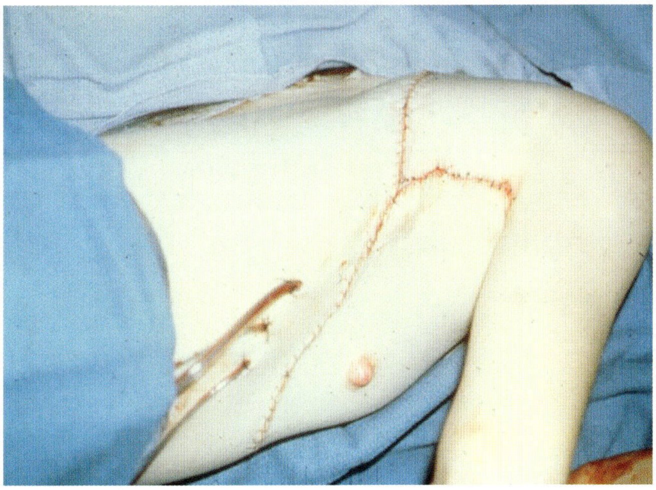

FIGURE 17.18 | Drains, wound closure after obliteration of cavity with muscle transposition.

- If the Clagett procedure fails and infection redevelops in the fluid, the pleural space should be drained. Repeating the Clagett procedure one to two times brings success of this procedure to 85% to 90%. If it fails after the third attempt, leave the pleural cavity open and pursue muscle transposition to fill the cavity (ie, free flap).
- If all attempts to close the space fail, the remaining cavity is left open and packed with sterile packing.

Results

Success of buttressed repair of BPF in our experience:

- Omentum has the highest success rate, around 92% (25 cases).
- Muscle success rate is about 64% (14 cases, 9 closed successfully).
- Of just two cases with pleural buttressing, neither successfully closed the BPF.

Successful management of the residual space in our experience:

- We have similar results with both primary closure with muscle and secondary closure with antibiotics (Clagett procedure). Both approaches have about 75% successful closure in our experience.

Late BPF—Transsternal Approach

- A transsternal approach is an option in patients who have had multiple transthoracic procedures (especially previously placed flaps into the pleural space that need to be protected), a long bronchial stump, or a BPF at the carina.
  - Perform a standard sternotomy and open the pericardium anteriorly and posteriorly to expose the carina (Figure 17.19).

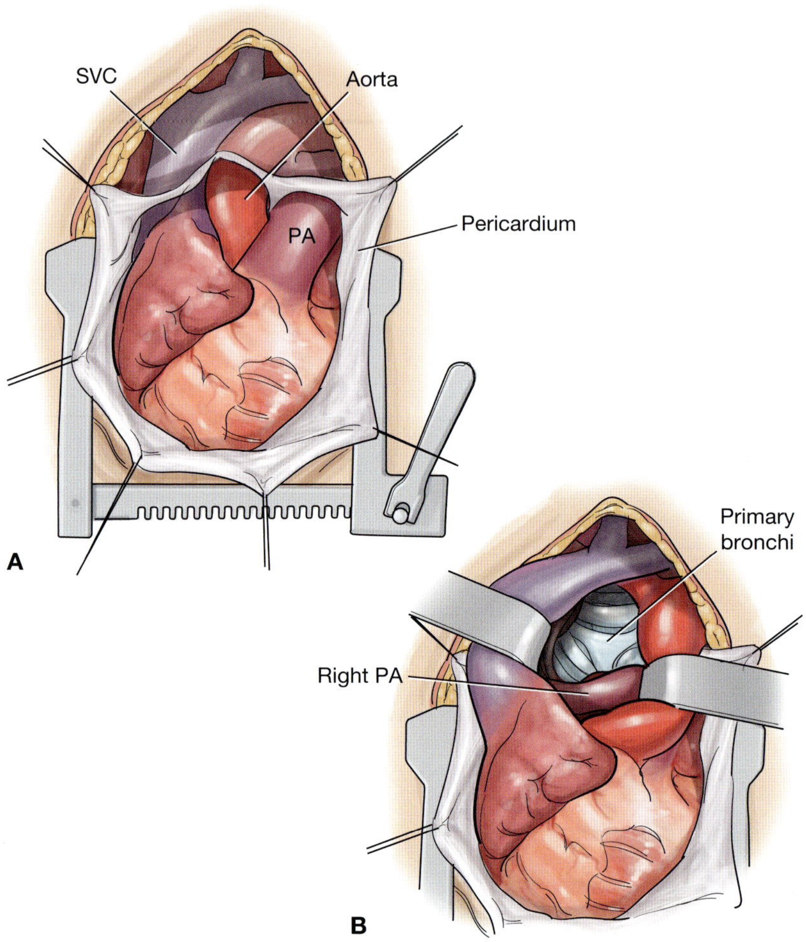

FIGURE 17.19 ▮ A. A full median sternotomy has been made and the anterior pericardium is open, exposing the great vessels (SVC, superior vena cava; PA, pulmonary artery). **B.** A wide incision of the posterior pericardium exposes both the bronchi and the lower trachea. (Reprinted from Ginsberg RJ, Saborio DV. Management of the recalcitrant postpneumonectomy bronchopleural fistula: the transsternal transpericardial approach. *Semin Thorac Cardiovasc Surg*. 2001;13:20-26, with permission from Elsevier. Copyright © 2001 W.B. Saunders Company. All rights reserved. Published by Elsevier Inc. All rights reserved.)

- Retract the superior vena cava and aorta, and mobilize the innominate vein to expose the bronchus.
- Carefully debride and close the bronchial defect with interrupted 4-0 Vicryl sutures. Cover the repair with thymus or mediastinal fat.
- Fill the residual pleural space with flaps or antibiotic instillation (Clagett procedure).
- Note, if the transsternal approach is too difficult to safely clear and close the bronchial defect, the proximal bronchus (healthy segment) may be divided, separated, and both ends (proximal and distal) closed with interrupted 4-0 Vicryl sutures and buttressed. The distal part of the bronchus, containing the BPF and fistulous tract, can then be addressed at a later date via thoracotomy (Figure 17.20).

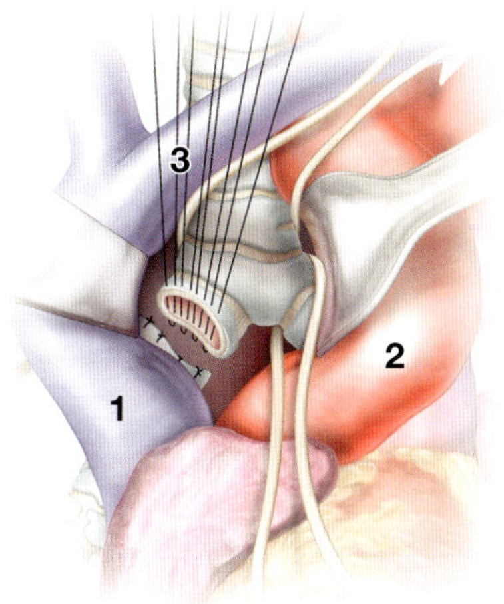

FIGURE 17.20 ▮ The proximal bronchus has been divided and closed with interrupted sutures. The distal stump with the bronchopleural fistula is closed. This distal stump can be resected via the sternotomy if feasible, or at a later date when dealing with the residual space via thoracotomy. (1-superior vena cava; 2-ascending aorta; 3-left innominate vein). (From Mercier O, de Perrot M, Keshavjee S. Transsternal repair of postpneumonectomy bronchopleural fistula. Mathisen DJ, Morse C, eds. *Master Techniques in Surgery: Thoracic Surgery—Lung Resections, Bronchoplasty*. Wolters Kluwer; 2015:469-476. Figure 48.3B.)

PEARLS AND PITFALLS

- BPFs are best avoided by handling the bronchus gently and precisely during the initial resection. Keep the stump short and avoid extensive lymphadenectomy and devascularization. Preserve the bronchial artery when possible.
- Prior radiation, postoperative ventilation, right pneumonectomy, preexisting infection, and steroids increase the risk of BPF.
- Early BPF (less than 7 days from the index operation) should be closed immediately if the good lung is healthy.
  - Protect the healthy lung with single-lumen intubation.
  - Repair the bronchus with absorbable suture and buttress with a muscle flap.
  - Fill the cavity with antibiotic solution.
- Intermediate or late BPFs (7-14 days or longer after the index operation) require adequate drainage and sepsis control, and they may be closed if conditions are optimal; otherwise, drain and perform delayed repair.
- Initial drainage should be for at least 10 days, and sepsis should be controlled before attempting the repair.
- For late BPF, widely open the pleural space and pack with antibiotic-soaked dressings daily. Once the infection is controlled and the patient is optimized, perform the bronchial repair and buttress. Fill the residual intrathoracic space with muscle or antibiotic solution.

Suggested Readings

1. Arnold P, Pairolero P. Chest wall reconstruction. *Plastic Reconstructive Surg*. 1997;98:804-810.
2. Deschamps C, Allen M, Miller DL, Nichols FC III, Pairolero PC. Management of post-pneumonectomy empyema and bronchopleural fistula. *Semin Thorac Cardiovasc Surg*. 2001;13(1):13-19.
3. Di Maio M, Perrone F, Deschamps C, Rocco G. A meta-analysis of the impact of bronchial stump coverage on the risk of bronchopleural fistula after pneumonectomy. *Eur J Cardio Thorac Surg*. 2015;48(2):196-200.
4. Puskas JD, Mathisen DJ, Grillo HC, Wain JC, Wright CD, Moncure AC. Treatment strategies for bronchopleural fistula. *J Thorac Cardiovasc Surg*. 1995;109(5):989-996.
5. Shrager JB, Wain JC, Wright CD, et al. Omentum is highly effective in the management of complex cardiothoracic surgical problems. *J Thorac Cardiovasc Surg*. 2003;125(3):526-532.
6. Wright CD, Wain JC, Mathisen DJ, Grillo HC. Post pneumonectomy bronchopleural fistula after sutured bronchial closure: incidence, risk factors and management. *J Thorac Cardiovasc Surg*. 1996;112(5):1367-1371.

Chapter 18

Tracheobronchoplasty for Tracheobronchomalacia

KATE KRAUSE
LANA Y. SCHUMACHER
CAMERON D. WRIGHT

Perioperative Considerations

- Patients must be carefully selected for surgery and should only be considered if severe symptoms (coughing, dyspnea, recurrent infections) match the radiographic and bronchoscopic findings of severe airway collapse. Patients with chronic obstructive pulmonary disease may provide a diagnostic challenge as their symptoms can be overlapping and confounding.
- Dynamic CT scan should demonstrate >50% collapse of the airway with forced expiration. If this is found, then the diagnosis should be confirmed with an awake bronchoscopy, looking for >90% collapse of the airway with normal expiration (not coughing). Bronchoscopy also allows for further assessment of the extent of the malacia and whether there is involvement of the left and right mainstem bronchi.
- There are no specific PFT findings which are diagnostic of tracheobronchomalacia but they should still be performed to assess for other pulmonary pathology and to evaluate the perioperative risk for operation.
- There are two anatomical classifications of tracheobronchomalacia:
  - Cartilaginous malacia results in is the classic, soft anterior tracheal cartilage.
  - Membranous malacia results in excessive forward displacement of the membranous wall—this is more common.
- The principle of tracheoplasty is to stabilize and add rigidity in the case of membranous malacia and to reconfigure the normal shape of the trachea in the case of cartilaginous malacia.
- Robotic-assisted approaches are being used in a few specialized centers, which avoids the morbidity of thoracotomy and allows for a high-definition view of the posterior airway. Initial data suggest robotic approaches are safe and technically feasible.

Anesthesia and Positioning

- Left lateral decubitus position with care to provide appropriate cushioning given prolonged case duration
- Thoracic epidural for postoperative pain control (if open approach) and intercostal nerve blocks (if robotic approach)
- A small left-sided double-lumen tube is used (#35).

Instruments and Equipment

- Open
  - Standard thoracotomy instrument tray
- Robotic-assisted approach
  - Four robotic arms/ports with one additional 12-mm port for the bedside assistant (Figure 18.1)

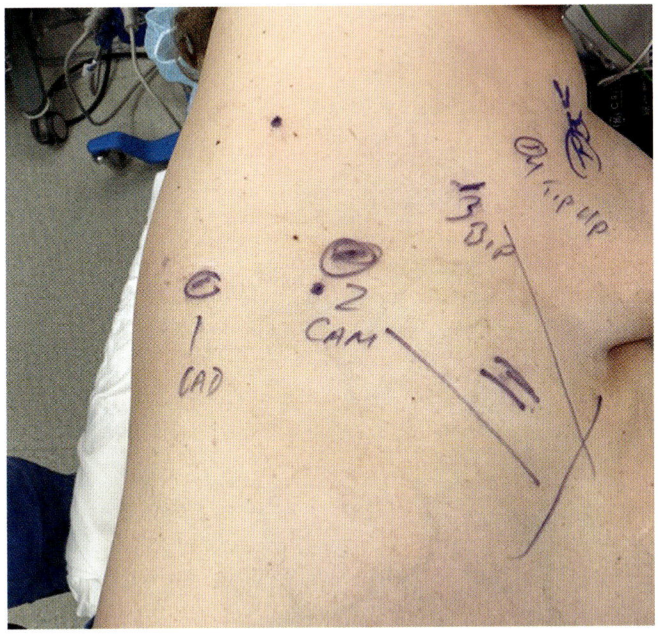

FIGURE 18.1 ▌ Robotic port placement.

- The material to stabilize the posterior tracheal membrane is not standardized. Our preference is either AlloDerm or a reinforced tissue matrix (OviTex) given concerns about possible mesh erosion. Polypropylene mesh is most commonly used although there are rare cases of mesh erosion, which are quite problematic to manage.
- Suture material for the tracheal splint is also varied and includes polypropylene, polyglactin 910, and polydioxanone—we favor polyglactin 910 (Vicryl).

Technique

Open

- Standard high right posterolateral thoracotomy in the fourth intercostal space for exposure of the intrathoracic trachea, bilateral main bronchi, and bronchus intermedius
- The mediastinal pleura is incised over the posterior trachea with care to avoid inadvertent injury to the right vagus nerve (Figure 18.2). The vagus nerve remains on the esophageal side of the dissection plane.

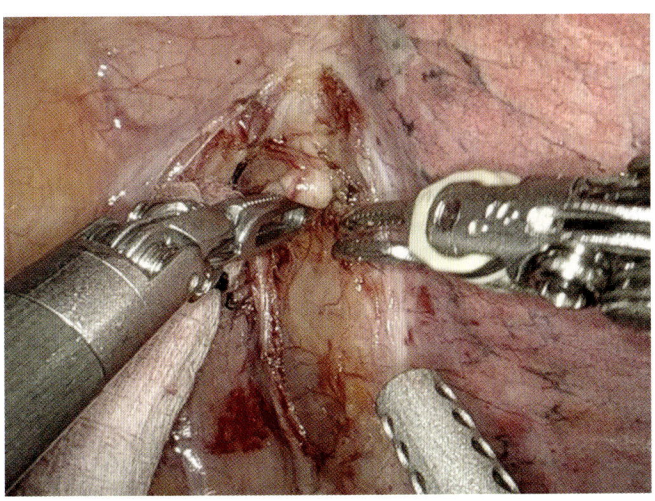

FIGURE 18.2 ▌ Beginning dissection of the inferior pulmonary ligament and the posterior pleura, allowing separation of the airway from the esophagus.

- The azygos vein is ligated to expose the posterior airway (Figures 18.3 and 18.4).

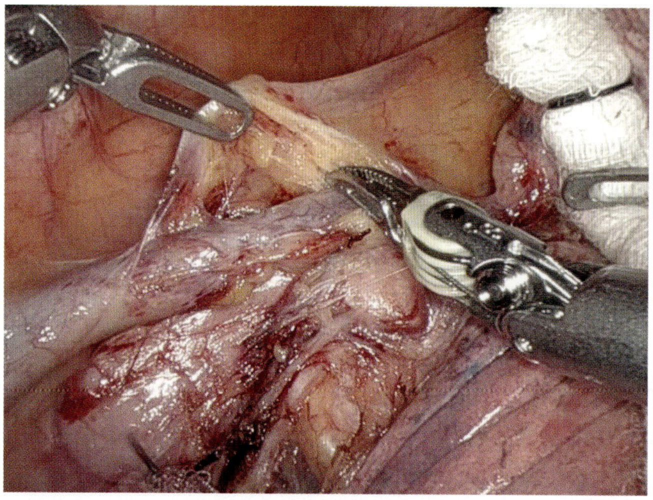

FIGURE 18.3 ▮ Dissection of the azygos vein.

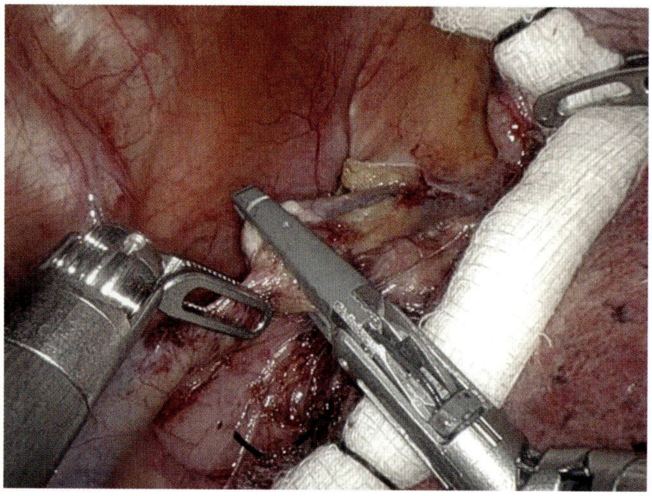

FIGURE 18.4 ▮ Division of the azygos vein with energy device.

- The posterior airway is exposed from the thoracic inlet to include the main bronchi bilaterally. The dissection extends down to the bronchus intermedius on the right and to the take-off of the left upper lobe on the right (Figure 18.5).

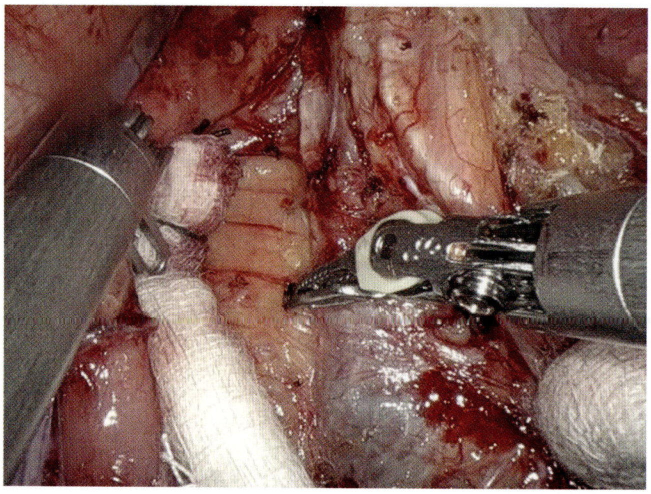

FIGURE 18.5 ▮ Exposure of the trachea.

- The splinting material is measured and cut to appropriate length depending on the extent of the tracheomalacia. Typically, three separate pieces are cut—one for the trachea and two for each main bronchi.

TIPS

- *In patients with cartilaginous malacia, the trachea is often widened with a redundant membranous wall, whereas patients with membranous malacia usually have a trachea of normal size (2.5 cm from side to side in the adult) and thus the membranous wall is not redundant, just hypermobile.*
- *When cutting the splint, it is important to estimate the degree of reduction in the width of the membranous wall that will re-create the D-shape of the trachea. This can be done by pinching the middle portion of the membranous wall together to achieve the appropriate shape and size, then measuring the distance between the lateral walls of the trachea. The typical width of the tracheal splint is 2.5 cm, while the main bronchi are usually 1.5 cm.*

- Suturing of the splint is begun by convention at the top of the intrathoracic trachea and then working down to the carina.
  - The lateral stitches catch the junction of the membranous wall and the cartilaginous wall for added strength (Figure 18.6).

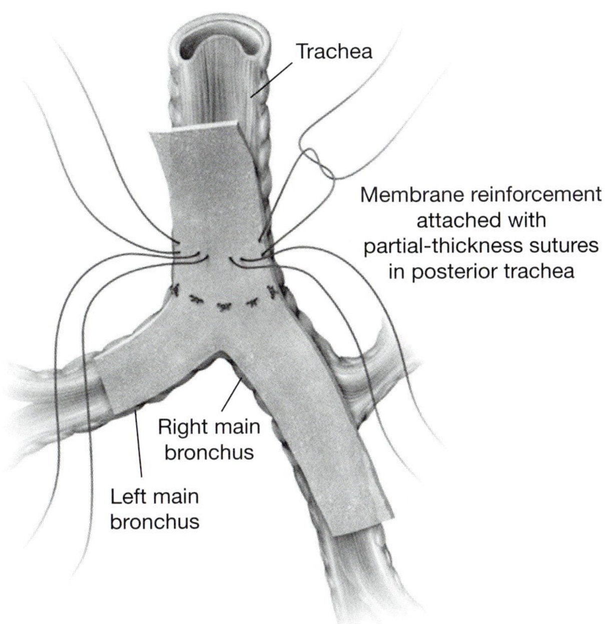

FIGURE 18.6 ▮ Artist's rendering of the concept of tracheobronchoplasty. The membranous wall splinting material is carefully sutured with partial thickness fine 4-0 sutures to the posterior membranous wall to stiffen the membranous wall and reconfigure the shape of the trachea. The strip of the splinting material is carefully measured such that when the sutures are tied, the trachea is reconfigured to a more normal shape (usually 2.5 cm). (Reprinted from Wright CD. Tracheal surgery: posterior splinting tracheoplasty for tracheomalacia. *Oper Tech Thorac Cardiovasc Surg*. 2015;20(1):31-45, with permission from Elsevier.)

  - The middle sutures are placed in a mattress fashion through the splint, then a partial thickness bite through the membranous wall and then back through the splint again (Figure 18.7).

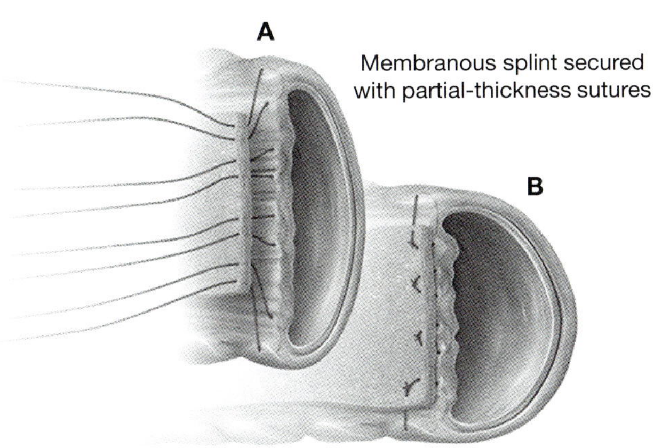

FIGURE 18.7 ▮ Cross-sectional diagram showing spacing of sutures. **A and B.** The lateral ones restore the D curve of the trachea and the central ones fix the redundant membranous wall to the splinting material. The sutures ideally do not penetrate the tracheal lumen. (Reprinted from Wright CD. Tracheal surgery: posterior splinting tracheoplasty for tracheomalacia. *Oper Tech Thorac Cardiovasc Surg*. 2015;20(1):31-45, with permission from Elsevier.)

    - All four sutures should be placed and snapped individually with hemostats for organization.
- The subsequent row of four sutures should be placed prior to tying as it is easier to position the splint for optimal placement of sutures when the preceding row is not already tied.
- Each row of four sutures is placed 5 to 7 mm apart, continuing down the trachea toward the carina.
- Ideally, all sutures are partial thickness in the airway.
- Alternating dyed and undyed sutures on adjacent rows can help prevent inadvertent errors when tying sutures from a given row.
- After completion of the trachea, the right bronchus is reinforced in a similar fashion with a row of three sutures followed by the left mainstem bronchus.
    - The left side is more difficult due to poor exposure deep in the mediastinum and the presence of the endotracheal tube.
    - In communication with the anesthesiologist, the cuff should be temporarily deflated and ventilation held when suturing the left main bronchus so as not to inadvertently puncture the cuff.
- At the end of the case, surveillance bronchoscopy is completed by withdrawing the endotracheal tube to the proximal trachea and inspecting the repair during inhalation and exhalation.
- Any airway narrowing should be identified and corrected immediately. It is not necessary to correct any tracheal sutures, which were mistakenly placed full-thickness through the membranous wall.
- A single chest tube is placed and the thoracotomy is closed in the routine fashion.

Special Considerations for Robotic-Assisted Approach

- Four robotic ports with one additional 12-mm port for the bedside assistant (Figure 18.1).
    - Robotic arms include: Cadiere forceps in the first arm, camera in the second arm, Maryland bipolar in the third arm, and a tip-up fenestrated grasper in the fourth arm.
    - Placement of robotic arm number one should take into consideration the patient's spine as too posterior of a location will make the dissection difficult if the Cadiere forceps is not able to move freely around the anterior vertebral body.
- The subcarinal nodal packet is dissected free from the carinal angle to facilitate optimal suture placement (Figures 18.8 and 18.9).

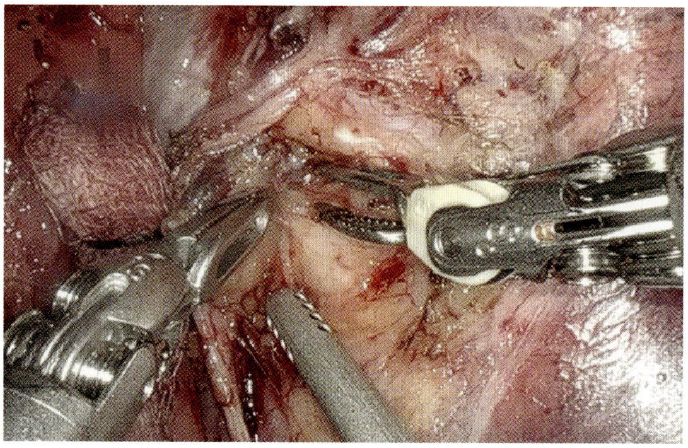

FIGURE 18.8 ▮ Beginning of subcarinal lymph node dissection.

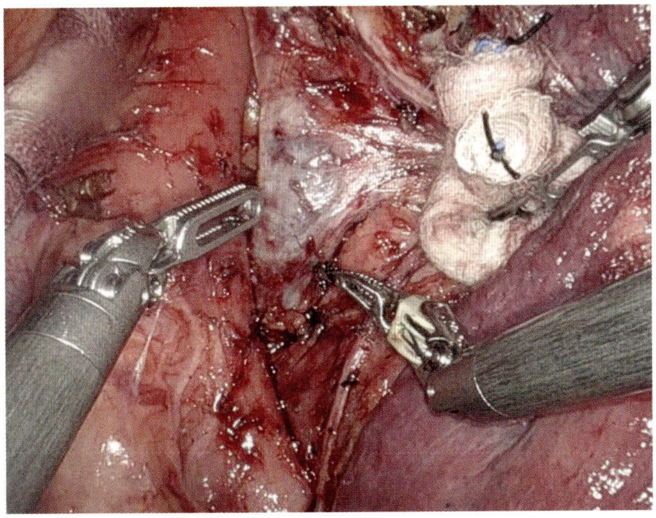

FIGURE 18.9 ▮ Completed lymph node dissection of the carina. Note the blue double-lumen endotracheal tube in the left main bronchus.

- The azygos vein is divided with a vascular staple load (Figure 18.4) or alternatively with a vessel sealer device and then oversewn on each end.
- The posterior trachea is exposed from the thoracic inlet to the bilateral mainstem bronchi with the Maryland bipolar cautery device (Figure 18.5).
- Gentle posterior retraction of the esophagus and rightward retraction of the right lung with rolled pieces of gauze will help nicely expose the left mainstem bronchi.
- 4-0 tracheal sutures are precut to 12 to 15 cm in length to facilitate intracorporeal suturing.
- The splint is sutured into place with rows of sutures on the main trachea and the bilateral bronchi.
  - As opposed to the open approach, improved visualization of the left-sided airway permits suturing of the left main bronchi first (Figures 18.10-18.15), followed by the trachea (Figures 18.16 and 18.17), then the right main bronchi (Figure 18.18).
  - All sutures are similarly placed in a mattress fashion with three sutures in each row on the bilateral bronchi and four sutures per row on the trachea.
  - The splint is sewn in three separate pieces. Additional interrupted sutures should be placed between the tracheal splint and each bronchial splint pieces at the level of the carina taking care not to narrow the orifice of the right upper lobe (Figure 18.20).
  - Completed repair (Figures 18.19 and 18.20)

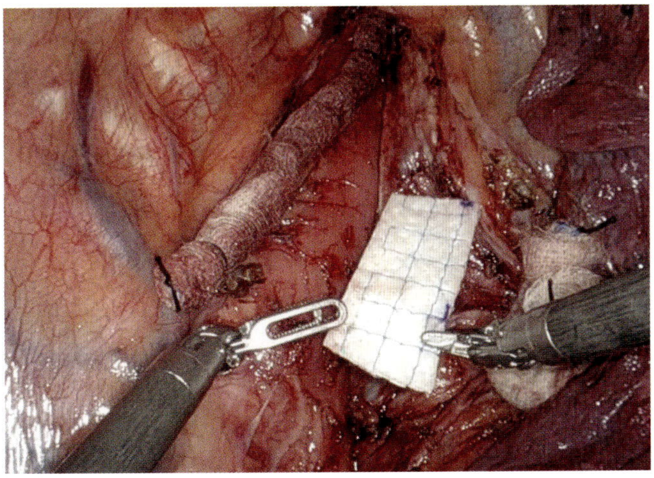

FIGURE 18.10 ▮ Reinforcing splint of the left main bronchus.

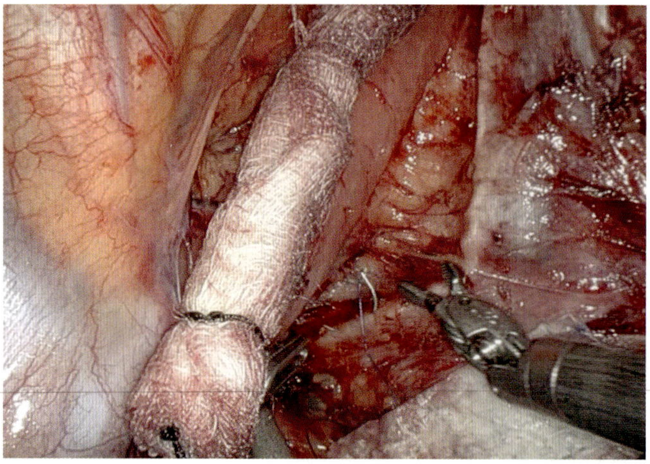

FIGURE 18.11 ▌ First suture placement on left main bronchus.

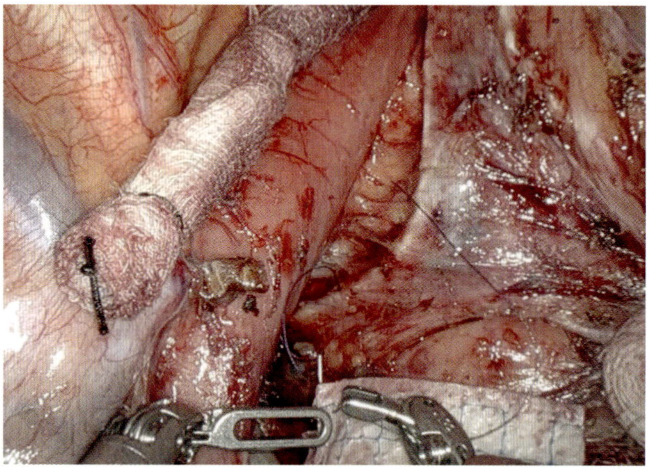

FIGURE 18.12 ▌ Mattress suture on left main bronchus.

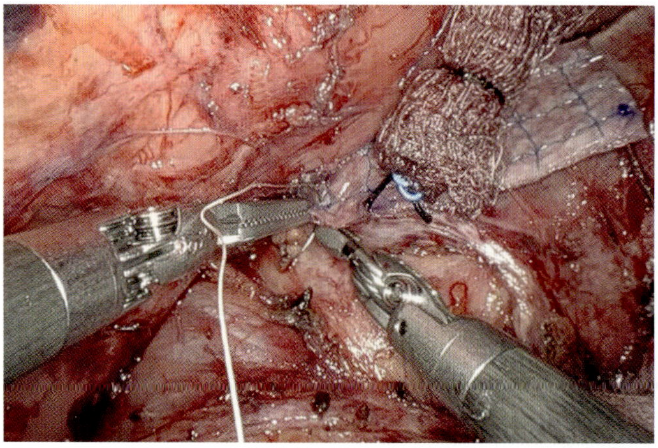

FIGURE 18.13 ▌ Beginning of medial sutures on left main bronchus.

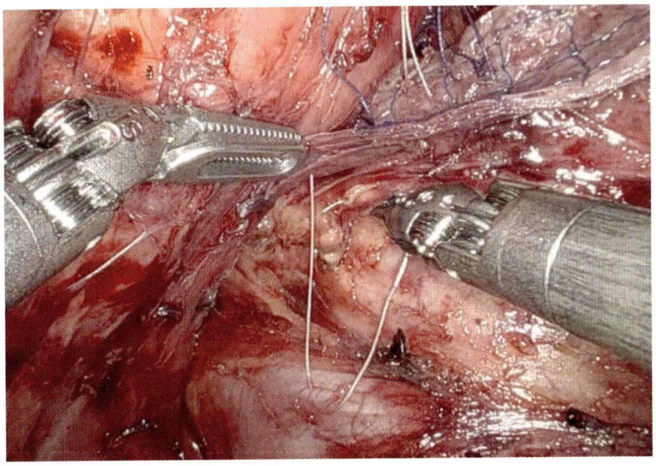

FIGURE 18.14 ▌ Medial left main bronchus sutures.

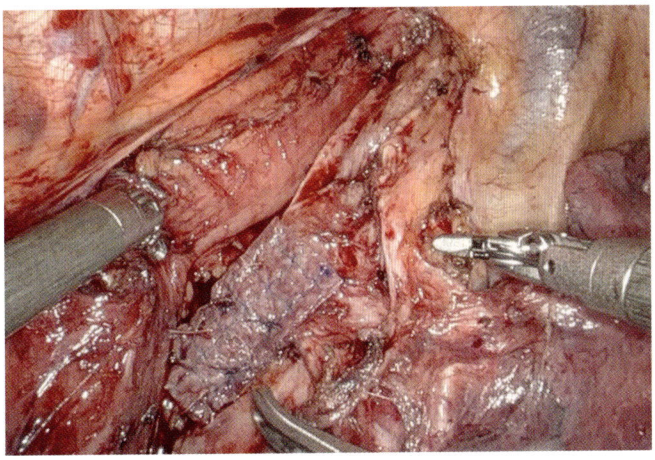

FIGURE 18.15 ▌ Completed left main bronchus repair.

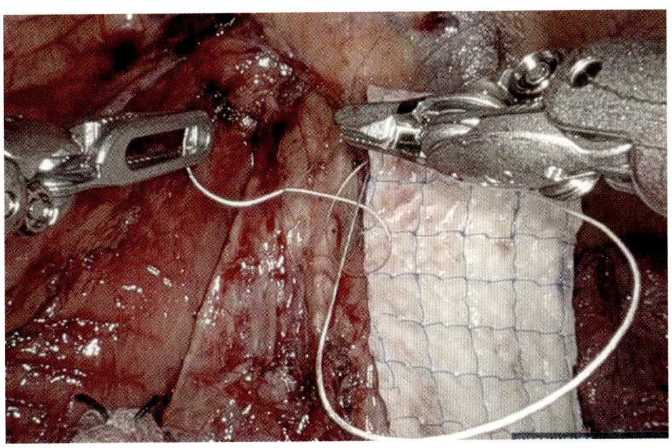

FIGURE 18.16 ▌ Beginning of tracheal repair.

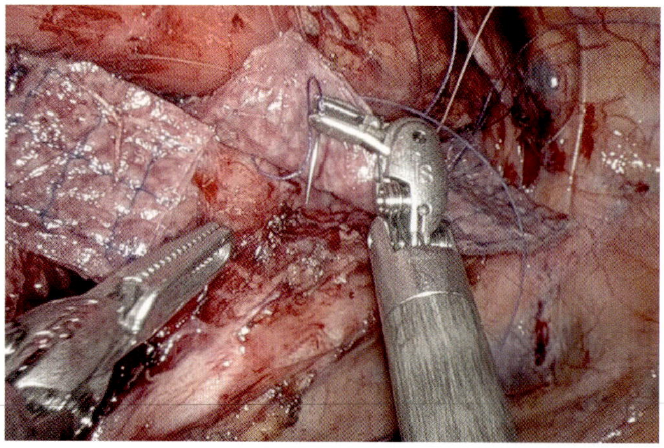

FIGURE 18.17 ■ Mattress suture on middle trachea.

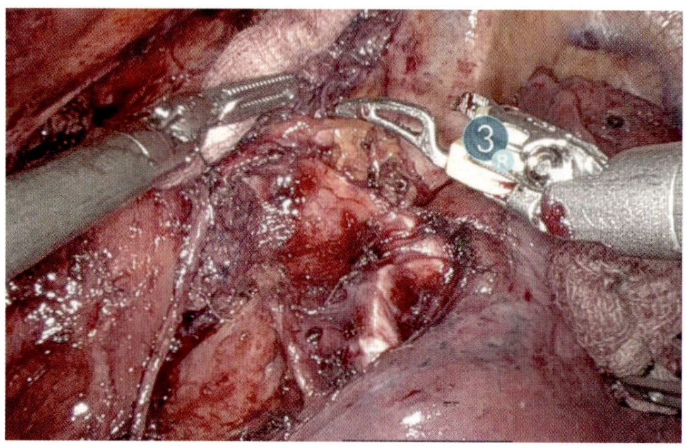

FIGURE 18.18 ■ Right main bronchus exposure.

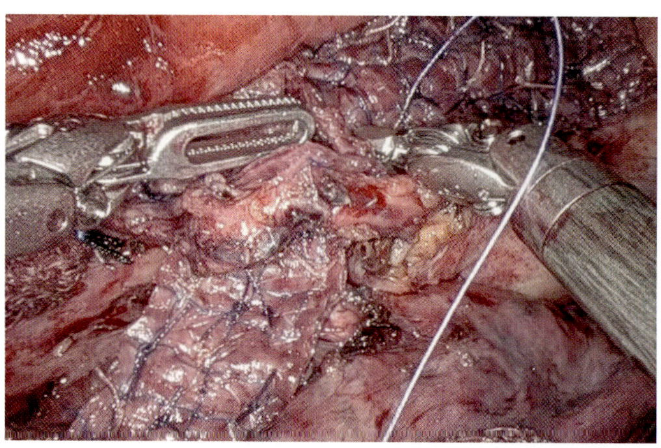

FIGURE 18.19 ■ Suture connecting all three splints together at the carina.

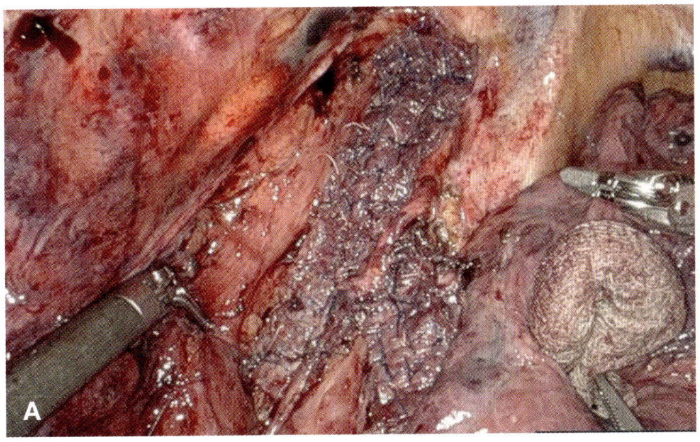

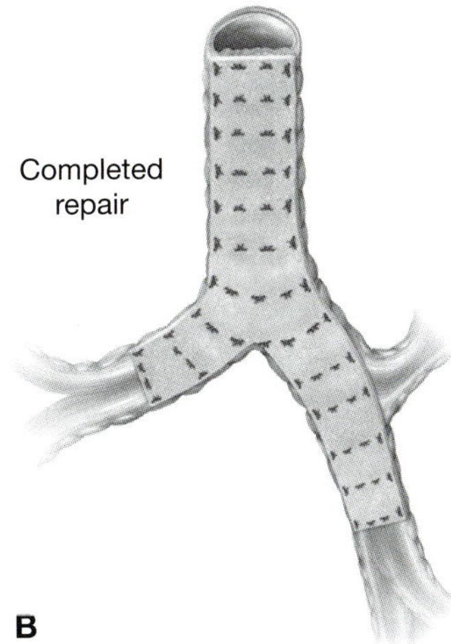

FIGURE 18.20 | **A.** Completed repair. **B.** Posterior view of the completed repair. The membranous wall is stabilized with the aid of the now closely apposed splinting material with multiple series of rows of four mattress sutures. The airway is now more rigid and collapses less during expiration. (**B.** Reprinted from Wright CD. Tracheal surgery: posterior splinting tracheoplasty for tracheomalacia. *Oper Tech Thorac Cardiovasc Surg*. 2015;20(1):31-45, with permission from Elsevier.)

Postoperative Care

- Patients are extubated in the operating room. Many patients require positive pressure during emergence from anesthesia.
- Monitoring in the ICU postoperatively for airway watch as difficulty clearing secretions is common for the first few days. Occasional therapeutic bronchoscopy is needed.
- Morbidity is most commonly attributed to atelectasis, difficulty clearing secretions, pneumonia, and respiratory failure though most patients recover uneventfully.
- Deconditioning preoperatively in the setting of severe symptoms may prolong recovery and lead to increased morbidity.

PEARLS AND PITFALLS

- With proper patient selection, patients will report near immediate improvement in their respiratory symptoms.
- The material to stabilize the posterior tracheal membrane is not standardized. Our preference currently is OviTex though polypropylene mesh is the most common.
- Suture material for fixation of the splint to the membranous wall of the trachea is also varied but we use polyglactin 910 (Vicryl).
- Because it is not uncommon to place full-thickness sutures into the airway when attempting to place a partial-thickness stitch, there is potential for introduction of bacteria next to the splint and thus a foreign body next to the airway. However, while absorbable sutures will eventually dissolve and eliminate a permanent foreign body in the airway, there is potential for weakening of the repair over time.
- When the lateral aspects of the trachea are dissected, it is important to avoid injury to the recurrent laryngeal nerve.
- Meticulous hemostasis during exposure of the trachea is important for optimal visualization while suturing the splint to the posterior wall of the trachea.
- Minimally invasive, robotic-assisted techniques provide excellent visualization of the posterior mediastinum and are especially advantageous with repair of the left mainstem bronchi. This is becoming increasingly common at specialized centers and has been found to be safe and effective in single-institution case series. A robotic approach is now preferred in our institution.
- The benefit of surgical treatment of tracheomalacia is measured by improvement of patient symptoms. Objective measures are still yet to be validated.

Suggested Readings

1. Wright CD, Grillo HC, Hammoud ZT, et al. Tracheoplasty for expiratory collapse of central airways. *Ann Thorac Surg*. 2005;80(1):259-266.
2. Wright CD. Tracheal surgery: posterior splinting tracheoplasty for tracheomalacia. *Operat Tech Thorac Cardiovasc Surg*. 2015:31-45.
3. Gangadharan SP, Bakhos CT, Majid A, et al. Technical aspects and outcomes of tracheobronchoplasty for severe tracheobronchomalacia. *Ann Thorac Surg*. 2011;91(5):1574-1581.
4. Lazzaro R, Patton B, Lee P, et al. First series of minimally invasive, robot-assisted tracheobronchoplasty with mesh for severe tracheobronchomalacia. *J Thorac Cardiovasc Surg*. 2019;157(2):791-800.
5. Lazzaro R, Patton B, Wasserman G, et al. Robotic-assisted tracheobronchoplasty: quality of life and pulmonary function assessment on intermediate follow-up. *J Thorac Cardiovasc Surg*. 2022;164(1):278-286.

Chapter 19

Nonintubated Thoracic Surgery

MARK R. KATLIC

Introduction

- General anesthesia and endotracheal intubation are a luxury rather than a necessity for many thoracic surgical operations (Figure 19.1).
- Patients with malignant pleural effusions, empyemas, pericardial effusions, diffuse lung disease, and multiple pulmonary nodules may be candidates for diagnostic and therapeutic video-assisted thoracic surgery (VATS) under local anesthesia and sedation.
- Anatomic lung resection is possible after a surgeon develops experience with pleural disease and lung biopsies.
- This technique eliminates the need for deep anesthesia and muscle paralysis and minimizes drying of airways and the small but real risk of tracheal trauma.
- It is useful for patients of any age or size or comorbid state, but thoughtful assessment and preparation is required.

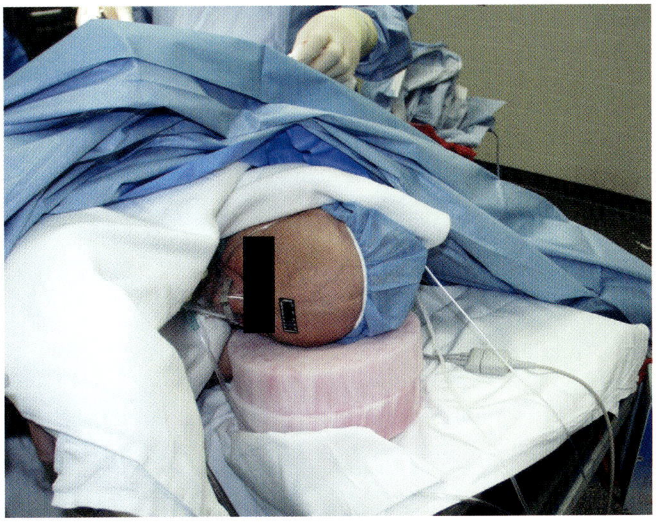

FIGURE 19.1 | The patient undergoing right video-assisted thoracic surgery under local anesthesia and sedation.

Perioperative Considerations

Selection Criteria (Table 19.1)

- This technique is not employed if patients are already intubated and ventilated or are hemodynamically unstable.
- Locating a solitary pulmonary nodule may be problematic, and creating a pericardial window in the absence of a coexisting pleural effusion is not recommended, as the expanded lung may get in the way.

TABLE 19.1 ▮ Patient Selection

General Anesthesia	Local Anesthesia/Sedation
Hemodynamic instability	Hemodynamic stability
Patient already intubated/ventilated	Large unilateral pleural effusion
Empyema, decortication anticipated	Empyema
Solitary pulmonary nodule	Diffuse lung disease, multiple nodules
Pericardial effusion	Pericardial effusion with coexisting pleural effusion
	Chronic hemothorax

- All patients with large pleural effusion, pleural mass, early or midstage empyema, diffuse lung disease, multiple lung nodules, or pericardial effusion with coexisting moderate-to-large pleural effusion are good candidates; in the last 25 years, the author has not used general anesthesia for any of these indications.
- Formal lung resection and mediastinal surgery are possible, usually with the use of bronchial blockers and supplemental techniques, but are not recommended until one has experience with the more straightforward indications described above.
- Advanced age is neither a contraindication (up to 104 years in our experience) nor is size (up to 181 kg in our experience) (Figure 19.2).

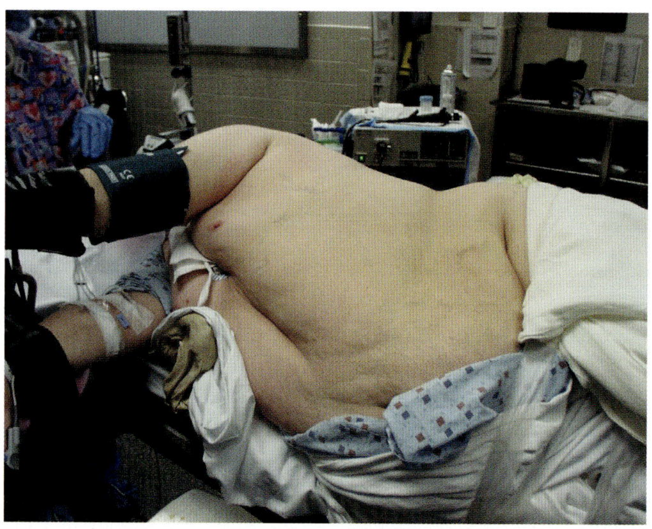

FIGURE 19.2 ▮ No age or weight is a contraindication to nonintubated thoracic surgery (172 kg man with multiloculated empyema).

- Many patients are American Society of Anesthesiologists Physical Status class 3 and 4 (Figure 19.3).
- Extensive comorbidities are not an absolute contraindication, as one can use less sedation and more local anesthetic in these instances.

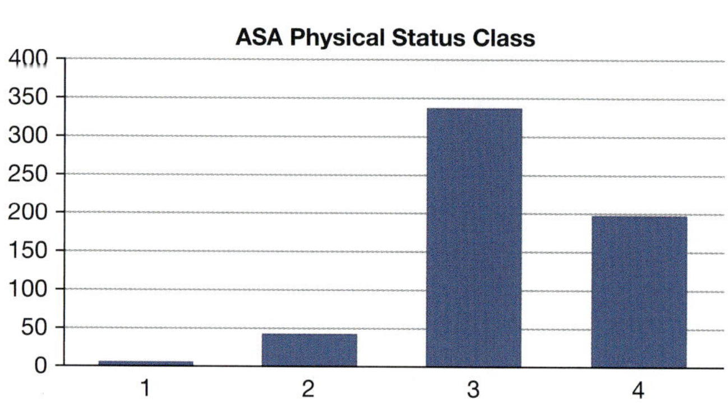

FIGURE 19.3 ▮ Most patients are American Society of Anesthesiologist Physical Status class III or IV.

Preparation

- Thoracic surgeons should be familiar with the basics of VATS, but no special skill is required.
- Robotic experience would only be necessary for formal lung or mediastinal resection, which is not being discussed here.
- Good local anesthesia is critical, and gentle manipulation of instruments and tissues is emphasized.
- As with any thoracic surgery, a careful personal preoperative review of all images, particularly computed tomography, is very important.
- The surgeon must be prepared to drain all discrete pleural collections, know if the pericardial effusion is loculated, and plan an optimal site for lung biopsy.
- The author teaches residents to locate these sites using fixed landmarks such as the carina, vertebral bodies, aortic arch, inferior pulmonary vein, and others.

Local Anesthesia

- Thoracic surgeons must be aware of the dose limitations of xylocaine.
- 1% xylocaine without epinephrine is employed, as the procedures are of short duration, and more concentrated solutions would limit the volume that could be administered (a potential problem if two or three port sites are required for a particular case).
- The limit of 1% xylocaine (10 mg/mL) is 4.5 mg/kg or about 30 mL for an adult man: 70 kg × 4.5 mg/kg = 315 mg; 315 mg ÷ 10 mg/kg = 31.5 mL.

Instruments and Equipment

- A minimum number of instruments is required (Figure 19.4A).

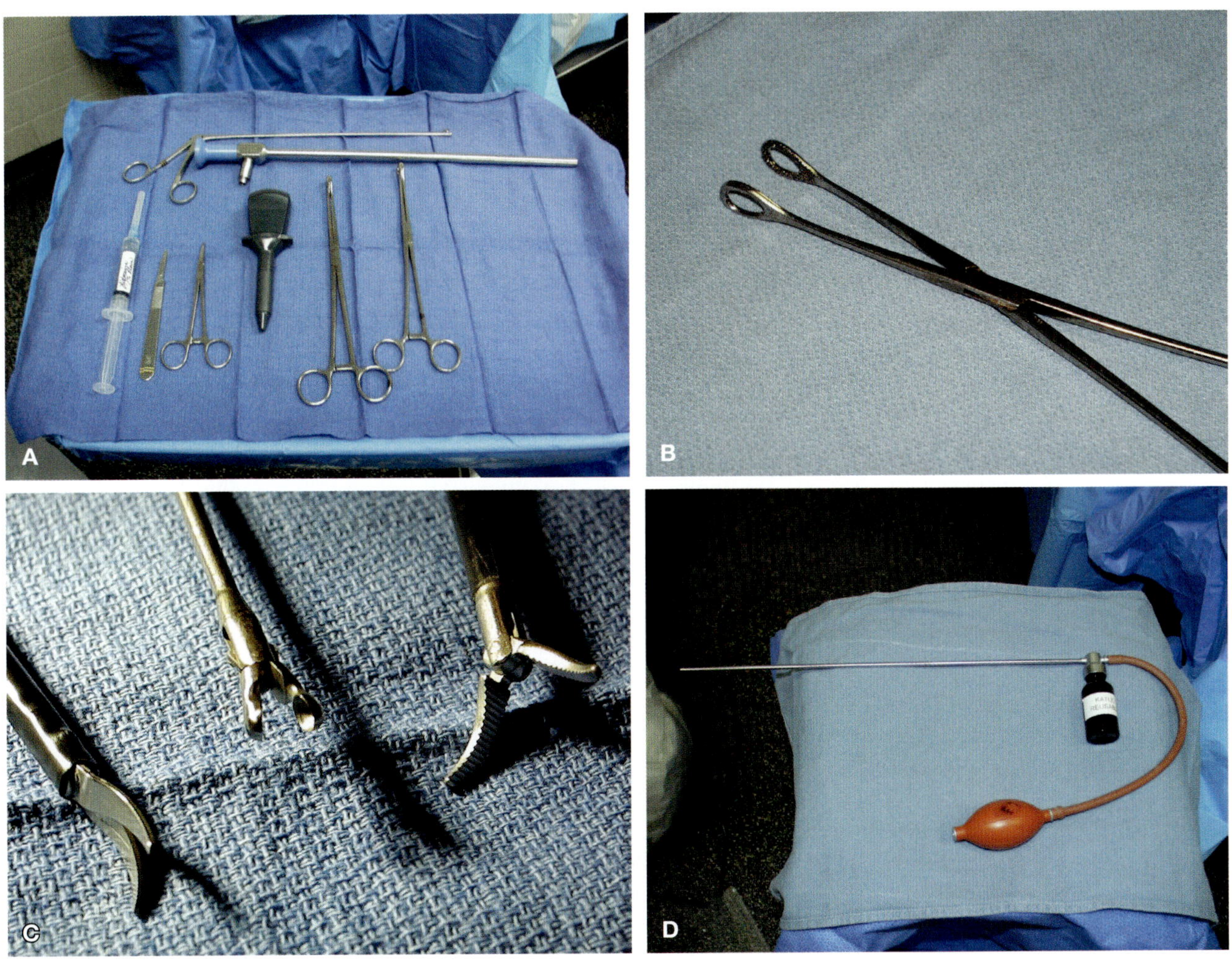

FIGURE 19.4 | **A.** Minimum instrument set needed for most procedures. **B.** Basic ring forceps will grasp lung atraumatically. **C.** Cup biopsy forceps and endoscopic scissors may be useful. **D.** Talc insufflator allows for controlled and selective insufflation of talc to promote pleurodesis.

- Due to the obligatory pneumothorax, we do not want to waste time: everything needed must be opened and on the scrub nurse's table before the pleural cavity is entered.
- 1% xylocaine, #15 scalpel, hemostat clamp for entry into the pleural cavity.
- 0° or 30° telescope, per surgeon preference.
- Atraumatic lung-grasping instruments (the author uses simple ring clamps) (Figure 19.4B).
- Cup biopsy forceps (Figure 19.4C).
- Endoscopic scissors if pericardial window is indicated (Figure 19.4C).
- Talc and insufflating device if pleurodesis is indicated (Figure 19.4D).
- Endoscopic stapler added if lung biopsy is indicated.
- 20, 24, or 28 French chest tube; 0 silk suture for chest tube.
- Pleural drainage container; the author uses Mini-Atrium Pleurovac© (Atrium Medical Corporation, Hudson, NH) if discharge home with tube is anticipated.
- 3-0 absorbable suture for subcutaneous fat, 4-0 absorbable suture for subcuticular skin closure, and clear dressings.

Positioning

- Full lateral position similar to any posterolateral thoracotomy or VATS (Figures 19.2 and 19.5).

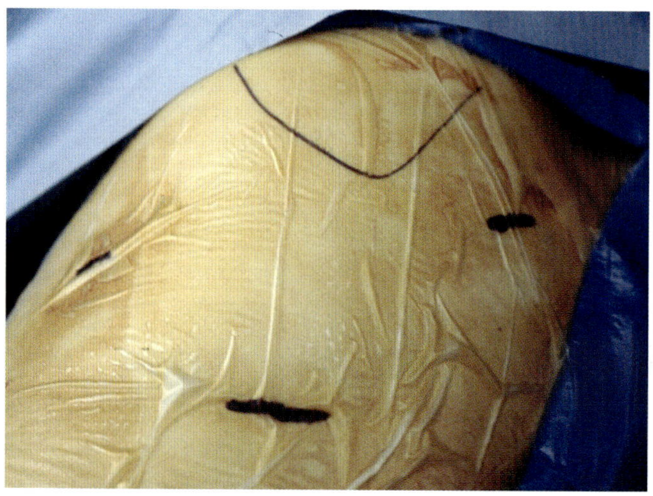

FIGURE 19.5 ▌ Left lateral position and three port sites for lung biopsy.

Technique

General Technique

- Patients are sedated with an individualized combination of midazolam, fentanyl, and propofol; ketamine may also be used. We allow our anesthesiology staff full discretion in this, having discussed the depth of sedation that we anticipate needing.
- Supplemental oxygen is administered via nasal prongs or facemask or both (Figure 19.6); bilevel positive airway pressure is continued if patients come to the operating room on it.
- Oxygen saturation, electrocardiogram, and blood pressure are monitored; end-tidal carbon dioxide may be assessed through a catheter tucked into an oral airway.
- Flexible bronchoscopy is carried out if indicated via the pharynx after direct xylocaine spray of the vocal cords, transtracheal puncture, or other local anesthesia.
- Local anesthesia (1% xylocaine without epinephrine, 10-30 mL depending on number of incisions) is infiltrated.
- We emphasize numbing skin and subcutaneous tissues first, then spreading dissection with a hemostat until ribs are easily palpated, then direct xylocaine infiltration of intercostal muscle and pleura, and then entering the pleural cavity more by repeated spreading dissection than pressure.
- The author emphasizes "spreading a hundred times if necessary." This is less stimulating to the patient; residents find that they can then place bedside chest tubes painlessly after learning the technique.
- Surgeons are impatient, but giving the xylocaine time to work is also important.
- We have not employed intercostal blocks or epidural analgesia, though others have, and this is acceptable.
- Carbon dioxide insufflation is not employed.

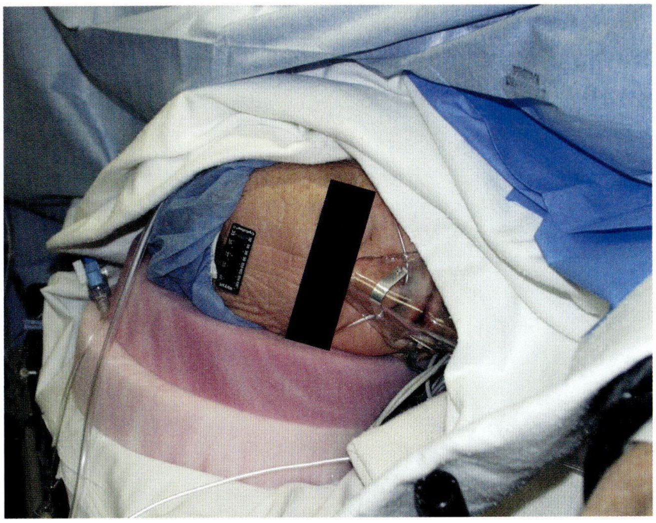

FIGURE 19.6 | Oxygen via both facemask and nasal prongs.

- Contingency plans for intubation or conversion to thoracotomy (not yet needed in our experience) include immediate placement of a chest tube via one port site and occlusive dressings to any others, then turning the patient supine for intubation. An alternative technique, also never used, would be placement of a laryngeal mask airway with the patient still in lateral position.
- Elective patients are discharged the same or next day, often with the chest tube attached to a Mini-Atrium Pleurovac©. The chest tube is then removed in the outpatient clinic when appropriate.

TIPS

- *Remember that the patient is spontaneously breathing.*
- *Have everything needed open and on the scrub table.*
- *Use plenty of local analgesia, within guidelines.*
- *Be patient, allow time for local anesthesia to work.*
- *Gentle handling of tissues, minimize torqueing the thoracoscope in the interspace.*
- *Do not waste time (there is a pneumothorax).*

Pleural Disease (Figures 19.7 and 19.8, Videos 19.1 and 19.2)

- One port is employed initially, with cup biopsy forceps and possible talc insufflation catheter passed along the outside of the short open trocar (Endopath©; Ethicon Endo-Surgery, Inc, Cincinnati, OH) (Figure 19.9).

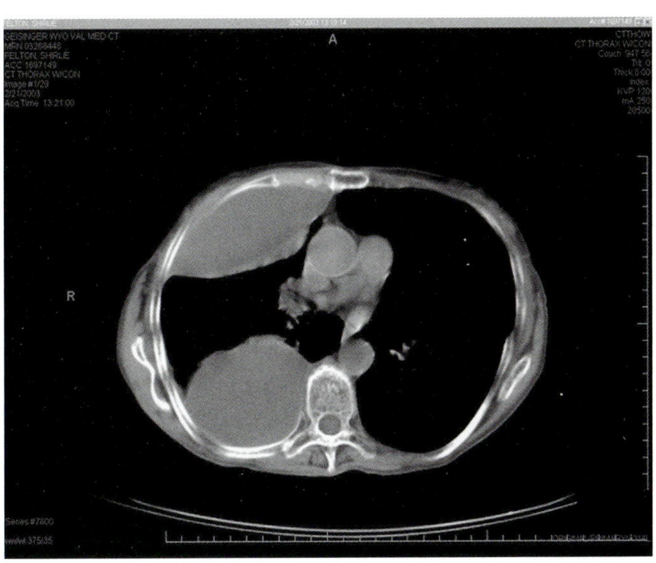

FIGURE 19.7 | Multiloculated malignant pleural effusion.

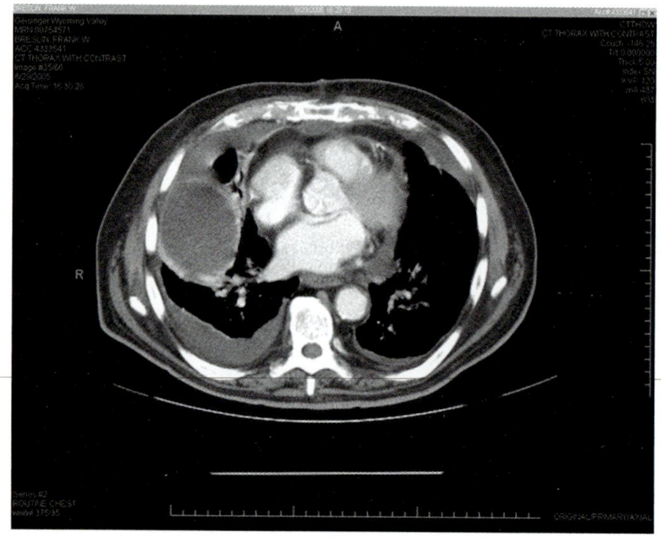

FIGURE 19.8 ▌ Loculated hemothorax following cardiac surgery.

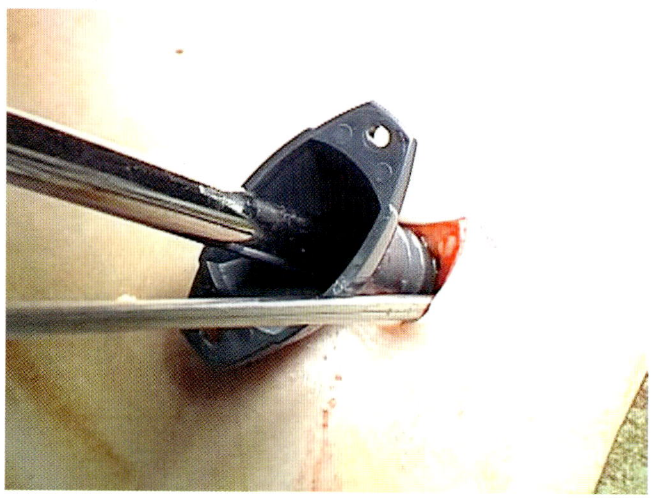

FIGURE 19.9 ▌ Several instruments may be passed via one port site. CO_2 insufflation is not employed.

- If the port site is "tight," the trocar may be withdrawn, leaving the 5- or 10-mm thoracoscope in place so that biopsies and talc insufflation may be performed under direct visualization.
- If adhesions exist, as in multiloculated empyema, a second or third site without trocar allows introduction of other instruments to disrupt adhesions.
- Sometimes it is possible for the surgeon to place a finger through each of two sites and, touching the undersurface of the ribs, connect the two openings, thereby allowing a ring clamp to be passed into the pleural cavity and be seen.
- Posteriorly, where the interspace is narrower, a small Richardson retractor may be placed into the intercostal space and "torqued" or twisted to widen the space; the ribs will not immediately return, allowing a full finger or stapler to be inserted.
- A PleurX© catheter (BD, Vernon Hills, IL) may be placed at the end of the case, whether or not talc has been introduced. The author uses these very selectively and preferring insufflated talc and discharge with a chest tube for 3 to 7 days, but this is a matter of surgeon choice.

Pericardial Window (Figure 19.10, Video 19.3)

- Select the side of the body with the coexisting pleural effusion if possible, as the lung is "accustomed" to being collapsed and is less likely to get in the way.
- With the lung out of the way, two port sites will suffice: the thoracoscope inferior to the tip of the scapula with a possible grasper alongside, and a separate anterior site over the pericardium for a #15 blade and then endoscopic scissors. If necessary, a third site in-between and superior allows retraction of the lung posterosuperiorly.
- A chest tube is left in the pleural space for several days.
- Only hemodynamically stable patients are offered this approach.

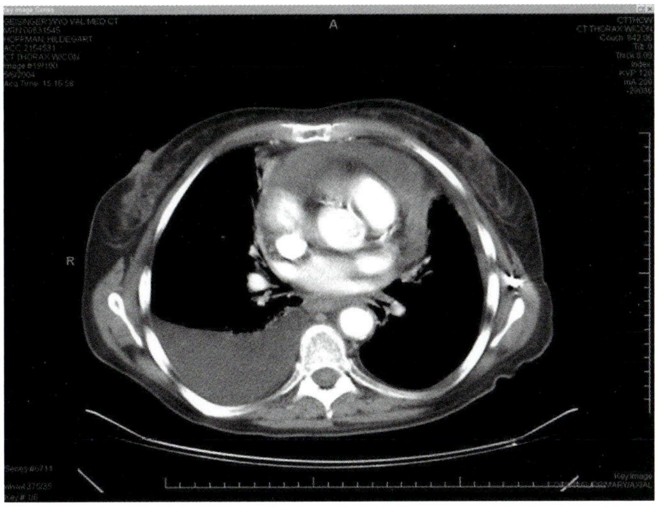

FIGURE 19.10 | Pericardial effusion with coexisting right pleural effusion.

Lung Biopsy (Figures 19.11 and 19.12, Video 19.4)

- Three port sites allow insertion of the telescope via the trocar, grasping ring forceps, and endoscopic stapler.

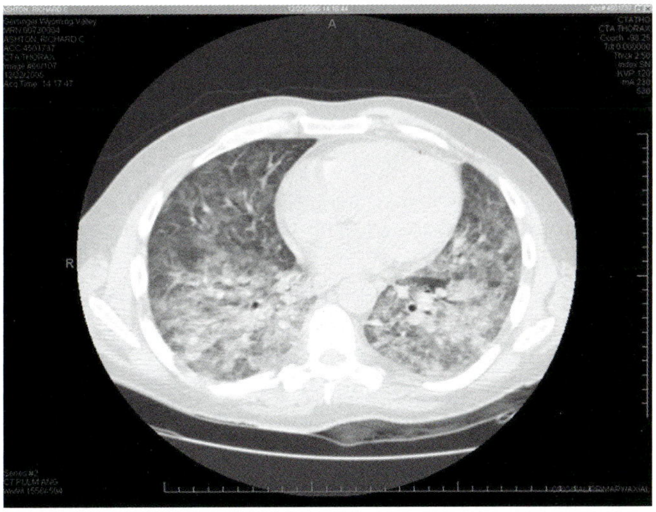

FIGURE 19.11 | Cytomegalovirus and pneumocystis pneumonia in a patient with human immunodeficiency virus.

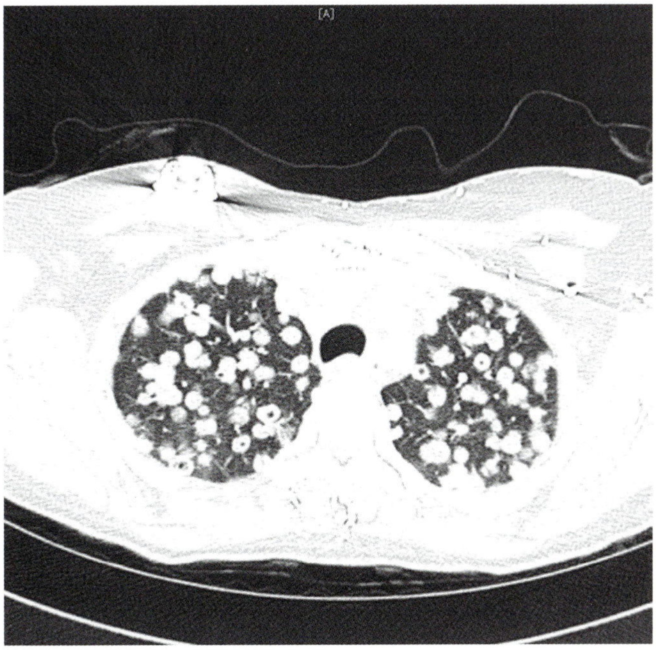

FIGURE 19.12 | Multiple lung nodules and multifocal adenocarcinoma.

- If the lung is fully expanded or if the patient coughs, the end of the stapler may be gently pressed down against the lung to push air out and transiently improve vision. This is generally long enough to allow the stapler to be passed beneath the ring forceps.
- Alternatively, a second ring forceps and the stapler may be passed through the same site, with the former briefly compressing the lung to allow better vision.
- Usually, any lobe may be selectively biopsied, but a solitary lung nodule could prove to be problematic to find.

Postoperative Care

- Patients may be discharged home the same or next day, with or without chest tube.
- Patients and/or family are taught how to empty the chest tube container if it fills.
- Patients are allowed to shower with the chest tube in place and are allowed full activity.
- If the chest tube has not been removed in the hospital, it is removed in the office as appropriate, eg, allowing 5 to 7 days for talc pleurodesis.

TIPS

Results in 576 cases (Tables 19.2 and 19.3)

- *Mean operating time was 26 minutes (range 8-111 min).*
- *No patient required intraoperative intubation.*
- *No conversion to thoracotomy.*
- *No epidural or nerve block analgesia.*
- *Diagnosis achieved in all cases of biopsy.*
- *Three patients (2.7% of 112) required a subsequent procedure for empyema.*
- *Twelve complications (cerebrovascular, atrial fibrillation, air leak, and urinary infection).*
- *No deaths due to operation.*
- *No patient had awareness or memory of operation.*

TABLE 19.2 ▮ Diagnoses

Malignant pleural effusion		224
Lung cancer	118	
Breast cancer	38	
Mesothelioma	12	
Ovarian cancer	10	
Colon	10	
Esophageal	6	
Lymphoma	6	
Endometrial	4	
Prostate	4	
Melanoma	3	
Gastric	2	

TABLE 19.2 ‖ Diagnoses (Continued)

Pancreatic	2	
Laryngeal	2	
Cholangiocarcinoma	2	
Sarcoma	1	
Other, 1 each (anal, tracheal squamous cell, renal cell, and pleomorphic)	4	
Benign pleural effusion		139
Chronic pleuritis	93	
Chronic pleuritis, radiotherapy	28	
Renal failure	10	
Ascites	8	
Empyema		112
Lung disease		56
Metastatic cancer	10	
Usual interstitial pneumonitis	9	
Interstitial disease	7	
Lung cancer	5	
Chronic aspiration pneumonia	4	
Granuloma	4	
Pneumoconiosis	3	
Bronchiolitis obliterans organizing pneumonia	3	
Cytomegalovirus pneumonitis	2	
Bacterial pneumonitis	2	
Chemotherapy toxicity	2	
Other, 1 each (aspergillus, primary amyloidosis, bronchiectasis, pneumocystis, and granulomatous pneumonitis)	5	
Chronic hemothorax		23
Pericardial effusion		10
Metastatic non-small cell lung cancer	6	
Metastatic small cell lung cancer	3	
Breast	1	
Mesothelioma		5
Chylothorax		2
Lung abscess		2
Pneumothorax		2
Mediastinal mass (metastatic breast cancer)		1
		576 total

TABLE 19.3 ▮ Operations

Drain effusion/pleural biopsy		368
With talc insufflation	302	
Without talc insufflation	66	
Drain empyema		112
Lung biopsy		56
Evacuate chronic hemothorax		23
Pericardial window		10
Treat chylothorax		2
Drain lung abscess		2
Treat pneumothorax		2
Biopsy mediastinal mass		1
		576 total

TIPS

- *The novice should start using this technique with malignant pleural effusions, then progress to early empyemas and pericardial window procedures, and then to complex empyemas and lung biopsies.*

PEARLS AND PITFALLS

- Patients tolerate these operations well, experiencing no pain or recall. Many who have previously undergone thoracentesis, or bedside chest tube, or general anesthesia prefer this approach.
- They awake quickly with few side effects and good respiratory strength.
- During the case, they tolerate the obligatory unilateral pneumothorax and up to an hour of operative time.
- The patient can be quite old, quite large, or quite sick and still undergoes successful VATS under local anesthesia/sedation.
- Multiple instruments or a finger may be passed via a single port site.
- The surgeon may make as many ports as necessary.
- Others have documented decreased operating room time, length of stay, and cost, plus increased patient satisfaction.
- Any thoracic surgeon can use this technique; it takes no special skill beyond VATS experience.

Suggested Readings

1. Bethune N. Pleural poudrage. A new technique for the deliberate production of pleural adhesions as a preliminary to lobectomy. *J Thorac Surg*. 1935;4:251-261.
2. Chen JS, Cheng YJ, Hung MH, Tseng YD, Chen KC, Lee YC. Nonintubated thoracoscopic lobectomy for lung cancer. *Ann Surg*. 2011;254(6):1038-1043.
3. Gonzalez-Rivas D, Bonome C, Fieira E, et al. Non-intubated video-assisted thoracoscopic lung resections: the future of thoracic surgery? *Eur J Cardio Thorac Surg*. 2016;49(3):721-731.
4. Hung WT, Hung MH, Wang ML, Cheng YJ, Hsu HH, Chen JS. Nonintubated thoracoscopic surgery for lung tumor: seven years' experience with 1,025 patients. *Ann Thorac Surg*. 2019;107(6):1607-1612.
5. Jacobaeus HC. The cauterization of adhesions in artificial pneumothorax treatment of pulmonary tuberculosis under thoracoscopic control. *Proc R Soc Med*. 1923;16(Electro Ther Sect):45-62.
6. Katlic MR. Video-assisted thoracic surgery utilizing local anesthesia and sedation. *Eur J Cardio Thorac Surg*. 2006;30(3):529-532.

7. Katlic MR. Video-assisted thoracic surgery utilizing local anesthesia and sedation: how I teach it. *Ann Thorac Surg*. 2017;104(3):727-730.
8. Katlic MR. Five hundred seventy-six cases of video-assisted thoracic surgery using local anesthesia and sedation: lessons learned. *J Am Coll Surg*. 2018;226(1):58-63.
9. Katlic MR, Facktor MA. Video-assisted thoracic surgery utilizing local anesthesia and sedation: 384 consecutive cases. *Ann Thorac Surg*. 2010;90(1):240-245.
10. Liu HY, Hsu HH, Tsai TM, et al. Nonintubated versus intubated uniportal thoracoscopic segmentectomy for lung tumors. *Ann Thorac Surg*. 2021;111(4):1182-1189.
11. Pompeo E. Awake thoracic surgery—is it worth the trouble? *Semin Thorac Cardiovasc Surg*. 2012;24(2):106-114.
12. Pompeo E, Mineo D, Rogliani P, Sabato AF, Mineo TC. Feasibility and results of awake thoracoscopic resection of solitary pulmonary nodules. *Ann Thorac Surg*. 2004;78(5):1761-1768.
13. Pompeo E, Tacconi F, Mineo D, Mineo TC. The role of awake video-assisted thoracoscopic surgery in spontaneous pneumothorax. *J Thorac Cardiovasc Surg*. 2007;133(3):786-790.
14. Wu CY, Chen JS, Lin YS, et al. Feasibility and safety of nonintubated thoracoscopic lobectomy for geriatric lung cancer patients. *Ann Thorac Surg*. 2013;95(2):405-411.
15. Zhang K, Chen HG, Wu WB, et al. Non-intubated video-assisted thoracoscopic surgery vs. intubated video-assisted thoracoscopic surgery for thoracic disease: a systematic review and meta-analysis of 1,684 cases. *J Thorac Dis*. 2019;11(8):3556-3568.

Chapter 20

Lung Transplantation

MARIA LUCIA L. MADARIAGA
PHILIP J. SPENCER

Perioperative Considerations

The success of lung transplantation relies on meticulous attention to patient selection (donor and recipient), technical excellence, and close collaboration with pulmonology and associated medical colleagues.

- Although various criteria have been previously published, the ultimate decision that a donor lung is acceptable for transplantation relies on surgeon judgment. Atelectasis should be carefully distinguished from pneumonia on computed tomography. Given the low lung organ utilization rate in the United States (~20%, compared to 60%-80% of livers and kidneys), a more aggressive approach with a low threshold for in-person evaluation of lung donors is warranted.
- Anastomotic technique varies from center to center. Despite the wide variation in anastomotic technique, particularly for the bronchus, the important principle is to achieve a well-vascularized, tension-free anastomosis while minimizing bronchial stump length. We present here several techniques practiced at high-volume centers.
- Indications for use of circulatory support during transplantation are center-specific. We present here the underlying principles that contribute to making this decision.
- Indications for use of ex vivo lung perfusion for the donor lung will not be discussed here.

Donor Operation

- **Bronchoscopy.** Normal anatomy should be confirmed with particular attention for a tracheal right upper lobe bronchus (pig bronchus). The presence, quality, quantity, and reaccumulation of secretions should be noted. Unfavorable signs include bile-tinged secretions (suggestive of aspiration) and reaccumulation of purulent secretions after suctioning (suggestive of ongoing infection).
- **Ventilation.** Tidal volumes should be within 6 to 8 mL/kg of ideal body weight. An easy bedside calculation for ideal body weight is to use ideal BMI = 22 kg/m^2 and solve for kilograms since donor height is known. Inspired FiO_2 should be kept to 50% or lower as the patient tolerates. Inspired FiO_2 should be increased to 100% about 5 minutes prior to recruitment breath and arterial blood gas sampling.
- **Aspiration precautions.** Nasogastric tube should be in place and maintained on suction.
- **Tactile and visual inspection.** After opening the chest, a thorough assessment of lung quality should be performed. The lungs should be smooth with no nodules, masses, or lacerations. Areas of atelectasis should be recruitable with Valsalva maneuver. The lungs should not be boggy or heavy (edema). Finally, compliance should be assessed by asking anesthesia to briefly disconnect the endotracheal tube from the ventilator. Good compliance will be evident by brisk deflation of the recruited lung upon disconnection from the ventilator.
- Prior to harvest, a mutual understanding should be reached with the heart procurement team about the line of division for the left atrium. This is facilitated by exposing Sondergaard's groove.
- After systemic heparinization, deliver pneumoplegia to the pulmonary artery via a cannula secured with a purse string. The cannula should be positioned such that pneumoplegia does not preferentially go to the right or left pulmonary artery. The left atrium should be opened immediately to allow the lung and heart to vent. The lung should be ventilated until the trachea is divided.

- Retrograde flush into each of the pulmonary veins can be accomplished in situ after the heart is removed, or on the back table. The flush exiting the pulmonary artery should eventually be clear without clots or blood. We deliver retrograde flush in situ using an 18-French Foley catheter with the balloon inflated to occlude the pulmonary vein ostia. Note in situ retrograde flush occurs while the lung is still being ventilated.
- Donor pneumonectomy is accomplished by dividing the inferior pulmonary ligaments and the posterior pleural attachments. Care is taken not to injure the esophagus. The trachea is palpated and the endotracheal tube is withdrawn into the neck. The lungs are recruited with Valsalva maneuver. Just after Valsalva is released, the trachea is clamped and divided. This ensures that the lungs are close to but not maximally inflated during transport (this is not applicable for cases where portable ex vivo lung perfusion is used). Leave the length of trachea and the length of the pulmonary artery long especially in cases where ex vivo lung perfusion is used. The donor descending aorta may need to be used to supplement for length of pulmonary artery.
- Avoid direct contact of ice on lungs.

Recipient Operation

- The need for extracorporeal membranous oxygenation (ECMO) should be determined. In some centers, venoarterial ECMO (VA ECMO) is used routinely for all cases. The advantage of this approach is that it allows controlled reperfusion of the freshly implanted lungs, and it allows for increased exposure especially for the left side since the heart has a higher tolerance for manipulation/retraction on support. The disadvantage of ECMO is the increased risk of bleeding due to systemic heparinization and inability to manage air without a reservoir. VA ECMO should be considered when the patient has pulmonary hypertension, high pCO_2, or if the patient develops hemodynamic instability when retracting the heart during the course of the operation. If planned VA ECMO is to be employed, a goal activated clotting time (ACT) of 180 to 220 s is sufficient, often requiring only 5,000U of systemic heparin compared with an ACT > 450 s for cardiopulmonary bypass. Utilizing central cannulation via the ascending aorta and right atrial appendage avoids a femoral cutdown, prevents the Harlequin syndrome, and allows for superior control having the cannulas immediately available in the field.
- Prior to operation, the decision should be made about which side should be implanted first (ie, if the left lung receives less perfusion than the right lung, the left lung should be transplanted first so that freshly implanted graft does not receive the majority of perfusion). If ECMO support is to be used, this decision is less important.

Instruments/Equipment and Monitoring

- Setup should include items needed for going on ECMO or cardiopulmonary bypass.
- Aquamantys is helpful for hemostasis.
- Satinsky clamps are used during vascular anastomoses.
- The sternum can be approximated with plates during chest closure.
- A pulmonary artery catheter, arterial line, and transesophageal echo should be placed.
- A double-lumen endotracheal tube is necessary.

Positioning and Preparation

- The patient is placed in supine position. It is important to be able to see the entire anterolateral chest well.
- We place the arms at 90° to the body and elevate using padded support.
- The entire anterolateral chest wall should be prepped into the field.
- The neck and groin are also prepped into the field in case access for emergent support is necessary.

Technique

- **Clamshell thoracotomy:** The second rib is attached anteriorly at the level of the angle of Louis. From this landmark, the fourth intercostal space can be found and palpated. The site of entry into the chest should be in the fourth intercostal space. Entry may sometimes occur in the fifth or third intercostal space; however, a lower entry provides less favorable exposure for the hilar dissection and anastomoses. The skin incision should follow the inframammary line to spare the breast tissue, curve slightly upwards in the midline, and end laterally at the anterior axillary line. Breast flaps may be needed to adequately expose the fourth intercostal space (and if performed, a drain should be left in this potential space at the end of the case). To enter the chest, the intercostal muscle is divided in half between the costal cartilaginous ribs to preserve blood supply to the cartilage. More laterally, the intercostal muscle is taken off the ossified ribs to minimize bleeding, and this plane right on top of the rib is followed to the posterior chest to just before the paraspinous muscle. The internal mammary artery is ligated and divided bilaterally before dividing the sternum. It is helpful to divide the sternum at a slight angle rather than at 90° to aid in reapproximation. Chest wall retractors are placed bilaterally.

- **Recipient pneumonectomy:** The pulmonary veins and pulmonary artery are dissected and divided with vascular staple loads, leaving a long stump on the recipient side. The bronchus is opened sharply with a blade. Hemostasis is achieved in the chest, paying particular attention to the divided inferior pulmonary ligaments and the subcarinal lymph nodes. Prophylactic clips along the cut inferior pulmonary ligament may prevent frustrating bleeding at the end of the case.
- **Stump preparation:** Allis clamps (for the pulmonary veins and bronchus) or Judd-Allis clamps (for the pulmonary artery) are used. The pulmonary veins and pulmonary arteries are retracted and mobilized into the pericardium (Figure 20.1). It is useful to open the pericardium anteriorly (which may already be open if the patient was placed on central VA ECMO) so that the surgeon's fingers can be inserted to help distinguish and divide the pericardial plane around the pulmonary veins and the pulmonary artery. The pulmonary veins are mobilized to the level of the left atrium circumferentially. Care should be taken when mobilizing the pulmonary artery stump not to injure the recurrent laryngeal nerve on the left or the superior vena cava on the right. Excessive mobilization and dissection around the bronchus is avoided to preserve its blood supply. The bronchus should be trimmed to within two rings from the carina so that the bronchial anastomosis can remain protected within the mediastinum rather than the pleural space. Bronchial artery bleeding is selectively controlled with cautery, minimizing ischemia to the bronchus stump. Once stump dissection is completed, it may be helpful to place a tourniquet or silk tie to retract the arterial and venous stumps anteriorly to improve visualization of the more posterior bronchus stump in preparation for anastomosis (Figure 20.2).

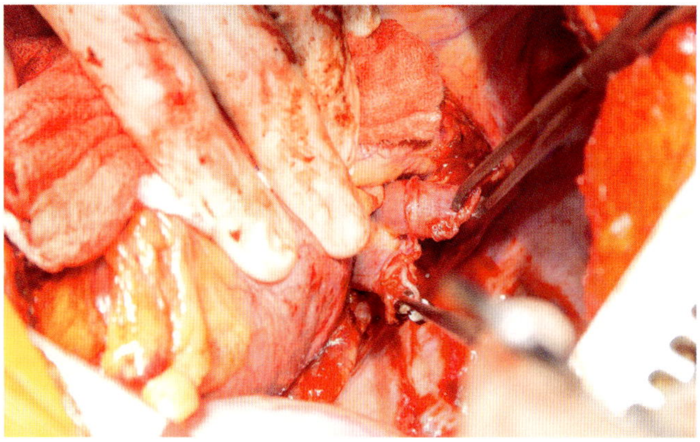

FIGURE 20.1 ▮ Stump exposure.

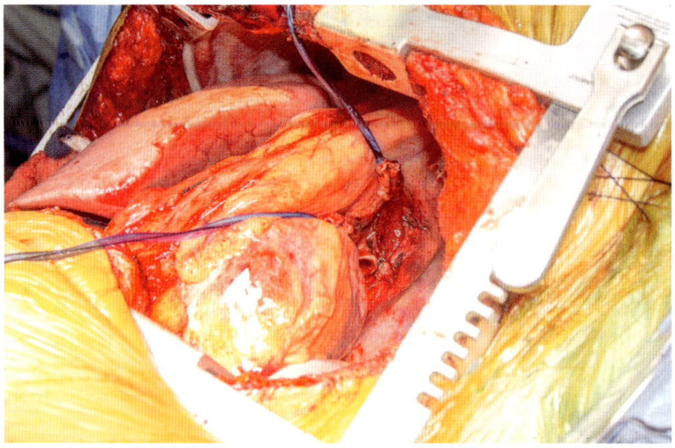

FIGURE 20.2 ▮ Left bronchus exposure.

- **Donor back table preparation:** The left and right lungs are separated with a stapler leaving the lungs inflated. The left atrial cuff is trimmed and the pericardial attachments are divided to increase mobility of the cuff. The pulmonary artery is skeletonized. The bronchus is opened with a knife. The airways should be suctioned to remove mucus and samples sent for microbiology culture. To minimize bronchus ischemia, the bronchus is trimmed to leave only one to two rings from the secondary carina and nodal tissue should remain undisturbed.
- **Implant:** The lung is brought onto the field. The bronchus anastomosis is performed first. There are many ways to perform the bronchial anastomosis—pick a method that is used at high-volume centers with a track record of success (Figure 20.3).

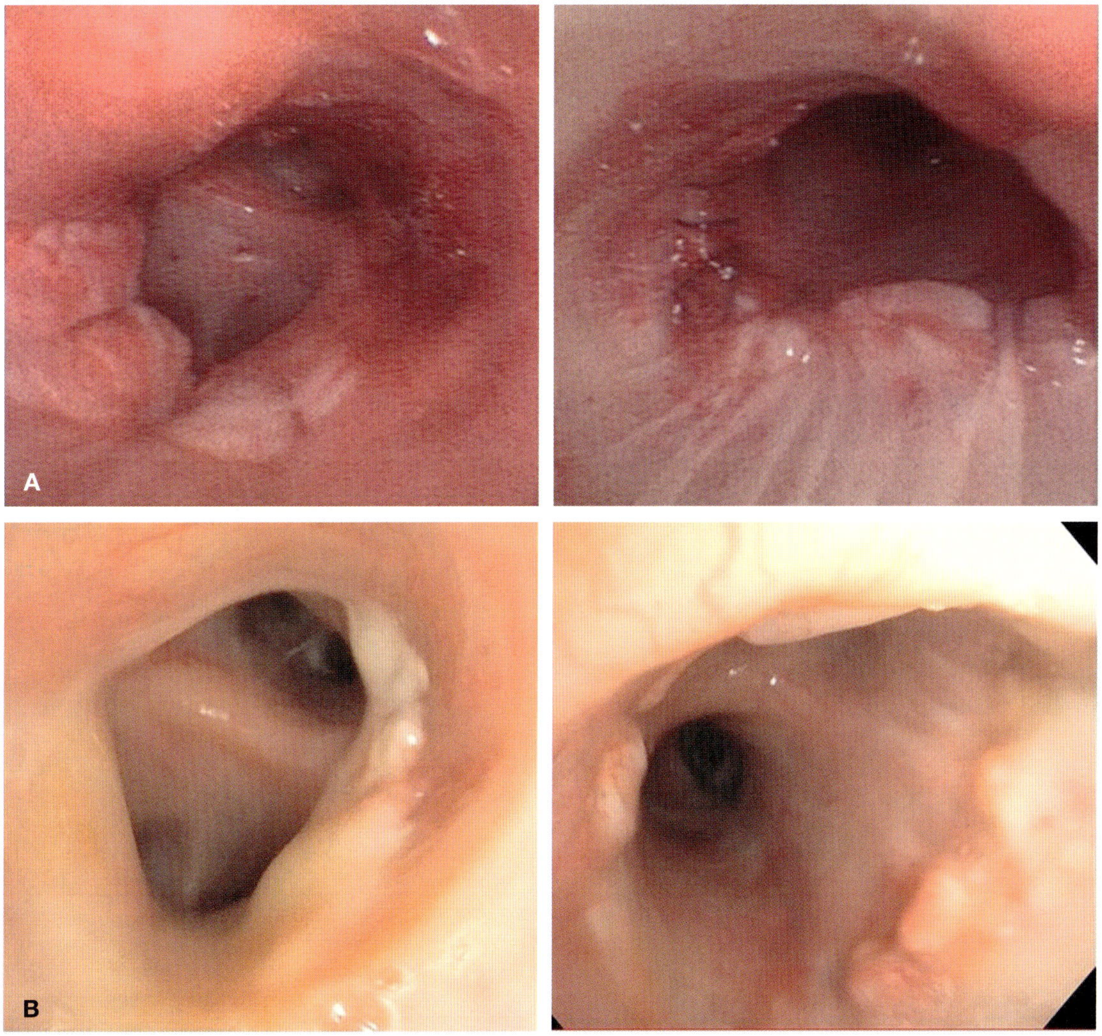

FIGURE 20.3 | Bronchial anastomosis **(A)** post operation and **(B)** 1 month post operation.

Options include (1) running 3-0 PDS membranous back wall and interrupted Vicryl cartilaginous front wall and (2) two running 3-0 polypropylene sutures anchored at the membrano-cartilaginous junction. The sutures should be placed 3 mm apart and 3 to 4 mm in depth to ensure adequate purchase and minimize ischemia. The anterior sutures should be placed around the first cartilage ring from the anastomosis. Air leak test is performed by submerging the anastomosis in saline and performing Valsalva maneuver. An additional measure of safety is to buttress healthy peribronchial tissue on the anterior aspect of the bronchial anastomosis to separate it from the pulmonary artery. The vascular anastomoses are then performed. A Satinsky clamp is placed on the left atrium and the pulmonary vein stumps are opened and trimmed. The anastomosis should be performed from left atrial muscle to left atrial muscle. Using a 4-0 polypropylene suture, the back wall is completed with a running everting mattress stitch that results in a smooth endovascular surface while the front wall can be a simple running stitch. A Satinsky clamp is then placed on the pulmonary artery. The donor pulmonary artery is inspected from the inside to ensure it is not twisted (seen by the first branches oriented superiorly). The length is trimmed so that the completed anastomosis will not kink. The anastomosis is performed with running 5-0 polypropylene. Both vascular anastomoses are left untied until after de-airing.

- **Reperfusion:** If the patient is on ECMO, ECMO flows are lowered slightly to allow blood flow into the lungs. The pulmonary artery clamp is released and the anastomosis is de-aired. Then the pulmonary vein anastomosis is inspected and de-aired with antegrade flow from the pulmonary artery prior to releasing the clamp and introducing retrograde flow from the left atrium. After adequate de-airing, the anastomotic sutures are tied. If the patient is not on ECMO, reperfusion is controlled by placing a partial bulldog clamp on the pulmonary artery distal to the anastomosis for 10 to 15 minutes prior to allowing full flow to the newly implanted lung. The above steps are repeated for the contralateral side. Some centers start ventilation prior to reperfusion. Ventilator settings should be set at low pressure, low FiO_2.
- **Closure:** The posterior and anterior hila are inspected for hemostasis. Chest tubes are placed. Interrupted figure-of-eight sutures are used to close the thoracotomy. Wire cerclage or a sternal plating system is used to close the sternum. The double-lumen endotracheal tube is switched for a single-lumen tube prior to transport to the ICU. Toilet bronchoscopy is performed and the anastomoses are inspected.

Circulatory Support During Lung Transplantation

- The tip box that follows describes the use of circulatory support during lung transplantation, including options and considerations.
- Note, some centers use circulatory support as routine practice.

TIPS

	Off-Pump	ECMO	Cardiopulmonary Bypass
Indications	Single lung transplant, stable hemodynamics, normal filling pressures and ventilation	Hemodynamic instability, pulmonary hypertension, high pCO_2	Concomitant cardiac procedure needed (eg, coronary artery bypass grafting), uncontrolled injury to left atrium
Configuration	Not applicable	Closed circuit Heparin not required Can be converted to cardiopulmonary bypass using same cannulas	Air-blood interface Systemic heparinization required Can be converted to ECMO using same cannulas
Pros	No coagulopathy, less time in operating room	Controlled lung reperfusion, potentially decreases primary graft dysfunction, increased exposure from maximizing heart retraction, allows minimal ventilator settings	Most flexibility in terms of exposure and conduct of operation
Cons	First implanted lung receives 100% of cardiac output Heart retraction may lead to hemodynamic instability, limiting exposure	Invasive Bleeding	Invasive Coagulopathy, bleeding, increased blood transfusions Increased inflammation Increased postoperative complications

Postoperative Care

- The patient is usually brought to the ICU intubated. Extubation should occur expeditiously within the first 1 to 2 days. Ventilator settings should minimize FiO_2 and pressure delivered.
- Removal of ECMO: Central VA ECMO should be removed. The patient usually will be able to come off VA ECMO. The patient may need to remain on VV ECMO peripherally, but this can be removed in the ICU within the first 1 to 2 days postoperatively.

- Primary graft dysfunction characterized by the development of noncardiogenic pulmonary edema usually occurs within the first 72 hours of transplantation. Treatment is supportive, with diuresis, protective lung ventilation, and, in severe cases, use of ECMO.

PEARLS AND PITFALLS

- To increase lung donor utilization, every potential organ donor should be evaluated during organ procurement as a potential lung donor. Lungs are often better during in-person evaluation than during reading the donor summary.
- Bilateral lung transplantation has significantly evolved over the past decades with meticulous attention to surgical technique. While minor variations are present between centers, the basic principles as outlined in this chapter remain constant.
- Clinical debate currently centers around indications for using ex vivo lung perfusion and whether circulatory support should be deployed for all lung transplant recipients. Ex vivo lung perfusion is costly but may expand the donor pool and one day improve organ health. Recent studies demonstrate the advantages of ECMO to regulate reperfusion injury.

Suggested Readings

1. Benazzo A, Schwarz S, Frommlet F, et al; Vienna ECLS Program. Twenty-year experience with extracorporeal life support as bridge to lung transplantation. *J Thorac Cardiovasc Surg*. 2019;157(6):2515-2525.e10. PMID: 30922636.
2. Boasquevisque CH, Yildirim E, Waddel TK, Keshavjee S. Surgical techniques: lung transplant and lung volume reduction. *Proc Am Thorac Soc*. 2009;6(1):66-78. PMID: 19131532.*The above papers outline the techniques performed at the highest-volume lung transplant centers in the world.*
3. Cypel M, Yeung JC, Hirayama S, et al. Technique for prolonged normothermic ex vivo lung perfusion. *J Heart Lung Transplant*. December 2008;27(12):1319-1325. PMID: 19059112. *This study is an excellent resource to understand the principles of ex vivo lung perfusion (EVLP) from one of the leading EVLP centers.*
4. Davis RD. Bilateral sequential lung transplantation. *Operat Tech Thorac Cardiovasc Surg*. 2007;12(1):57-72.
5. Munshi L, Keshavjee S, Cypel M. Donor management and lung preservation for lung transplantation. *Lancet Respir Med*. 2013;1(4):318-328. PMID: 24429157.
6. Parekh K, Patterson GA. Technical considerations in adult lung transplantation. *Semin Thorac Cardiovasc Surg*. 2004;16(4):322-332. PMID: 15635536. *This paper provides a thoughtful review of the technical decisions in lung transplantation.*
7. Schwarz S, Hoetzenecker K, Klepetko W. Procedural mechanical support for lung transplantation. *Curr Opin Organ Transplant*. 2021;26(3):309-313. PMID: 33782246. doi:10.1097/MOT.0000000000000873. *This group routinely performs lung transplantation using circulatory support.*
8. Sundaresan S, Trachiotis GD, Aoe M, Patterson GA, Cooper JD. Donor lung procurement: assessment and operative technique. *Ann Thorac Surg*. 1993;56(6):1409-1413. PMID: 8267453. *Optimizing donor lung management before and during lung procurement is key to achieving good posttransplant outcomes.*

SECTION II Mediastinum/ Diaphragm

Chapter 21

Thoracic Outlet Syndrome and First Rib Resection: Supraclavicular, Transaxillary, and Minimally Invasive Approaches

BRETT L. BROUSSARD
DEAN DONAHUE

SUPRACLAVICULAR FIRST RIB RESECTION

Perioperative Considerations

- Thoracic outlet syndrome (TOS) is considered a disease of compression and may be associated with the subclavian artery, vein, or brachial plexus (Figure 21.1).

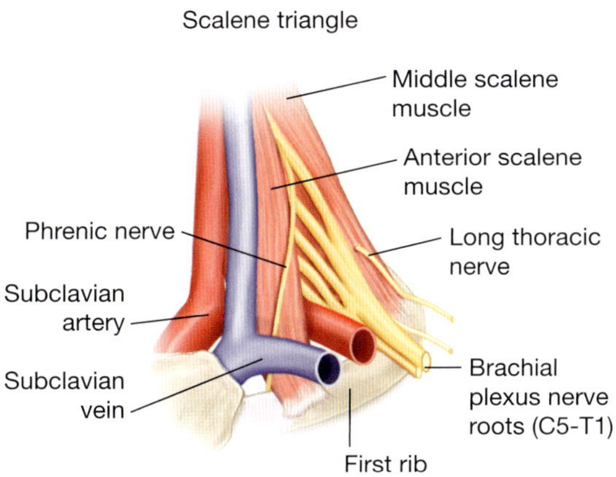

FIGURE 21.1 | The anatomy of the first rib related to the anterior/middle scalene muscles and the neurovascular structures of the thoracic outlet. (From Thompson RW, Vemuri C. Chest wall/pleural space/diaphragm: thoracic outlet syndrome—supraclavicular thoracic outlet decompression. In: Mathisen DJ, Morse CR, eds. *Master Techniques in Surgery: Thoracic Surgery—Transplantation, Tracheal Resections, Mediastinal Tumors, Extended Thoracic Resection*. Wolters Kluwer, 2015:85-99. Figure 10.1.)

- The primary tenet of surgery for TOS centers around relieving compression of the thoracic outlet by removing the first rib and all other fibrous attachments (anterior/middle scalene, etc.) that may tether the subclavian artery/vein or brachial plexus.
- Choosing an approach to undergo TOS decompression and first rib removal is based on surgeon experience/comfort, but etiology of the disease should also be considered.

Indications

- Indications for surgery can vary by etiology.
- The advantages of the supraclavicular approach include more extensive anterior/middle scalenectomy with good visualization of the phrenic nerve, complete exposure of the first rib, extensive exposure of the brachial plexus, exposure of cervical ribs and C7 transverse process, and access to subclavian vessels for repair/reconstruction if needed.

Preoperative Testing

- The workup prior to surgery will depend on etiology.
- We prefer computed tomography with specific TOS protocol (with intravenous contrast) to evaluate bony structures, surrounding muscle and vascular compression.

Instruments and Equipment

- Typical open instrument tray should suffice with some specialized additions listed below.
- 5-mm Kerrison Rongeur.
- Nerve root retractor, 5 in × 4.25 in × 0.5 in.
- Cervical Cloward retractor, 13 mm.
- Extended protected needle tip electrocautery.
- Bipolar forceps with pointed tip and heavy tip.
- Nerve stimulator.

Positioning (Figure 21.2)

- The head should be supported with a low-profile pillow or gel cushion such as the doughnut.
- A slight 45° turn should be applied to the head away from the surgical side.
- The skin should be protected from all intravenous tubing and electrocardiogram leads.
- The hands and wrists should be in a neutral thumbs-up position, and we recommend placing a rolled blue towel in the hand as support.
- The operative side shoulder should then be supported with a stack of towels raising it off the bed, which allows opening of the costoclavicular space.
- The table is then configured into a semi-Fowler position with the back in a 30° incline with the legs flat or with a slight decline to relieve tension in the lower back.
- The patient is prepped from the chin to the umbilicus including both sides of the neck and shoulder to shoulder.
- Although rare, the sternum should be accessible in the event where sternotomy is needed for more proximal vascular control.

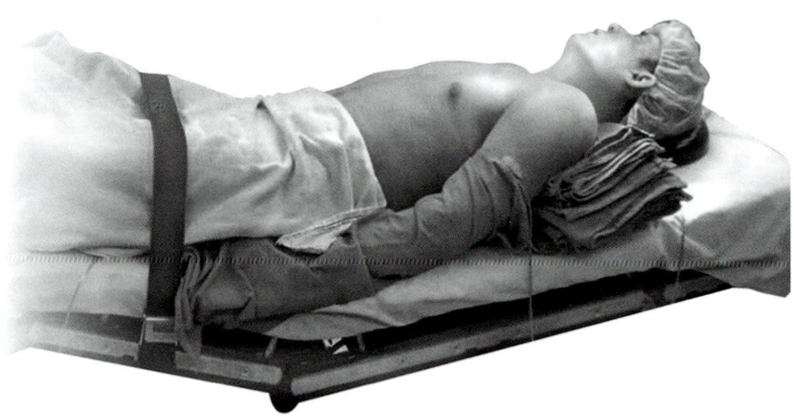

FIGURE 21.2 ▌ The patient is placed in a semi-Fowler position with a stack of towels under the operative side shoulder to open the costoclavicular space. (Reprinted from Broussard BL, Donahue DM. Surgical technique: supraclavicular first rib resection. *Thorac Surg Clin*. 2021;31(1):71-79, with permission from Elsevier.)

TIPS

- *It is useful to have a discussion with anesthesia colleagues regarding positioning and no use of neuromuscular blockage after induction of anesthesia.*
- *Preservation of cutaneous nerves, omohyoid muscle, and unnamed vascular structures is attempted throughout the case.*
- *It is ideal to remove as much anterior scalene as possible without damaging the phrenic nerve.*
- *The posterior rib should be transected medial to the transverse process to completely free the T1 nerve root.*
- *All fibrous attachments to the subclavian artery and brachial plexus should be mobilized.*

Technique

Incision and Initial Dissection (Figure 21.3)

- A 4- to 5-cm skin incision is made with the medial starting point on the lateral border of the sternocleidomastoid (SCM) muscle.
- The incision should be 1 to 2 cm above the clavicle.
- The subcutaneous tissue is then divided along with the platysma.
- Subplatysmal flaps are created for 2 to 3 cm in all directions using skin hooks to retract the platysma.

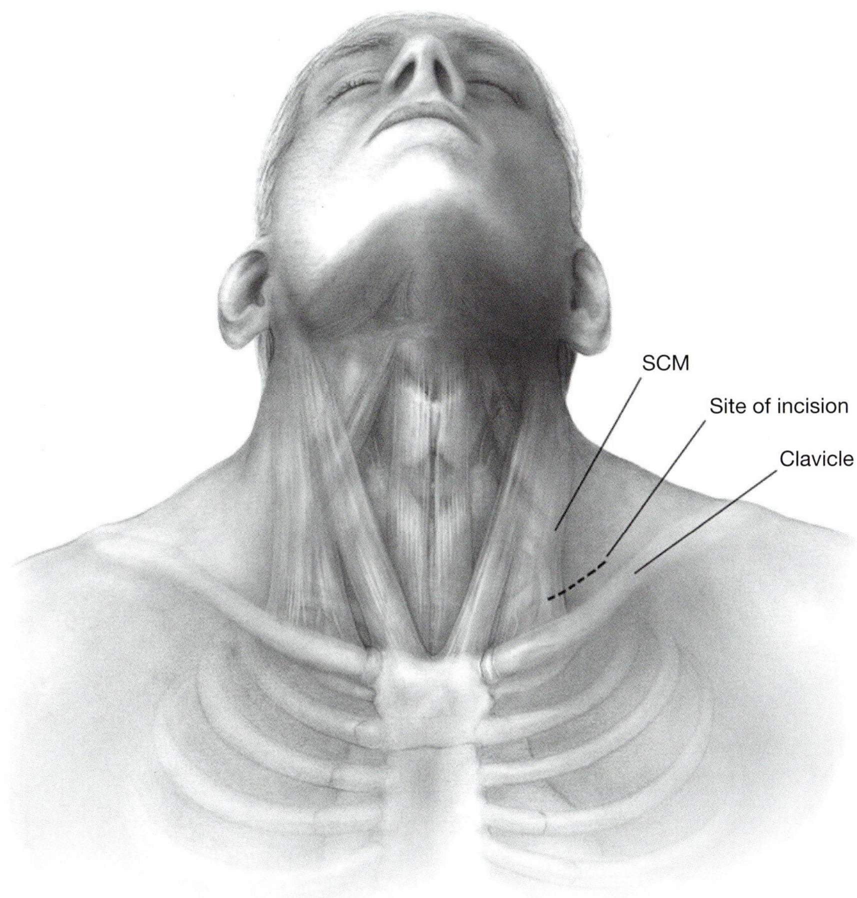

FIGURE 21.3 | A supraclavicular incision is made from the lateral border of the sternocleidomastoid muscle (SCM) laterally toward the shoulder. This incision is 1 to 2 cm above the clavicle. (Reprinted from Broussard BL, Donahue DM. Surgical technique: supraclavicular first rib resection. *Thorac Surg Clin*. 2021;31(1):71-79, with permission from Elsevier.)

Mobilization of the Scalene Fat Pat and Omohyoid Muscle (Figure 21.4)

- The scalene fat pat is mobilized from medial to lateral beginning at the lateral edge of the SCM.
- Cutaneous nerve branches and vessels should be preserved and mobilized with the pad.
- The omohyoid muscle should be identified running parallel to the incision. This should be circumferentially dissected, and a vessel loop is used around it for retraction assistance.
- Once caudal to the omohyoid, lateral mobilization of the fat pad should continue, but electrocautery may be switched to bipolar dissection as the anterior scalene is approached.
- A silk stitch can be placed into the fat pad once it is mobilized and used a retraction.

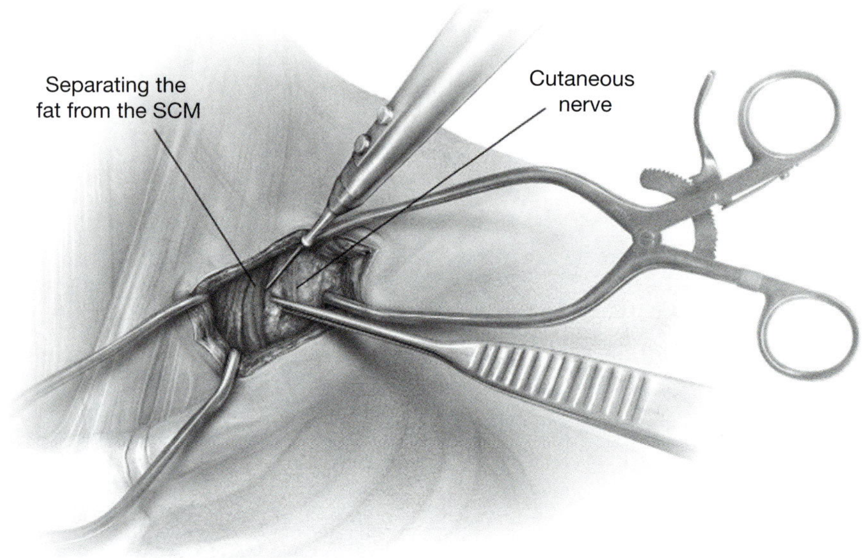

FIGURE 21.4 ▌ The scalene fat pad is mobilized from a medial to lateral direction. (Reprinted from Broussard BL, Donahue DM. Surgical technique: supraclavicular first rib resection. *Thorac Surg Clin*. 2021;31(1):71-79, with permission from Elsevier.)

Anterior Scalene Division (Figure 21.5)

- Finger palpation can be used to help guide identification of the anterior scalene muscle and the subclavian artery.
- The anterior scalene is typically deep and slightly medial to the lateral edge of the SCM.
- Once identified, the anterior surface of the anterior scalene should be carefully dissected as this is where the phrenic nerve typically runs.
- A nerve stimulator (current setting 0.5-1 mA; frequency setting 30 Hz) can be used to help identify the phrenic nerve.
- The anterior scalene is then dissected circumferentially down to the insertion at the tubercle on the first rib.
- The subclavian artery runs posterior to the anterior scalene and is protected during this mobilization.
- The anterior scalene is then partially divided off the first rib. Complete division is avoided at this time to aid in the cephalad division.
- The cephalad division is then done as high as possible with special care to not injure the phrenic nerve and its C5 contribution. The caudal portion is then completed, and this portion of muscle is removed.

Brachial Plexus and Subclavian Artery Dissection

- The subclavian artery is then mobilized anteriorly and posteriorly with special care to protect the dorsal scapular branch. This typically originates 1 to 2 cm from the anterior scalene muscle.
- The trunks of the brachial plexus are then identified on the ventral surface of the middle scalene muscles. There is typically dense connective tissue here, and its removal around the plexus is essential to the conduct of the operation.

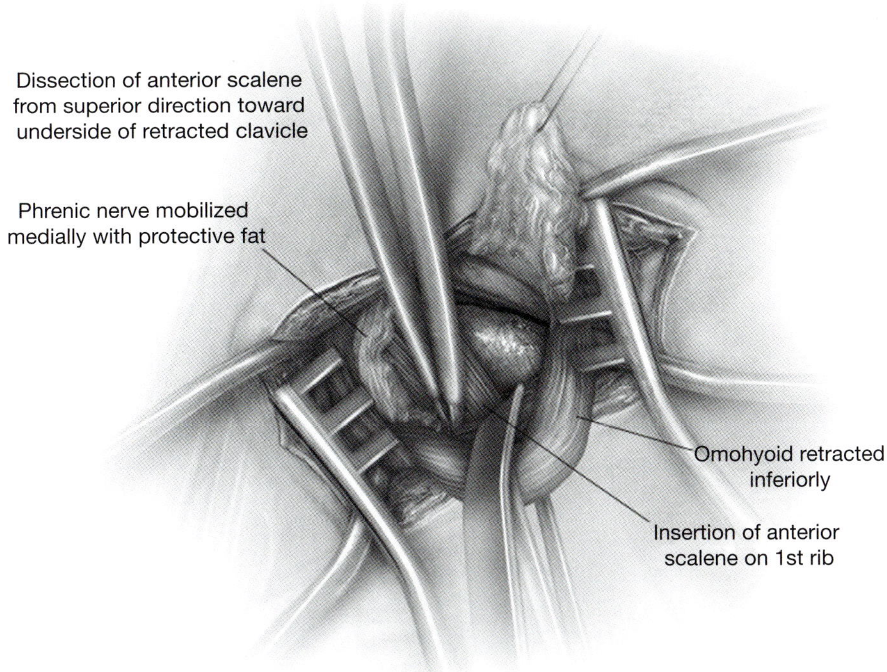

FIGURE 21.5 ▌ The anterior scalene muscle is mobilized and transected. Special care is made such that the phrenic nerve is protected during this mobilization. (Reprinted from Broussard BL, Donahue DM. Surgical technique: supraclavicular first rib resection. *Thorac Surg Clin*. 2021;31(1):71-79, with permission from Elsevier.)

- The orientation of the trunks is typically oblique with the middle trunk lying more dorsal than the upper trunk and the lower trunk further dorsal than the middle trunk.
- Atraumatic forceps with scissors or fine-tip bipolar can be used to carry out this dissection. All fibrous tissue and scalene fibers should be dissected free from all three trunks of the plexus and the subclavian artery.

Middle Scalene Division and Posterior Rib Exposure (Figure 21.6)

- The middle scalene typically lies posterior to the trunks of the brachial plexus, and the posterior portion of the first rib can be palpated deep to the middle scalene.
- The middle scalene must be taken off the posterior rib typically with bipolar energy as the dorsal scapular nerve and long thoracic nerve penetrate the middle scalene. For this reason, it is important to divide the fibers only 1 to 2 cm above the insertion on the rib.
- The posterior inner curve of the rib can have dense attachments, which will need to be freed and divided.
- These can be in the form of costoseptal or costoseptalcostal ligaments, which can be a site of entrapment of the T1 spinal nerve.

Intercostal Muscle and Costotransverse Ligament Division

- Along the lesser curve of the rib, blunt dissection can be performed to separate the Sibson fascia from the underside of the rib.
- An extended flat protected tip electrocautery is then used to divide the intercostal muscles. The tip is bent to a 45° angle and eventually a 90° angle to completely divide the intercostal muscles.
- The cautery is then used at a 15 to 20° angle to divide the costotransverse ligaments between the neck of the rib and the transverse process.

Division of the First Rib (Figure 21.7)

- The posterior rib is divided first between the head and neck of the rib medial to the tip of the T1 transverse process. A 5-mm Kerrison Rongeur is used to divide the rib from the inner curve toward the outer curve.
- The rib is then retracted caudally to improve exposure of the anterior rib.

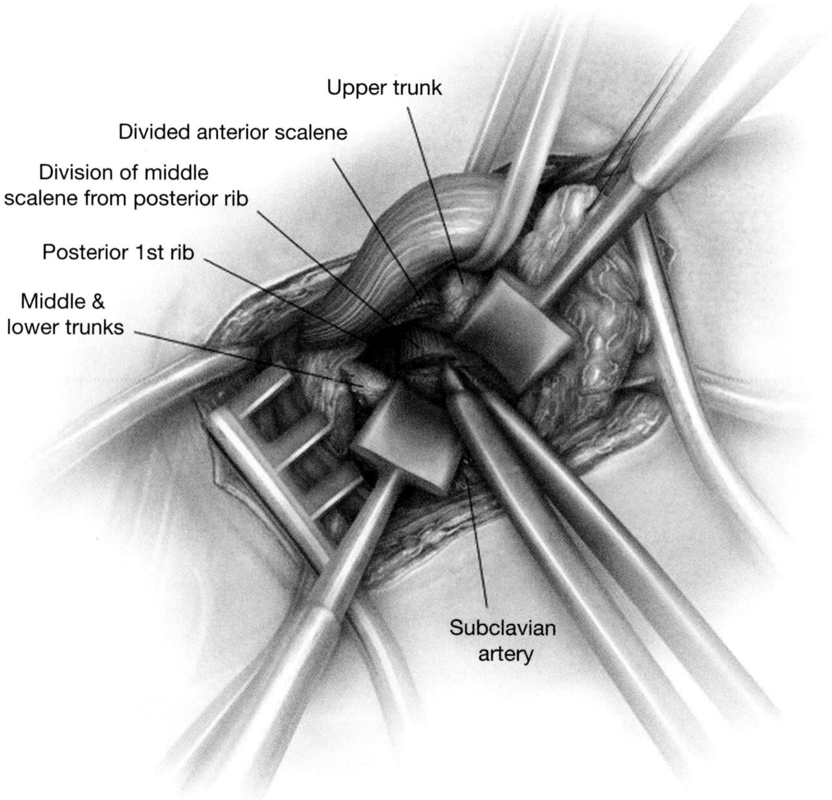

FIGURE 21.6 ▌ The middle scalene muscle is divided off the posterior rib, dorsal from the brachial plexus. (Reprinted from Broussard BL, Donahue DM. Surgical technique: supraclavicular first rib resection. *Thorac Surg Clin*. 2021;31(1):71-79, with permission from Elsevier.)

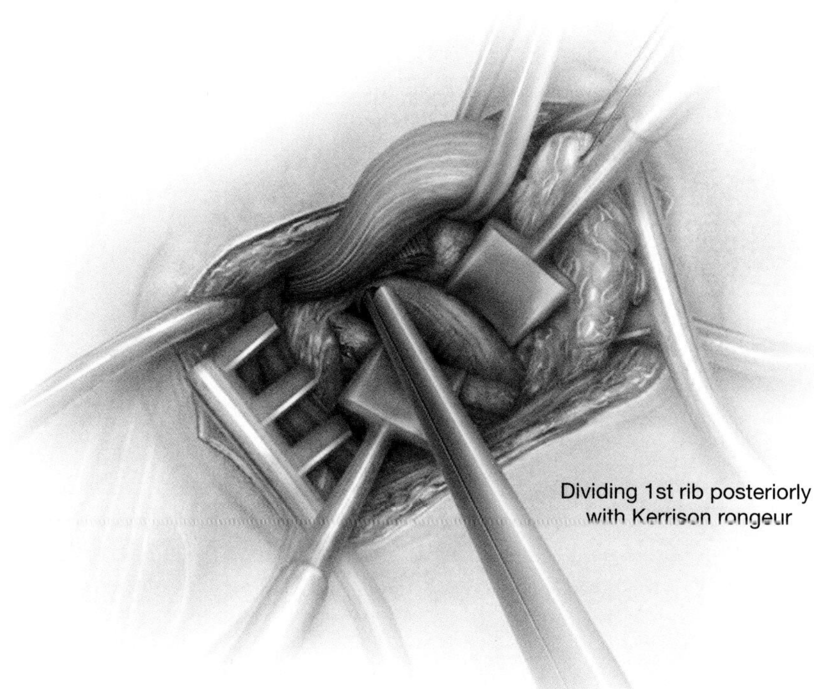

FIGURE 21.7 ▌ The posterior rib is cut using a 5 mm Kerrison Rongeur. The rib is transected medial to the transverse process at the neck of the rib. (Reprinted from Broussard BL, Donahue DM. Surgical technique: supraclavicular first rib resection. *Thorac Surg Clin*. 2021;31(1):71-79, with permission from Elsevier.)

- The same Kerrison is then used to divide the anterior rib from the outer curve toward the inner curve.
- Once complete, the rib should be completely free and carefully removed from the surgical field.
- A 14-French red rubber catheter is then placed into the pleural space and will be used to evacuate any pneumothorax once the platysma muscle is nearly closed.
- Prior to closing the platysma, a 15-French round drain is placed into the wound via a lateral stab incision and positioned posteriorly with the tip in the pleural space.

Postoperative Care

- A chest radiograph is performed in the recovery room and repeated the morning after surgery. Lung expansion, the presence of pleural effusion/apical capping, and the level of the diaphragm should be evaluated.
- Postoperative analgesia is controlled with a patient-controlled analgesia (PCA) system and ketorolac intravenously (if age and comorbidities allow).
- On postoperative day 1, the patient is transitioned to oral pain medicine.
- A high-fat diet is encouraged on postoperative day 1, and monitoring of the surgical drain for quality and quantity of fluid is important. If a chyle leak is present, the fluid may change to a milky/pink consistency. This can almost always be managed conservatively with a low-fat diet for 2 to 3 weeks depending on the volume of output. If the output is very low (<100 mL/d), the drain can be removed.
- The patient should use the hand and arm as tolerated and not put the appendage in a sling. Range-of-motion exercises are started on postoperative day 1 and encouraged to be done three times per day.
- Physical therapy can be considered but not started for 4 to 6 weeks after surgery.

PEARLS AND PITFALLS

- Gentle tissue retraction and dissection is key to avoid unwanted tension of neurovascular structures.
- Nerve stimulator can be helpful in identifying and avoiding injury to the phrenic nerve.
- The transection of the posterior rib should be medial to the transverse process.

TRANSAXILLARY FIRST RIB RESECTION

Perioperative Considerations

- Advantages of the transaxillary approach include good access to the subclavian vein, minimal retraction on the brachial plexus, and improved cosmesis given an axillary scar.

Positioning (Figure 21.8)

- The patient is positioned in the lateral decubitus position with the operative side up. A beanbag or institutional preference may be used to secure the patient to the operating room table.
- The arm on the operative side is prepped circumferentially, and the patient is draped.
- A Machleder retractor is secured to the bed, and after the operative side arm is extensively padded, the arm is secured to the Machleder retractor with coband.

TIPS

- *Intermittent relaxation on the upward retraction is necessary to avoid prolonged tension on the neurovascular structures.*
- *Elevation of tissue directly off the rib is key to avoid injury to structures or entering the pleural space.*
- *Further rib removal with rongeur may be warranted to smooth edges and to remove more rib posteriorly.*

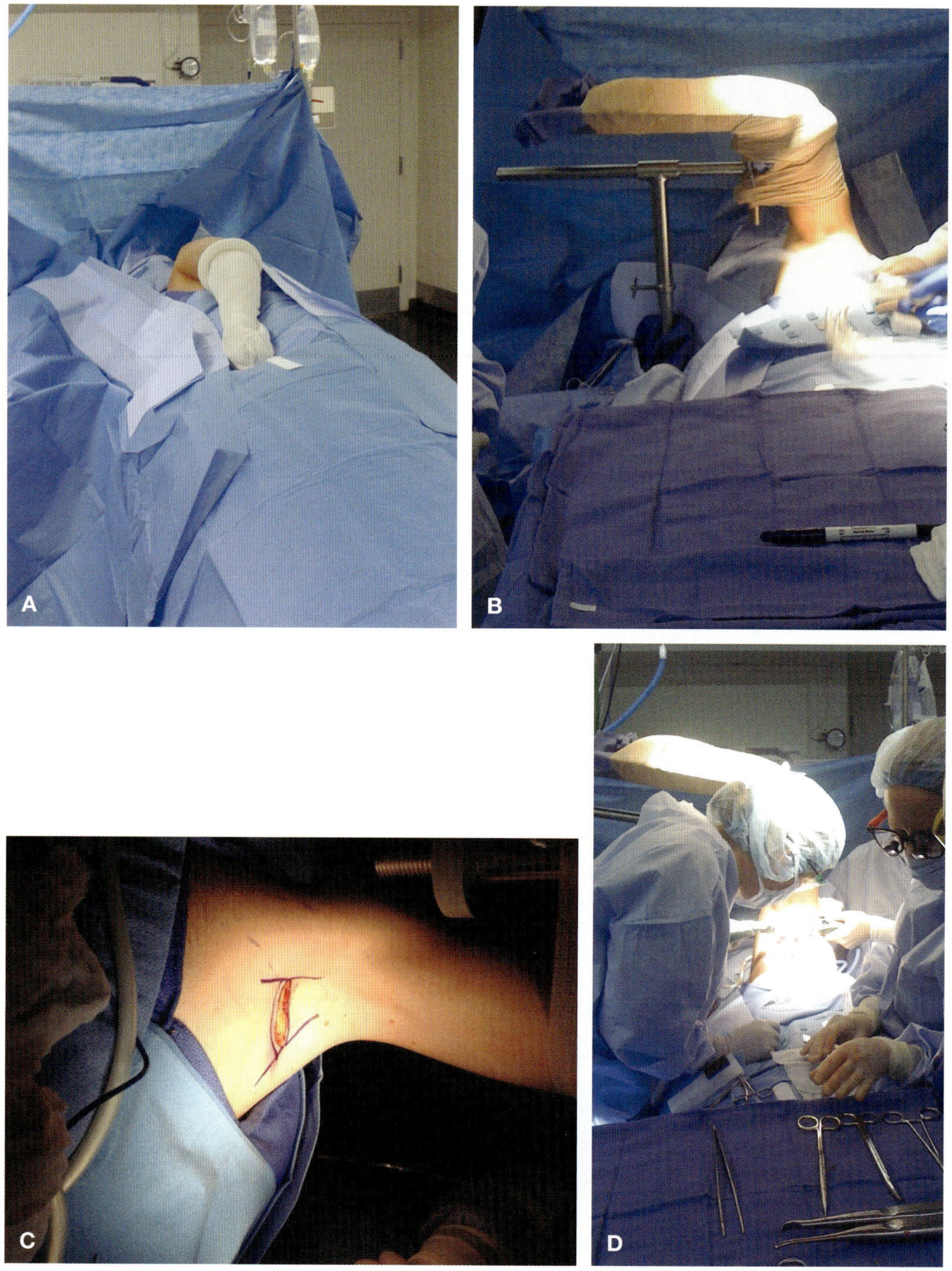

FIGURE 21.8 ▌ A-D. The patient is placed in the lateral decubitus position. The arm is prepped into the surgical field. An axillary incision is made from the lateral border of the pectoralis major toward the latissimus dorsi. (From Freischlag J, Glebova N. Thoracic outlet syndrome: transaxillary approach. In: Mathisen DJ, Morse CR, eds. *Master Techniques in Surgery: Thoracic Surgery: Transplantation, Tracheal Resections, Mediastinal Tumors, Extended Thoracic Resections*. Wolters Kluwer; 2015:109-115. Figure 12.1.)

Technique

Incision and Initial Dissection

- Incision is made at the inferior aspect of the hairline between the posterior border of the pectoralis major and the anterior border of the latissimus dorsi muscles.
- Electrocautery and blunt dissection are used to dissect to the chest wall, ligating lymphatics that may be encountered along the way.
- A self-retaining retractor such as a Weitlaner is used at the skin, and the arm is elevated by raising the Machleder retractor. A Deaver retractor and a lighted retractor (St. Marks retractor) is then used on either side to assist in visualization of the deep axillary structures.

- The upward tension on the arm is frequently relaxed throughout the case while the wound is packed to minimize stretch on the brachial plexus.

Identification of Vascular Structures (Figure 21.9)

- It is crucial to identify the subclavian vein and artery and their relation to the first rib.
- It is helpful to palpate the pulse of the subclavian artery. Once found, the vein is anterior to the artery with the anterior scalene between the two structures.
- The brachial plexus is located posterior to the artery and typically not dissected via this approach due to poor visualization.
- Blunt dissection is used to sweep away tissue around the vein and artery.

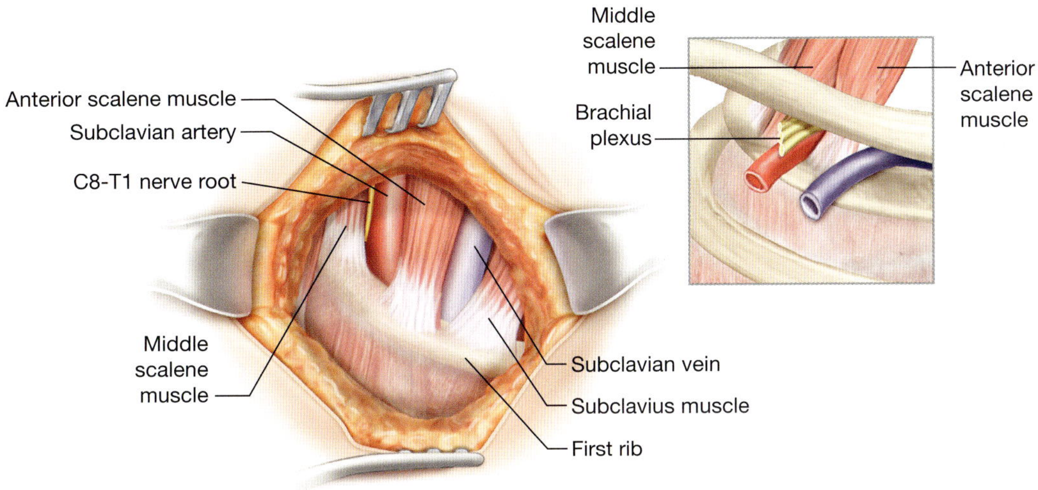

FIGURE 21.9 | The neurovascular structures are identified as they course over the rib from the transaxillary view. (From Dilosa KL, Humphries MD, Venous and arterial thoracic outlet syndrome. In: Hawn MT, ed. *Operative Techniques in Surgery*. 2nd ed. Wolters Kluwer; 2023: 1901-1910. Figure 6.9.10A.)

First Rib Dissection (Figure 21.10)

- A periosteal elevator is used to clear the intercostal muscle fibers off the inferior aspect of the rib.
- A small blunt elevator is then used along under surface of the rib to push the pleura and lesser curve attachments away from the rib.

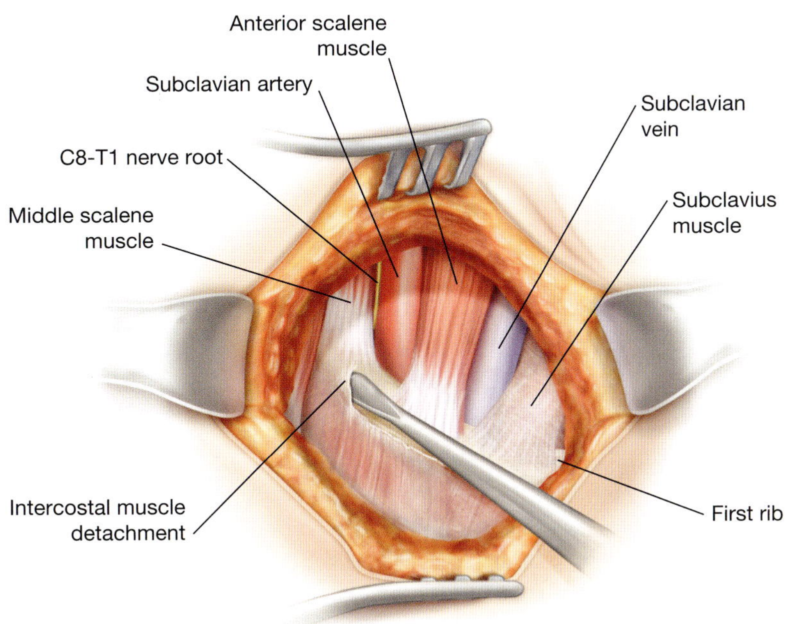

FIGURE 21.10 | A periosteal elevator is used to mobilize the soft tissue attachments to the rib. (From Arnaoutakis GJ, Reifsnyder T, Freischlag JA. Neurogenic thoracic outlet syndrome exposure and decompression: transaxillary. In: Mulholland MW, Albo D, Dalman R, Hawn MT, Hughes S, Sabel MS, eds. *Operative Techniques in Surgery*. Wolters Kluwer; 2015: 1862-1868. Figure 6.8.3.)

- The subclavius muscle is then located along the anterior aspect of the rib next to the subclavian vein. The muscle is divided sharply away from the rib.
- The anterior scalene muscle is then encountered between the artery and the vein. A right-angle clamp is used to lift muscle fibers up and away from the artery, and the muscle is divided sharply (Figure 21.11).

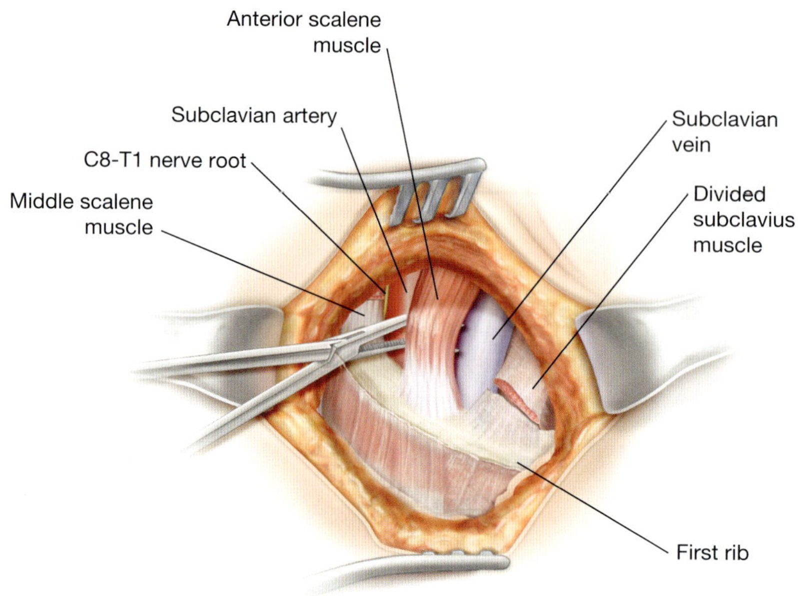

FIGURE 21.11 ▌ The anterior scalene muscle is sharply divided off the first rib. (From Arnaoutakis GJ, Reifsnyder T, Freischlag JA. Neurogenic thoracic outlet syndrome exposure and decompression: transaxillary. In: Mulholland MW, Albo D, Dalman R, Hawn MT, Hughes S, Sabel MS, eds. *Operative Techniques in Surgery*. Wolters Kluwer; 2015: 1862-1868. Figure 6.8.5.)

- A periosteal elevator is then used to lift the middle scalene away from the rib.
- A right-angle clamp can again be used to evaluate the extent of mobilization.
- The rib is first divided anteriorly using a bone cutter next to the subclavian vein (Figure 21.12).

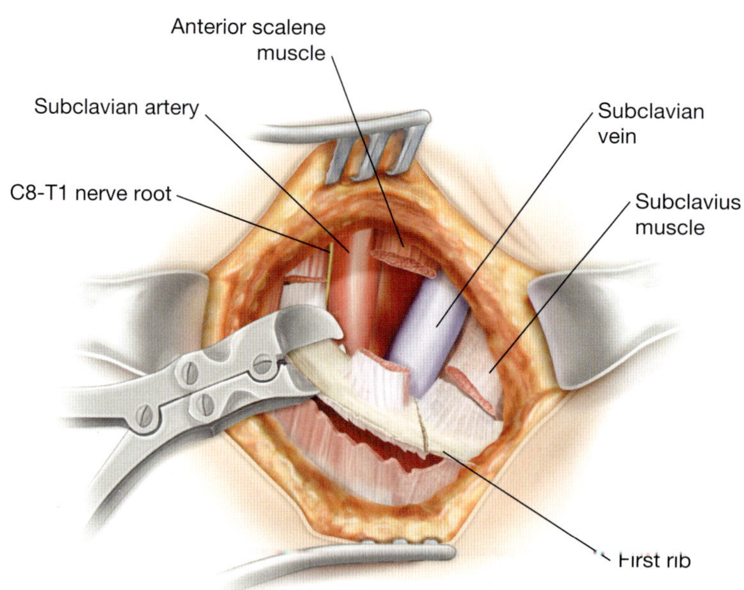

FIGURE 21.12 ▌ The first rib is then cut anterior and posteriorly with the bone cutter. (From Arnaoutakis GJ, Reifsnyder T, Freischlag JA. Neurogenic thoracic outlet syndrome exposure and decompression: transaxillary. In: Mulholland MW, Albo D, Dalman R, Hawn MT, Hughes S, Sabel MS, eds. *Operative Techniques in Surgery*. Wolters Kluwer; 2015: 1862-1868. Figure 6.8.7.)

- With inferior traction placed on the anteriorly divided rib, the rib is divided posteriorly with special care to not injure the brachial plexus. A rongeur can then be used to remove any remaining bony edges and smooth surfaces of the remaining rib so they are away from the neurovascular structures.
- The field is then filled with saline and positive pressure breaths given to evaluate for pneumothorax. If pneumothorax is suspected, a chest tube can be placed through a separate incision.

Postoperative Care

- Postoperative care is similar to supraclavicular approach in that chest radiograph is obtained in the recovery room and PCA is initially used for analgesia. This is transitioned to oral pain medicine on the first postoperative day.
- The patient can be discharged from the hospital once pain is controlled with oral medication and chest tube has been removed (if placed at operation).

PEARLS AND PITFALLS

- Blunt dissection of the pleura away from the rib is key to avoiding pleural injury.
- Visualization can be difficult in this approach, and the surgeon should ensure all vascular structures are cleared away from the rib prior to transection.
- Brachial plexus neurolysis may be difficult due to poor visualization through this approach.

ROBOTIC MINIMALLY INVASIVE APPROACH

Perioperative Considerations

- The expansion of minimally invasive surgery, in particular robotic surgery, has many benefits with regard to thoracic surgery, which can be applied to first rib resection.
- These benefits center around improved visualization for the surgeon, improved dexterity in dissection (when compared to the video-assisted thoracoscopic approach), avoidance of supraclavicular scar, and potential for improved long-term outcomes.

Instruments and Equipment

- Our institution uses a Da Vinci Xi robot surgery platform (Intuitive Surgical).
- Robotic instruments used:
  - 0° endoscope plus
  - Three 8-mm robotic ports
  - 10-mm AirSeal assistant port
  - One robotic hook monopolar
  - One Prograsp
  - One curved biopolar dissector
  - 10-in Kerrison Rongeur or Midas-Rex drill with drill bit and shaft cover (Medtronic, Minneapolis, MN)
- Other items
  - Laparoscopic grasper
  - Suction irrigator
  - Kittner roll gauze sponge (Carefree Surgical, New Castle, CA)

Positioning

- General anesthesia is induced, and a double-lumen endotracheal tube is placed.
- As with other approaches, anesthesia should use short-acting neuromuscular blockade at induction and avoid further use throughout the case.
- The patient is positioned in the lateral decubitus position with the side being operated on facing upward.

TIPS

- *The anterior and posterior ports should not extend too far anterior or posteriorly as this will limit access to the area where the rib will need to be transected.*
- *Use a laparoscopic grasper to tap on the anterior and posterior aspect of the rib to ensure good access.*
- *The anterior portion of the rib can usually be divided with monopolar cautery as this area is usually cartilaginous.*
- *A 10-in Kerrison Rongeur or the Midas Rex drill system can be used to transect the posterior portion of the rib.*
- *Careful understanding of the thoracic outlet anatomy must be mastered and constantly evaluated prior and during the procedure.*

Technique (Figure 21.13 and 21.14)

Port Placement

- The posterior port is first marked just inferior or slightly posterior to the scapular tip. The anterior port marked anterior to the anterior axillary line in the fourth intercostal space. The camera incision is marked between those two ports and slightly inferior.
- The camera port is placed first and ensures placement into the pleural space and allows visualization of the ribs and neurovascular anatomy. The posterior and anterior ports are then placed under direct visualization.
- An assistant port is also placed under direct visualization anterior and inferior on the chest in approximately the ninth intercostal space. A 10-mm AirSeal port is used here.

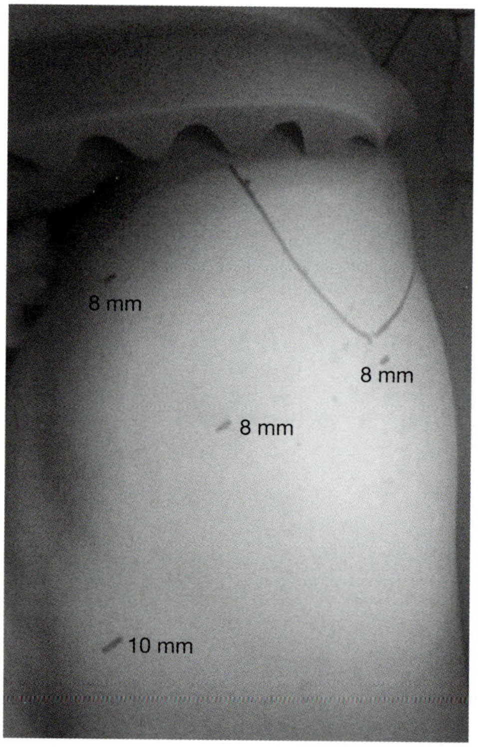

FIGURE 21.13 | Configuration of port placement for transthoracic robotic first rib resection. (Reprinted from Burt BM, Palivela N, Karimian A, Goodman MB. Transthoracic robotic first rib resection: twelve steps. *JTCVS Tech*. 2020;1:104-109, with permission from Elsevier. Published by Elsevier Inc. on behalf of The American Association for Thoracic Surgery.)

Division of the Intercostal Muscle and Mediastinal Pleura

- Monopolar energy on the robotic hook cautery is used to make a pleurotomy, which provides access to divide the intercostal muscle from the lateral border of the rib.
- This is extended posteriorly and anteriorly to the border of the mammary artery and vein.
- The mediastinal pleura is then bluntly peeled off the inferior aspect of the first rib with occasional use of monopolar hook cautery.
- This step is helpful in defining the medial extent of the rib, which sets up division of the rib.

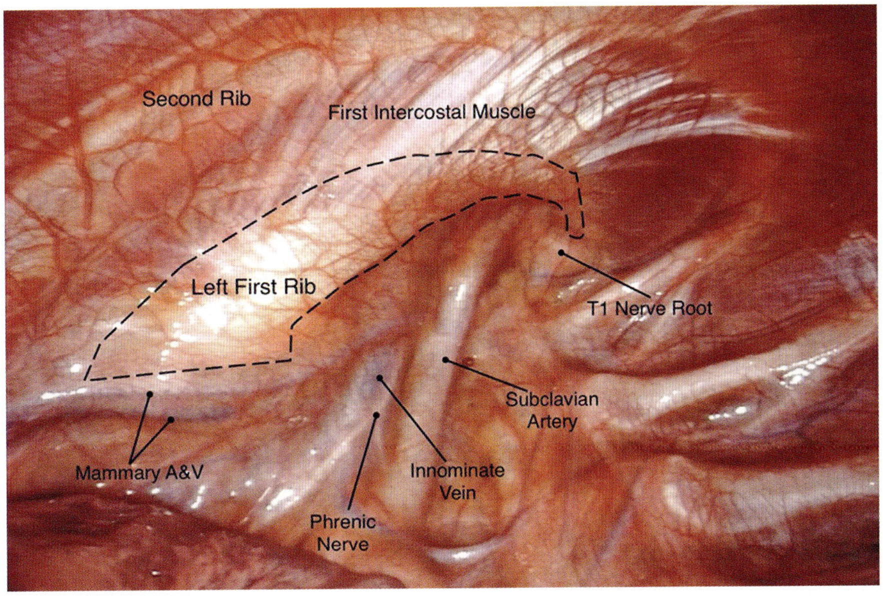

FIGURE 21.14 ▌ Anatomy of the first rib and neurovascular structures of the thoracic outlet from an intrathoracic perspective. (Reprinted from Burt BM, Palivela N, Karimian A, Goodman MB. Transthoracic robotic first rib resection: twelve steps. *JTCVS Tech*. 2020;1:104-109, with permission from Elsevier. Published by Elsevier Inc. on behalf of The American Association for Thoracic Surgery.)

Division of Costal Cartilage and Posterior Rib Dissection

- In the anterior aspect of the rib, the soft costal cartilage can be found and divided with hook cautery monopolar energy. The suction irrigator can be useful to clear the opaque smoke produced by desiccated cartilage.
- The drill can be used if there is ossification of the cartilage.
- Dissection posteriorly is continued with further removal of the first intercostal muscle on inferior/lateral surface of the rib. This is done with the bipolar dissector given the proximity to the T1 nerve root posteriorly. A prograsp is used in the surgeon's left hand to retract tissue. This will be used to gently retract the T1 nerve root from the anterior/inferior portion of the posterior rib.

Bedside Division of the Posterior Rib

- All robotic ports are decoupled from the robot. The posterior port is typically used for the drill or Kerrison. The suction irrigator is placed in the anterior port.
- The rib is then divided posteriorly medial to the transverse process.

Division of the Serratus Anterior, Anterior/Middle Scalene, and Subclavius Muscle

- The rib is now divided anteriorly and posteriorly, which allows medial reflection of rib into the chest, which exposes the superior attachments.
- A prograsp is used in the left hand to retract the rib, and the bipolar dissector is used along with blunt dissection to take the muscle attachments off the superior surface.
- The middle scalene muscle is then divided from the posterior portion of the rib in a similar fashion. The subclavian artery and brachial plexus will be located just anterior to the middle scalene muscle.
- The subclavius muscle is then separated from the insertion on the first rib in a similar fashion. The costoclavicular ligament is also located and divided in this step. In venous TOS cases, these bands can be dense.
- The anterior scalene muscle is then encountered and divided at its insertion on the first rib. Once divided, the rib should be free of attachments and placed to the side for removal.

Venolysis and Brachial Plexus Neurolysis

- With the rib now removed, the nerve and vascular structures can be accessed.
- Near circumferential dissection of the subclavian vein with bipolar and blunt dissection can be used to free scarring from around the vein.

- In neurogenic cases, the trunks of the brachial plexus can be dissected with removal of the fibrous bands that surround them.
- The subclavian artery can be dissected free of the plexus anteriorly.

Removal of First Rib

- A long ringed forcep is used through the assistant port to grasp the rib and remove it from the chest.
- When looking caudally, the surgeon can also witness the diaphragm contracting, thus verifying the phrenic nerve is functional.

Postoperative Care

- Analgesia and range of motion considerations are similar to the supraclavicular and transaxillary approaches.
- Only a chest tube is placed postoperatively in the robotic approach, but high-fat diet and assessment for chyle leak is still recommended.

PEARLS AND PITFALLS

- When placing the anterior and posterior ports, ensure they are not too anterior or too posterior. This will limit access to the respective extents of the rib.
- It remains important to divide the rib posteriorly medial to the transverse process.
- It is imperative to have an excellent grasp of the thoracic outlet anatomy from the intrapleural perspective to avoid vascular or nerve injury.
- Venolysis and neurolysis should be completed to the maximal extent to achieve optimal patient outcomes.
- The surgeon should consider some limitations in this approach regarding the extent of the anterior scalenectomy and brachial plexus neurolysis.

Suggested Readings

1. Panda N, Hurd J, Madsen J, et al. Efficacy and safety of supraclavicular thoracic outlet decompression. *Ann Surg*. 2023;278(3):417-425.
2. Broussard BL, Donahue DM. Surgical technique: supraclavicular first rib resection. *Thorac Surg Clin*. 2021;31(1):71-79.
3. Urschel HC. The transaxillary approach for treatment of thoracic outlet syndromes. *Semin Thorac Cardiovasc Surg*. 1996;8(2):214-220.
4. Burt BM, Palivela N, Karimian A, Goodman MB. Transthoracic robotic first rib resection: twelve steps. *JTCVS Tech*. 2020;1:104-109.

Chapter 22
Sternoclavicular Resection

TIMOTHY M. MILLINGTON

Perioperative Considerations

Preoperative Planning

- Septic arthritis of the sternoclavicular (SC) joint is a rare condition, comprising less than 1% of septic arthritis cases.
- The principal associated medical comorbidity is diabetes mellitus, although intravenous drug use, central venous catheter infection, immunodeficiency, and antecedent trauma are also common.
- Localized pain, swelling, and erythema should be evaluated with CT imaging of the chest, and percutaneous sampling of fluid collections is diagnostic in most cases. About 75% of cases are due to *Staphylococcus aureus*.
- Mediastinitis, localized abscess, or osteomyelitis mandates immediate surgical intervention. In more indolent cases, nonoperative management with intravenous antibiotics or limited incision and drainage is occasionally attempted, but the failure rate likely exceeds 80% (Figure 22.1).

Instruments and Equipment

- In addition to basic general surgical instruments and retractors, a variety of different sized and shaped rongeurs facilitate bony debridement.
- Choice of saw depends on surgeon preference and extent of planned resection. The clavicle may be divided with a Gigli saw or oscillating saw. If a significant portion of the manubrium is resected, then a sternal saw or Lebsche knife may be used instead of the oscillating saw.
- If an oscillating saw is chosen to divide the clavicle, then an appropriately sized malleable retractor is required to protect the underlying vascular structures.
- Instruments to control and repair a major vascular injury must be readily available. A sternal saw should be available in case an urgent sternotomy is needed.
- A vacuum-assisted closure system may be used for more severe infections as an alternative to primary closure.

Patient Positioning

Semi-Fowler Position

- Arms tucked with joints in neutral position and pressure points well padded
- Rolled towel or gel pad placed behind shoulders to slightly extend the neck
- Head rotated slightly away from operative side
- Imperative to prep skin from chin to upper abdomen in the unlikely event that an urgent sternotomy is required

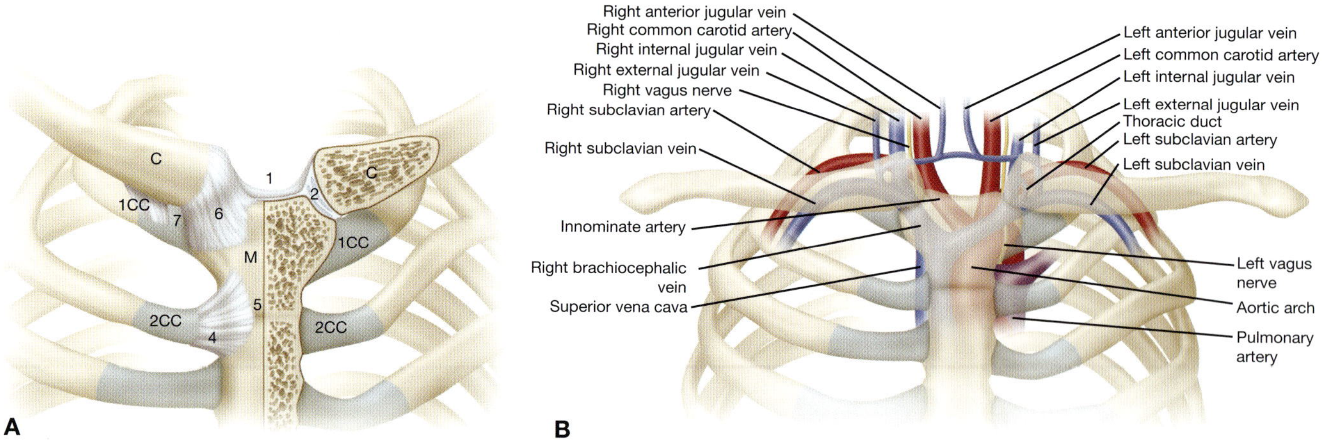

FIGURE 22.1 ▌ A and B. Anatomy of the sternoclavicular (SC) joint and underlying vascular structures. 1, interclavicular ligament; 2, SC joint disk; 4, costochondral capsule; 5, sternum; 6, SC joint capsule; 7, costoclavicular ligament; C, clavicle; CC, costochondral cartilage; M, manubrium. (Reprinted with permission from Hsu JE, Keener JD. Disorders of the sternoclavicular joint. In: Lieberman JR, ed. *AAOS Comprehensive Orthopaedic Review 3.* Vol 2. 3rd ed. American Academy of Orthopaedic Surgeons; 2020:795-803.)

TIPS

- *Debridement limited to arthrotomy of the SC joint and drainage is unlikely to resolve an infection adequately.*
- *If no osteomyelitis of the manubrium is present, then resection of the joint and rongeur debridement of the manubrial aspect of the joint capsule may be adequate.*
- *If osteomyelitis of the first or second ribs is present, then debridement of these costosternal joints is necessary.*
- *Mediastinitis, extensive abscess, and rib involvement are associated with failure of primary closure, and in these cases, wet-to-dry packing or vacuum-assisted closure should be considered.*
- *See also Figures 22.2-22.4*

Technique

- Curvilinear incision following the involved clavicle and then directed inferior along the middle/border of the sternum
- Platysma is divided and pectoralis major muscle and sternocleidomastoid are freed from the clavicle and sternum with electrocautery.
- Meticulous blunt mobilization posterior to the manubrium at the sternal notch is performed and carried laterally along the posterior aspect of the clavicle to free it from the underlying vascular structures.
- The clavicle is divided distal to the area of presumed infection with an oscillating saw or Gigli saw, again emphasizing mobilization and protection of posterior vascular structures prior to division.
- If limited debridement of the manubrium is planned, then the SC joint may be divided with electrocautery. The manubrial aspect of the SC joint is then debrided with rongeurs until healthy-appearing tissue is encountered. Intraoperative cultures should be taken.
- If a more extensive resection is planned, then a right angle–shaped osteotomy is made in the manubrium with the sternal saw or Lebsche knife to permit en bloc removal of the clavicle and SC joint.
- If indicated, additional mediastinal debridement is performed including removal of the heads of the first and occasionally second ribs.
- Resection bed is further debrided with a pulse irrigator. Edges of cut bone are smoothed with a rasp.
- If extensive purulence or poorly perfused tissue is present, then delayed closure or secondary intention may be planned. In most cases, a vacuum-assisted closure device is appropriate, although nonadherent foam should be placed over any exposed subclavian vessels. In heavily contaminated cases, wound packing with wet-to-dry gauze is preferred.

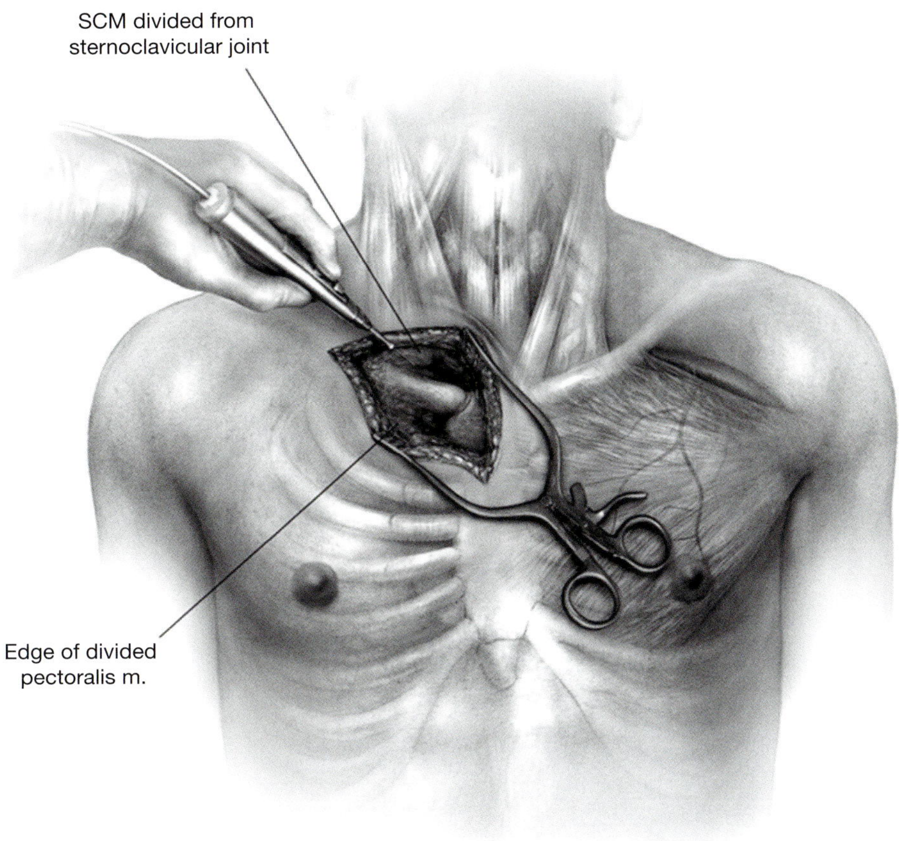

FIGURE 22.2 ▌ A curvilinear incision is made following the course of the clavicle and manubrium, and the sternoclavicular joint is cleared of soft tissue anteriorly. SCM, sternocleidomastoid muscle. (Reprinted from Jackson RS, Carter YM, Blair Marshall M. Surgical management of the infected sternoclavicular joint. *Operat Tech Thorac Cardiovasc Surg*. 2013;18(1):42-52, with permission from Elsevier.)

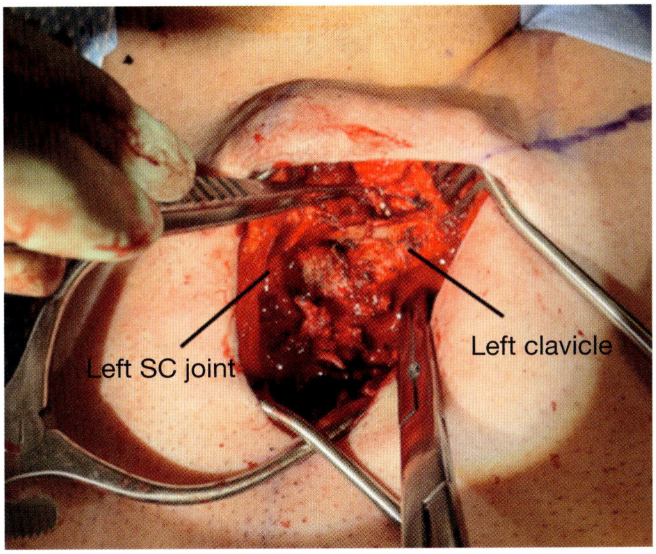

FIGURE 22.3 ▌ After careful blunt dissection hugging the clavicle and avoiding the vascular structures, an instrument is placed posteriorly to guide the saw. SC, sternoclavicular.

- In most cases, primary closure may be attempted. Pectoralis major muscle is mobilized deeply by dividing its attachments to the chest wall and superficially by elevating a subcutaneous flap from the surface of the muscle.
- If a smaller defect is present, then the upper third of the pectoralis major may be separated in line with the muscle fibers to create a flap. For larger defects, the entire muscle is advanced medially.
- The pectoralis flap is anchored to the cut edge of the sternocleidomastoid muscle superiorly and medially to fascial tissue overlying the manubrium.
- Closed suction drains are placed adjacent to the muscle flap and the overlying soft tissue and skin is closed in layers (Figure 22.5).

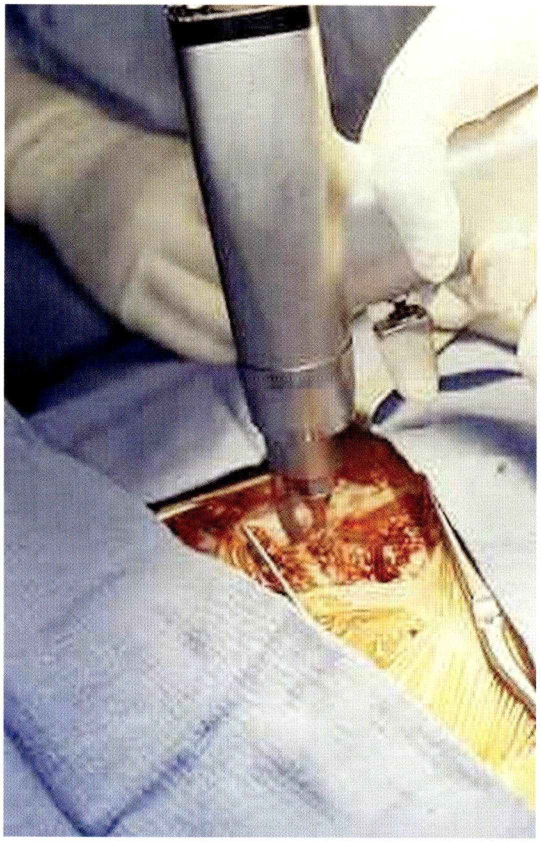

FIGURE 22.4 ▌ An oscillating saw may be used to divide both the clavicle and the manubrium and is therefore the most versatile option, although the choice of saw depends on surgeon preference. (From Grunenwald D. Surgical resection of superior sulcus lesions. In: LoCicero J, ed. *Shields' General Thoracic Surgery*. 8th ed. Wolters Kluwer; 2019:527-546. Figure 38.20.)

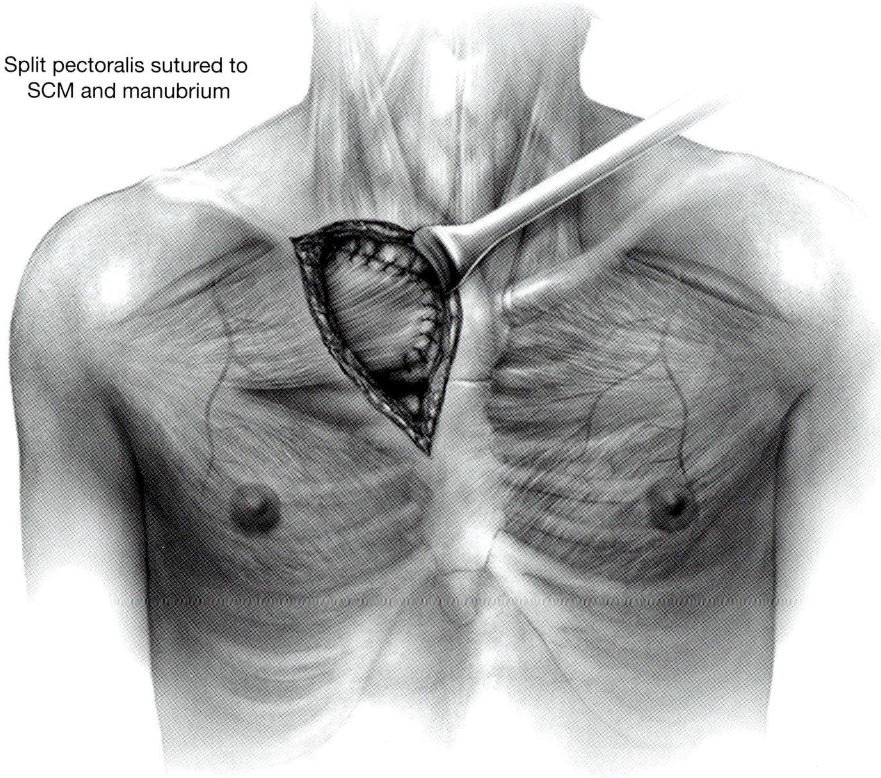

FIGURE 22.5 ▌ The upper portion of the pectoralis muscle is used to provide soft-tissue coverage and is anchored to the cut sternocleidomastoid muscle (SCM) and presternal fascia. (Reprinted from Jackson RS, Carter YM, Blair Marshall M. Surgical management of the infected sternoclavicular joint. *Operat Tech Thorac Cardiovasc Surg*. 2013;18(1):42-52, with permission from Elsevier.)

Postoperative Care

- Postoperative chest radiograph is indicated to rule out unanticipated pneumothorax. A daily radiograph is not necessary.
- If the wound is closed primarily, then drains should be left in place until output is scant (<30 mL per day) and serosanguinous in character. If a vacuum-assisted closure system is used, it should be changed at minimum every third day. This can typically be done at the bedside unless further debridement is anticipated.
- Antibiotics are determined by pre- and intraoperative culture results and should be continued for 14 days postoperatively.
- Early ambulation and physical therapy focusing on shoulder range of motion is imperative. Sternal precautions are not necessary in most cases.
- Follow-up after discharge should focus on physical therapy and signs of recurrent or persistent infection.

PEARLS AND PITFALLS

- Injuries to the subclavian vein or artery during blunt dissection around the clavicle are uncommon. Most can be temporized with direct pressure on the site of injury and endovascular control by balloon occlusion via either a retrograde or antegrade approach.
- Smaller injuries due to avulsion of a branch vessel can be oversewn. Larger injuries can often be repaired endovascularly with a stent graft.
- Only in very rare cases is proximal control through a median sternotomy (right) or high anterolateral thoracotomy (left) necessary.

Suggested Readings

1. Ali B, Barlas V, Shetty AK, Demas C, Schwartz JD. The preferred treatment of sternoclavicular joint infections: a systematic Review. *Cureus*. 2020;12(8):e9963.
2. Ali B, Shetty A, Qeadan F, Demas C, Schwartz JD. Sternoclavicular joint infections: improved outcomes with myocutaneous flaps. *Semin Thorac Cardiovasc Surg*. 2020;32(2):369-376.
3. Jackson RS, Carter YM, Blair Marshall M. Surgical management of the infected sternoclavicular joint. *Operat Tech Thorac Cardiovasc Surg*. 2013;18(1):42-52.
4. Kachala SS, D'Souza DM, Teixeira-Johnson L, et al. Surgical management of sternoclavicular joint infections. *Ann Thorac Surg*. 2016;101(6):2155-2160.

Chapter 23

Chest Wall Resection and Reconstruction: Minimally Invasive Surgery/ Thoracotomy

YOLONDA L. COLSON
JAMES S. ALLAN
PAUL W. FURLOW

Perioperative Considerations

- Prior to chest wall resection, functional status should be assessed preoperatively in a manner similar to that performed for pulmonary resections.

TIPS

Chest pain is the most important sign of local invasion.

- The oncologic goal of chest wall tumor resection is wide local excision of the tumor with negative margins, as positive margins are a strong predictor of local recurrence (Table 23.1).

TABLE 23.1 | Tumors of the Chest Wall

Primary benign chest wall tumors	Typically, slow-growing, asymptomatic, and painless
Bone	Osteochondroma, chondroma
Soft tissue	Fibrous dysplasia, desmoid tumors, etc.
Neural	Neurofibroma, neurilemmoma
Primary malignant chest wall tumors	Typically, more progressive, symptomatic, and painful
Bone	Chondrosarcoma, Ewing sarcoma, osteosarcoma, and plasmacytoma (spine)
Soft tissue	Synovial sarcoma, malignant fibrous histiocytoma, liposarcoma, rhabdomyosarcoma, and other
Neural	Malignant peripheral nerve sheath tumors
Lung cancer invasion of chest wall	T3: Invasion of the chest wall T4: Invasion of the vertebral body With clear chest wall involvement, en bloc thoracectomy and lung resection indicated
Metastasis to the chest wall	Thyroid, breast, kidney, and other hematogenous tumor seeding

- Involved or compromised skin and soft tissue should be resected en bloc with the specimen.
- Margins of 1 to 2 cm are sufficient for benign tumors or low-grade malignancies.
- Typically, a 4 cm margin is required for high-grade, aggressive, or infiltrative malignancies.
- Rib invasion should be assessed preoperatively by physical exam and radiographic imaging and evaluated directly intraoperatively, as adjacent ribs may require resection to obtain adequate margins.
  - Computed tomography (CT) scan is optimal for assessment of vascularization, large vessel proximity, calcifications, ossification, and cortical invasion, while magnetic resonance imaging is best suited for involvement of the bone marrow and spine.
  - Positron emission tomography/CT is used for staging and for monitoring treatment response for almost any high-grade malignant chest wall tumor.
- The reconstructive goal is to restore chest wall rigidity with minimal deformation, prevent lung herniation, protect mediastinal organs, and prevent paradoxical breathing by preserving respiratory mechanics.
- A thorough surgical history is obtained, and the patient is inspected for scars that may indicate compromise of potential soft tissue flaps.
- Large full-thickness defects generally require mesh with or without titanium plating and coverage with soft tissue (primary repair, skin graft, or soft tissue flap).
- Complex resections and reconstructions should be managed by a multidisciplinary team of clinicians, often including thoracic surgeons, thoracic anesthesiologists, orthopedic surgeons, and reconstructive plastic surgeons.

TIPS

- *Resection of three or more ribs generally requires prosthetic coverage unless covered by the scapula.*
- *Smaller defects at the tip of the scapula can lead to entrapment of the scapula and should also be covered.*

Instruments and Equipment

- Mesh
  - Ideal prosthetic material
    - Rigid—to prevent paradoxical movement.
    - Inert—to allow in-growth of fibrous tissue and reduce risk of infection.
    - Malleable—to fashion the desired shape at the time of operation.
    - Radiolucent—to allow radiographic follow-up and surveillance for recurrence.
  - Synthetic
    - Polypropylene (Marlex) or polytetrafluoroethylene (PTFE/Gore-Tex)
      - Nonabsorbable synthetic woven mesh.
      - Semirigid and relatively easy to manipulate.
      - Easy to sew.
      - Easy to remove (useful when high likelihood of redo resection or repeat thoracotomy).
      - Polypropylene is water permeable, whereas PTFE is water tight.
    - Polymethylmethacrylate (PMMA)
      - Increased rigidity though still malleable for custom contouring.
      - More cumbersome to manipulate.
      - More prone to fracture.
      - In our experience, felt to be slightly higher risk of infection and is only used in sterile fields.
      - Frequently fashioned as PMMA "sandwich" inside a top and bottom layer of synthetic (often polypropylene) or biologic mesh.

TIPS

Synthetic mesh is contraindicated in contaminated wounds or in at-risk fields (eg, adjacent to bowel or liver, within mucormycotic spaces).

- Bioprosthetic
  - Acellular dermal matrix (allograft or xenograft).
  - Incorporate and vascularize at the site of implantation and therefore do not require excision and can be used in infected or at-risk fields.
  - Decreased rigidity makes them less optimal for the reconstitution of chest wall mechanics.
  - Used in cases where synthetic mesh is contraindicated (eg, high infection risk, abutment of hollow viscera or liver).
  - Unlike synthetic mesh, biologic mesh can safely be in contact with visceral surfaces.

TIPS

Bioprosthetic mesh is expensive.

- Metallic
  - High rigidity and durability.
  - More difficult to handle given degree of rigidity and sharpness at the edges.
  - Uncommonly used at our institution except for select complex rib and sternal reconstructions.
  - Angled 5-mm or 10-mm thoracoscope.
  - Thoracoscopic camera port of appropriate size.
  - Standard video-assisted thoracoscopic surgery (VATS) instrument tray.
  - Thoracoscopic stapling device with assorted staple cartridges if there is potential for lung resection.
  - Intraoperative consultation with vendor representative from hardware manufacturer.
    - Titanium plates (preformed or customizable) of various sizes and thicknesses.
    - Screws (self-drilling or predrilled).
    - Powered and manual screwdrivers.
    - May require power drill if using non-self-drilling screws.
  - Allograft/homograft
  - Ensure availability of necessary equipment for all involved surgical teams.

Anesthesia and Patient Positioning

- General anesthesia with a double-lumen endotracheal tube (or bronchial blocker) to allow for single lung ventilation contralateral to the tumor.
- Complex cases will necessitate a Foley catheter for intraoperative fluid management and postoperative monitoring.
- Patients should receive perioperative antibiosis suitable to the patient's allergies and clinical history as well as subcutaneous deep venous thrombosis (DVT) prophylaxis.
- Patient positioning will depend on the location of the tumor and planned tissue flap creation.

TIPS

Intraoperative repositioning may be needed for soft tissue flap harvesting and should be discussed perioperatively with all consultants.

- Supine with arms out allows access to the anterior chest wall—from the sternum medially to the midaxillary lines bilaterally.
- Lateral decubitus with ipsilateral arm extended 90° to 120° anteriorly at the shoulder allows access to the lateral chest wall—from the posterior axillary line medially to the sternum and the spine laterally.
- Prone positioning permits access to the posterior chest wall.

Technique

- To minimize local recurrence, en bloc resection of the chest wall tumor as well as all involved adjacent tissue is necessary.
- The extent of resection is guided by the diagnosis and indication for surgery (Table 23.2).

TABLE 23.2 ▌Oncologic Principles for Chest Wall Tumor Resection

Indication for Chest Wall Resection	Resection Margin Principles
Benign tumors	• Tumor removal with negative margins • Do not resect skin or muscle if not clearly indicated • Wider margins may be required in selected cases (eg, concern for undiagnosed malignancy, desmoid tumors)
Primary malignant tumors	• Complete en bloc resection with wide negative margins is paramount to reducing recurrence and improving survival • Typically, en bloc resection with 4-cm-wide negative margins • Margins must include skin, soft tissue, ribs, sternum, vertebrae, and any other involved structures
Lung cancer invasion of chest wall	• En bloc chest wall and pulmonary resection • Chest wall margins should include 1 rib above and 1 rib below the tumor with a lateral margin of 3-4 cm • In select cases where morbidity from resection may be excessive, 1 cm margins in all directions may be considered
Metastasis to the chest wall	• If surgery is indicated, negative margins are typically acceptable • Resection of chronic wounds or infections should be widely resected and covered with a highly vascularized soft tissue flap (eg, pedicled omental flap)

Video-Assisted Thoracoscopic Surgery

- Often used as an adjunct to thoracotomy for incision planning and intrathoracic assessment of the ribs, pleura, lung, diaphragm, mediastinum, and spine (Figure 23.1).

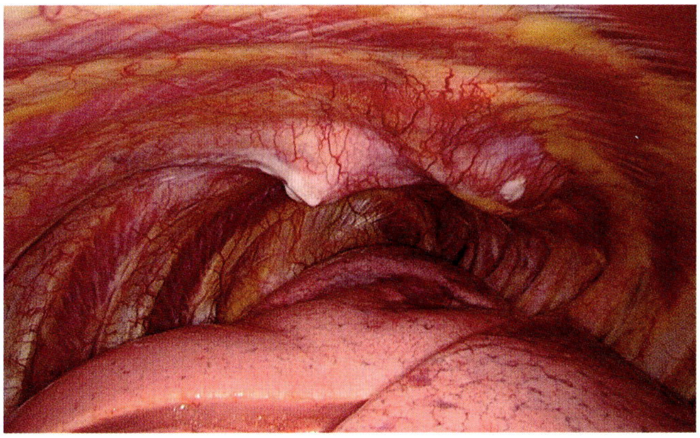

FIGURE 23.1 ▌ Thoracoscopic evaluation of a 32-year-old man with a biopsy-proven osteosarcoma of the left chest wall involving ribs 3 to 7. Note the utility in angled visualization of the extent of the mass from within the pleural space.

- The location of the camera port incision is dictated by the location of the tumor, though typically it is positioned within the seventh, eighth, or nineth interspace at the anterior or midaxillary line.
- A 5-mm endoscopic "peanut" or curved ring forceps is used to retract the lung, examine the pleural space, and assess the intrathoracic extent of the tumor.
- When assessing the extent of the tumor, pay specific attention to rib involvement (count ribs), lateral extension, lung invasion, and encroachment on the mediastinum, superior sulcus, spine, or diaphragm.

Thoracotomy

- Preparing for incision
  - Palpate the tumor and use a skin marker to approximate the location (rib spaces) and size of the tumor (rib involvement).

TIPS

Thoracoscopic assessment guides thoracotomy incision placement.

- Plan the incision with input from all involved surgical teams by considering margins and coverage strategies (Figure 23.2).

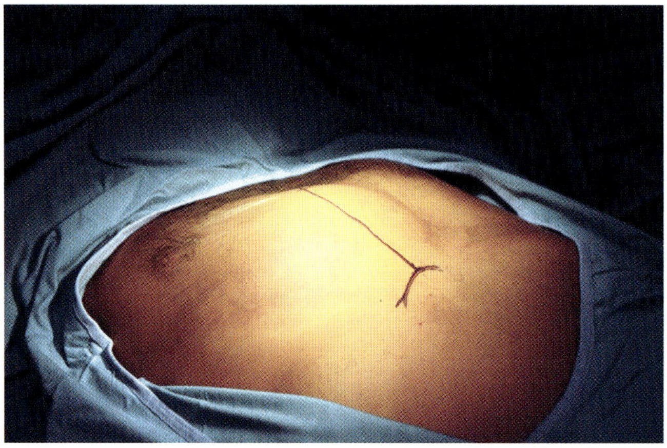

FIGURE 23.2 ▌ Chest wall resection incisional preparation. Right-sided anterior chest wall mass in a man with history of neurofibromas shown here with marking pen delineating the planned extent of longitudinal incision to provide exposure for margins in all directions.

- Previous surgical incisions in the operative field should be considered when designing the incision and when planning for soft tissue coverage, as flap integrity can be compromised by prior dissections.

TIPS

Ensure that the predrawn sketch of the planned incision is approved by all involved surgical teams prior to making incision.

- Resection
  - After thoracoscopic assessment and determination of operative strategy, sharp incision is made and soft tissue dissection is carried down to the deep thoracic fascia using electrocautery.

TIPS

Consider retracting or mobilizing latissimus rather than dividing as it may be necessary for reconstruction.

- During dissection, continually monitor the margins and be mindful of the location and vascular supply of the planned reconstructive flap, if applicable.
- If the incision allows for access to the scapula, we routinely free it from the chest wall to allow for manual counting of the ribs. If need be, the thoracoscopic camera can be reinserted for orientation and margin verification.

- Once the chest wall is reached circumferentially at the expected margins, begin the resection where exposure is favorable (eg, work anterior to posterior for posterior lesions, etc.) (Figure 23.3).

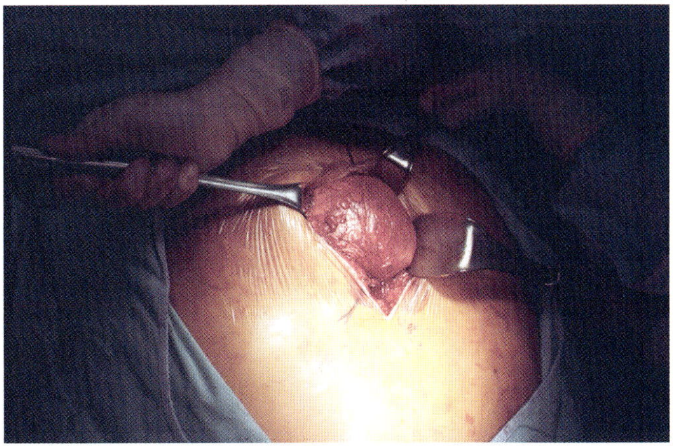

FIGURE 23.3 ▌ Circumferential exposure of the anterior chest wall mass after dissection to the deep thoracic fascia.

TIPS

To optimize margins, use thoracoscopy when visualization via thoracotomy is limited.

- Once the upper, lower, and lateral extent of the planned margins is agreed upon, the ribs, intercostal muscles, and neurovascular bundles are ligated and divided in a standard fashion (Figure 23.4).

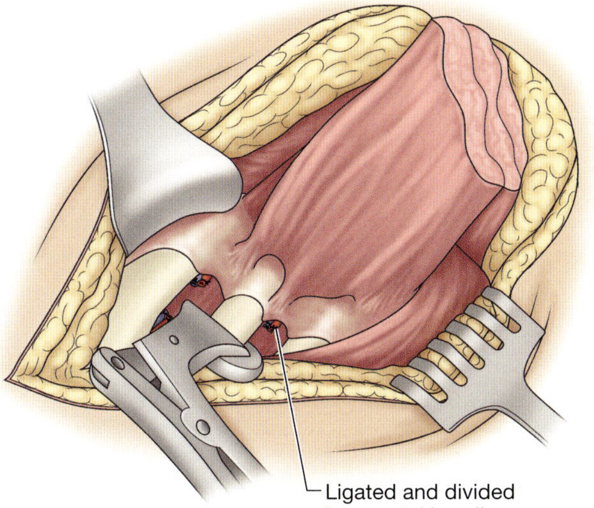

FIGURE 23.4 ▌ Costotomy during full thickness chest wall resection. The sliding rib cutter is placed flush around the superior aspect of the most upper rib to be resected where margins have been deemed adequate. Subsequent costotomy should follow the line of the expected margin. The ligated neurovascular bundles are shown.

- The cephalad and caudad margins are formed by using electrocautery to enter the pleura above the most upper rib to be removed and above the rib just below the lowest intercostal muscle to be removed, respectively.
- Great care is taken to establish hemostasis at this point, as ongoing bleeding from the chest wall will make for a more difficult thoracectomy and, if planned, pulmonary resection.

TIPS

Benign tumors limited to soft tissue may not require rib removal.

- For posteromedial lesions near the spine, lateral division of the rib is performed first followed by exposure of the costotransverse joint by division of the erector spinae muscles and tubercular ligament. Disarticulation of the rib is then performed by aggressively rocking the rib back and forth with a curved heavy periosteal elevator wedged between the vertebral transverse process and tubercle of the rib.
- Resection of the transverse process risks difficult-to-control bleeding adjacent to the intervertebral foramen as well as dura mater disruption with cerebrospinal fluid leak and therefore should only be resected if the undersurface of the head of the rib is infiltrated by tumor.
- If resection of additional structures within the chest is not required, the thoracectomy specimen can be removed for pathological assessment (Figure 23.5).

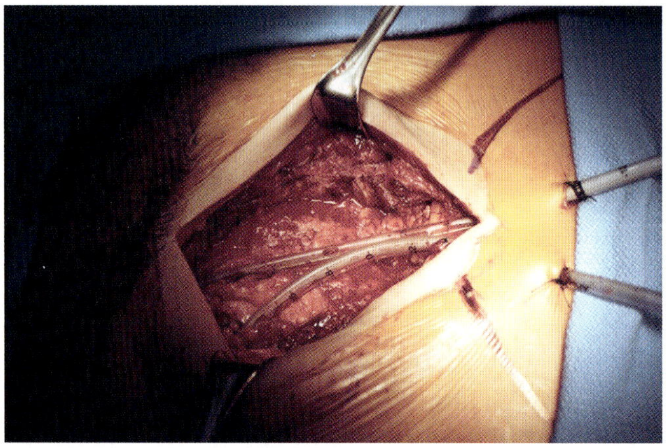

FIGURE 23.5 ▮ Resultant chest wall defect after thoracectomy. 24-French argyle chest tubes seen placed within the defect allowing for drainage and lung re-expansion.

TIPS

Send cultures of any tissue concerning for infection, paying special attention to bone and prior indwelling foreign bodies.

- If intrathoracic resection is required (eg, locally advanced lung cancer), the thoracectomy is placed within the pleural space and gently manipulated to provide exposure for subsequent pulmonary, diaphragmatic, vertebral, or mediastinal resections.
- For extensive chest wall invasion, wide pulmonary wedge resection with linear staplers performed through either the thoracotomy or VATS port may be required to allow for safe completion of thoracectomy, lobectomy, and nodal dissection.
  - Prior to reconstruction, a tube thoracostomy is often placed and positioned for postoperative monitoring (Figure 23.5).

TIPS

Only perform pulmonary wedge resections through disease-free parenchyma.

  - Negative pressure wound dressings have been used to delay complex repair if frozen margins are questionable, though this is uncommon in our practice. We strongly advise against delayed closure in the presence of synthetic mesh.

Reconstruction (Skeletal Stabilization and Soft Tissue Coverage)

- Mesh reconstruction
  - Using measured dimensions or a handmade paper template of the defect, the mesh is trimmed and fashioned with an additional 2 to 3 cm of mesh added circumferentially to aid in suture fixation.

- The mesh is then secured as an underlay to durable tissue on all sides of the defect using heavy nonabsorbable sutures placed above the superior rib, below the first remaining intercostal muscle inferiorly, and to all available bone or cartilage stumps medially and laterally (Figure 23.6).

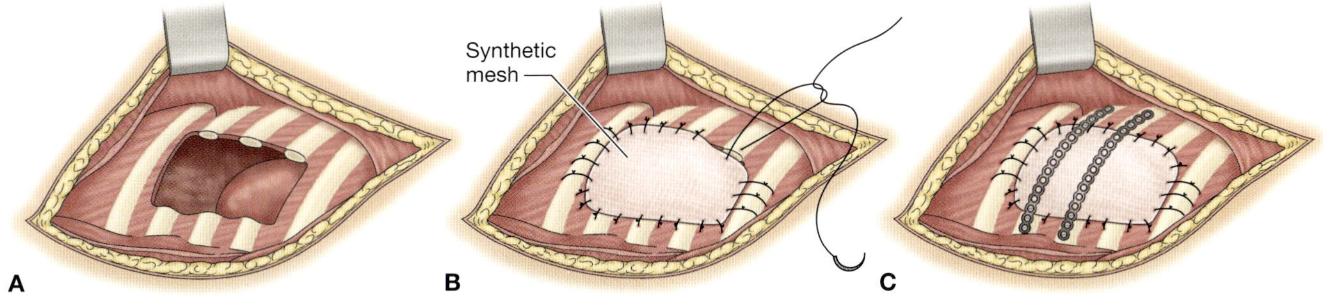

FIGURE 23.6 ▌ Anterior chest wall reconstruction. **A.** The chest wall defect after resection spanning three rib spaces. **B.** A Gore-Tex patch fixed to the edges of the defect with nonabsorbable sutures. **C.** Skeletal reconstitution with bridging titanium struts screwed to the bone edges and customized to mimic the contour of the absent anterior ribs.

- We typically fix the mesh with heavy nonabsorbable horizontal mattress sutures to help balance the tension circumferentially.
- For added rigidity, a PMMA "sandwich" can be made by sizing two pieces of polypropylene mesh 1 cm larger than the defect, spreading out a layer of PMMA on the surface of one piece of polypropylene and then covering the PMMA with the second piece of polypropylene (Figure 23.7).

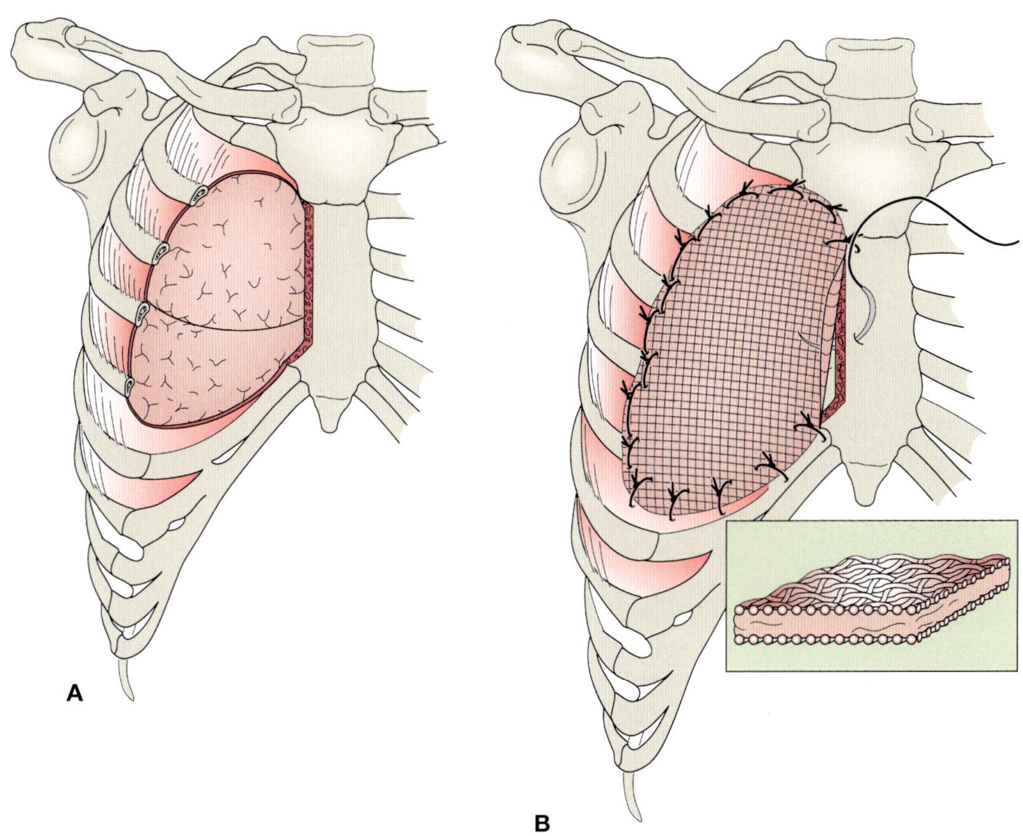

FIGURE 23.7 ▌ Marlex methylmethacrylate sandwich technique for chest wall reconstruction. **A.** Upper anterior chest wall defect resulting from resection of ribs 2 to 5 and a portion of sternum. **B.** Marlex methylmethacrylate prosthesis being sutured in place. Heavy and nonabsorbable sutures either encircling the ribs or passed through the sternum are used to anchor the prosthesis in place. Inset: Detail of prosthesis showing sandwich of hardened methylmethacrylate between two sheets of Marlex. (From Reddy RM. Nonneoplastic thoracic disease. In: Dimick JB, ed. *Mulholland & Greenfield's Surgery*. 7th ed. Wolters Kluwer; 2022:1339-1372. Figure 80.9.)

TIPS

Suturing two pieces of polypropylene together with nonabsorbable suture and injecting activated PMMA between the two mesh layers has been described.

- The prosthetic sandwich is then molded to the desired contour, immediately after creation before it hardens. The mesh is then fixed to the surrounding bone and cartilage in the same manner as simple patch reconstruction (Figure 23.8).

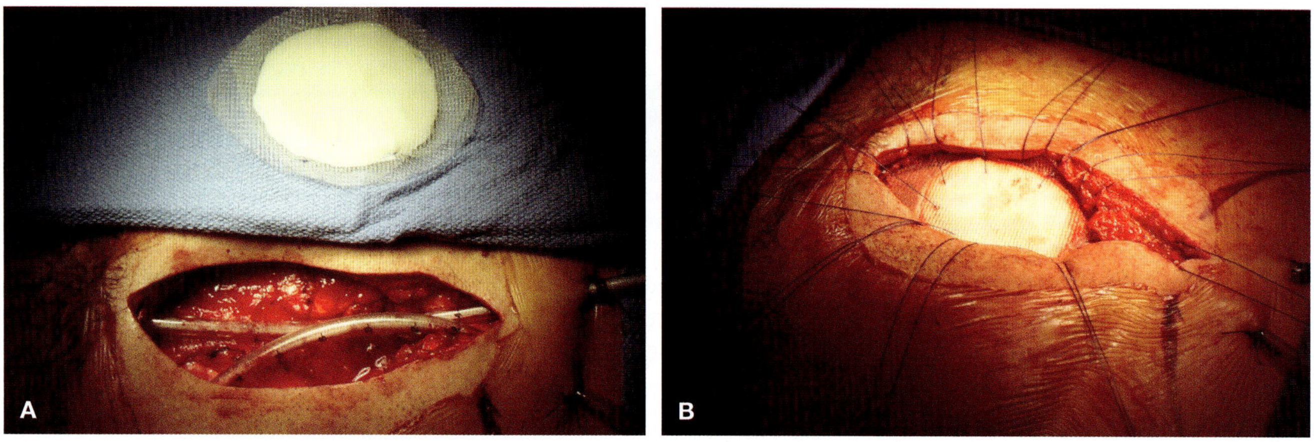

FIGURE 23.8 ▮ Polymethylmethacrylate "sandwich" reconstruction of an anterior thoracectomy. **A.** Two polypropylene layers are sized to be under even tension when incorporated within the defect. A layer of activated PMMA is spread between the two layers of polypropylene and fashioned to the desired contour (not shown). **B.** The PMMA "sandwich" is fixed to the bone and cartilage on all sides with horizontal mattress stitches using nonabsorbable suture. Note the tension spread evenly across the patch.

Reinforcement with Titanium Struts

- If titanium struts are used to replace the excised ribs, a mesh is still placed deep to them to exclude the pleural space.
- There are a variety of rib plating platforms, but the steps generally include (1) selecting the desired size and thickness of the strut, (2) molding to the desired contour, (3) selecting or cutting the appropriate length, (4) and fastening to the bone at both ends (self-drilling screws, predrilled screws, or rib clips).
- Typically, 3 to 4 rib screws are required on each side of the strut to ensure secure anchoring.
- Detailed instructions for the system used at each institution should be clearly explained and monitored by the manufacturer's representative.

TIPS

Generally, select screws 2 mm longer than the thickness of the rib to account for the depth of the plate and to avoid injury of structures deep to the rib.

Soft Tissue Coverage

- A detailed outline of the soft tissue flaps available for chest wall reconstruction describing anatomy, clinical indications, advantages/disadvantages, and operative techniques is outside the scope of this chapter and has been covered in great depth elsewhere (see Suggested Readings section).
- Table 23.3 is provided for an overview of chest wall soft tissue coverage options.

TABLE 23.3 | Options for Soft Tissue Coverage in Chest Wall Reconstruction

Soft Tissue Flap	Flap Type	Insertion	Origin	Vascular Supply	Common Uses
Pectoralis major	Muscle, myocutaneous	Intertubercular groove of the humerus	Sternal surface, ribs, and costal cartilage 2-6	Thoracoacromial artery, perforators from internal thoracic and intercostal arteries	Upper sternal defects, upper ventral and dorsal chest wall, axilla, neck
Latissimus dorsi	Muscle, myocutaneous	Intertubercular groove of the humerus	Iliac crest, ribs 9-12, spines of T7-T12, lumbar vertebrae, sacral vertebrae	Thoracodorsal artery, perforators from intercostal and lumbar arteries	Commonly used due to size and pedicle length. Lateral, midposterior, and anterior
Serratus anterior	Muscle flap, myocutaneous (with pectoralis major or latissimus dorsi)	Scapula	Ribs 1-8	Serratus branch of thoracodorsal artery, long thoracic artery	Commonly used within the chest. Lateral chest wall, lateral posterior (with latissimus dorsi), and lateral anterior (with pectoralis major)
Rectus abdominis	Muscle, myocutaneous	Costal cartilages 5-8	Pubic crest	Internal mammary and inferior epigastric arteries	Anteroinferior chest wall. Lower sternum, anterior lower chest wall
Omentum	Pedicled greater omental flap	Inferior stomach	Transverse colon	Right omental branch of the right gastroepiploic artery	Versatile. Commonly used in infected or irradiated fields (eg, sternal infections), basilar defects (eg, diaphragm)

- Flap choice is based upon the location and geometry of the defect, integrity of the potential muscles used, previous radiation or operations, and patient morbidities.
- To prevent severe wound complications, space occupying healthy soft tissue should always be placed over rigid skeletal reconstructions.
- To mitigate seroma or hematoma formation, round silicone drains are typically placed between the mesh and the flap as well as at the site of the flap harvest.

TIPS

Awareness of flap blood supply is critical to preservation of a viable and effective muscle flap during chest wall dissection and resection.

Special Circumstances

- Sternum
  - Infection after sternotomy or intravenous drug use is the most common indication for sternal resection and requires complete debridement of the involved tissue.
  - Sternal tumors, most commonly sarcomas (especially chondrosarcomas), require radical resection with 3- to 5-cm macroscopic margins with en bloc removal of all involved deep structures.
    - Total sternectomy: manubrium, sternal body, medial 1/3 of clavicles.
    - Subtotal sternectomy: sternal body.
    - Partial sternectomy: manubrium or lower 1/3 of sternal body.

TIPS

Manubrial resections are performed carefully to avoid injury to the nearby phrenic nerves and underlying vascular structures.

- Large sternal defects typically require rigid fixation and soft tissue coverage.
- Smaller bony defects (ie, <5 cm) do not necessarily require reconstruction, unless located in an area of particular vulnerability (eg, smaller sternal defects).
- The principles of sternectomy and reconstruction are similar to that of thoracectomy and reconstruction.
  - After the sternum is exposed, the pectoralis major attachments are divided and the muscles are raised to expose the lateral boarders of the sternum.
  - Sternal notch dissection is carried out, the retrosternal space is developed, and the xiphoid is exposed up to the costal cartilages.
  - After determining margins (one intercostal space away from the upper and lower limits of the tumor), the intercostal spaces are dissected out with electrocautery and the internal thoracic arteries are identified, ligated, and divided.
  - The perichondrium is removed, and the costal cartilages are divided with a sternal saw (Figure 23.9).
  - For a subtotal sternectomy, a sternal saw is used to divide the sternum just above the second intercostal space.

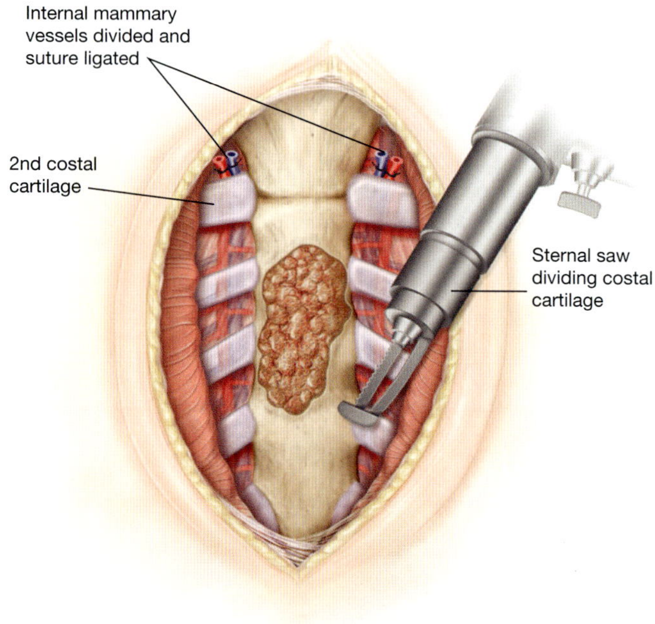

FIGURE 23.9 ▮ The sternum is fully exposed, with complete dissection of the intercostal spaces. The internal mammary arteries have been ligated. Division of the costochondral cartilage is performed with a sternal saw. (From Fein E, Morse CR. Sternal resection/reconstruction. In: Mathisen DJ, Morse C, eds. *Master Techniques in Surgery: Thoracic Surgery—Transplantation, Tracheal Resections, Mediastinal Tumors, Extended Thoracic Restrictions*. Wolters Kluwer; 2015:173-181. Figure 17.3.)

TIPS

Oscillating saws permit accurate and safe cuts. Use malleable retractors or large right-angle clamps to protect underlying structures.

- For a total sternectomy, the dissection and bony division proceeds superiorly to the first rib and laterally along 1/3 of the clavicles.
- Skeletal reconstruction of the sternum proceeds largely like that of the chest wall (Figure 23.10).

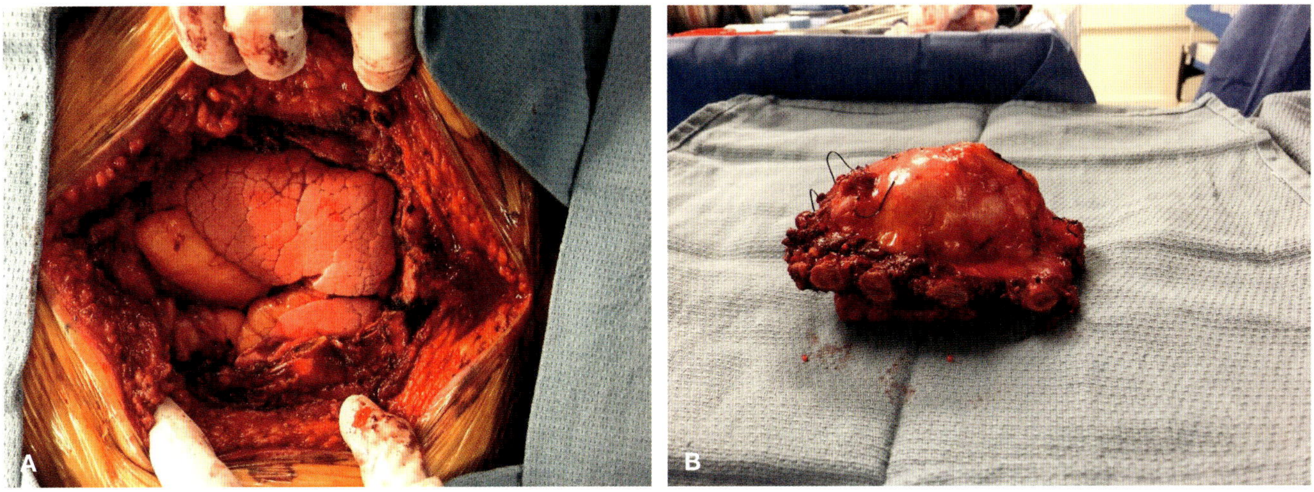

FIGURE 23.10 ▮ Subtotal sternectomy. **A.** Sternal defect after resection of the sternum, lower half of the manubrium, and 2-cm margin of all adjoining costal stumps in a 71-year-old female with a sternal mass. **B.** En bloc resection specimen diagnosed as choroid sarcoma of the sternum with negative margins. Reconstruction was performed with a Gore-Tex mesh covered by a gentamicin-infused polymethylmethacrylate plate (not shown).

- Polypropylene-PMMA "sandwich," iliac crest allograft, or titanium struts are most commonly used to recapitulate skeletal rigidity and are fixed to bony limits of the sternal defect.
- An omental flap may be harvested and placed on top of the prosthesis as sternal tumors may have been irradiated or sternectomy is often performed for infection (Figure 23.11).
- A drain is then placed between the omental flap and the prosthesis.

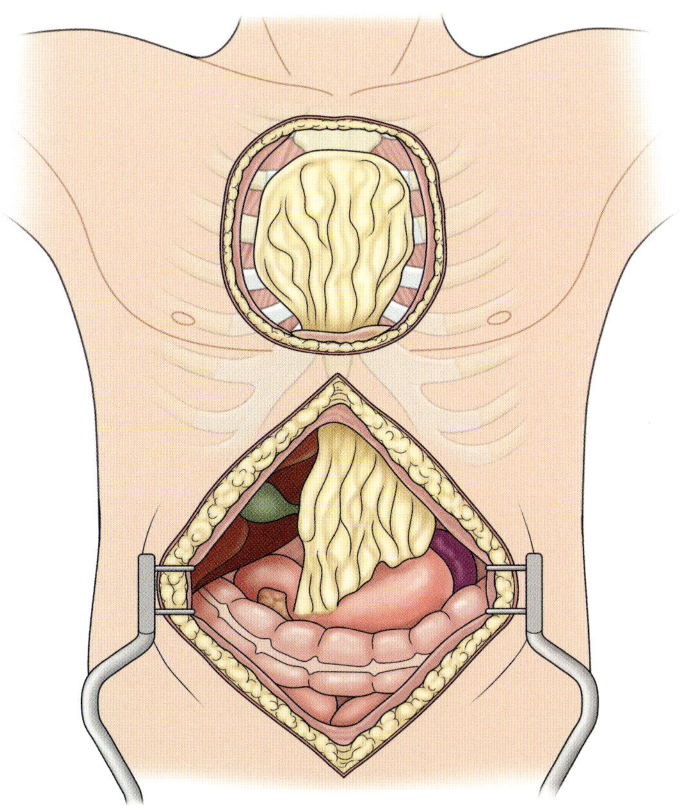

FIGURE 23.11 ▮ Omental flap placement after sternal reconstruction. An upper midline laparotomy is made for creation of a pedicled omental flap, which is passed into the mediastinum and up into the sternal defect.

- Over a second drain, the pectoralis muscles are reapproximated to the costal cartilage and presternal fasica in the midline. The soft tissue is then reapproximated with running absorbable suture, and the skin is closed with a running subcuticular monocryl suture.
- For large defects, a muscle or myocutaneous flap reconstruction with a pectoralis major advancement flap is often preformed.

Spine

- Chest wall resections requiring spinal resection are performed with the help of spine surgeons as staged operations with en bloc removal of the specimen.
- These posterior chest wall defects often will not require skeletal reconstruction.
- If mesh is needed for a large defect, we prefer PTFE in the region of the spine.

Diaphragm

- Chest wall defects with diaphragmatic involvement require structural reconstitution of both the chest wall and diaphragm.
- With small defects, one mesh can often be used to cover both the chest wall and diaphragm.
- With larger defects, two pieces of mesh can be used, one for the chest wall and one for the diaphragm, and should be stitched together with heavy nonabsorbable suture where they intersect.

Postoperative Care

TIPS

The most feared complications after chest wall reconstruction arise due to altered respiratory mechanics.

- Analgesia is paramount in promoting effective pulmonary toilet and early ambulation to prevent respiratory compromise secondary to pneumonia and venous thromboembolism, respectively.
- Postoperative DVT prophylaxis is essential to preventing venous thromboembolic events in this susceptible patient population. Daily low molecular weight heparin (Lovenox) or subcutaneous heparin three times a day can be held until the first postoperative day if there is concern for bleeding.
- Early chest physiotherapy coupled with physical and occupational therapy to mitigate changes in chest wall mechanics and preserve pulmonary function.
- To prevent seroma and aid in monitoring of hematoma formation, drains should be left indwelling until low output (20-40 mL/d).
- In the presence of osteomyelitis, intravenous antibiotics are indicated for 6 to 8 weeks and narrowed according to culture data.
- Flap perfusion should be monitored closely while hospitalized—often under the guidance of the plastic surgery team.

PEARLS AND PITFALLS

- Chest wall tumor diagnosis made by symptomatology, imaging, and often biopsy will guide the planned extent of resection.
- Multidisciplinary communication crucial for successful complex chest wall resections and reconstructions.
- The final extent of en bloc chest wall resection is determined intraoperatively by careful assessment via thoracoscopy and/or thoracotomy.
- Large chest wall defects require skeletal reconstruction with mesh and/or titanium struts to restore rigidity, protect intrathoracic organs, and preserve respiratory mechanics.
- Well-vascularized soft tissue coverage of rigid prosthetics is vital to a successful reconstruction.
- Pain control, postoperative mobilization, chest physiotherapy, and DVT prophylaxis are essential to the prevention of complications after chest wall resection and reconstruction.

Suggested Readings

1. Clemens MW, Butler CE, Mehran MJ. *Surgical Management of Chest Wall Tumors*. In: Collins KA, ed. *UpToDate*. Accessed September 10, 2021.
2. Mathisen DJ, Morse CM. Sternal resection/reconstruction. In: Mathisen DJ, Morse CM, Fischer JE, eds. *Master Techniques in Surgery: Thoracic Surgery—Transplantation, Tracheal Resections, Mediastinal Tumors, Extended Thoracic Resections*. Wolters Kluwer; 2015:173.
3. Puma F, Vannucci J. Chest wall resection/reconstruction for tumors. In: Mathisen DJ, Morse CM, Fischer JE, eds. *Master Techniques in Surgery: Thoracic Surgery—Transplantation, Tracheal Resections, Mediastinal Tumors, Extended Thoracic Resections*. Wolters Kluwer; 2015:149.
4. Rocco G. Anterior chest wall resection and reconstruction. *Oper Tech Thorac Cardiovasc Surg*. 2013;18(1):32-41.
5. Sanna S, Brandolini J, Pardolesi A, et al. Materials and techniques in chest wall reconstruction: a review. *J Vis Surg*. 2017;3:95.

Chapter 24

Sympathectomy for Hyperhidrosis and Ventricular Dysrhythmias

JAMES S. ALLAN
CYNTHIA L. MILLER

Perioperative Considerations

- Minimally invasive thoracoscopic thoracic sympathectomy is indicated for the treatment of focal upper body hyperhidrosis (palmar and axillary). It is also indicated for sympathetically driven ventricular dysrhythmias.
- Sympathectomy for facial sweating and blushing carries a high risk of Horner syndrome, and for this reason, our group prefers not to offer this procedure.
- The appropriate level(s) and length of sympathectomy are a subject of debate and depend upon the primary indication for the procedure.
- For palmar hyperhidrosis, a sympathectomy is typically performed from mid-second rib to the top of the fourth rib. This corresponds roughly to a T2-T3 sympathectomy. Many feel that the inclusion of the T4 ganglion is needed for optimal control of axillary hyperhidrosis.
- For sympathetically driven ventricular dysrhythmias, a sympathectomy is performed from the middle of the first rib down to the top of the fifth rib, thereby encompassing the lower portion of the stellate ganglion down through the T4 ganglion.
- Open approaches to upper thoracic sympathectomy (via posterior, supraclavicular, anterior thoracic, or transaxillary approaches) provide limited exposure and increased risk of debilitating muscular pain/dysfunction, scarring, and Horner syndrome.
- Bilateral VATS sympathectomy offers superior visualization and smaller incisions. It is typically a well-tolerated outpatient procedure that can be accomplished in under an hour.
- Patients who report the highest satisfaction are those with severe palmar hyperhidrosis causing significant functional impairment and social embarrassment.
- Patients should expect to have some compensatory hyperhidrosis, which usually presents as focal hyperhidrosis below the T4 dermatome in at least two-thirds of patients. The location and degree are largely idiosyncratic. However, longer sympathectomies may result in a greater degree and incidence of compensatory hyperhidrosis, whereas shorter sympathectomies run the risk of compromising the primary goal of the procedure.
- Rare complications of sympathectomy include infection, bleeding, unintended injury to adjacent structures, possible need for nonelective conversion to open surgery, postoperative air leak, Horner syndrome, Harlequin syndrome, gustatory sweating, reduction in maximal heart rate/bradycardia, and orthostasis.

Instruments and Equipment

- Two operating ports to accommodate 5-mm instruments
- 5-mm 0° straight thoracoscope
- Long, protected-tip cautery

- 5-mm endoscopic peanuts
- 5-mm endoscopic scissors
- Two 18-French Blake drains to serve as temporary thoracostomy tubes
- Two water seal chest drainage systems

Preparation and Positioning

- General anesthesia is obtained and the patient is intubated using a left-sided, double-lumen endotracheal tube.
- Beginning on either side, the lung is isolated and the patient is placed in a lateral decubitus position with the arm abducted 90° and supported to expose the axilla (Figure 24.1).

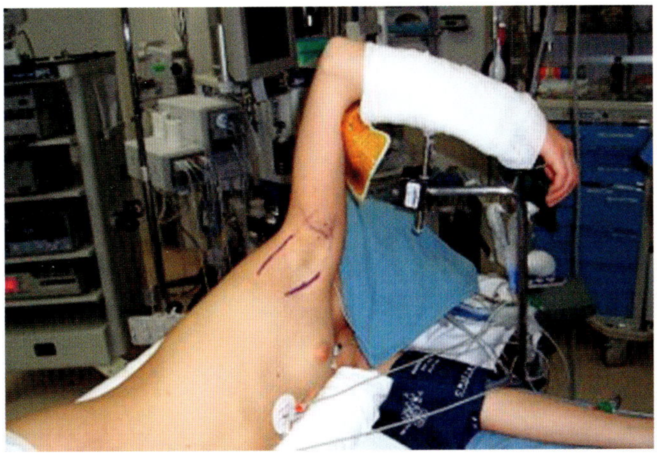

FIGURE 24.1 ▌ Position for right video-assisted thoracoscopic surgery sympathectomy.

TIPS

For focal hyperhidrosis, the operator can start with either side. If the procedure is being done for ventricular dysrhythmias, the left side is the more important side to complete, as it provides more of the sympathetic innervation to the heart.

- The table is placed in steep reverse Trendelenburg position and rotated toward the patient's anterior aspect.
    - This allows the isolated lung to lie inferiorly and anteriorly, facilitating exposure to the sympathetic ganglion chain running across the heads of each rib.

TIPS

Use of this positioning provides superior exposure and lower risk of ulnar neuropathy compared to supine positioning with arms extended over the head. CO_2 insufflation of the pleura space is not typically needed.

- Teaching and assisting are easiest if the operating surgeon and assistant both stand at the anterior side of the patient.
- At the conclusion of the first side, the position is reversed. The patient is placed on the opposite side, prepped, and draped.

Technique

Port Placement

- After prepping and draping the chest, back, and axilla, ports are placed high on the lateral chest wall just inferior to the axilla (Figure 24.2).

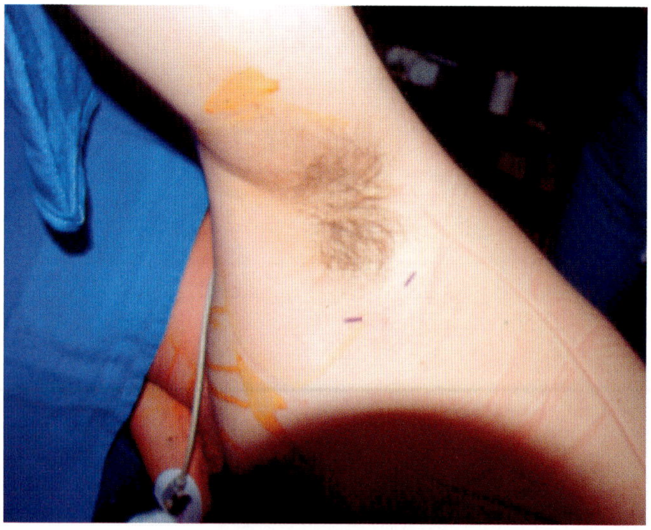

FIGURE 24.2 ▮ Location of ports for left video-assisted thoracoscopic surgery sympathectomy.

- One port should be just posterior to the pectoral muscle.
- The other port should be just anterior to the latissimus dorsi muscle.

- A 5-mm 0° straight thoracoscope is inserted through the anterior port.
- With good lung isolation and patient positioning, as above, the operative site should be easily visualized. If necessary, a 5-mm endoscopic peanut can be used through the posterior port to gently compress and manipulate the lung.
- The relevant anatomy should be identified (Figures 24.3-24.5). Small cautery burns may be made on either side of the sympathetic chain at each rib level where sympathectomy is to be performed. By bracketing the chain with these marks, the operation can be easily completed even if the operative field becomes blood stained.

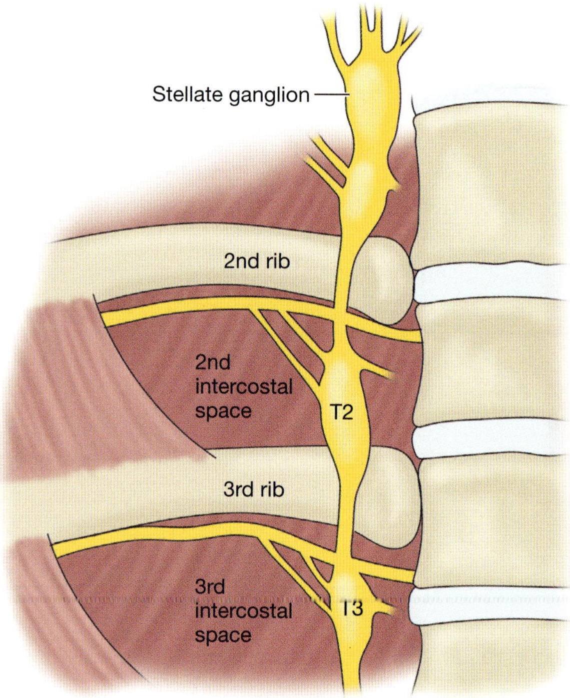

FIGURE 24.3 ▮ Anatomic diagram of right superior thoracic sympathetic chain. Note that lower portion of the stellate ganglion typically overlies the head of the first rib. ICS, intercostal space; G, ganglion.

Ablation of T2 to T3 Ganglia for Palmar and Axillary Hyperhidrosis

- Using a long protected-tip cautery through the posterior port, the sympathetic chain is divided at the middle of the second rib.

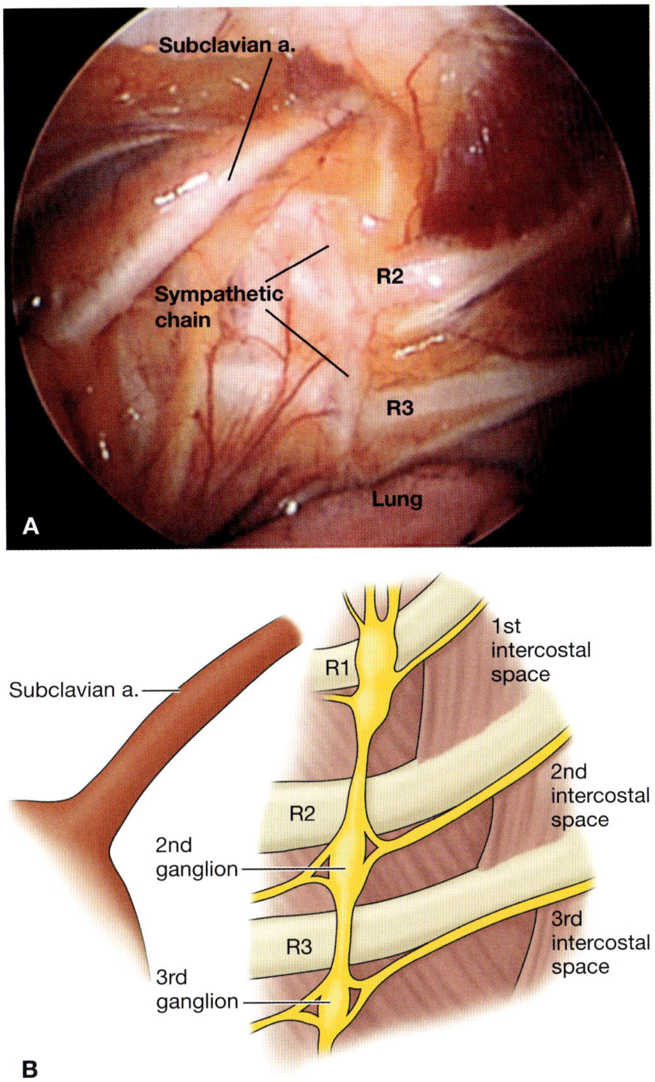

FIGURE 24.4 | A. Thoracoscopic view of the left superior posterior mediastinum. The sympathetic chain runs just under the parietal pleura over the rib heads. The first rib is not typically seen in its entirety but can be palpated with an endoscopic peanut. **B.** Schematic diagram of the left superior posterior mediastinum. a, artery; R1, first rib; R2, second rib; R3, third rib. (**B.** Reprinted from Baumgartner FJ. Surgical approaches and techniques in the management of severe hyperhidrosis. *Thorac Surg Clin*. 2008;18(2):167-181, with permission from Elsevier.)

TIPS

Care should be taken not to linger with the cautery when dividing the chain over the second rib to avoid risk of transmitting cautery energy cephalad toward the region of the stellate ganglion. A cautery setting of ~25 is typical.

- A cautery line is extended laterally from the initial division of the chain along the middle of the second rib for about 5 cm to divide any accessory sympathetic fibers ("accessory nerve fibers of Kuntz"), which might run parallel and lateral to the main body of the sympathetic chain. These nerve fibers are often not visible.
- Using cautery, the sympathetic chain is then ablated down to the top of the fourth rib. An additional level (T4) may be ablated for improved control of the axilla, if desired.

TIPS

There is no need to dissect out the chain or remove it. This just increases the risk of bleeding or unintended injury. Cautery ablation in situ is sufficient and permanent. Also, some of the ganglion chain may be obscured by underlying or overlying crossing veins. These veins do not need to be dissected out or otherwise manipulated. Because unipolar cautery creates a zone of injury around the cautery tip, the surgeon can simply skip over portions of the chain associated with crossing veins and continue the ablation immediately below the vein.

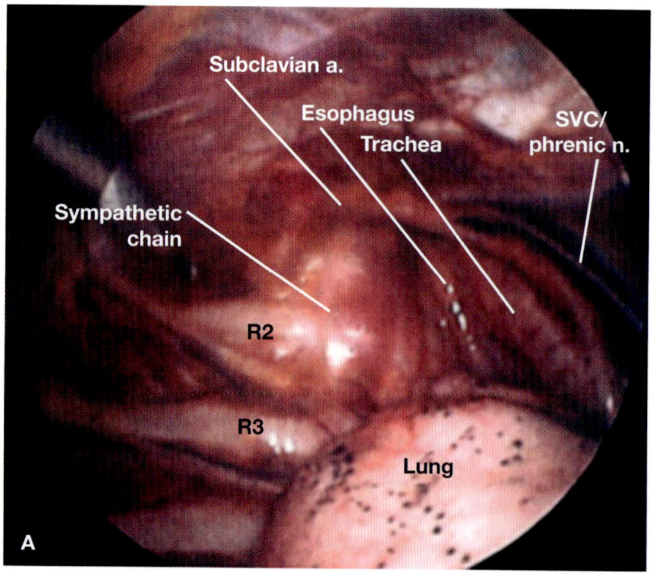

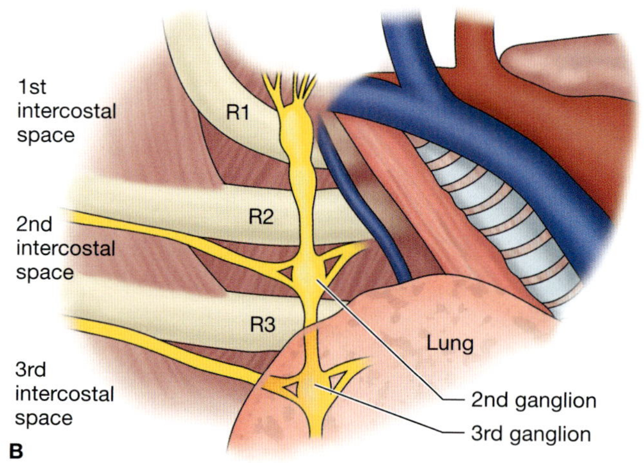

FIGURE 24.5 ▌ A. Thoracoscopic view of the right superior posterior mediastinum. The sympathetic chain runs just under the parietal pleura over the rib heads. The first rib is not typically seen in its entirety but can be palpated with an endoscopic peanut. **B.** Schematic diagram of the right superior posterior mediastinum. a, artery; n, nerve; R1, first rib; R2, second rib; R3, third rib; SVC, superior vena cava. (**B.** Reprinted from Baumgartner FJ. Surgical approaches and techniques in the management of severe hyperhidrosis. *Thorac Surg Clin*. 2008;18(2):167-181, with permission from Elsevier.)

Ablation of Lower Stellate to T4 Ganglia for Dysrhythmias

- The initial division of the sympathetic chain is carried out across the middle of the first rib. The intention is ultimately to ablate the lower portion of the stellate ganglion without injuring the upper portion of the ganglion. Injury to the upper portion of the ganglion will result in Horner syndrome. This initial division can be done with an endoscopic scissors to minimize the chance of transmitted cautery energy reaching the upper portion of the ganglion.

TIPS

Patients undergoing high sympathectomies should be clearly informed about the higher risk of Horner syndrome and this specific complication should be described on the consent form. Please note that the stellate ganglion and its components are not readily identifiable and rarely has the stylized appearance that is depicted in anatomic drawings. Also, there is some patient-to-patient variation in the location and appearance of the ganglion, which can make precise identification of the different functional areas of the ganglion almost impossible, even in expert hands.

- As described previously, a cautery line is extended laterally from the initial division of the chain along the middle of the second rib for about 5 cm to divide any accessory sympathetic fibers ("accessory nerve fibers of Kuntz"), which might run parallel and lateral to the main body of the sympathetic chain. These nerve fibers are often not visible.
- The sympathetic chain is then ablated down to the top of the fifth rib.

Completion of Procedure

- After completion of the first sympathectomy, the posterior port site is closed and a temporary pleural drain is placed through the anterior port site.
- With the drain attached to −20 cm H_2O of suction using a standard water seal suction system, the lung is reinflated, and the patient is repositioned for the left-sided sympathectomy.
- An identical procedure is performed on the left.
- With both sides completed, the patient is repositioned supine and both lungs are reinflated.
- Once all air is evacuated from both pleural spaces, both pleural drains can be removed, provided that there is no ongoing air leak or active bleeding.
- Some bupivacaine at both port sites may be used for local pain control.

Postoperative Care

- A postoperative chest radiograph is obtained to evaluate for residual pneumothorax. A tiny stable pneumothorax is often seen due to incomplete evacuation of air from the pleural space.
- Once the patient's clinical condition and chest radiograph are satisfactory, the patient can be discharged home.
- Patients should be instructed to expect some pain at the incision sites, as well as some pleuritic pain in the chest and back. Ice packs along with standing acetaminophen and ibuprofen are usually sufficient, with narcotic for breakthrough pain.
- Outpatient follow-up 1 to 2 weeks after surgery is appropriate. A follow-up chest radiograph may be done.

PEARLS AND PITFALLS

- Proper positioning (lateral decubitus, steep reverse Trendelenburg, rolled anteriorly, with arm abducted 90°) displaces the lung away from the operative site high in the back of the chest.
- Good lung isolation greatly facilitates the procedure. A properly positioned left-sided double-lumen tube is essential. The operative lung should be denitrogenated by ventilation with 100% oxygen prior to isolation for optimal operative conditions.
- It is not necessary to dissect out the sympathetic chain or manipulate crossing veins. This increases the risk of bleeding and conversion to an open procedure. Because unipolar cautery creates a zone of injury around the cautery tip, the surgeon can simply skip over portions of the chain associated with crossing veins, while still achieving a complete ablation.

Suggested Readings

1. Baumgartner FJ. Surgical approaches and techniques in the management of severe hyperhidrosis. *Thorac Surg Clin*. 2008;18(2):167-181.
2. Cerfolio RJ, De Campos JR, Bryant AS, et al. The Society of Thoracic Surgeons expert consensus for the surgical treatment of hyperhidrosis. *Ann Thorac Surg*. 2011;91(5):1642-1648.
3. Gossot D, Toledo L, Fritsch S, Célérier M. Thoracoscopic sympathectomy for upper limb hyperhidrosis: looking for the right operation. *Ann Thorac Surg*. 1997;64(4):975-978.
4. Hsia JY, Chen CY, Hsu CP, Shai SE, Yang SS. Outpatient thoracoscopic limited sympathectomy for hyperhidrosis palmaris. *Ann Thorac Surg*. 1999;67(1):258-259.
5. Kwong KF, Hobbs JL, Cooper LB, Burrows W, Gamliel Z, Krasna MJ. Stratified analysis of clinical outcomes in thoracoscopic sympathicotomy for hyperhidrosis. *Ann Thorac Surg*. 2008;85(2):390-394. discussion 393-394.
6. Krasna MJ. Thoracoscopic sympathectomy: a standardized approach to therapy for hyperhidrosis. *Ann Thorac Surg*. 2008;85(2):S764-S767.
7. Li X, Tu YR, Lin M, Lai FC, Chen JF, Dai ZJ. Endoscopic thoracic sympathectomy for palmar hyperhidrosis: a randomized control trial comparing T3 and T2-4 ablation. *Ann Thorac Surg*. 2008;85(5):1747-1751.
8. Ram R, Lowe NJ, Yamauchi PS. Current and emerging therapeutic modalities for hyperhidrosis, part 1: conservative and noninvasive treatments. *Cutis*. 2007;79(3):211-217.
9. Sciuchetti JF, Corti F, Ballabio D, Angeli MC. Results, side effects and complications after thoracoscopic sympathetic block by clamping: the Monza clinical experience. *Clin Auton Res*. 2008;18(2):80-83.
10. Tan V, Nam H. Results of thoracoscopic sympathectomy for 96 cases of palmar hyperhidrosis. *Ann Thorac Cardiovasc Surg*. 1998;4(5):244-246.
11. Walling HW, Swick BL. Treatment options for hyperhidrosis. *Am J Clin Dermatol*. 2011;12(5):285-295.

12. Weksler B, Luketich JD, Shende MR. Endoscopic thoracic sympathectomy: at what level should you perform surgery? *Thorac Surg Clin*. 2008;18(2):183-191.
13. Wolosker N, Yazbek G, Ishy A, de Campos JRM, Kauffman P, Puech-Leão P. Is sympathectomy at T4 level better than at T3 level for treating palmar hyperhidrosis? *J Laparoendosc Adv Surg Tech A*. 2008;18(1):102-106.
14. Vannucci F, Araújo JA. Thoracic sympathectomy for hyperhidrosis: from surgical indications to clinical results. *J Thorac Dis*. 2017;9(suppl 3):S178-S192.
15. Vaseghi M, Barwad P, Malavassi Corrales FJ, et al. Cardiac sympathetic denervation for refractory ventricular arrhythmias. *J Am Coll Cardiol*. 2017;69(25):3070-3080.

Chapter 25
Pectus Excavatum Repair

NUMA P. PEREZ
ASHOK MUNIAPPAN
DANIEL P. DOODY

Perioperative Considerations

- The severity and morphology of pectus excavatum, the patient's age, the rigidity of the chest wall, and any past chest wall surgery determine the number of supporting bars.
- For the typical chest wall reconstruction, thoracoscopy should always be performed to safely guide the tunneler and hardware through the anterior mediastinum and avoid injury to the underlying pericardium and heart.
- For severe defects, sternal retraction improves visualization of the anterior mediastinum and enhances the safety of the mediastinal dissection.
- A multimodal pain management strategy has helped to improve patient experience and address the perioperative and postoperative pain associated with the surgery.
- A preoperative bowel regimen is initiated shortly before surgery as opioid-induced constipation is a common problem complicating postoperative recovery.

TIPS

Patients with an allergy or sensitivity to nickel or nickel-containing jewelry require custom titanium bars.

Instruments and Equipment

- Video-assisted thoracoscopy equipment, including a 4-mm, 70° thoracoscope
- Zimmer Biomet Pectus System container (including an introducer, measuring templates, bar implants of assorted lengths ranging from 7 to 17 in, handheld bar benders, a bar flipper, horizontal stabilizers). The tabletop bar bender, wrapped separately, should be available.
- 22 G wire, wire cutter, Berry sternal needle holder, or similar sternal wire twisting clamp
- A reinforced, braided, ultra–high-molecular-weight suture with a polyethylene core and a polyester jacket may be needed to secure the pectus bars if stabilizing bars are not appropriate for the patient.
- A sternal elevator system, along with penetrating bone reduction clamp
- Cryoablation equipment if indicated, and the patient has been consented prior to surgery

TIPS

In January 2021, the FDA approved cryoablation for localized analgesia in children and adolescents 12 years of age and older to expand previous approval of cryoablation in adults.

Anesthesia and Patient Positioning

- If not using cryoablation, thoracic epidural placement before anesthesia induction
- If using cryoablation, isolated lung ventilation with a double-lumen endotracheal tube or bronchial blocker is indicated.
- The patient is positioned supine; two gel rolls are placed longitudinally beneath the posterior thorax to elevate the chest wall (Figure 25.1).

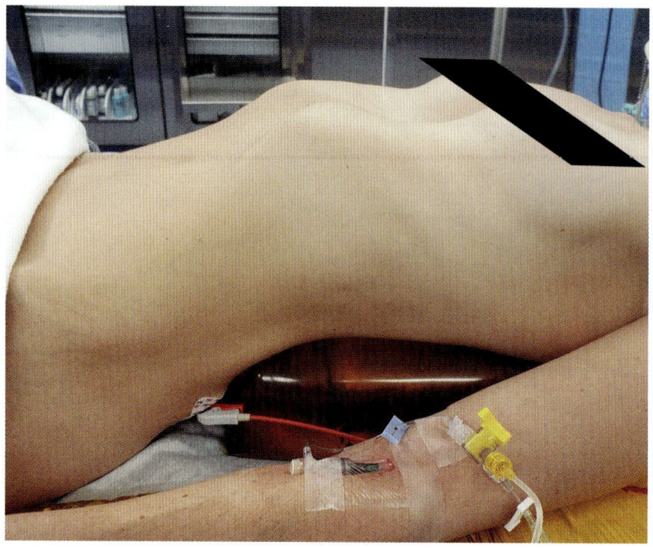

FIGURE 25.1 | Patient positioning.

- Both arms are tucked at the patient's side to avoid brachial plexus injury. The positioning provides surgical access to the anterolateral chest walls where the primary surgical dissection is performed for hardware placement. Joints are in neutral position and pressure points well padded.
- The lower body is secured to the operative table to avoid patient movement during bed positioning.

Technique

- If multiple bars are to be placed, the surgeon must decide whether they will be placed in adjacent intercostal spaces or farther away, which aids in choosing between oblique or separated transverse incisions on the lateral chest walls (Figure 25.2).

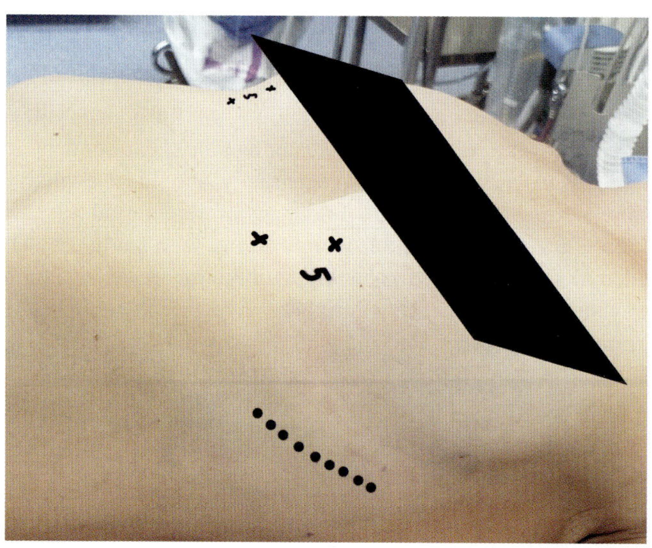

FIGURE 25.2 | Preoperative marking.

- Following the skin incisions, the dissection continues through the subcutaneous tissues using electrocautery.
- The serratus anterior muscle is identified. A subcutaneous pocket is created above this muscular fascia by dissecting along the areolar tissue plane (Figure 25.3).

- If the intercostal space of the superior bar is above the inferior margin of the pectoralis major muscle, the lateral margin of the pectoralis muscle is elevated from the chest wall to expose the ribs and intercostal musculature (Figure 25.3).

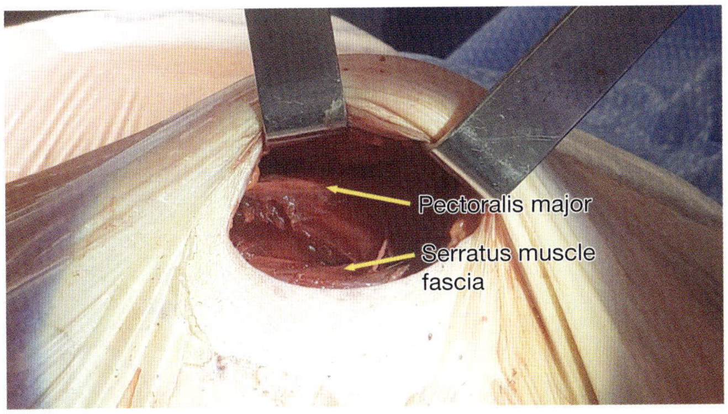

FIGURE 25.3 | Dissection of pocket.

- A small incision is made on the right lateral chest, one or two intercostal spaces below the expected placement of the lowest bar, and a 5-mm thoracoscopic port is placed and connected to the gas insufflator. The intrathoracic pressure is set at a pressure of 8 mm Hg and a flow of 6 L/min. The thoracoscope is then introduced.
- Two small stab incisions are made at the lateral borders of the sternum at the point of maximum depression, and a bone reduction or spinal perforating clamp is placed and secured to the sternal body (Figure 25.4). The sternum can now be elevated by affixing the clamp to the sternal elevator (Figure 25.5). This leads to increased retrosternal space (difference in length of yellow arrow, Figure 25.6A and B).

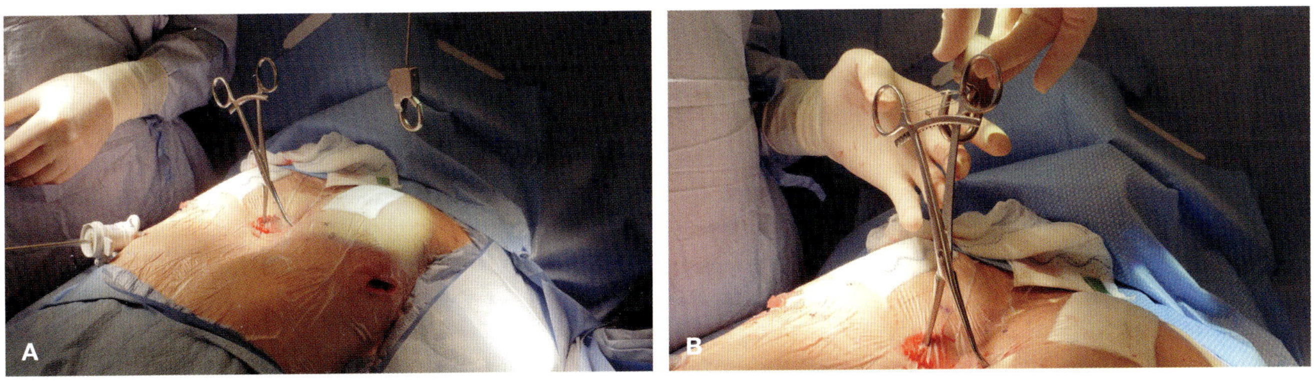

FIGURE 25.4 | Placement of bone reduction clamp **(A and B)**.

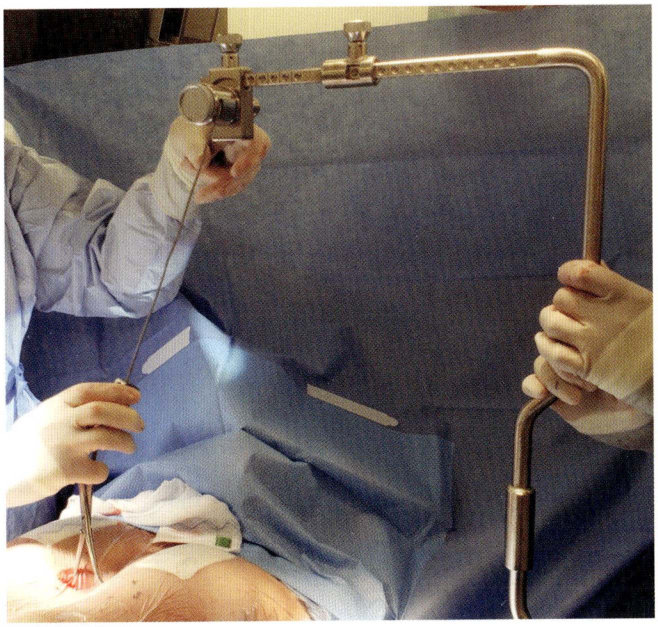

FIGURE 25.5 | Sternal elevation.

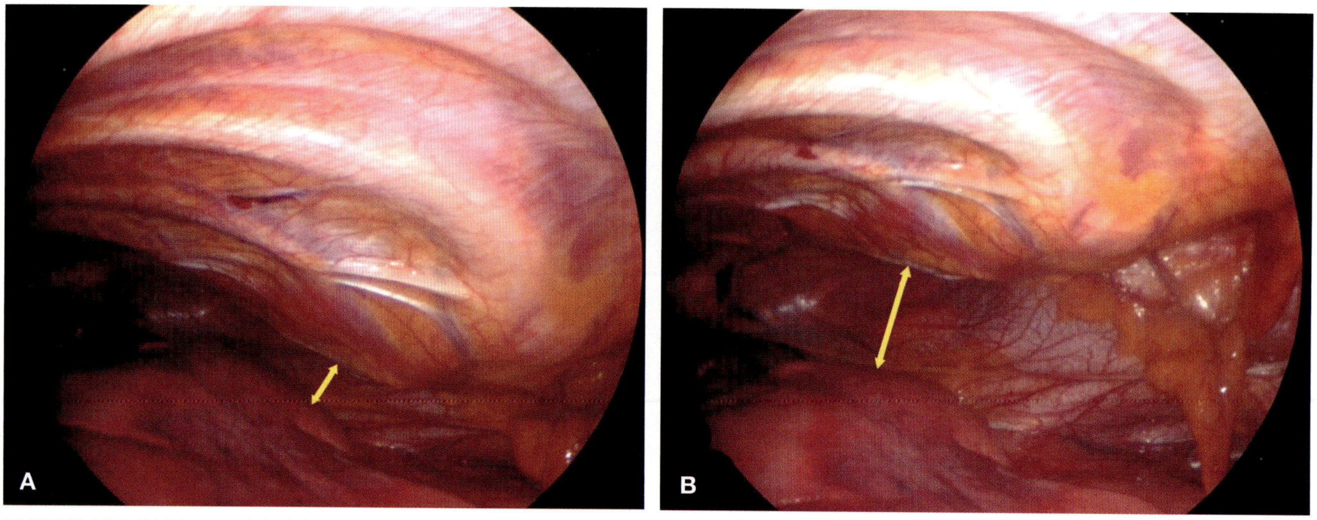

FIGURE 25.6 ▮ Video-assisted thoracic surgery view of retrosternal space before **(A)** and after **(B)** sternal elevation (double sided arrow indicating distance between posterior sternum and anterior border of mediastinal contents).

- If the patient has elected to have cryoablation for perioperative and postoperative analgesia, a double-lumen endotracheal tube or bronchial blocker would be placed with position confirmed by bronchoscopy.
  - The right lung is isolated and deflated.
  - The cryoablation probe is introduced through a separate incision in the chest wall from the camera port, but ideally within the same skin incision as the subcutaneous pocket.
  - Cryoablation is applied to the third to eighth intercostal bundles.
  - Take care to avoid accidental contact of the cryoprobe to the lung's visceral pleura, which could result in injury and a postoperative air leak.
  - A port must be placed into the left hemithorax for thoracoscopic-directed placement of the cryoablation probe if using cryoablation.
  - Like the right side, the third to eighth left intercostal bundles are ablated.
- Under thoracoscopic guidance, a curved clamp is introduced into the right hemithorax in the intercostal space at the top of the pectus ridge. Depending on the size of the patient and the severity of the pectus depression, an introducer of an appropriate size is inserted into this space (Figure 25.7A and B).

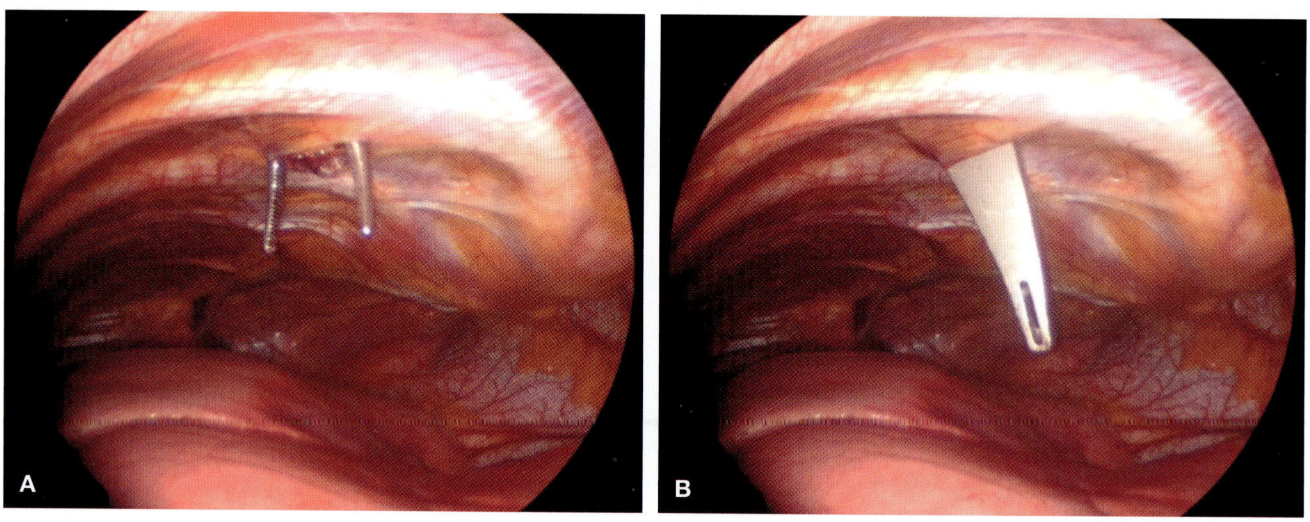

FIGURE 25.7 ▮ Insertion of pectus bar introducer **(A and B)**.

- The introducer is used to develop a retrosternal tunnel through the anterior mediastinum connecting both pleural spaces (Figure 25.8). Care is taken to avoid cardiac injury; sternal elevation makes this critical dissection simpler and safer.

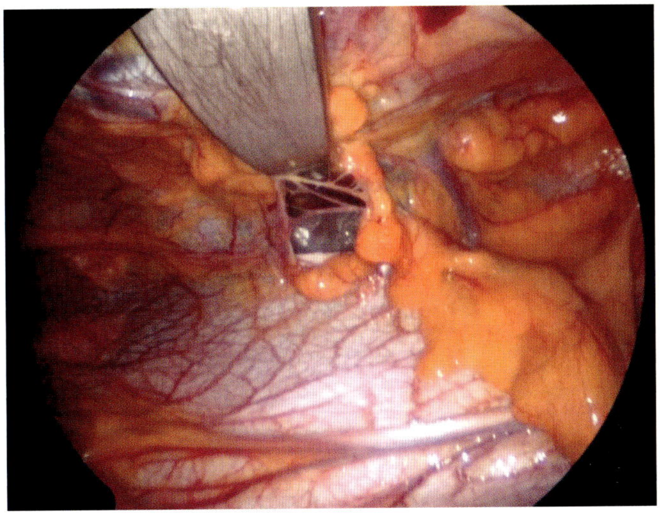

FIGURE 25.8 | Retrosternal blunt dissection using pectus bar introducer.

- Once the tip of the introducer is palpated at the left pectus ridge opposite the entry site on the right side, the introducer is brought out through the intercostal space. The left-sided surgical team often helps direct the introducer into the appropriate space.
- A sufficient length of umbilical cord tape is passed through the eyelet at the tip of the introducer that has exited the left hemithorax. Withdrawing the introducer brings the umbilical cord tape across the chest and out the right side. The tape is divided into two, with one tape used to guide the pectus bar across the chest while the second tape is reserved as a safeguard in the event the first tape breaks (Figure 25.9).

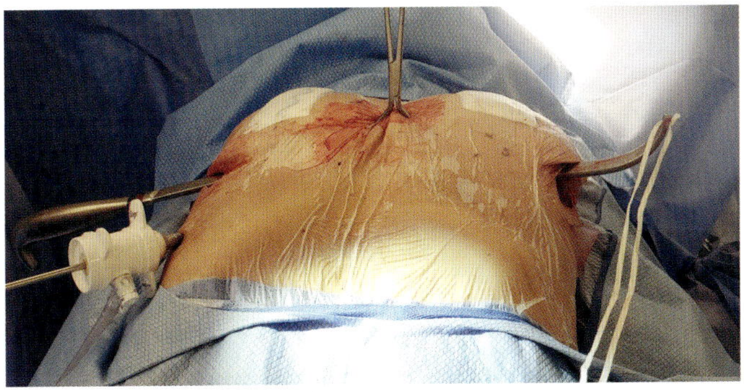

FIGURE 25.9 | Bar introducer traversing bilateral chest with umbilical cord tape at the tip.

- If placement of a second bar is indicated, the previous steps are repeated at the appropriate location along the chest wall.
- The measuring salmon-colored aluminum templates are used to decide the appropriate bar length and the shape needed for correction of the defect.
- Using the tabletop and handheld bar benders, the bar(s) is (are) bent to the desired shape. The pectus bars are shaped to the individual's chest wall contour to account for the sternal depression and the lateral supporting chest wall contour.
- One of the two umbilical cord strings placed as a guide after the intrathoracic dissection on the left side is tied securely to the eyelet at the tip of the pectus bar. The umbilical cord tape is then drawn under vision from the left chest through the anterior mediastinum and out the right chest with the bar in a U-configuration (Figure 25.10).
- Once the bar is centered on the chest wall (Figure 25.11), the thoracoscope is withdrawn to prevent damage to the scope's shaft, and the bar flippers are used to turn the bar into the inverted U placement (Figure 25.12).
- If placement of a second bar is indicated, the previous steps are repeated for the second bar.
- Once the bar(s) is (are) in place (Figure 25.13), the sternal elevator is released to gauge the adequacy of the repair and to ensure that the pressure of the anterior chest does not result in the lateral portion of the bar splaying outwards and off the lateral chest wall.

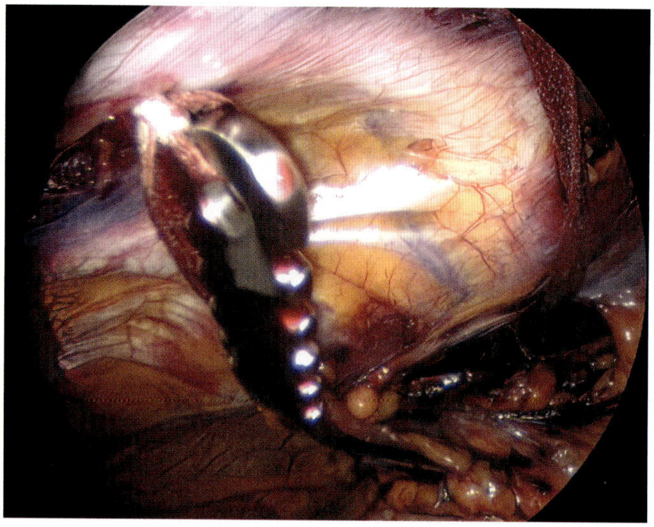

FIGURE 25.10 | Umbilical cord tape guiding pectus bar across the chest.

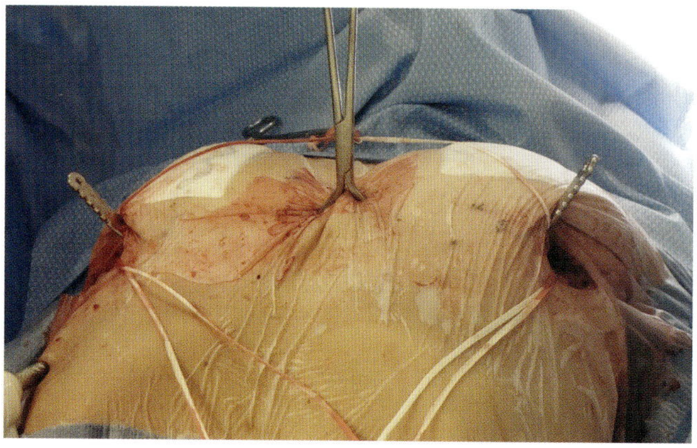

FIGURE 25.11 | Pectus bar exiting through the anterolateral chest.

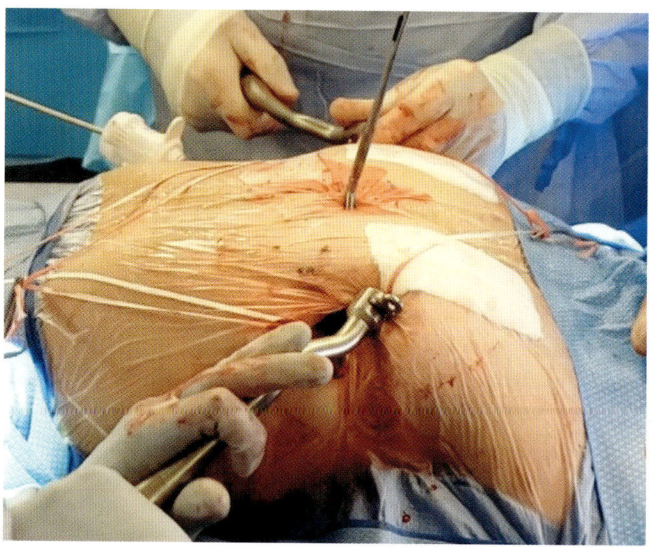

FIGURE 25.12 | Rotating pectus bar into place.

- The bars may require further correction to ensure that the ends are appropriately against the lateral chest wall (neither deeply embedding into the intercostal space nor elevating off the lateral chest wall). This reshaping of the pectus bar can be accomplished by turning the bar upwards into the U-configuration and using the handheld bar bender to adjust the bar's shape.
- The bars are now in place. If a single bar is used, stabilizing bars are placed on both sides. If two or more bars are placed in adjacent intercostal spaces, the authors place one stabilizer per bar on opposite sides.
- Securing the elongated stabilizing bar:
  - A 22 G wire is fitted under the edge of the pectus bar and advanced medially.
  - The horizontal stabilizer is fitted onto the end of the bar and advanced medially, taking care to leave at least one bar groove exposed for wire placement (Figure 25.13). The curved shape of the lateral chest may leave a relatively short segment to fit the elongated stabilizing bar.

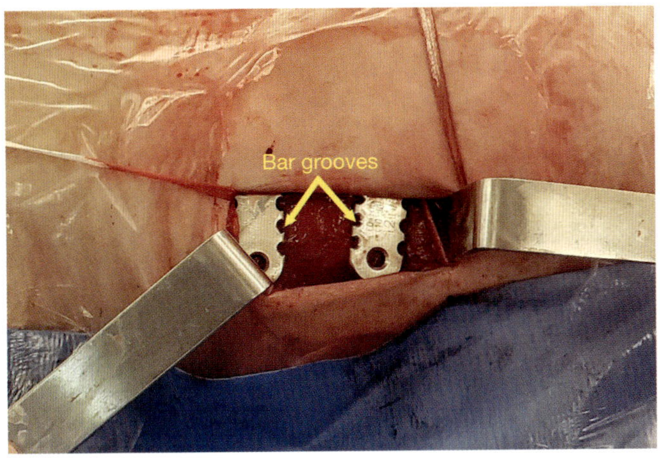

FIGURE 25.13 | Two pectus bars in place.

  - One end of the wire is brought over the stabilizer across to the other side and folded under the bar. The same is done with the other end of the wire, thus forming an X over the stabilizer (Figure 25.14).
  - The wire is then brought around the lower end of the pectus bar and initially twisted by hand. The final tightening of the wire is performed using the Berry sternal needle–holding clamp.
  - The twisted tail is cut to a sufficient length to be folded under the bar to prevent it from causing local soft-tissue and skin discomfort (Figure 25.14).

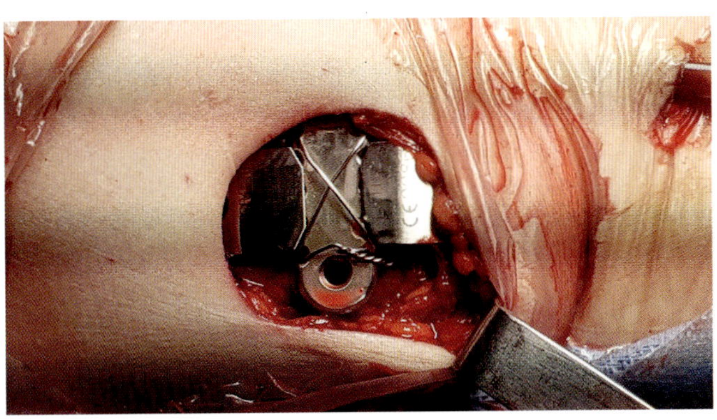

FIGURE 25.14 | Horizontal stabilizer in place secured using 22 G wire.

- The side without an elongated stabilizer is secured using an ultra–high-molecular-weight polyethylene-polyester suture placed around the pectus bar and adjacent rib. Typically, two figure-of-8 sutures are placed under thoracoscopic guidance (Figure 25.15A and B).

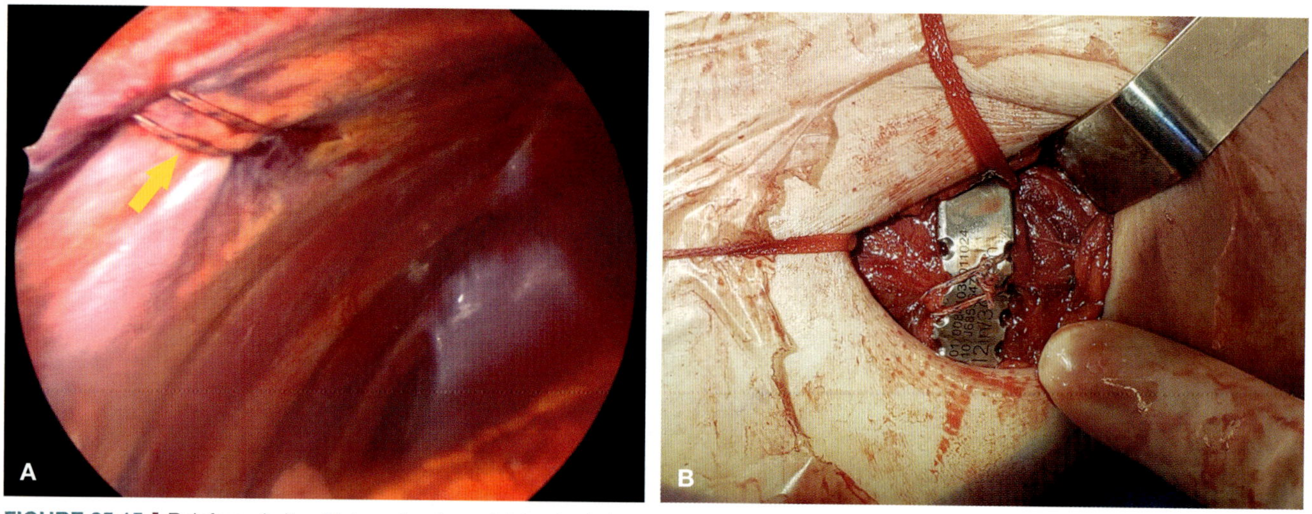

FIGURE 25.15 ▌ Reinforced ultra–high-molecular-weight polyethylene-polyester (arrow, suture around rib) **(A)** and pectus bar **(B)** in figure-of-8 configuration.

- The pectus hardware is further secured to the serratus muscle fascia using 0-Vicryl sutures, with at least three sutures placed within each hardware eyelet (two eyelets in stabilizer bar and one at the end of the pectus bar).
- The thoracoscope is removed from the right chest, and a 16-French chest tube is advanced through the port into the right chest and connected to a chest drainage system at −20 cm H_2O suction.
- The wounds are closed in layers, approximating the subcutaneous tissue in layers and the skin with a running subcuticular or dermal stitch.
- The patient is placed in the Trendelenburg position and airplaned with the left side down. The anesthesia team administers several large inspiratory breaths to expand the atelectatic lungs and promote CO_2 evacuation via the right-sided chest tube.
- When no further air leak is seen in the chest drainage system, the chest tube is removed during an inspiratory hold, and the port site is closed.
- While a persistent air leak is uncommon in the initial surgery, if an air leak does persist, the chest tube is left in place during the postoperative recovery until the leak resolves.

Postoperative Care

- The most critical issue following pectus excavatum repair is pain control. This can be augmented by intraoperative administration of cryoanalgesia. In the authors' practice, cryoanalgesia requires 1 to 2 days before maximal effect. Other pain management methods are needed in the immediate postoperative period.
- If cryoablation is inappropriate or consent is not received for its use, we prefer a combination of thoracic epidural analgesia (bupivacaine and hydromorphone or bupivacaine and fentanyl) and scheduled analgesics (acetaminophen, intravenous ketorolac, and gabapentin). Lorazepam may be given if anxiety is contributing to a heightened pain response.
- Most patients remain on this pain protocol until postoperative day 2 when the epidural is capped and then removed if the patient transitions successfully to an oral opioid program. Ketorolac is similarly stopped, and an oral nonsteroidal anti-inflammatory drug (NSAID) is started.
- The pain control regimen above is accompanied by an aggressive bowel regimen, antinausea medication, and acid-reducing medication.
- Most patients are discharged home on postoperative day 3. Anteroposterior and lateral chest x-rays are obtained before discharge. The lateral film is particularly important in determining bar position after surgery if there is a future concern for bar rotation.
- Most patients are directed to avoid strenuous activities and organized sports for 8 to 12 weeks after surgery to decrease the risk of bar rotation.

PEARLS AND PITFALLS

- In the preoperative period, a straightforward discussion of postoperative pain and the different pain management options with the patient and their family is key in setting appropriate expectations and improving patient experience.
- Preoperative testing for metal allergies of individuals with multiple food or environmental allergies, known atopy, or atopic dermatitis (ie, eczema) is performed, even if they do not have a known nickel allergy.
- Sternal elevation has been beneficial for safe retrosternal dissection and bar placement.
- The pectus bars should be shaped to the individual's chest wall contour to account for the sternal depression and the shape of the lateral supporting chest wall.
- Optimal postoperative results (Figure 25.16A and B) are dependent on the placement of the correct number and size of bars through the appropriate intercostal space(s).
- The use of the elongated stabilizers and ultra–high-molecular-weight polyethylene-polyester sutures, when appropriate, minimizes the risk of postoperative bar rotation.
- In patients undergoing redo pectus excavatum repair or with a history of chest surgery, postoperative air leaks are common and expected in the early recovery period. In those cases, it is our practice to leave chest tubes to suction drainage after surgery.
- A multimodal pain control approach (eg, cryoablation, thoracic epidural, PCA, gabapentin, or pregabalin) can achieve adequate postoperative pain control. It is important to be aware of the morbidities associated with pain management and employ additional strategies to address these related problems (eg, acid suppressant to prevent NSAID-induced gastritis, bowel regimen to prevent opioid-induced constipation).
- Timing of bar removal is assessed on an individual patient basis, primarily keeping in mind the development level of the chest wall. In general, removal can be considered after 1 to 2 years in younger patients (<18 years old), and 3 to 4 years for older patients with stiffer chest walls.

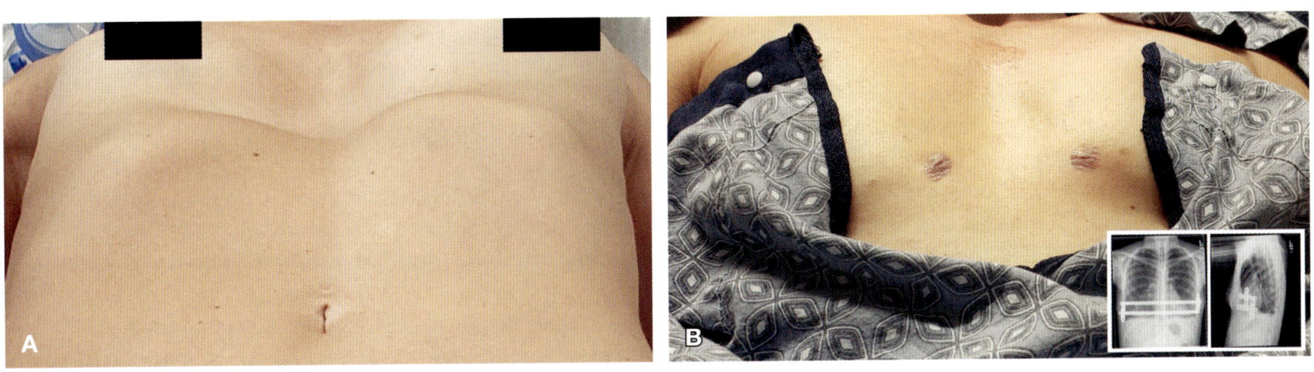

FIGURE 25.16 ❙ Before **(A)** and after **(B)** surgery with radiographs confirming bar position.

Suggested Readings

1. Cramm SL, Luckhurst C, Galls A, et al. Thoracic epidural-based Enhanced Recovery After Surgery (ERAS) pathway for Nuss repair of pectus excavatum shortened length of stay and decreased rescue intravenous opiate use. *Pediatr Surg Int*. 2021;37(9):1191-1199.
2. Graves CE, Moyer J, Zobel MJ, et al. Intraoperative intercostal nerve cryoablation during the Nuss procedure reduces length of stay and opioid requirement: a randomized clinical trial. *J Pediatr Surg*. 2019;54(11):2250-2256.
3. Zimmer Biomet. *Pectus Excavatum Correction Guide Website*; 2017. Accessed June 29, 2024. https://assets.ctfassets.net/rc4arfpyhdpw/5Va8N5P5Wk87FvWf1Y9Ew5/bcbc63f8cd8ee6aefae3203759e989ce/pectus_brochure.pdf
4. Nuss D, Kelly RE Jr, Croitoru DP, Katz ME. A 10-year review of a minimally invasive technique for the correction of pectus excavatum. *J Pediatr Surg*. 1998;33(4):545-552.

Chapter 26

Diaphragmatic Plication

DANNY WANG
ASHOK MUNIAPPAN

Preoperative Considerations

- Preoperative imaging (chest x-ray, ultrasound, CT) is required for diagnosis and helpful for identifying the level of the diaphragm and port placement.
- Pulmonary function testing (PFT) is obtained for preoperative planning (single-lung ventilation) and demonstrating the extent of restrictive disease that is worse with lying supine. Symptoms are often more pronounced than PFT abnormalities.
- Optimizing medical comorbidities contributing to respiratory insufficiency such as heart failure, reactive airway disease, smoking, and especially obesity may resolve symptoms without the need for surgery. Surgery is never offered for the asymptomatic patient.

Anesthesia and Positioning

- General anesthesia with double-lumen endotracheal tube is necessary for a minimally invasive thoracic approach (helpful but not mandatory for an open approach).
- For a transthoracic approach, the patient is positioned in lateral decubitus position with the paralyzed diaphragm facing up.
- For a laparoscopic approach, the patient remains supine with arms out. A footboard is applied to permit steep Trendelenburg position.
- Preoperative thoracic epidural for postoperative pain management is considered if a thoracotomy is utilized and for patients with very poor functional status.
- The stomach is decompressed with an orogastric tube to improve intraoperative visualization and reduce risk of injury.
- The patient must have adequate neuromuscular blockade before attempting plication.

TIPS

- *Steep Trendelenburg position may assist with caudal displacement of the abdominal viscera and better visualization of the diaphragm.*
- *For an open transthoracic approach, consider making an incision in the central tendon for visualization of both sides of the diaphragm when suturing.*
- *For thoracic approaches, release of the inferior pulmonary ligament greatly improves working space.*
- *For abdominal approaches, inducing a capnothorax through intentional perforation of the diaphragm or a small pleural catheter will equalize the abdominal and thoracic pressures, allowing for easier retraction of the diaphragm.*
- *Both intra- and extracorporeal knot-tying may be used based on surgeon preference and experience with minimally invasive approaches but pledgets should always be used whenever able.*

Technique

Open Transthoracic

- An anterior thoracotomy, sparing the latissimus dorsi muscle, through the sixth or seventh intercostal space provides adequate exposure. A separate port for a 5- or 10-mm 30° thoracoscope can help with visualization and lighting.
- Takedown of the inferior pulmonary ligament greatly improves working space.
- An accordion technique is used to create pleats and remove redundancy from the diaphragm (see Figure 26.1).

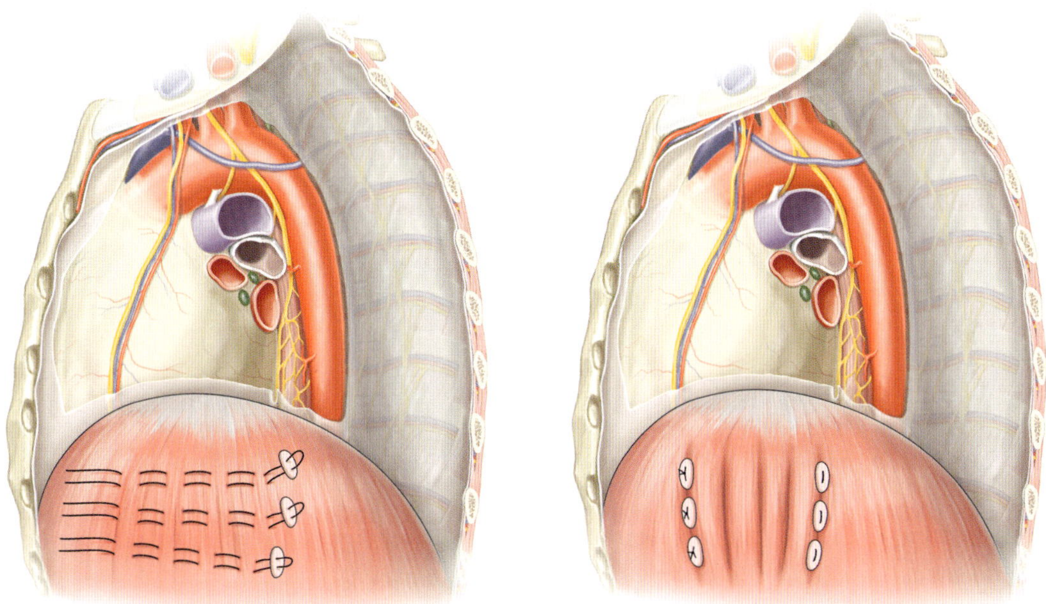

A B

FIGURE 26.1 | Accordion plication technique. **A.** Mattress sutures are placed with bites oriented along the posterior-to-anterior axis. **B.** Completed repair. (Modified from Kwon MH, Morse CR. Plication/thoracotomy/ VATS. In: Mathisen DJ, Morse C, eds. *Master Techniques in Surgery: Thoracic Surgery—Transplantation, Tracheal Resections, Mediastinal Tumors, Extended Thoracic Resections*. Wolters Kluwer; 2015:183-189. Figure 18.1.)

- Interrupted sutures through the pleats run from posterior to anterior (or vice versa) with a pledget preloaded in the middle. The knot is tied on the pledget.
- Sutures are placed sequentially and parallel to each other, working from medial to lateral until the whole diaphragm has been traversed.
- Additional sutures may be necessary to gather up any remaining redundancy or laxity.

Thoracoscopic

- The camera port is generally placed along the eighth interspace around the mid- to posterior axillary line (see Figure 26.2 for port placements).
- In the three-port technique, two working ports are placed along the anterior and posterior fifth interspace.
- An anterior mini-thoracotomy may be used in a two-port technique with traditional instruments. Ideally, rib spreading would be avoided.
- Multiple techniques may be used based on working space and experience of the surgeon including but not limited to the accordion technique, interrupted U-stitches/horizontal mattress sutures, imbrication sutures, and continuous running sutures. A caveat for a running suture is that a single point of failure (either suture fatigue or unraveling of the knot) can result in complete recurrence (see Figure 26.3).

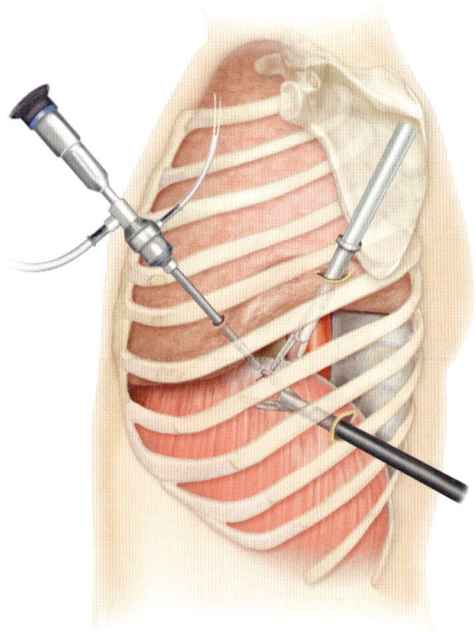

FIGURE 26.2 | Video-assisted thoracic surgery diaphragmatic plication port placement. The camera port is placed in eighth interspace at the mid- to posterior axillary line. The working ports are placed along the anterior and posterior fifth interspace. The level of the camera port may be adjusted based on the level of the diaphragm. (Modified from Kwon MH, Morse CR. Plication/thoracotomy/ VATS. In: Mathisen DJ, Morse C, eds. *Master Techniques in Surgery: Thoracic Surgery—Transplantation, Tracheal Resections, Mediastinal Tumors, Extended Thoracic Resections*. Wolters Kluwer; 2015:183-189. Figure 18.2.)

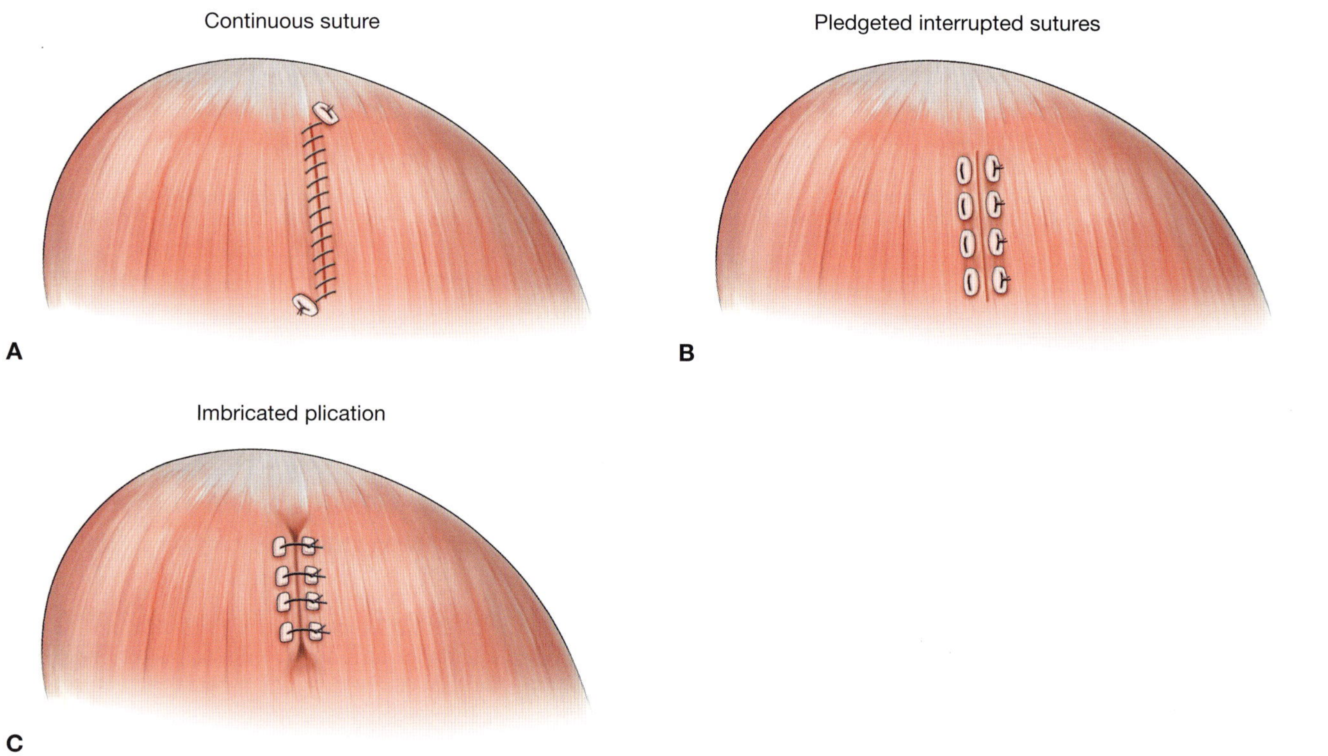

FIGURE 26.3 | Alternative schema for plication. **A.** Continuous running suture. **B.** Interrupted horizontal mattress. **C.** Imbricated sutures. (Modified from Kwon MH, Morse CR. Plication/thoracotomy/ VATS. In: Mathisen DJ, Morse C, eds. *Master Techniques in Surgery: Thoracic Surgery—Transplantation, Tracheal Resections, Mediastinal Tumors, Extended Thoracic Resections*. Wolters Kluwer; 2015:183-189. Figure 18.3.)

Laparoscopic

- Four 12-mm ports are used with two assistant ports placed parallel to midline on the contralateral side to the hemidiaphragm elevation and two working ports placed above the umbilicus on the ipsilateral side (see Figure 26.4).

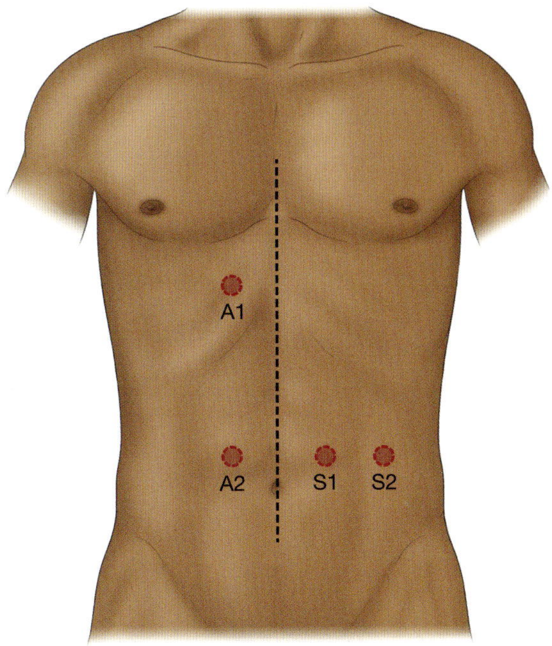

FIGURE 26.4 ▌ Port placement for left-sided laparoscopic diaphragmatic plication. The two assistant ports (A1 and A2) are placed on the patient's right side around 2 to 4 cm off midline. The camera port is placed 2 to 4 cm above the umbilicus. The two surgeon's ports (S1 and S2) are placed 2 to 4 cm above the umbilicus on the patient's left side.

- The diaphragm may be retracted caudally either using retraction stitches or inducing a capnothorax through perforation of the diaphragm or insertion of a thoracic port.
- Placement of a chest tube may allow for venting of the capnothorax as needed and adjustment of the intraabdominal and intrathoracic pressures as necessary.
- Right-sided laparoscopic diaphragmatic plication should be avoided as the liver prevents adequate exposure of the diaphragm.
- Posterior plication of the diaphragm is performed starting centrally and advancing posteriorly using interrupted U-stitches. Retraction of the central stitches will allow for better exposure of the posterior diaphragm (see Figure 26.5).
- Anterior plication of the diaphragm is achieved through weaving U-stitches that are placed from the posterioanterior direction until the diaphragm is flat and taut (see Figure 26.6).

Robotic Transthoracic

- The camera port is generally placed under direct visualization at the posterior axillary line in the fifth or sixth interspace (see Figure 26.7 for port placements).
- Two 8-mm working ports are placed a hands width anterior and posterior to the camera port.
- An assistant port is placed midway between the anterior working port and camera port in the same interspace or one level above.
- The robotic boom is placed on the ipsilateral side as the disease facing the feet.
- Plication using any number of techniques may be performed (see Figure 26.8).

Robotic Transabdominal

- The camera port is placed at least 2 cm above the umbilicus (see Figure 26.9 for port placements).
- A 12-mm assistant port is placed lateral to the umbilicus on the ipsilateral side.
- Two working ports are placed with one on each side of the camera port to triangulate the diaphragm.
- Similar to the laparoscopic approach, a capnothorax should be induced through perforation of the diaphragm.
- Plication using any number of techniques may be performed.

Postoperative Care

- The orogastric tube is removed prior to extubation.
- A chest tube is left for evacuation of pneumothorax or capnothorax. Early trial of water seal and removal of chest tube will aid with pain control.

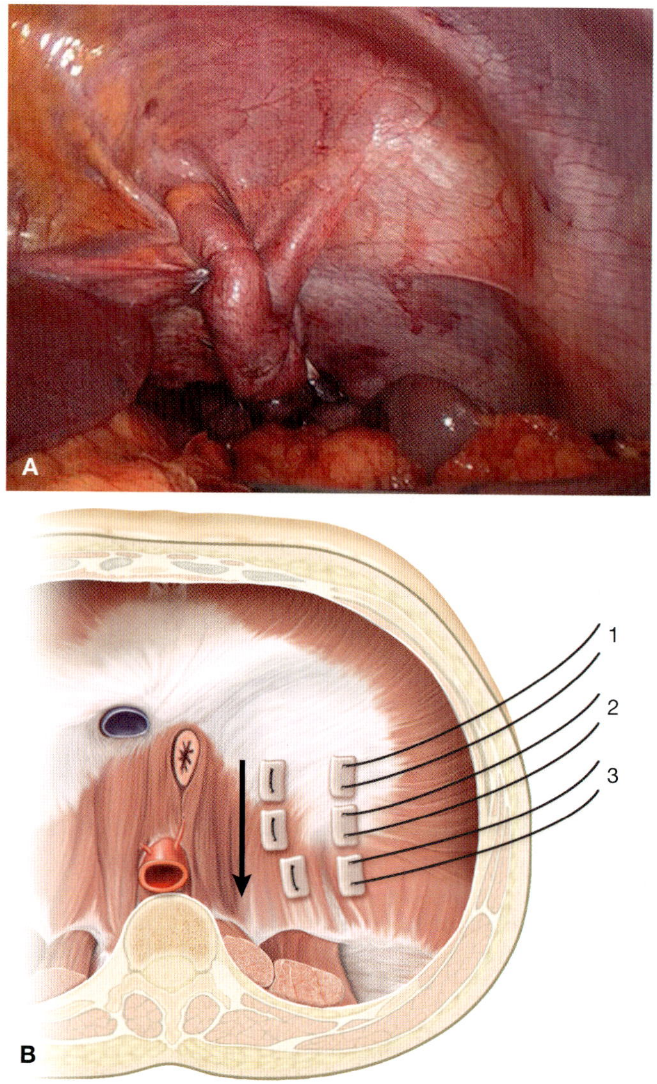

FIGURE 26.5 ▌ Laparoscopic plication of the posterior diaphragm. **A.** Completion of the posterior plication demonstrating a taut posterior portion of the diaphragm. **B.** U-stitches are placed sequentially starting centrally and advancing posteriorly. (From Podgaetz E, Andrade RS. Laparoscopic diaphragmatic plication. In: Mathisen DJ, Morse C, eds. *Master Techniques in Surgery: Thoracic Surgery—Transplantation, Tracheal Resections, Mediastinal Tumors, Extended Thoracic Resections*. Wolters Kluwer; 2015:191-199. Figure 19.3D and E.)

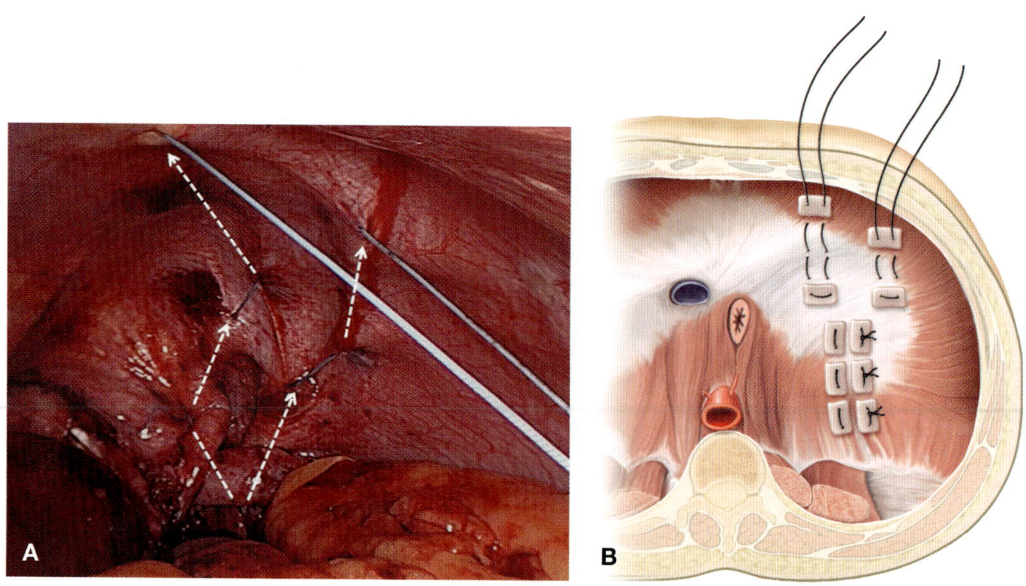

FIGURE 26.6 ▌ Laparoscopic plication of the anterior diaphragm. **A.** Weaving U-stitches are placed in the posteroanterior direction. **B.** Suturing scheme for posterior diaphragm. U-stitches are placed sequentially starting centrally and advancing posteriorly. (From Podgaetz E, Andrade RS. Laparoscopic diaphragmatic plication. In: Mathisen DJ, Morse C, eds. *Master Techniques in Surgery: Thoracic Surgery—Transplantation, Tracheal Resections, Mediastinal Tumors, Extended Thoracic Resections*. Wolters Kluwer; 2015:191-199. Figure 19.4.)

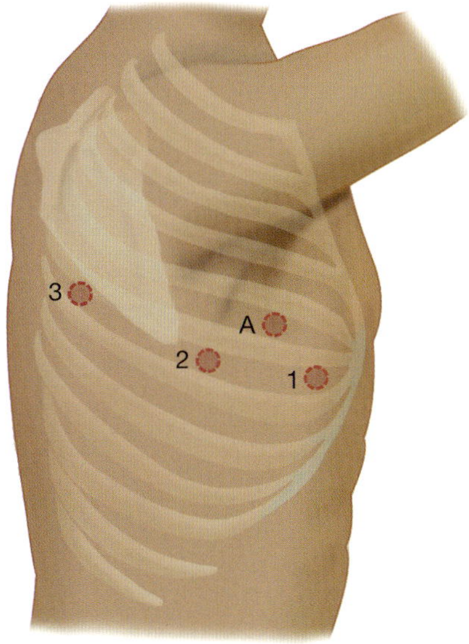

FIGURE 26.7 ▮ Port placement for a robotic transthoracic approach for a right diaphragmatic plication. The patient is placed in the lateral decubitus position. The camera port (#2) is placed in the posterior axillary line of the fifth or sixth interspace. The working ports are placed 8 to 10 cm anterior and posterior to the camera port in the same interspace. The assistant port (A) is placed between the camera port and anterior working port in the same interspace or one interspace above.

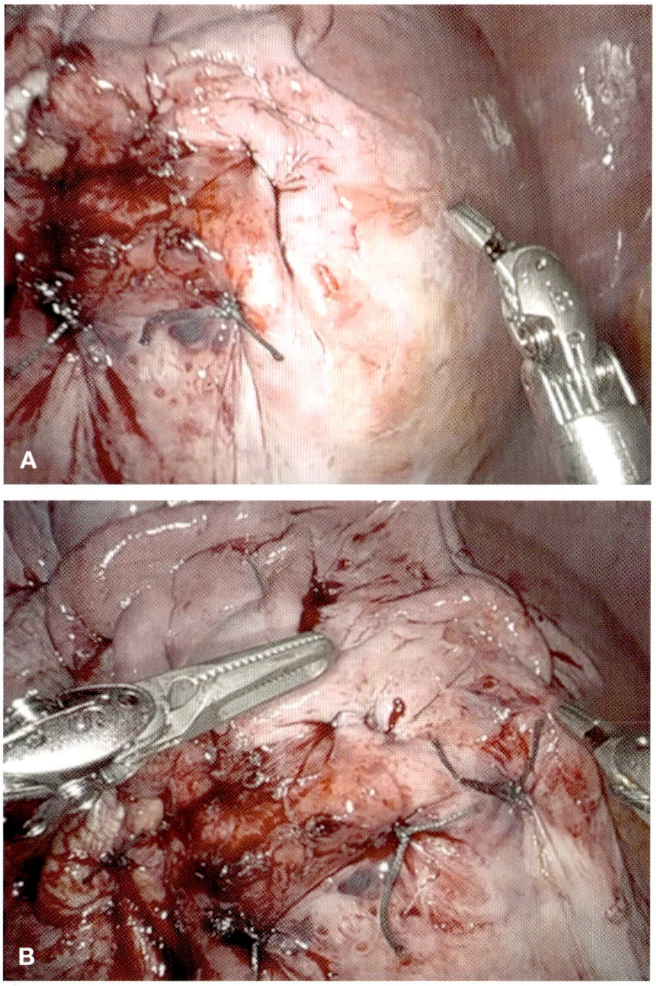

FIGURE 26.8 ▮ Accordion technique during robotic transthoracic diaphragmatic plication. **A.** Partially completed rows of accordion plication. **B.** Completed plication. (Courtesy of: Dr. Lana Schumacher-Beal, Massachusetts General Hospital.)

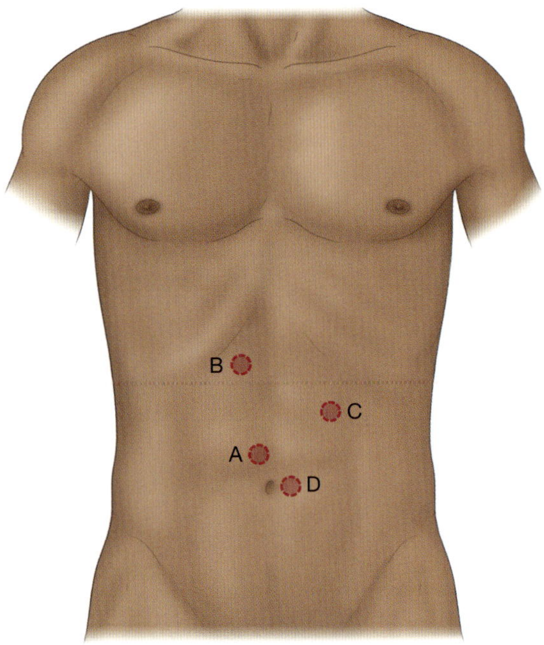

FIGURE 26.9 ❙ Port placement for robotic transabdominal approach for a left diaphragmatic plication. The camera port (A) is placed 2 to 4 cm above the umbilicus, roughly ¼ from the umbilicus to the xiphoid process. The working ports (B and C) are triangulated around 8 to 10 cm on either side of the camera port. The assistant port (D) is placed 2 to 4 cm lateral to the umbilicus.

- Immediate postoperative chest x-ray should be performed to assess for new baseline diaphragm position and lung expansion.
- Consider patient-controlled analgesia for early postoperative pain control.
- Diet may be swiftly advanced as tolerated. Pain medications should be transitioned to oral formulations with timely discontinuation of patient-controlled analgesia or epidural.
- Patients should receive adequate nausea control and cough suppression to prevent undue stress on the diaphragm and plication.

PEARLS AND PITFALLS

- Knowing the level of the diaphragm preoperatively may guide and adjust location of the incision or port placement.
- Consider different approaches in patients with prior abdominal or thoracic surgical history or disease.
- Abdominal approaches for right-sided diaphragmatic plication are more challenging due to the liver. Adequate posterior and lateral exposure are also more difficult to achieve during abdominal approaches.
- Always use pledgeted, large caliber, nonabsorbable suture (Prolene, Ethibond).
- For friable or poor quality tissue, consider a series of interrupted stitches and even spacing of stitches in multiple dimensions to ensure equally distributed tension.
- Always take full-thickness bites of the diaphragm while being cognizant of the structures on the other side of the diaphragm (liver, spleen, stomach, bowel, lung).
- All redundancy must be removed from the diaphragm to maximize lung volume and symptomatic relief.
- Postoperative slow return of bowel function, abdominal pain/distension, and signs of anemia should raise concern for injury to abdominal organs.

Suggested Readings

1. Kwon MH, Morse CR. Plication/Thoracotomy/VATS. In: *Master Techniques in Surgery: Thoracic Surgery—Transplantation, Tracheal Resections, Mediastinal Tumors, Extended Thoracic Resections*. 1st ed. Wolters Kluwer; 2014.
2. Podgaetz E, Andrade RS. Laparoscopic diaphragmatic plication. In: *Master Techniques in Surgery: Thoracic Surgery—Transplantation, Tracheal Resections, Mediastinal Tumors, Extended Thoracic Resections*. 1st ed. Wolters Kluwer; 2014.
3. Schumacher L, Zhao D. Outcomes and techniques in robotic diaphragmatic plication. *J Thorac Dis*. 2020;13(10):6113-6115.
4. Zwischenberger BA, Kister N, Zwischenberger JB, Martin JT. Laparoscopic robot-assisted diaphragm plication. *Ann Thorac Surg*. 2016;101(1):369-371.

Chapter 27

Four Approaches to Thymectomy: Robotic/Video-Assisted Thoracoscopic Thymectomy/Sternotomy/Transcervical

JOSEPH B. SHRAGER

GENERAL PERIOPERATIVE CONSIDERATIONS

- Thymectomy may be performed for myasthenia gravis (MG), or for thymic tumors when the widest possible margins are desired (although there is a trend toward thymomectomy with only 2 to 3 cm of normal thymus as a margin, rather than total thymectomy, for smaller tumors in the absence of MG).
- Thymectomy for MG (with or without tumor) must be an "extended thymectomy," encompassing all tissues between the phrenic nerves and down to the diaphragm, as well as the entirety of both cervical horns.

TIPS

The surgeon operating for MG must be committed to performing a true, extended thymectomy, whatever approach he/she uses.

- I always obtain an MG serum panel preoperatively in thymoma patients, to identify those who may have subclinical MG, which would dictate performance of an extended thymectomy even for a small tumor.
- Referrals for these operations have increased since randomized data showing the benefits of thymectomy in MG were published in 2016.
- While in the randomized study, extended thymectomy via median sternotomy was used, most experienced surgeons believe that one of the minimally invasive approaches allows an equivalent extended thymectomy. A meta-analysis published by my group suggests this is true.
- All patients with MG must have their disease optimized preoperatively by medication ± intravenous (IV) immunoglobulin or plasmapheresis. We aim to have prednisone weaned to ≤20 mg daily to minimize wound problems.
- On the morning of surgery, MG patients must take all their MG medications.
- For all the approaches, the critical issues are performing a true, extended thymectomy while avoiding injury to the phrenic nerve(s) and bleeding from the innominate vein.

TIPS

Obtain a serum MG panel in all thymoma cases to rule out subclinical MG, which would dictate performing an extended thymectomy.

THYMECTOMY BY MEDIAN STERNOTOMY

Perioperative Considerations

- While sternotomy can be a bit of a setback for a patient with severe MG, for the vast majority, it is very well tolerated. There should therefore be no hesitation to choose this approach if less experienced and for larger and invasive tumors.
- The three downsides of sternotomy are about 1 day extra length of stay; about 4 to 6 weeks increased time to return to moderate-heavy physical activity; and the small but nonzero risk of sternal wound infection.

Anesthesia and Patient Positioning

- General anesthesia with double-lumen endotracheal tube.
- Supine, bump beneath shoulders, and arms tucked.
- For giant tumors that may require extension into a thoracotomy, keep ipsilateral arm abducted.

Instruments and Equipment

- Standard thoracic surgical instrumentation including long, insulated Debakey forceps, long insulated monopolar cautery, Kittners, and titanium clips.

Technique

It is difficult to demonstrate the technique of extended thymectomy by sternotomy in images/photos. We therefore provide limited images. The images shown for video-assisted thoracoscopic surgery (VATS)/robotic thymectomy in the section that follows will demonstrate also the structures that are dissected during thymectomy by sternotomy.

- For MG, a total extended thymectomy is the goal, corresponding to a "T3b" thymectomy according to the Thymectomy Classification of the Myasthenia Gravis Foundation of America.
- Some advocate partial upper sternotomy, but I find this limits exposure substantially without reducing pain significantly.
- Pick a side to begin on (the side the tumor leans toward, in a thymoma case—the left side for this description). Airplane the table slightly toward that left side (surgeon on the opposite side of table) and incise the mediastinal pleura on the left, ~5 mm posterior to the posterior sternal table, parallel to the sternum (Figure 27.1).
- Continue this first anterior mediastinal pleural incision from caudal to cephalad, and as you approach within a few centimeters of the innominate vein, stop, retract the divided pleura and underlying heart toward the surgeon, and identify the phrenic nerve at midchest level.

TIPS

Make two mediastinal pleural incisions, one anteriorly just behind the sternal edge and one posteriorly just anterior to the phrenic nerve. Everything between these comes out.

- Trace the phrenic nerve from the pleural-space side, progressively cephalad, to get an initial feel for its course.

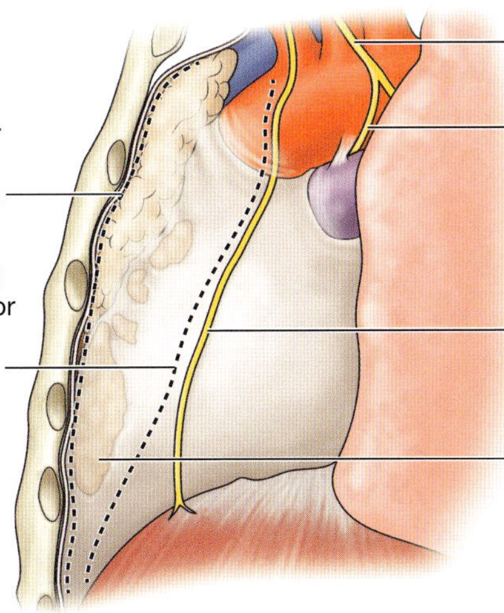

FIGURE 27.1 | View from the left chest (not surgeon's view) demonstrating the anterior (first) and posterior (second) mediastinal pleural incisions. Extended thymectomy involves removal of the pleura and all fat/thymus between these incisions, across the midline, down to the diaphragm, and the two upper horns.

TIPS

The phrenic nerves become more anterior and medial as they are traced from caudal to cranial. At the cranial end, they are therefore easy to injure.

- Go back to the cephalad end of this left-sided dissection. Establish a clean plane of dissection on the surface of the leftward half of the innominate vein and find the left internal mammary vein and trace it toward the sternum. Take all the fatty/thymic tissue from the mammary vein medially, toward the ultimate specimen, constantly keeping the phrenic in mind/view. Some small clips are generally used in this area so as not to cauterize close to the nerve.

TIPS

One always leaves a small amount of fat on the nerves just lateral to the innominate vein and medial to the internal mammary veins; one cannot remove every fat globule in this area without putting the nerve at risk.

- Now find again the phrenic nerve at the level of the internal mammary vein and then incise the mediastinal pleura (just a thin layer here) about 5 mm anterior to nerve, progressing from cephalad to caudal. This is the second, posterior incision of the mediastinal pleura (Figure 27.1). The cautery should be set on a low setting during this portion, and the assistant can help greatly by tenting up the mediastinal pleura off of the pericardium with a pediatric suction tip or right angle. Take this division all the way down to the level of the diaphragm.
- Use cautery, Kittner, or sharp dissection to strip all the fatty, thymic, and pleural tissues off of the pericardium from near the nerve, medially/anteriorly with the developing specimen.

TIPS

Small branches of the pericardiophrenic vessels run anteriorly from the phrenic nerves. If they are cauterized close to the nerve, the energy will conduct to and perhaps injure the nerve. These are best handled with tiny clips and sharp division.

- Move to the opposite side of the chest, and carry out the same steps: airplane the table to the right, incise the mediastinal pleura anteriorly just below the sternum (Figure 27.2), trace the phrenic nerve, identify the innominate and mammary veins, then divide the mediastinal pleura more posteriorly, just anterior to the nerve along its course (Figure 27.2), then sweep all the fatty/thymic/pleural tissue medially.

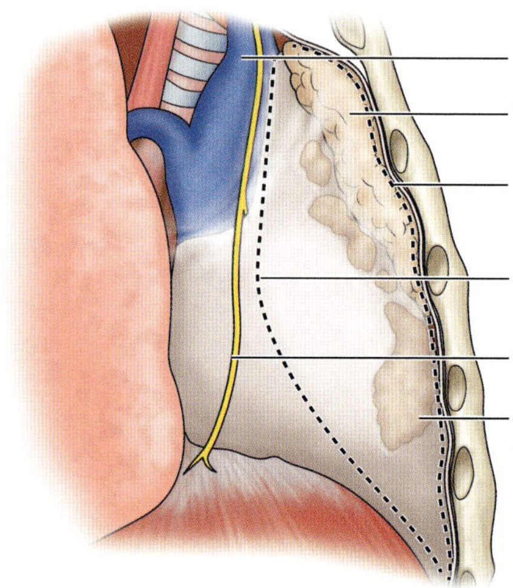

FIGURE 27.2 | View from the right chest (not surgeon's view) demonstrating same points as in Figure 27.1.

- Now go down to the level of the diaphragm. Dissect all the fatty tissues from the diaphragm (the pericardiophrenic fat pads) and from the anterior surface of the pericardium off of the diaphragm at the caudal aspect of the dissection and then begin to take the fatty/thymic tissue off the pericardium from caudal to cephalad for a few centimeters. In most patients, this is a very nice filmy plane (Figure 27.3).
- Go back to the superior (cephalad) end of the dissection. Identify the superior thymic horns that typically are two distinct structures coursing anterior to the innominate vein, toward the thyroid gland.
- Trace each horn up by blunt and cautery dissection, staying directly on the capsule of each horn, until it fades into the thyrothymic ligament (you are there when you see a small vascular pedicle as the horn narrows to a thin structure and you approach the thyroid gland) (Figure 27.4). Control and divide each ligament with cautery or between ligatures.

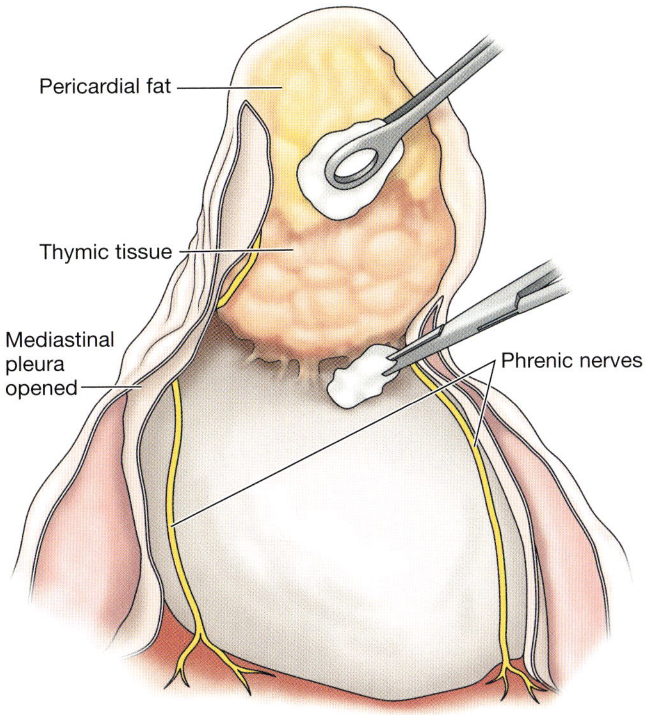

FIGURE 27.3 ■ The thymus and all associated fatty tissue is dissected from the level of diaphragm, cephalad, using blunt dissection with Kittner or cautery dissection in this filmy plane.(Technical assistance with figures by Winston Trope, BS.)

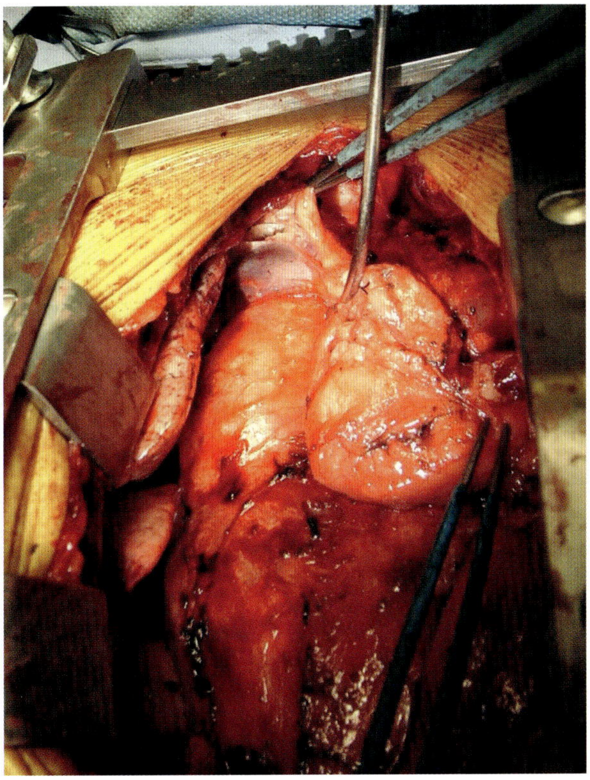

FIGURE 27.4 ■ The right upper horn is shown being dissected up into the neck. (Technical assistance with figures by Winston Trope, BS.)

TIPS

Occasionally, one of the two, or a third, superior horn courses aberrantly, posterior to the innominate vein. Be alert for this and dissect it out as necessary.

- Flip the horns inferiorly, and identify the thymic veins that drain from the body of the gland into the caudal aspect of the innominate vein. Ligate and divided these (Figure 27.5).

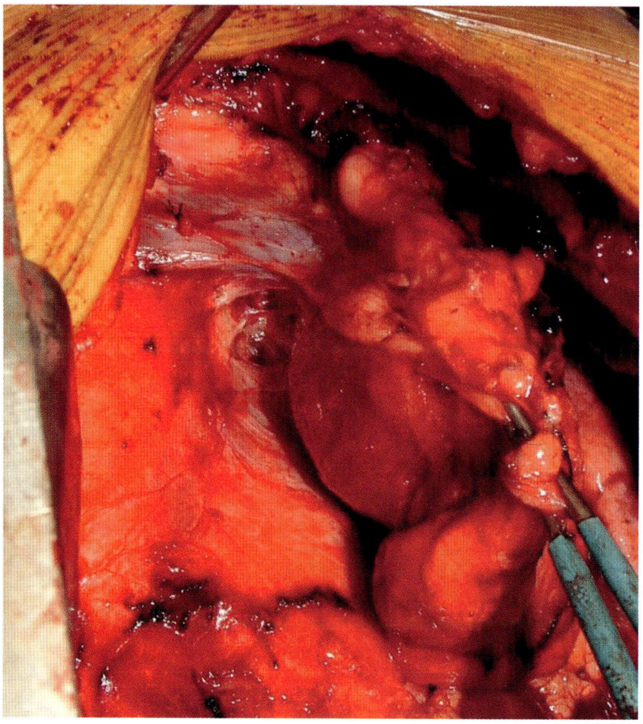

FIGURE 27.5 ▍ With the right horn now flipped down, the innominate vein is better exposed, and thymic veins draining into the innominate are controlled. Note one already controlled with silk (the right pleura remains closed in this case of a left-sided tumor, in a patient without myasthenia gravis). (Technical assistance with figures by Winston Trope, B.S.)

TIPS

There are almost always 2 or 3 thymic veins—so focus on finding more after you have found only one!

TIPS

It is always better, when dissecting the innominate vein, to be directly *on the plane of the vessel. While this feels more "dangerous," it is in fact safer and will allow you to mobilize the vessel and identify its branches more expeditiously.*

- You are now ready to complete the mobilization of the gland/tumor from the pericardium, from caudal to cephalad. This plane is typically filmy and easily taken with cautery—sometimes Kittner or larger ball sponges on ring clamps are effective to bluntly mobilize the tissue off the pericardium (Figure 27.3).
- In tumor cases, the slightest hint of adherence to the pericardium should push you to open the pericardium and take it en bloc with the specimen (Figure 27.6B, robotic). Similarly, any suggestion of invasion of the innominate vein or lung is managed with en bloc resection (Figure 27.6A).

There is close to zero downside to doing this, including resecting the vein entirely. Phrenic nerve division (Figure 27.6C) and great vessel resection/reconstruction (Figure 27.6D) have more potential impact on the patient but must be done when there is clear invasion.

- Ask the anesthesiologists to give an IV equivalent dose of pyridostigmine about 30 minutes prior to closure.

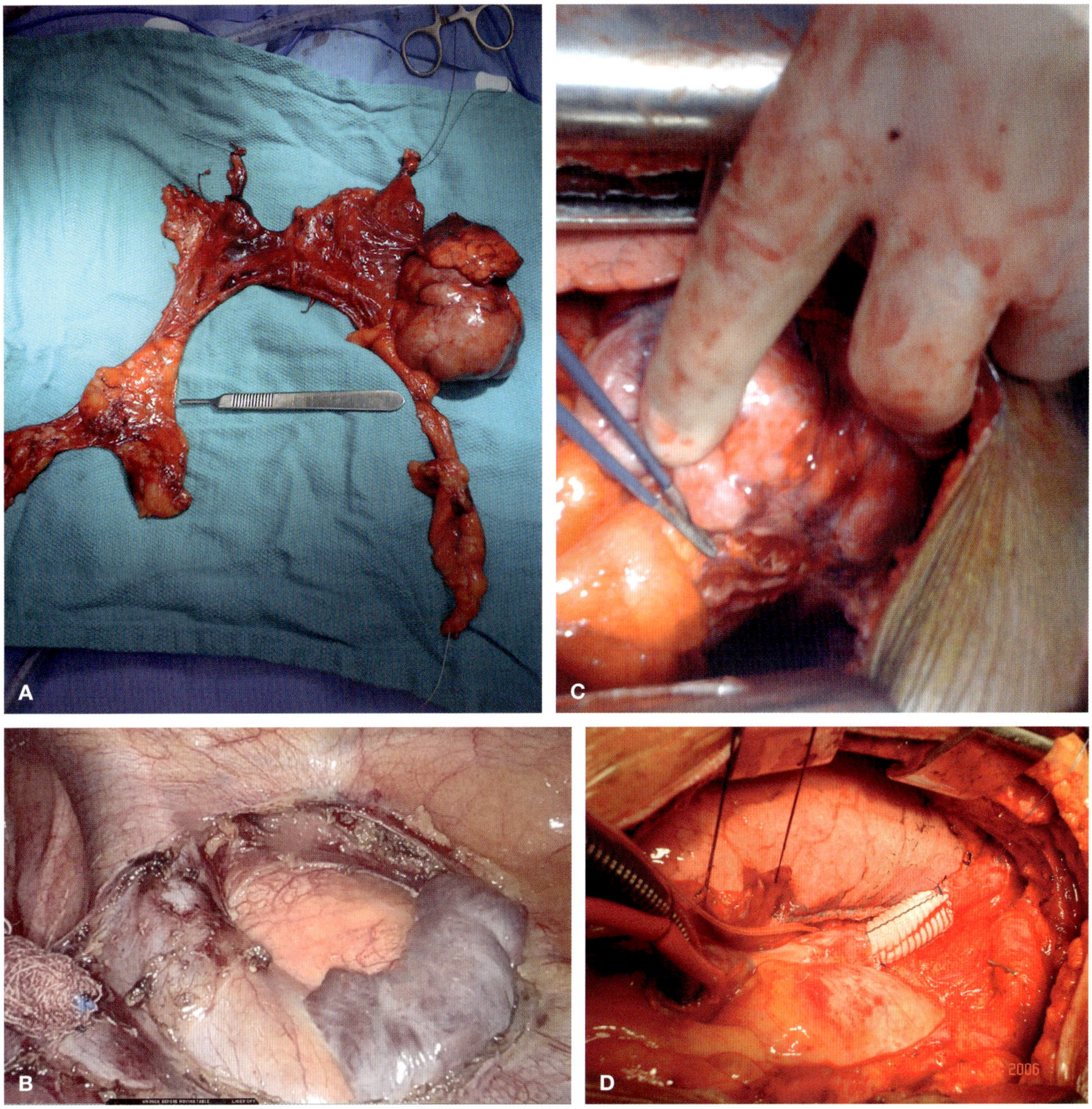

FIGURE 27.6 | A-D. Invasive thymoma cases showing en bloc resection of various structures. **A.** Thymoma/myasthenia gravis (MG) specimen with en bloc wedge of the left upper lobe. **B.** Pericardial defect after thymoma (no MG) case, which required patch/repair after pericardial and right phrenic nerve resection (robotic approach). **C.** Left-sided thymoma involving the left phrenic nerve, which required resection. **D.** Thymoma/MG case requiring circumferential superior vena cava resection, after the reconstruction. (Technical assistance with figures by Winston Trope, BS.)

TIPS

If a portion of pericardium has been resected, which it seems might entrap the atrium or allow cardiac herniation, one can either open the sac fully as one would for a cardiac procedure or repair the defect with Gor-Tex or bovine pericardium.

- I prefer 2 straight chest tubes, passed from the upper abdomen just off midline, through the mediastinum, and then with the tips at each apex directed posteriorly.

Postoperative Care

- MG patients should take their first postoperative dose of oral pyridostigmine about 3 hours after the end of anesthesia. And we typically give 100 mg IV hydrocortisone × 1 dose at midnight after the operation if they have been on steroids. They then restart their home steroid dose orally the next morning.
- We check bedside forced vital capacity twice daily and consider intervening with ramped-up MG treatments if these fall by 20% or there are other increasing signs of weakness.
- I am a great believer in early mobilization: out of bed to chair the evening after a morning operation. Ambulate no later than the next morning. Foley out first morning.
- Minimize lab tests. If no concern for bleeding, one set of labs on morning of postoperative day (POD) 1 is typically all that is needed. This lets the patients get better sleep!
- I ask patients to "make believe there is a huge plate of glass running through your body from side-to-side: you should not move your arms back through this plate of glass, or above your chin" until I see them at the approximately 3 week postoperative visit (to reduce stress on the sternotomy).

PEARLS AND PITFALLS

- When there is a tumor approaching the phrenic nerve on one side, we prefer to dissect that side first, so that if that phrenic nerve requires resection, one can then be particularly careful not to injure the opposite nerve.
- If a tumor immediately abuts or frankly involves a phrenic nerve on one side, that nerve must be sacrificed en bloc with the tumor (Figure 27.6C), if the patient is expected to tolerate losing that nerve. I try to perform an immediate diaphragm plication in that situation (easier on the right than on the left, for obvious reasons).
- One knows one has reached the extreme cephalad end of the upper thymic horns when they dissipate into a vascular bundle that seems to emerge directly from the inferior edge of the thyroid.
- Even the pericardiophrenic fat pads have been proven to not infrequently contain small nests of thymic tissue, so they should be resected in MG patients. Removing them as separate specimens can reduce the bulk and aid ease of manipulation of the main specimen as dissection proceeds.
- We use 3 wires in the manubrium and at least 5 in lower intercostal spaces—this has resulted in zero sternal dehiscences.

THYMECTOMY BY VIDEO-ASSISTED TRANSCERVICAL APPROACH

Perioperative Considerations

- This operation is only performed for nonthymomatous MG. Although very experienced users have reported it for very small thymomas, I cannot recommend that.
- The original transcervical thymectomy (TCT) was performed "blindly," with an intern or medical student trying to pull up on the sternum, and this was clearly not an extended thymectomy.
- The subsequent innovations of the substernal retracting blade and the addition of video visualization via the neck incision allow a true, extended thymectomy to be performed.

TIPS

The Cooper thymectomy blade and 5-mm thoracoscope allow a T3B thymectomy to be performed via the neck.

- This operation is frequently performed as an outpatient, its main advantages being almost zero impact on pulmonary function and usually only 3 to 4 days before return to full normal activities.
- TCT is likely harder to learn to do well than VATS/robotic approaches, since the technique/instrumentation is not as familiar to thoracic surgeons as VATS/robotics.

TIPS

TCT is truly the most minimally invasive of all the approaches to thymectomy—often done as an outpatient.

Anesthesia and Patient Positioning

- General anesthesia via single-lumen endotracheal tube. No need for lung isolation.
- Supine, arms tucked.
- Inflatable shoulder roll, neck maximally extended, head resting on a "doughnut."
- Prep entire sternum in case of rare need for sternotomy.

TIPS

TCT can only be easily performed on a patient who is nonobese and who is able to extend their neck fully.

Instruments and Equipment

- Cooper Thymectomy retractor (substernal blade) and RuleTrac sidebars and crossbars to attach it to.
- Standard thoracic surgical instrumentation, plus:
  - 5-mm 30° videoscope
  - Kaiser-Pilling Thoracoscopic instrument set (or other diverse set that includes curved ring clamps)
  - Small ball sponges to place within jaws of the various ring clamps
  - Hook cautery
  - Long, thin Penrose drains to use to attach army-navy retractors to the corners of the table for exposure
- Both surgeon and assistant wear a headlight at the start. This becomes unnecessary once the video camera can be introduced beneath the sternum.

Technique

TIPS

It is useful to look at the preoperative computed tomography scan to get a sense of whether the innominate vein is a "high" one or not. This will be helpful to know as you approach the vein during the dissection.

- A 4 to 5 cm curvilinear incision is made one pinkie breadth above the clavicular heads and through the jugular notch, in Langer lines (Figure 27.7).
- Subplatysmal flaps are raised superiorly to the thyroid cartilage and inferiorly to the sternum with cautery.

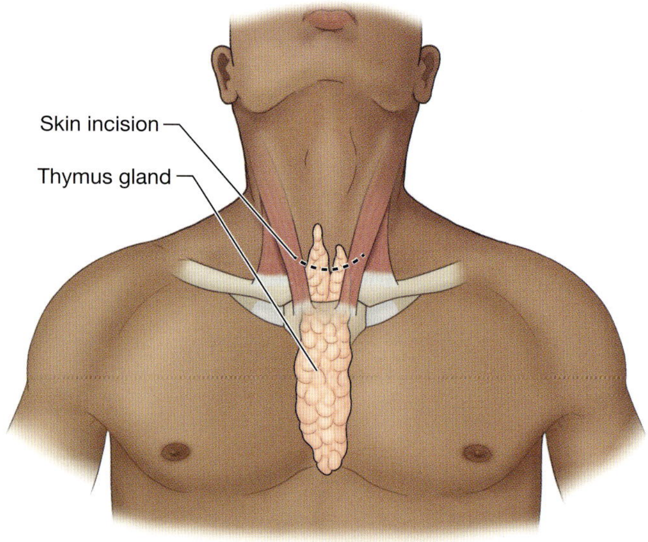

FIGURE 27.7 | Transcervical thymectomy incision.

- The strap muscles are separated longitudinally in the midline with cautery, from the level of the thyroid cartilage to the sternum.
- The cleido-cleido ligament is divided, taking care not to enter the capsule of the gland that sits just beneath.
- Identify one of the upper thymic horns by blunt and careful cautery dissection just posterior to the strap muscles on either side (Figure 27.8A).

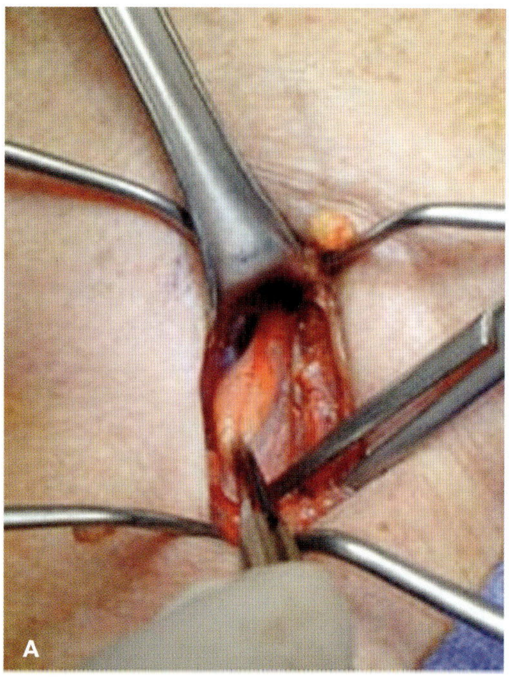

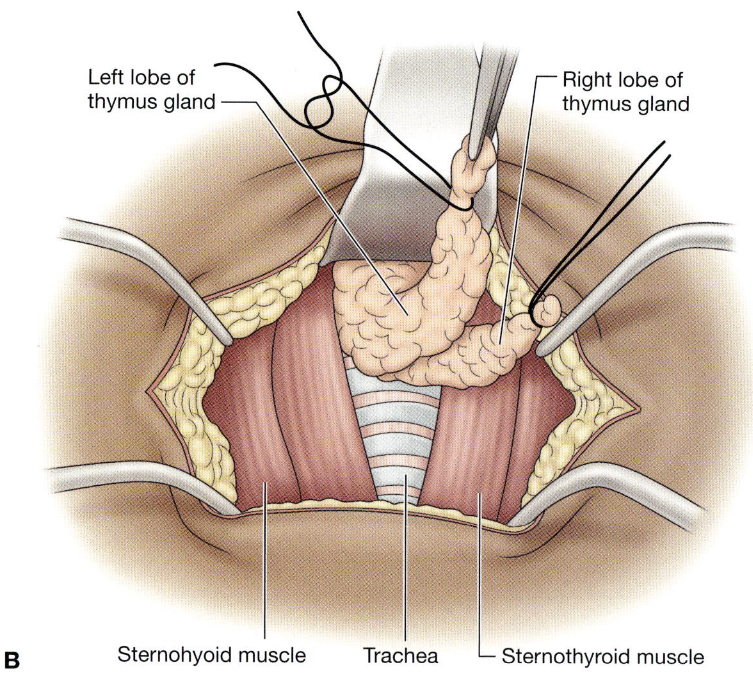

FIGURE 27.8 | **A and B.** Dissecting out the upper horns. (**A.** Technical assistance with figures by Winston Trope, BS.)

TIPS

The upper thymic horns are identifiable from the surrounding cervical fat by a slightly darker, pinker color than the yellower fat, and by the smoother contour created by the capsule that surrounds the gland.

- Once one upper horn is found, dissect it cephalad to its disappearance into the thyrothymic ligament and divide it there (with cautery or ligature on ligament). Then place a long 0 (zero) silk tie, leaving arms long and of equal length, around a solid part of that horn within 2 cm of its tip. Place a Kelly clamp on these silk arms.

TIPS

The capsule around the horns is typically fairly firm, allowing much of the dissection of them to be done bluntly, with a pediatric sucker tip, then dividing remaining bands with cautery.

- Trace down the medial side of whichever horn is found first until reaching the body of the gland, then over to the other side, and back up to identify the opposite horn. Dissect and place a silk tie on this horn as you have on the other (Figure 27.8B).
- Using the two silk ties you have placed on the horns to retract the gland as you dissected on the lateral edges of the body of the gland as far into the mediastinum as possible without at this point placing the retractor. Be alert to a high-riding innominate vein.
- Dissect on the superficial surface of the gland in the midline until you reach the substernal plane; then use finger dissection deeply into the mediastinum, superficial to the gland.

TIPS

Do not enter the plane between the strap muscles and the sternum as you finger dissect into the mediastinum. This will be bloody and make you unhappy. Stay directly on the capsule of the gland.

- Now, place the sidebars, the crossbar, and the Cooper thymectomy blade beneath the sternum.
- Allow the patient to "hang" from the substernal retractor by pulling up on it forcefully and locking it in place while deflating the bag beneath the shoulders (Figure 27.9A and B).
- It is often helpful at this point to place army-navy retractors at each corner of the neck incision, clipped via long Penrose drains to the corners of the table near the patient's head. This improves the view via the neck incision into the mediastinum, until the point that the videoscope begins to be employed.

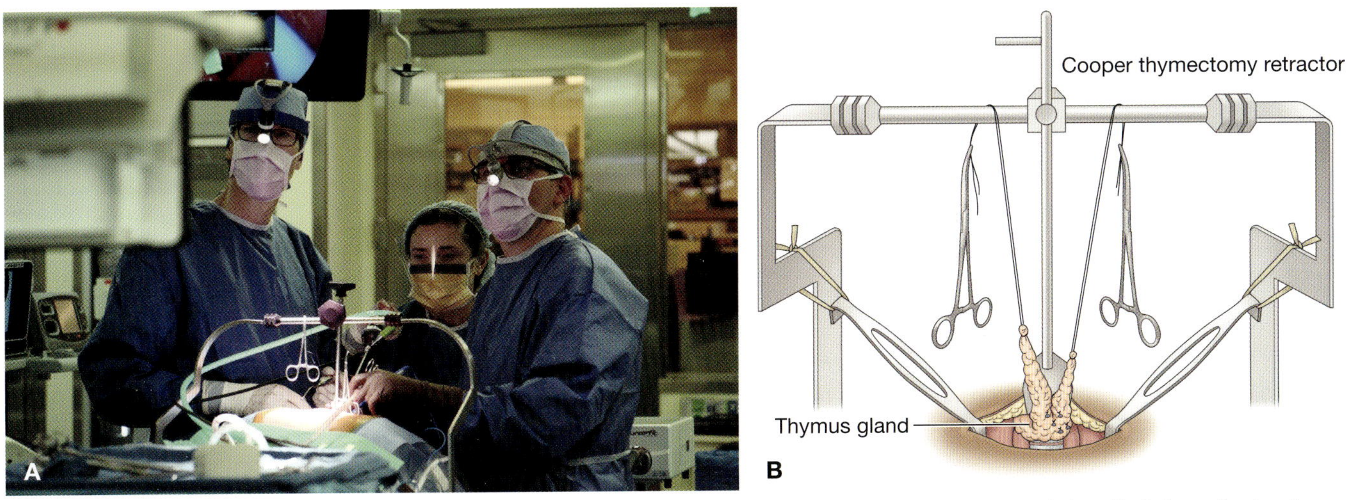

FIGURE 27.9 ▮ A and B. Arrangement of the sternum-elevating retractor. **A.** Photographic view from the patient's feet. **B.** Schematic view from the patient's head. (**A.** Technical assistance with figures by Winston Trope, BS.)

TIPS

The procedure from the point of placing the sternal retractor onward is performed with the primary surgeon seated and assistant standing.

- Flip the silk ties on the horns, with their associated Kelly clamps, up over the crossbar. This allows you to dissect on the posterior aspect of the gland until you see the innominate vein (Figure 27.9A and B).
- Clear the entire surface of the vein sharply, and identify the 2 to 3 draining thymic veins.
- It is critical that these are divided between ligatures (00 silk), so no bleeding is caused as instruments/ball sponges are passed through this avenue during the remainder of the dissection into the mediastinum (Figure 27.10A and B).

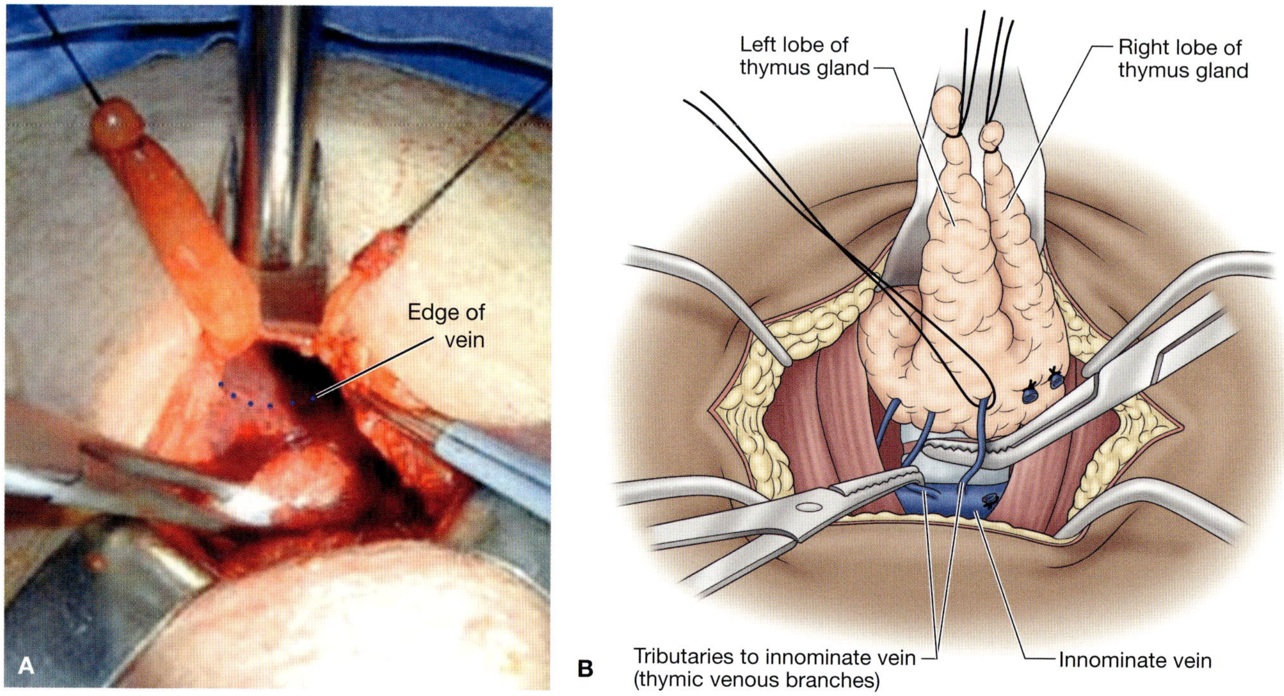

FIGURE 27.10 ■ **A and B.** Identifying the innominate vein and controlling veins that drain thymus into the innominate vein with silk ties. (**A.** Technical assistance with figures by Winston Trope, BS.)

- The 5-mm 30° video camera is placed for the remainder of the dissection via the neck incision, adjacent to the operating surgeon's instruments, by the assistant.
- Once past the vein, take the dissection posterior to the gland, directly onto the surface of the pericardium, as far down into the chest as possible. This is generally a clean plane easily dissected bluntly with ball sponges on ring clamps (Figure 27.11A and B).
- Next, do the same dissection anterior to the gland, separating the gland from the anterior chest wall with ball sponges on ring clamps. There are usually a few small feeding arterioles off of the internal mammary, which can be either cauterized or clipped/divided.

TIPS

When working on the right side of the gland, retract the sutures on the upper horns toward the left and vice versa. This countertraction is critical. But don't pull so hard that you tear off an upper horn.

- Now, separate the right side of the gland from the right mediastinal pleura, proceeding from cephalad to caudal, with ball sponges on ring clamps—essentially dragging the thymus and surrounding fat bluntly off of the pleural membrane toward the midline. As one approaches the phrenic nerve, one will typically reach a "bare area" where there is no longer any tissue on the pericardium. This denotes the extent of the initial lateral dissection on the right. This dissection is easiest if the mediastinal pleura is maintained intact.

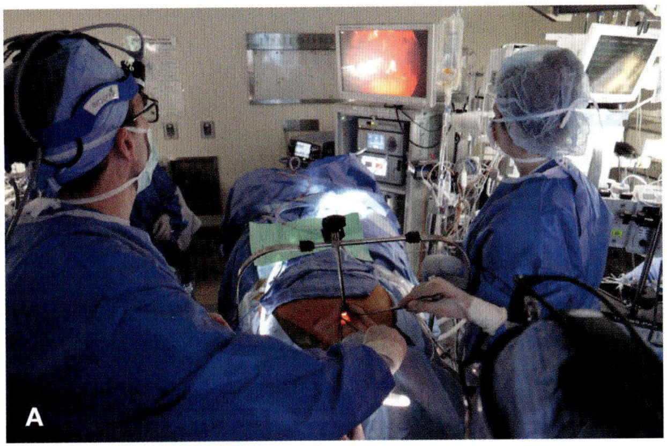

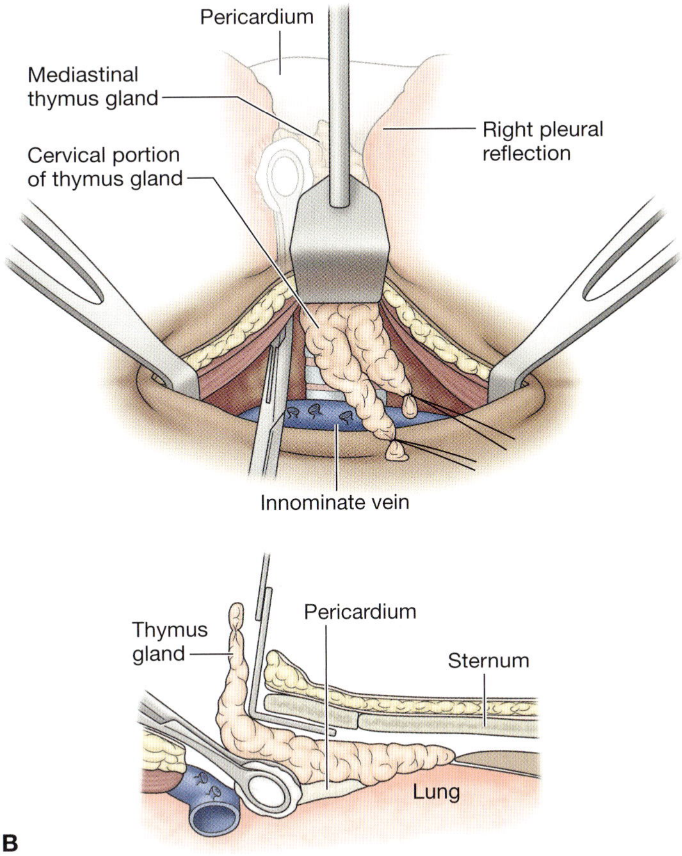

FIGURE 27.11 ▌ **A and B.** Dissecting the body of the thymus and surrounding fat progressively deeper into the mediastinum (under video guidance in **A**). (**A.** Technical assistance with figures by Winston Trope, BS.)

TIPS

During the lateral dissections, have the anesthesiologists intermittently hold ventilation to allow clear identification of the pleural membranes and create more space for visualization near the phrenic nerve.

- On the left, the left side of the gland is then separated from left phrenic nerve and pericardium, in similar fashion.
- Some remaining attachments to the diaphragm in the midline are often all that is left to fully free the main specimen and remove it through the neck (Figure 27.12).

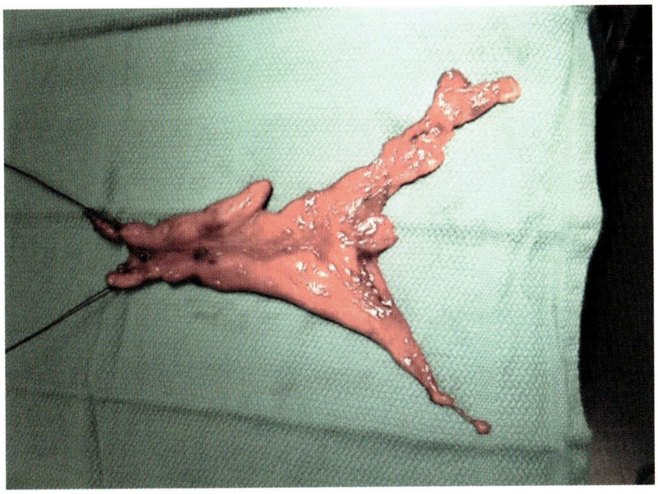

FIGURE 27.12 ▌ A typical video-assisted transcervical thymectomy specimen with both intracapsular thymus and surrounding mediastinal/pericardial fat. (Technical assistance with figures by Winston Trope, BS.)

TIPS

After removal of the main specimen, which includes the entire intracapsular thymus and the bulk of the surrounding mediastinal fat, go back to remove any small bits of fat that may remain (which may contain thymic rests) in piecemeal fashion.

- To remove the small areas of mediastinal fat that may remain, and the pericardiophrenic fat pads, open the pleurae widely bilaterally, safely anterior to the phrenic nerve, below the level of the innominate vein. Retracting the pleura medially after incising it allows one to fully trace the phrenic nerve and remove any fat that may remain near the nerve, with or without pleura that it may be attached to.
- Opening the pleura also allows one to reach all the way down into each chest to remove the pericardiophrenic fat pads on each side.
- Assure hemostasis, place a red rubber catheter into the substernal space, and remove the thymectomy blade to allow the sternum to fall to its usual position.
- Close the strap muscles around the red rubber catheter and evacuate remaining air while removing it on intermittent suction as the anesthesiologists give a large positive pressure breath.
- Close the platysma and skin with running absorbable sutures.

Postoperative Care

- Some surgeons send these patients home on the day of surgery. I prefer to keep them overnight to monitor for MG exacerbation.
- The only complication of any frequency is a small seroma beneath the incision, which rarely needs to be drained.

PEARLS AND PITFALLS

- If you cannot find the upper horns at the start of the procedure, it is essentially impossible to complete this operation transcervically. In that case, conversion to a partial upper, or complete, sternotomy is indicated.
- Tearing off one horn during retraction will make the procedure more difficult to complete transcervically, but it can typically be done using one horn only to retract with, and retracting the other side by grasping the main specimen with a curved ring clamp.
- The dissection off of the phrenic on the right tends to be easier than on the left. On the left, a tongue of thymic tissue tends to extend toward the aortopulmonary window, and lymph nodes in this area can be confusing and cause some oozing. I therefore always open the left pleura and trace the phrenic in detail in this area while removing tissue well down to the nerve.

THYMECTOMY BY TRANSTHORACIC ROBOTIC AND/OR VATS APPROACHES

Perioperative Considerations

- *It is my opinion that a true extended thymectomy cannot be performed by a unilateral VATS or robotic approach.* One needs a bilateral surgical approach, or at least bilateral visualization (via a contralateral thoracoscope) of the phrenic nerve, in order to allow complete resection of fatty/thymic tissue to near the nerve without a high risk of injuring it.
- Any of these approaches can be performed either robotically or using traditional thoracoscopic instrumentation. I believe, however, that the robot provides particular advantages for thymectomy over standard VATS because of the small spaces and awkward angles for the thoracoscopic instruments. At a minimum, if using VATS, one must insufflate gas to create space. There is no doubt the operation is just easier with the robotic wrists.

TIPS

In my opinion, safe and extended VATS or robotic thymectomy requires some sort of bilateral approach.

- The options for a bilateral approach include:
  - True bilateral approach, with 3-port VATS or robotic approach on one side and 4-port approach on the opposite side.
  - Operation via a 4-port VATS or robotic approach on one side only (I prefer right), with only a videoscope on the left, to allow visualization of that nerve while the dissection is performed from the right side (if using the robot, this image can be shown using the "tile" feature). *This* "tiled bilateral approach" *is what is shown in the images that follow.*
  - My preference has evolved in most cases to the true bilateral approach, typically with a preliminary dissection by VATS on the left, so the robot does not need to be moved and redocked midprocedure, then most of the work done from the right with the robot. This "true bilateral approach" is described in the section that follows in the text, but a unilateral right approach is shown in the images.

Anesthesia and Patient Positioning

- General anesthesia with double-lumen endotracheal tube.
- Supine, with a bump longitudinally positioned beneath the right side, and the right shoulder hanging off the edge of the table to prevent clash with a robotic arm.
- Prep entire sternum in case of rare need for sternotomy.

Instruments and Equipment

- For left VATS: 5-mm 30° videoscope, Hunter endoscopic grasper, hook cautery, endoKittner, and specimen retrieval bag. We have not found it necessary to add to costs by using expensive energy devices.
- For the right robotic approach: Cadiere grasper, hook cautery, bipolar cautery forceps, specimen retrieval bag, and rare need for robotic clip.

Technique

TIPS

These operations proceed much more quickly if one uses primarily the hook cautery for the dissection, using mainly the hook's blunt portion, in a spatula manner, reserving the bipolar forceps cautery only when one must dissect very close to one of the phrenic nerves.

- **Begin with 3-port left VATS.** Have the anesthesiologists drop the left lung. Place a 5-mm port at inferior axillary hair line, just posterior to the pectoralis edge, and insufflate; place a 5-mm port about 3 ribs lower (midsternal level) in the same line; place a 12-mm port in the inframammary fold just lateral to midclavicular line.

TIPS

Always place the most cephalad port first on the left. Otherwise one risks placing the first port into *the heart—which has been known to occur.*

- Place the camera via the middle port and work alternatively with the hook cautery and grasper via the upper and lower ports.
- Begin by removing the entire left pericardiophrenic fat pad, and remove it via a bag as a separate specimen.
- Trace the phrenic nerve, dividing the mediastinal pleura and fatty/thymic tissue with the hook cautery on a low setting, proceeding from caudal to cephalad, staying about 5 mm from the nerve. The endoKittner can be helpful to then strip this tissue further anteriorly, away from the nerve toward the ultimate specimen.
- At the upper end of this dissection, identify the left internal mammary vein and trace it down to the left side of the innominate vein. Take all fatty/thymic tissue from about 5 mm from the nerve and mammary vein toward the ultimate specimen.
- Move rightward along the innominate vein until you reach the left upper thymic horn crossing anterior to the vein into the neck. This can be preliminary dissected from the left, but full dissection of it is typically saved for the right robotic approach later in the procedure.
- Dissect all the left-sided fatty/thymic tissue from caudal to cephalad off of the pericardium, using hook and endoKittner, until reaching approximately the midline.
- Divide the left mediastinal pleura anteriorly and begin the dissection of the fatty thymic tissue off of anterior chest wall, in the typical filmy plane, with the hook, until reaching approximately the midline. Take care not to injure the left internal mammary artery or vein.
- If the specimen is particularly large and fatty and it seems as though it will be difficult to manipulate and maintain intact, I sometimes "carve" off the leftward half of the body of the thymus and associated fat from this side and remove it as a separate specimen, before moving to the right-sided approach.

TIPS

If the specimen is large and fatty (typically in an obese patient), remove much of the left side of the specimen separately (in addition to the left pericardiophrenic fat pad), from the left, to facilitate the later dissection from the right. Typical-sized specimens are left intact and ultimately removed entirely from the right side (apart from the pericardiophrenic fat pad).

- Reinflate the left lung, remove the ports, and close the left-sided incisions. Leave a small tube if any chance of having injured lung.
- **Move to the right robotic approach**: Have the anesthesiologists drop the right lung. Place an 8-mm robotic at the level of the midsternum at the anterior axillary line and insufflate; place a second 8-mm port at least 5 cm more cephalad, near the inferior edge of the axillary hair line, just posterior to the pectoralis edge; place a third 8-mm port in the inframmary fold just lateral to the midclavicular line; place a 12-mm thoracoscopic assistant port more posteriorly, triangulated between the two more caudal robotic ports.

TIPS

Occasionally, a patient will become hypotensive with insufflation. Inform the anesthesiologists when you first insufflate, and release the pressure and reinsufflate at a lower pressure if there is hypotension.

- Place the robotic camera via the middle robotic port. The dissection on this side is almost exclusively with the hook cautery via more caudal arm and the Cadiere grasper via more cephalad arm. The assistant helps by retracting with a Hunter via the assistant port.

TIPS

An action with the hook cautery that includes alternately bluntly "pushing" the thymic tissue anteriorly off of the pericardium and cauterizing—taking care to use the nonsharp curved part of the instrument for the "pushing" action—allows this operation to move along quickly. Only rarely does one need to change out the two main instruments used.

- Begin on this side by removing the right pericardiophrenic fat pad as a separate specimen as you already did on the left.
- Trace the right phrenic nerve, dividing the mediastinal pleura and fatty/thymic tissue with the hook cautery on a low setting, proceeding from caudal to cephalad, staying about 5 mm from the nerve (Figure 27.13). The assistant port can be used to pass the endoKittner, which can be helpful to then strip this tissue further anteriorly, away from the nerve toward the ultimate specimen.
- At the upper end of this dissection, identify the right internal mammary vein and trace it down to the right side of the innominate vein. Take all fatty/thymic tissue from about 5 mm from the nerve and mammary vein, medially/leftward toward the ultimate specimen (Figure 27.13).

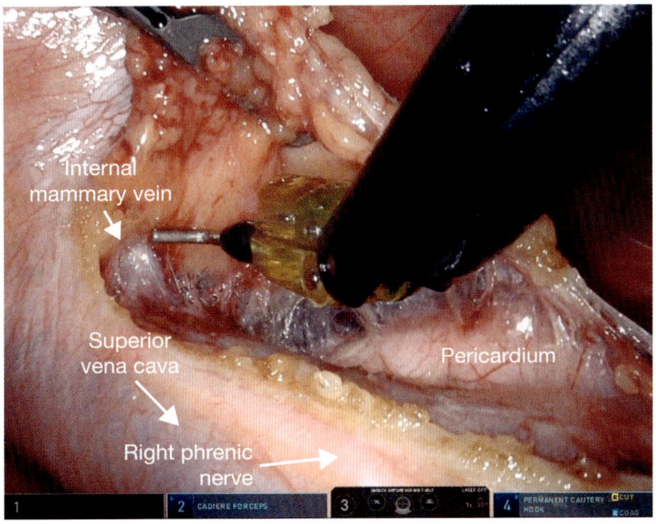

FIGURE 27.13 ▌ Separate the thymus/fat off of the right phrenic nerve (here shown near junction of superior vena cava and innominate vein) up to the level of the right internal mammary vein. (Technical assistance with figures by Winston Trope, BS.)

- Open the right mediastinal pleura anteriorly, just lateral to the mammary pedicle as it runs along the chest wall, and then dissect in the filmy substernal plane from right to left, leaving some tissue in place (Figure 27.14). Ideally, open this fully as late as possible to preserve the benefits of unilateral gas insufflation as long as possible.

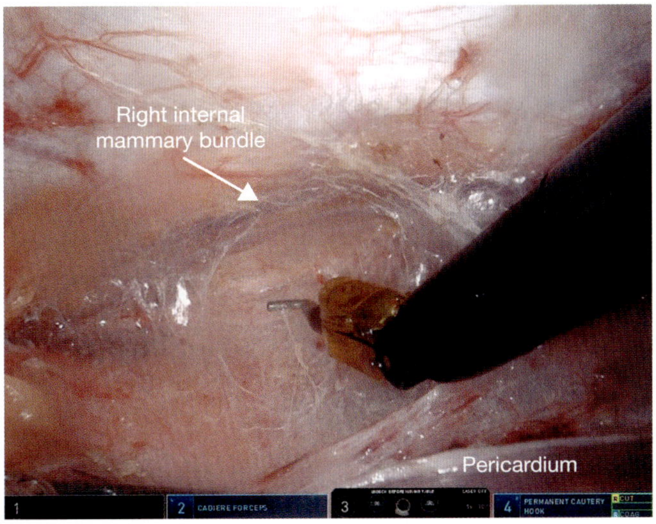

FIGURE 27.14 ▌ After incising the mediastinal pleura near the chest wall, just caudal/medial to the right internal mammary vessels, dissect from right to left in the retrosternal filmy plane. (Technical assistance with figures by Winston Trope, BS.)

- Move leftward along the innominate vein until you identify the right upper thymic horn crossing anterior to the vein into the neck (Figure 27.15). Dissect it either now or later (see below).

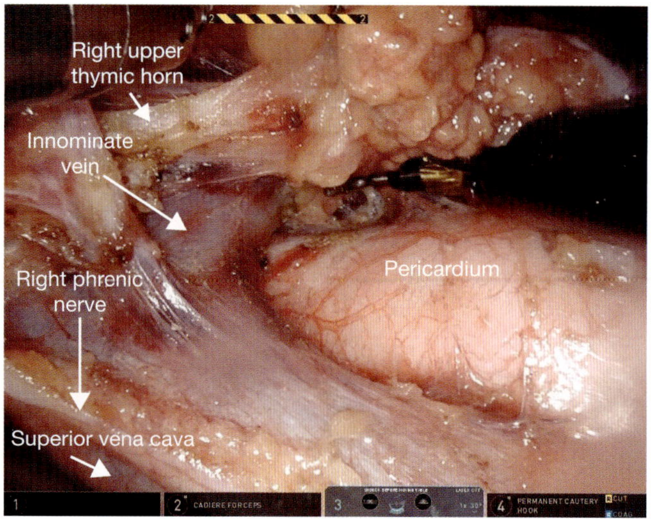

FIGURE 27.15 ▮ Expose the innominate vein at its junction with the superior vena cava, then dissect the thymus from it, working from right to left, until you meet the right upper horn. (Technical assistance with figures by Winston Trope, BS.)

- Usually one will encounter at least one draining thymic vein at about this point. If smaller, these can be cauterized aggressively, staying at least 5 mm from the main vein, without risk of bleeding. If large, they should be controlled with robotic clips and then sharply divided.
- Dissect all the right-sided fatty/thymic tissue from caudal to cephalad and right to left off of the pericardium (Figure 27.16), until reaching the plane of dissection that had previously been created on the pericardium during the preliminary left VATS (or not, if using the "tile" approach). Open the left pleural membrane just anterior to the nerve, using "tile," if not already done.

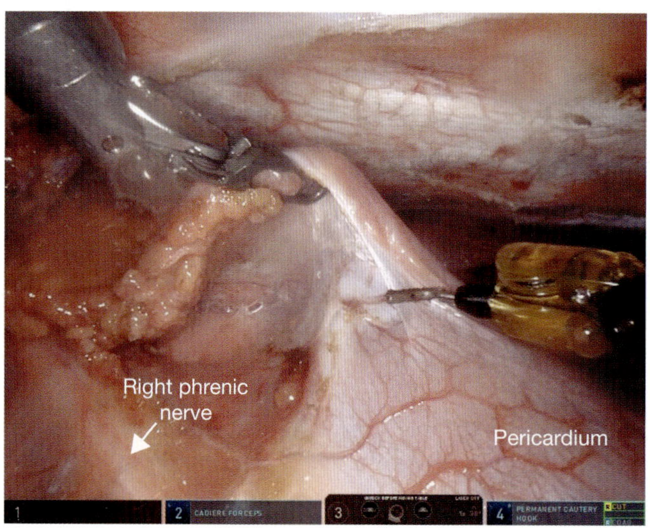

FIGURE 27.16 ▮ Dissect the thymus/fat off of the pericardium caudal to cephalad. (Technical assistance with figures by Winston Trope, BS.)

- Divide the left mediastinal pleura anteriorly (if not already done via a preliminary left approach), a few millimeters posterior to the anterior chest wall (Figure 27.17). Take care not to injure the left internal mammary artery or vein.

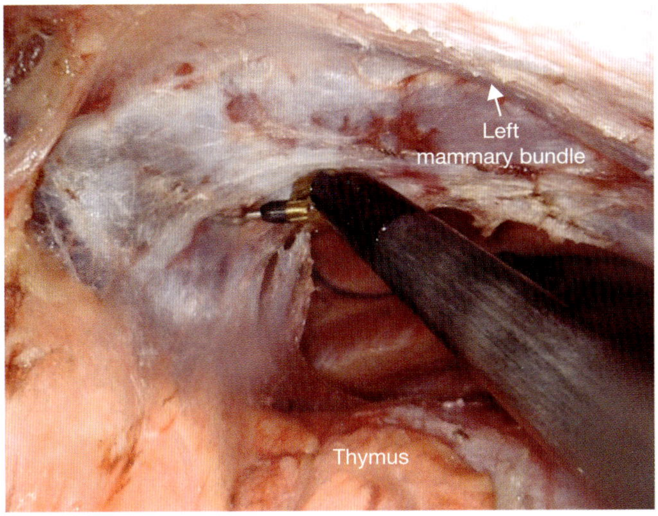

FIGURE 27.17 | Divide the left mediastinal pleura anteriorly. (Technical assistance with figures by Winston Trope, BS.)

TIPS

In tumor cases, the tumor itself must never be directly touched or vigorously retracted. The tumor should only be gently pushed (in the direction that facilitates tension on the tissue being divided) through adjacent fatty and normal thymic tissue, so as not to risk breaching its capsule.

- Go back to the level of the innominate vein and, if not already done, complete tracing first the right, then the left upper thymic horns all the way up to their disappearance into the thyrothymic ligaments, which can be divided with careful cautery. Flip the horns down with the specimen.

TIPS

The complete removal of the upper thymic horns is the most challenging part of a robotic thymectomy. It requires mobilizing progressively further cephalad along each horn with cautery, by passing the horn back and forth between the assistant's Hunter grasper and the surgeon's Cadiere, until the thyrothymic ligament is clearly reached. This is the portion that most requires the bedside assistant. The mammary vein often needs also to be retracted and in rare cases divided between clips.

- There typically remain some attachments between the posterior aspect of the gland and the pericardium at this point. Complete the division of this tissue, control and divide any thymic vein that might remain, and remove the specimen in a large endobag via the assistant 12-mm port.
- The port itself must be removed, and the fascia stretched or even divided with cautery for several millimeters, to allow removal of the bag with specimen.
- Place a 24-French chest tube anterior to the hilum of the right lung, to the apex of the chest, via the most caudal robotic incision. Reinflate the lungs vigorously, close the port sites, and keep the chest tube on suction initially to evacuate all gas.

TIPS

If a tumor unexpectedly invades the pericardium, or even the innominate vein, these can fairly easily be removed en bloc with the tumor by the robotic approach—but my recommendation is that if these are suspected preoperatively, to perform the operation by median sternotomy.

Postoperative Care

- These VATS/robotic patients typically stay two nights.
- We prophylax and monitor for an MG exacerbation exactly as described above for the median sternotomy approach.
- The chest tube is watersealed or removed on POD 1. Be alert for chylothorax, which I have seen in a couple of these patients.

PEARLS AND PITFALLS

- See Pearls and Pitfalls for sternotomy technique, above. Additionally:
- The robotic approach is an excellent one for smaller noninvasive tumors and for nonthymomatous MG; I prefer median sternotomy for tumors over approximately 4.5 cm in size or with suspected invasion of surrounding structures.
- If a tumor sits clearly to the left of midline and/or may involve a left-sided structure, perform the robotic portion from the left rather than from the right.
- For nonthymomatous MG, I still prefer the VATS-assisted transcervical approach in thinner patients who can extend their neck, because of the ease of recovery for the patients. The VATS/robotic approaches occasionally incur intercostal neuralgia for 1 to 3 months, though rarely permanent.

SUMMARY

Any of these approaches to thymectomy are reasonable to employ, but it is an advantage to be comfortable with all three, to apply in different situations:

- The minimally invasive approaches—particularly the transcervical approach—have obvious advantages in terms of recovery time, and they appear to have the same MG remission rates as the sternotomy approach, when performed by surgeons experienced with the techniques.
- A surgeon should always use the approach that he/she is most comfortable with. The key is that a thymic surgeon must be committed to achieving in MG patients a complete and extended thymectomy, removing not only the intracapsular thymus but also all surrounding mediastinal fat to the phrenic nerves laterally and the diaphragm inferiorly.
- For tumors, there must be minimal manipulation ("no touch") and zero hesitation to resect adherent structures en bloc to assure complete resection.

Acknowledgments

I thank Winston Trope for extraordinary help with getting the images for this chapter into shape; and Donna Minagawa for a good deal of administrative help surrounding this chapter.

Suggested Readings

1. Jaretzki A, Barohn RJ, Ernstoff RM, et al. Myasthenia gravis: recommendations for clinical research standards. Task Force of the Medical Scientific Advisory Board of the Myasthenia Gravis Foundation of America. *Ann Thorac Surg*. 2000;70(1):327-334.
2. Jaretzki A III, Wolff M. Maximal thymectomy for myasthenia gravis. Surgical anatomy and operative technique. *J Thorac Cardiovasc Surg*. 1988;96(5):711-716.
3. Shrager JB, Brinster ND, Yousuf O, et al. Outcomes after 151 extended transcervical thymectomies for myasthenia gravis. *Ann Thorac Surg*. 2006;85:1863-1869.
4. Solis-Pazmino P, Baiu I, Lincango-Naranjo E, et al. Impact of the surgical approach to thymectomy upon complete stable remission rates in myasthenia gravis: a meta-analysis. *Neurology*. 2021;97(4):e357-e368.
5. Ruckert JC, Ismail M, Swierzy M, et al. Thoracoscopic thymectomy with the da Vinci robotic system for myasthenia gravis. *Ann N Y Acad Sci*. 2008:1132-11329.
6. Wolfe GI, Kaminski HJ, Aban IB, et al. Randomized trial of thymectomy in myasthenia gravis. *N Engl J Med*. 2016;375(6):511-522.

Chapter 28

Extended Superior Vena Cava Resection

MICHAEL F. REED
JONATHAN RICE
OLIVIA ZIEGLER

Perioperative Considerations

TIPS

- *Thorough preoperative planning including adequate pulmonary function testing*
- *Incision (posterolateral thoracotomy vs median sternotomy or clamshell) should be based on tumor location.*
- *Vascular control prior to SVC dissection*
- *Make note of phrenic nerve involvement and attempt preservation whenever possible.*
- *Intrapericardial control of the right PA if needed*
- *Heparin administration prior to clamping*
- *Reverse Trendelenburg positioning upon SVC clamping*
- *Shunt SVC if prolonged clamping is expected*

Anesthesia and Patient Positioning

- General anesthesia with double-lumen endotracheal tube or bronchial blocker to allow for single-lung ventilation
- Utilization of capnometer and pulse oximeter for continuous systemic oxygenation monitoring
- Urinary catheter to monitor for appropriate fluid resuscitation during the operation
- Large-bore intravenous or central line placed in the femoral vein. Preexisting long-term central venous catheters in the subclavian or jugular venous system need to be removed prior to operative intervention to facilitate superior vena cava (SVC) resection.
- For posterior right upper lobe tumors, a right posterolateral thoracotomy in the fourth or fifth intercostal space, with the patient in the lateral decubitus position, is ideal. Although possible from this approach, the dissection and control of the left brachiocephalic (innominate) vein is technically demanding.
- For anterior compartment mediastinal lesions with SVC involvement, as well as some anterior right upper lobe tumors, median sternotomy or right hemiclamshell is the optimal approach with the patient in the supine position. These incisions provide excellent exposure of the anterior mediastinum, entire length of the SVC with extension into the right atrium, and right and left brachiocephalic vein.

Technique

- Immediately following entry, palpation of the tumor and its involvement of the SVC should be evaluated. Vascular control should be obtained prior to extensive dissection of the tumor off the SVC. This will help prevent, or control, dramatic bleeding if inadvertent injury to the SVC occurs during dissection (Figure 28.1).

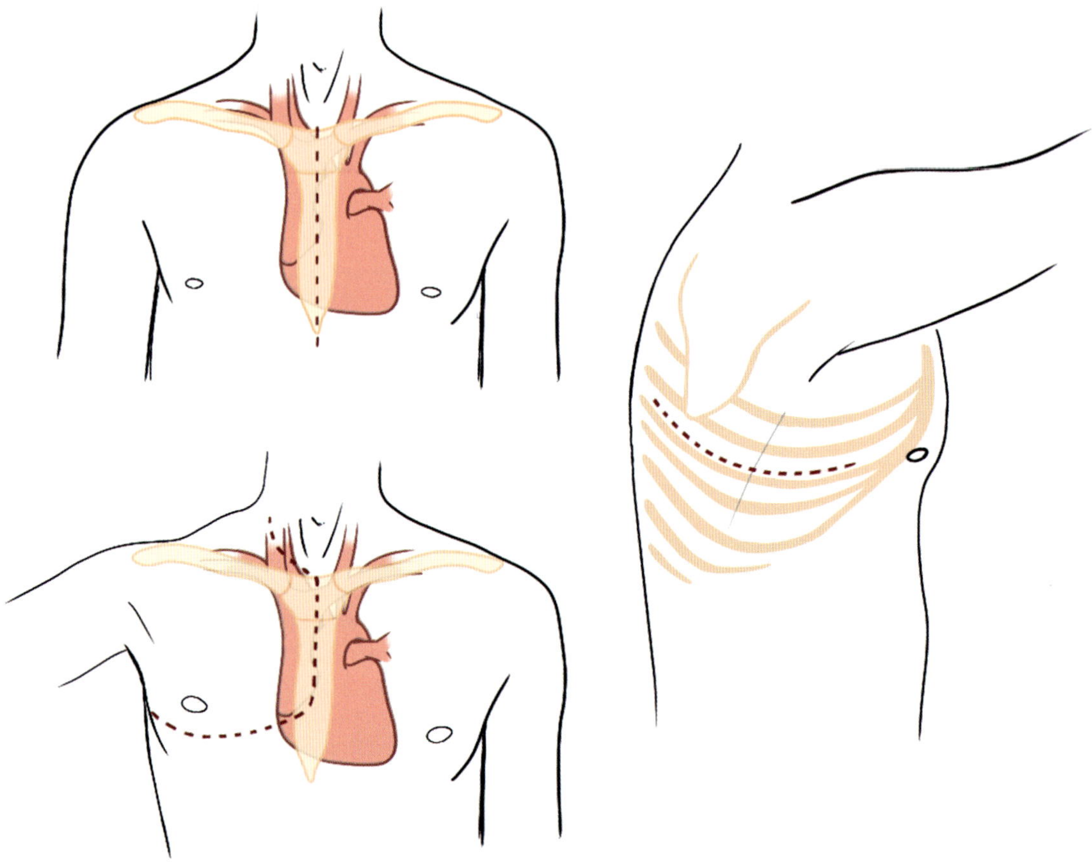

FIGURE 28.1 ▌ Common surgical incisions for potential superior vena cava resection and reconstruction. (Courtesy of Dr. Olivia Ziegler.)

- Proximal control of the SVC and left brachiocephalic vein should be obtained first (Figure 28.2).
- Phrenic nerve and its involvement should be noted (Figure 28.2).
- For right upper lobe lesions, first isolate and divide the superior pulmonary vein (Figure 28.2).
- After this, a logical next step would be to isolate the right pulmonary artery (PA) and subsequently the truncus arteriosus branch to the right upper lobe. At this point, depending on the location of the lesion, intrapericardial PA control can be obtained.
- Once the right upper lobe PA is divided, visualization of the distal SVC is optimized beneath the azygos vein. This view allows the surgeon to gain vascular control of the distal SVC at this point (Figure 28.3).
- If proximal control was not obtained earlier, it is now recommended to place umbilical tapes around the proximal and distal extent of the SVC and the left brachiocephalic vein (Figure 28.3).
- If greater mobilization of the SVC is needed, division of the azygos vein is straightforward from this viewpoint and will allow for further mobility of the SVC.
- Once vascular control of the SVC has been obtained, further dissection of the primary tumor can be done safely.
- Evaluate the extent of invasion of the primary lesion into the SVC. Determine if resection and reconstruction is required, or if primary repair with a patch closure is feasible.
- If the primary lesion invades less than 50% of the circumference of the SVC, a side biting or partial occluding clamp is a good option to undertake partial excision of the wall of the SVC.

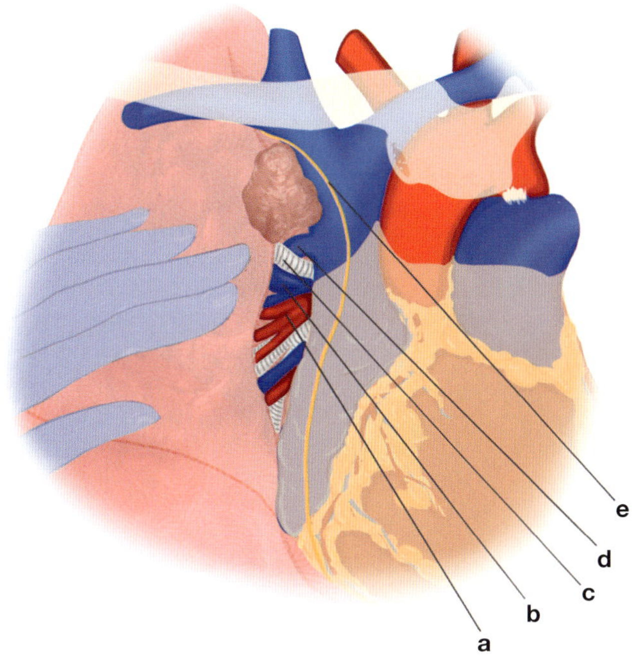

FIGURE 28.2 | Right upper lobe (RUL) mass with involvement of the superior vena cave (SVC). RUL pulmonary artery **(A)**; RUL pulmonary vein **(B)**; RUL bronchus **(C)**; azygos vein **(D)**; and phrenic nerve on SVC **(E)**. (Courtesy of Dr. Olivia Ziegler.)

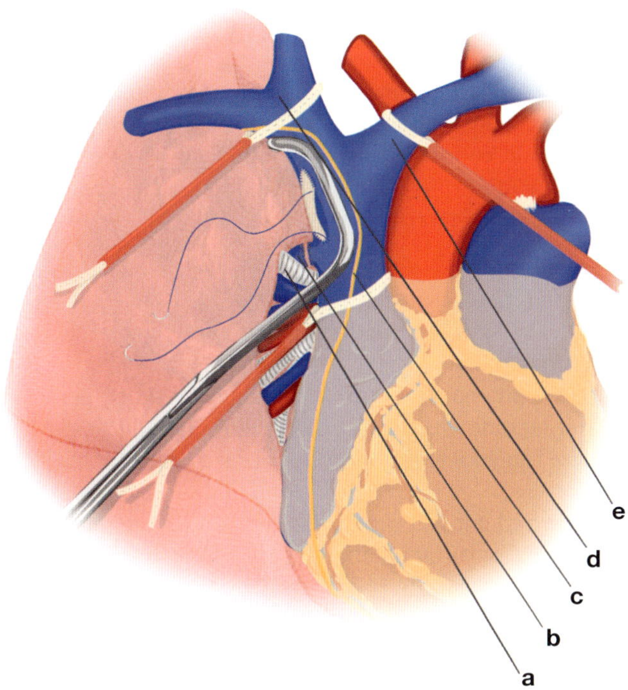

FIGURE 28.3 | Patch repair of superior vena cava (SVC) when less than 50% of SVC involvement of the repair. RUL bronchus **(A)**; azygos vein **(B)**; SVC **(C)**; right brachiocephalic vein **(D)**; and left brachiocephalic vein **(E)**. (Courtesy of Dr. Olivia Ziegler.)

- Once the primary lesion has been resected, it is recommended to consider intraoperative frozen section to verify negative margins.
- For a resection that involves less than 50% circumference of the SVC, its reconstruction can either use autologous or bovine pericardium for patch closure to avoid narrowing or kinking.
- If the lesion invades greater than 50% of the circumference of the SVC, it is recommended that the involved SVC be resected and reconstructed. The use of polytetrafluoroethylene (PTFE), as well as autologous or bovine pericardial tube, bovine pericardial prosthesis, cryopreserved arterial allografts, and other conduits, has been described (Figure 28.4).
- If resection and reconstruction is to occur, prior to vascular clamping of the SVC and left brachiocephalic vein, 5000 units of heparin is administered and the operating table is placed in reverse Trendelenburg position.

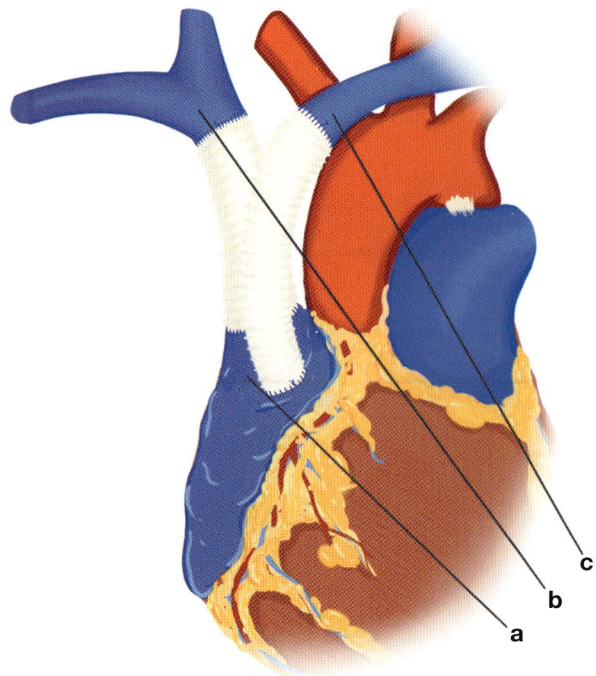

FIGURE 28.4 ▮ Bilateral brachiocephalic vein replacement with graft. This configuration should be avoided due to the creation of low flow states in both conducts, which risks occlusion of both grafts. Right atrium **(A)**; right brachiocephalic vein **(B)**; and left brachiocephalic vein **(C)**. (Courtesy of Dr. Olivia Ziegler.)

- SVC shunting has been described, but most reconstructions should be achieved within a 60-minute clamp time. Complete occlusion of the SVC is generally well tolerated by the patient without a shunt. Blood pressure should be maintained with intravenous volume and vasopressors as needed.

Types of Reconstruction

- Trunk replacement
- Left brachiocephalic vein replacement
  - If the right brachiocephalic is occluded preoperatively, then conduit creation can occur to the left brachiocephalic vein.
  - If this reconstruction is planned, median sternotomy should be performed. Access to the proximal extent of the left innominate vein is challenging via right posterolateral thoracotomy.
  - It is optimal to utilize ringed PTFE graft to reduce the risk of kinking of the graft after the sternotomy is closed.
  - The anastomosis is carried out in a similar fashion as trunk replacement. The distal anastomosis can be performed at the cavoatrial junction, at the right atrial appendage, or directly to the right atrium.
- Right brachiocephalic vein replacement
  - Performed from either sternotomy or right posterolateral thoracotomy
  - Conduit is less prone to kinking due to vertical nature of the path from the right brachiocephalic vein to the cavoatrial junction or the right atrium.
  - Again, the anastomosis is performed in a circular fashion using 4-0 or 5-0 polypropylene. The anastomosis to the right brachiocephalic vein is completed first. This can be technically challenging due to the short nature of the right innominate vein.
  - After the proximal anastomosis is performed, the distal anastomosis can be placed at the cavoatrial junction, at the right atrial appendage, or directly to the right atrium in a running fashion. De-air and flush the graft with heparinized saline prior to completing the anastomosis.
  - Bilateral individual reconstruction of the left and right innominate vein has been reported; however, it is not commonly performed due to the creation of a low flow state in both individual grafts. This can lead to a scenario of conduit occlusion. Compression of the two conduits is also a risk (Figure 28.4).

PEARLS AND PITFALLS

- Prior to obtaining vascular control of the SVC, it can be hazardous to perform dissection of the tumor involving the SVC due to the risk of massive bleeding. It is better to first obtain proximal and distal control of the SVC, and left and right brachiocephalic veins with umbilical tapes or vascular loops before extensive dissection.
- If a vascular wall clamp is used for partial SVC wall excision and patch repair, have proximal and distal control prior to excision because the SVC can retract out of the partial occluding clamp after the mass is excised.
- Isolated left brachiocephalic vein replacement should occur via sternotomy because proximal anastomosis is challenging from a right posterolateral thoracotomy.
- Bilateral brachiocephalic vein replacement should be avoided due to creation of low flow state in both conduits, which risks occlusion of both grafts.
- Postoperative anticoagulation can be converted from intravenous to oral once chest tube drainage has diminished and the patient is tolerating a diet.

Suggested Readings

1. Jones D. Technique of superior vena cava resection for lung carcinomas. *Oper Tech Thorac Cardiovasc Surg*. 2008;13(4):274-282.
2. Spaggiari L, Thomas P, Magdeleinat P, et al. Superior vena cava resection with prosthetic replacement for non-small cell lung cancer: long-term results of a multicentric study. *Eur J Cardio Thorac Surg*. 2002;21(6):1080-1086.
3. Ohata N, Nakahara R, Ui A, Matsuguma H. Azygos flap as a novel method for superior vena cava reconstruction. *Interact Cardiovasc Thorac Surg*. 2010;11(5):519-521.
4. Xu X, Qiu Y, Pan H, Mo L, Chen H, He J. Resection of the sidewall of superior vena cava using video-assisted thoracic surgery mechanical suture technique. *J Thorac Dis*. 2016;8(3):612-616.

Chapter 29

Thoracic Duct Ligation

AUSTIN KLUIS
EITAN PODGAETZ

Perioperative Consideration

- The thoracic duct (TD) is a valved, tubular (~3 mm diameter), lymphatic conduit in the posterior mediastinum.
- The anatomy of the TD is "constant only in its variability."
- Typically:
  - Originates from the cisterna chyli (CC), which lies anterior to L1-2 and ascends cephalad, right-sided, anterolateral to the vertebral bodies
  - The duct enters the chest via the aortic hiatus. Above the diaphragm, the duct lies posterolateral to the esophagus, lateral to the aorta, and medial to the azygos vein.
  - The duct crosses midline to the left around T4-5 and empties into the confluence of the left subclavian and internal jugular vein.
- TD is chiefly responsible for transporting chyle from its origin at the CC to the venous system at the confluence of the left subclavian and internal jugular vein.
  - Chyle is formed from dietary long chain triglycerides as well as lymph, immunoglobulins, and T-lymphocytes, which explains the detrimental immunological and dietary sequelae of a prolonged leak.
  - Ingested fats and lymph from the intestines and stomach are absorbed by peritoneal lymphatics and transported to the CC as chyle, anywhere from 2 to 4 L/d.
- While intrathoracic procedures rarely cause chyle leaks, they remain the most common indication for TD ligation.
  - Nontraumatic chylothorax is typically a result of malignancy or infection.
  - Esophagectomy is the most common iatrogenic cause of chyle leak.
- Chest tube output that turns cloudy and increases in volume with enteral nutrition raises suspicion for chylothorax.
  - Fluid analysis with triglyceride >100 mL/dL or presence of chylomicrons is confirmatory of chyle.
- Initial conservative management includes total parenteral nutrition, bowel rest, and fluid/electrolyte repletion.
- Octreotide may lower total chylous output but rarely resolves the leak.
- While volumes <500 mL/d are deemed low volume, volumes >1000 mL/d are considered high output leaks and should be entertained for earlier intervention.
- Surgery is indicated after 3 to 5 days of failed conservative management.
- High output injuries include damage to the CC, large tributaries, and the TD itself.
- Proximal supradiaphragmatic ligation of TD is the most predictable approach.
- We avoid dyes such as methylene blue as they stain the field and make surgery more difficult.
- Enteral fat loading prior to and intraoperatively can aid in identification of the leak.
- Suspicion of infradiaphragmatic leak by lymphangiogram may be best approached through abdomen by ligating the CC.
- Surgery has a >90% effectiveness in resolution with minimal morbidity.

- Relative contraindications: Failed prior surgical ligation, hostile chest, unstable spine injury, severe multiple organ injury, severe comorbidities precluding single lung ventilation, locally unresectable advanced tumor
- Inability for patient to tolerate single-lung ventilation may prompt laparoscopic or embolization techniques.
  - Diagnostic lymphangiography may help identify location of leak and help decide surgical approach especially after failed ligation and if suspected leak is intra-abdominal.

TIPS

High-volume leaks should be surgically addressed right away rather than awaiting conservative management.

Anesthesia and Patient Positioning

- Dual-lumen endotracheal tube
- Left lateral decubitus position
- Breaking of the table to increase surface area and intercostal space
- Blood type/cross and perioperative antibiotics within 1 hour of incision
- Arterial line for close BP monitoring
- Two large-bore peripheral IV access

Instruments and Equipment

Standard

- Major chest tray (thoracotomy tray)
- Thoracoscopic tray (30° camera)
- Knot pusher
- Carter-Thompson suture passer
- Extra-small Alexis wound protector
- Large right-angle clamp (Mixter or DeBakey-Semb)

Prep and Drape

- Chlorohexidine scrub
- Ioban drape
- Field view includes supraclavicular area, costal margin, and spine to nipple line

Drains and Dressing

- 28-French straight chest tube
- Drainage atrium (Pleur-evac)

Technique

- The TD is approached in the right chest regardless of chylothorax laterality as ligation needs to occur caudal to leak, including all potential collaterals, and thus the ligation of the intrathoracic duct at its proximal portion above the diaphragm.
- We recommend mass ligation of the TD as duct dissection or attempt to skeletonize has a high risk of injury.

Thoracoscopic Thoracic Duct Ligation

Different techniques to ligate the TD have been described:
- Single suture ligation of the TD, incorporating the azygos vein and lymphatics
- Skeletonizing the TD and applying two 5-mm clips 5 cm apart; a figure-of-8 suture incorporating all tissue is used in difficult exposure cases.

- Skeletonizing the TD and clipping/suture ligating in multiple locations along the TD
- Grabbing the tissue between the azygos vein and aorta with a DeBakey forceps and broadly suture ligating, three sutures at 2-cm increments, 2 cm above the esophageal hiatus of the diaphragm. No dissection.

Authors' Preferred Technique

The authors' preferred technique is noted in the sections that follow.

Anesthesia and Position

- General anesthesia with a double-lumen endotracheal tube for proper right lung isolation
- The patient is positioned in left lateral position with the bed extended at the break to maximize the thoracic space.
- Preoperative administration of lipids with a nasogastric tube (heavy cream, melted butter, or olive oil) can aid in identification of the leak when attempt of repair is undertaken. When ligating the TD, such preparation is not necessary as there is no need to identify the actual site of the leak as the goal is mass ligation.

Access

- Camera site (12-mm port): anterior axillary line, eighth intercostal space
- Working port: sixth intercostal space with extra small wound protector

Exposure

- Surgeon and assistant both stand at patient front with lateral decubitus positioning. We utilize a 30° camera.
- Chest is examined, chylothorax drained.
- Single-lung ventilation allows for right lung to be deflated and retracted anterosuperior for posterior mediastinum exposure.
- The inferior pulmonary ligament may be divided if necessary for increased exposure.
- The diaphragm may be manipulated caudally with sponge stick or retracted with a figure-of-8 suture at the most caudal and anterior part of the chest.
- We perform intercostal nerve blocks from the outside with a mixture of Marcaine and liposomal bupivacaine for long-lasting analgesia.
- In cases after esophagectomy, one must be very gentle to retract the gastric conduit with a sponge stick, cautious not to compress the right gastroepiploic artery.

Dissection

- Ligation must be below the leak at the level of the inferior pulmonary ligament (T10-11) right above the diaphragm.
- The azygos vein, aorta, esophagus, and vertebral bodies are identified (Figure 29.1).

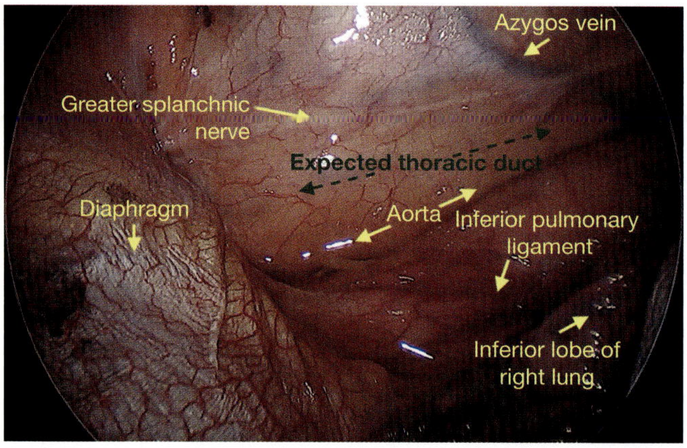

FIGURE 29.1 ▌ Caudal posterior mediastinum with the diaphragm now in view. The inferior pulmonary ligament is visualized and is at the level of T10-T11 and is a landmark for incision.

- The azygos vein is identified, and an incision is made in the parietal pleural just lateral to it right on top of the vertebral bodies spanning the length between the intercostal veins ~2 cm (Figure 29.2).

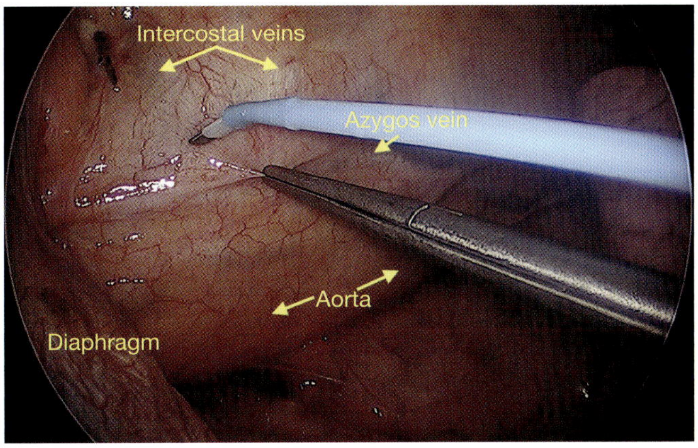

FIGURE 29.2 | The parietal pleura is grasped, and an incision is made just lateral to the azygos vein. The incision spans the distance between the intercostal veins, which is approximately 2 cm.

- Care is taken to ensure the incision is made medial to the greater splanchnic nerve.
- The intervertebral disc will be visualized. The greater splanchnic nerve and azygos vein are preserved (Figure 29.3).

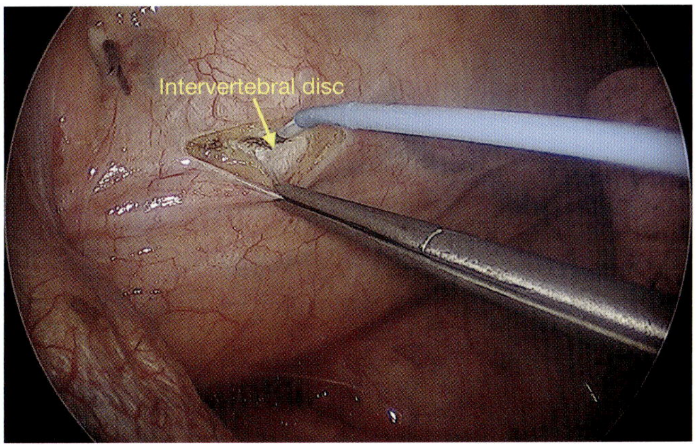

FIGURE 29.3 | The incision is made, and the intervertebral disc is revealed as the posterior boundary of the dissection. Care is taken to not incise the azygos or intercostal veins.

- The aorta is identified, and a parietal pleural incision is made on the right lateral aspect of the aorta at the same level of the initial incision (Figure 29.4).

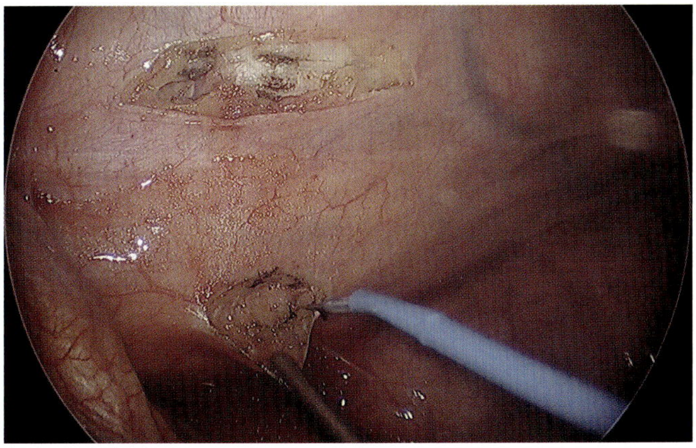

FIGURE 29.4 | The aorta is identified, the parietal pleural grasped, and an incision is made just lateral to the aorta at the same level as the initial incision.

- A blunt right-angle clamp is utilized to dissect the tissues above the aorta off the spine in an attempt to connect both incisions, which will bluntly encircle the TD, azygos vein, and any present lymphatics (Figure 29.5).

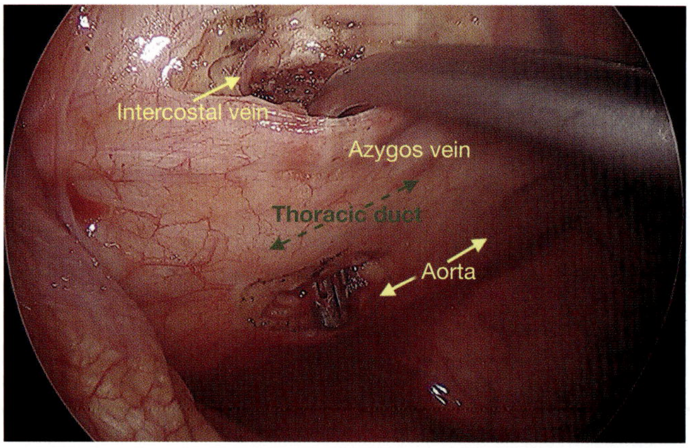

FIGURE 29.5 ▮ A blunt right-angle clamp is utilized to dissect the tissues between the incisions and connect them, encircling the thoracic duct, azygos vein, and all present lymphatics. The intervertebral disc is the posterior landmark, and the dissection should be done in a fashion to incorporate all tissue anterior to it.

Ligation

- A 0-silk tie is passed and can be used to retract as subsequent passes with the right angle are used for further dissection with care to not injure the intercostal arteries (Figure 29.6).

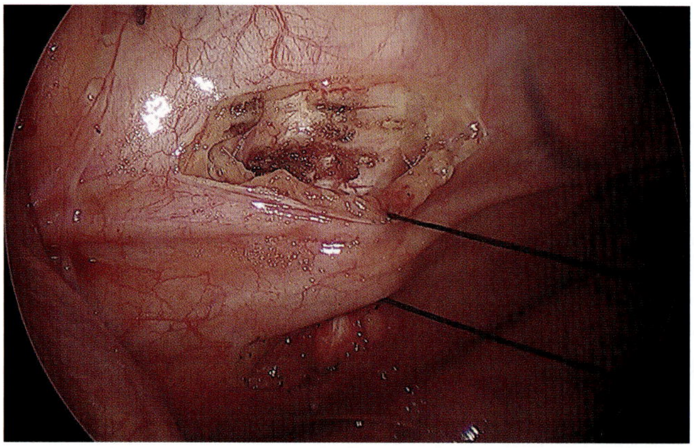

FIGURE 29.6 ▮ Once the tissue has been encircled with the blunt right-angle clamp, 0-silk suture is passed and used to retract and visualize all incorporated tissue. Deemed satisfactory, a second 0-silk suture is passed to incorporate all tissue in preparation for double ligation.

- The tissue encircled in the silk may then be tied down to effectively ligate the TD. Two separate ligatures are used and spaced approximately 1 cm in between (Figure 29.7).

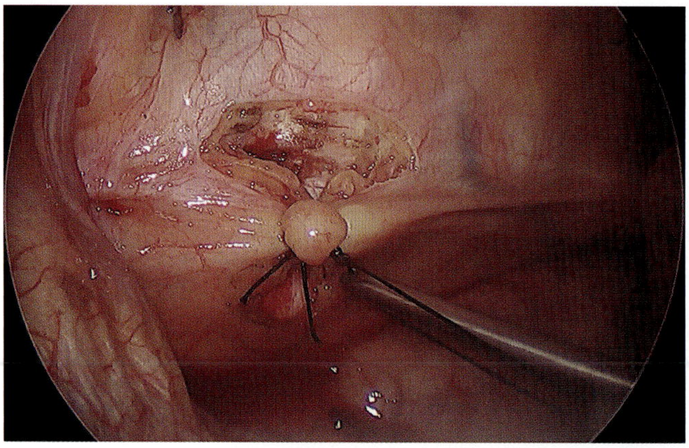

FIGURE 29.7 ▮ All encircled tissue is doubly ligated with 0-silk suture utilizing a knot pusher. The ligated tissue will contain the azygos vein, thoracic duct, and associated lymphatics.

- No division is performed following suture ligation.
- Clips can also be utilized but provide no better ligation that a simple silk ligature while having potential to injure the duct or other structures and make the leak worse.
- Mass ligation allows pleural buttressing, adding strength to the ligation improving efficacy.

TIPS

Blunt clamp dissection with mass ligation is a safe technique for chyle leaks.

Closure

- Chest tube placed through camera port site and secured in standard fashion. Chest tube is placed on water seal only.

TIPS

We do not use suction on the chest tubes and allow water seal drainage only.

Thoracic Duct Ligation via Thoracotomy

- Angled visualization, magnification, and size of incision are all superior with thoracoscopy and thoracotomy should be avoided unless it is unsafe due to prior operations, inflammation, or resources are unavailable.
- Right posterolateral thoracotomy is performed through the sixth/seventh intercostal space, dividing the latissimus dorsi while preserving the serratus anterior.
- Diaphragm retraction can be achieved with a heavy stitch through a future chest tube site.
- Tactile feedback is superior with this approach and palpation can be used to easily identify the aorta and the spine. Additionally, palpation allows assurance that all tissues within this plane are included in the ligation.
- The dissection and ligation maneuvers are identical to that of the video-assisted thoracic surgery approach.
- Chest tube is placed under direct visualization and the ribs are approximated in a figure-of-8 fashion with pericostal sutures and the remainder of the thoracotomy closed in layers with absorbable suture.

Laparoscopic CC Ligation for Refractory Chylothorax

Anesthesia and Position

- General anesthesia with a single-lumen endotracheal tube
- The patient is positioned in supine position with arms tucked
- Patient securely fastened to table as steep reverse Trendelenburg position is utilized for visualization

Access

- A standard foregut 5-mm port approach

Exposure

- Surgeon and assistant stand on opposite sides; a 30° camera is utilized.
- Abdomen is examined for any evidence of chylous drainage.
- The liver is retracted through the right most lateral port and secured in place with a Nathanson liver retractor.
- The gastrohepatic ligament is divided and the stomach is retracted toward patient left upper quadrant.
- We perform transversus abdominis nerve blocks from the outside with a mixture of Marcaine and liposomal bupivacaine for long-lasting analgesia.

Dissection

- The right lateral aspect of the of the aorta is exposed at the level of the celiac trunk with clipping of fatty tissue between the aorta and right crus.
- The right crus is then skeletonized and dissection is carried out laterally to the inferior vena cava (IVC).
- Once the IVC has been exposed, it is retracted laterally to expose the CC, which typically lies posteromedial to the IVC at this level.

Ligation

- Suture ligation with heavy silk as well as clips are used to ligate all fatty tissue between the right crus and IVC effectively ligating the CC.

Closure

- The fascia of the ports >10 mm are closed using 0 PDS and a Carter-Thompson device. The ports are removed, and the skin is closed in standard fashion.
- Typically, no drain in left in place.

Interventional Radiology Embolization

Centers with expertise in interventional radiology can attempt TD embolization percutaneously.

- Bilateral pedal or groin lymphangiogram is utilized to opacify the TD (Figure 29.8).

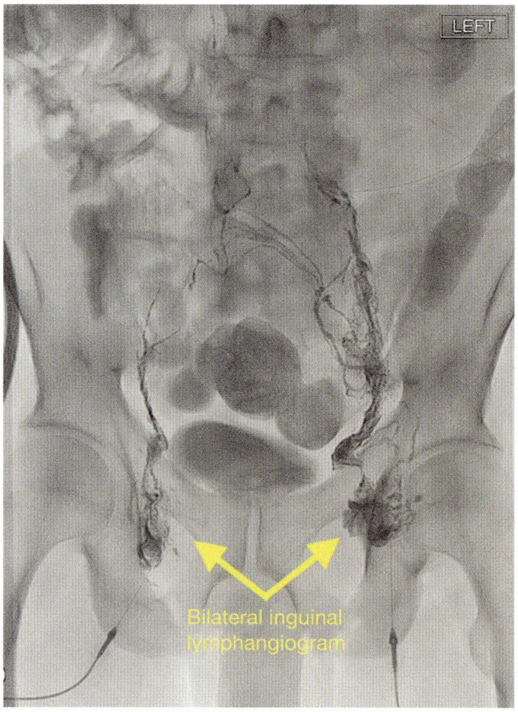

FIGURE 29.8 ▮ Bilateral groin lymphangiogram used to determine location of thoracic duct.

- A target duct is selected inferior to the CC for cannulation and right transabdominal approach under fluoroscopic guidance is utilized to avoid the aorta.
- The duct is cannulated, positioned confirmed with wire, and a catheter is placed.
- Contrast is then injected through the catheter to identify the location of the leak and the TD is embolized caudally to the leak (Figure 29.9).

Postoperative Care

- Patient is preferably extubated after the procedure.
- Chest tubes remain on water seal without applying suction.

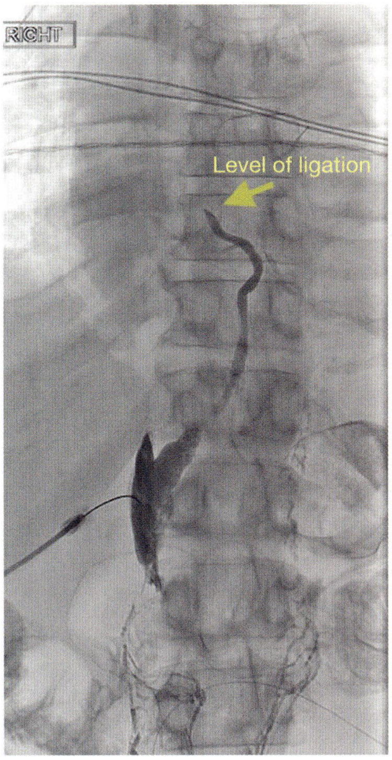

FIGURE 29.9 ▌ Lymphangiogram of the thoracic duct demonstrating intraluminal contrast demarcating the successful site of ligation.

- Aggressive pulmonary hygiene is encouraged including the following: Frequent ambulation, incentive spirometry, vibratory positive expiratory pressure, hyperinflation therapy, bronchodilators, chest physiotherapy, and mucolytics as needed.
- Postoperative day 1: CXR, resume low-fat diet, deep vein thrombosis prophylaxis, and chest tube to water seal
- If chest tube output remains serosanguineous or serous after 2 days of low fat to regular diet, then it is safe to remove the chest tube once output is below 200 mL/24 h.

PEARLS AND PITFALLS

- Recognize variations in anatomy and help plan future interventions.
- Perform TD ligation caudal to leak.
- Prophylactic TD ligation does not always prevent postoperative chylothorax.
- Careful dissection and understanding of the anatomy to avoid bleeding from intercostal arteries, injury to diaphragm, or lung parenchyma. In postesophagectomy cases, careful manipulation to the gastric conduit is critical.

Suggested Readings

1. Ahmed SU, Sancheti MS, Pickens A. Thoracoscopic thoracic duct ligation. *Oper Tech Thorac Cardiovasc Surg*. 2012;17(4):292-301.
2. Chen E, Itkin M. Thoracic duct embolization for chylous leaks. *Semin Intervent Radiol*. 2011;28(1):63-74.
3. Icaza OJ Jr, Andrews K, Kuhnke M. Laparoscopic ligation of the thoracic duct in management of chylothorax. *J Laparoendosc Adv Surg Tech*. 2002;12(2):129-133.
4. Phang K, Bowman M, Phillips A, Windsor J. Review of thoracic duct anatomical variations and clinical implications. *Clin Anat*. 2014;27(4):637-644.

SECTION III Esophageal

Chapter 30

Antireflux Surgery/ Fundoplication (Partial/ Complete): Minimally Invasive/Open Surgery

CAMERON T. STOCK
ELLIOT L. SERVAIS

Perioperative Considerations

- Gastric fundoplication can be performed alone or often in the setting of another procedure: such as paraesophageal hernia repair or Heller myotomy.
- All patients being considered for an antireflux procedure should undergo workup with esophageal manometry, 24-hour pH probe, and an upper endoscopy. A barium swallow and/or axial imaging can also be used as part of the preoperative evaluation.
- The type of wrap should be tailored to the patient's symptoms and concomitant surgical procedures. Significant motility disorders of the esophagus should prompt consideration of a partial fundoplication procedure.
- If you plan to perform an upper endoscopy prior to laparoscopic abdominal entry, minimize insufflation of the stomach to avoid gastric and small bowel dilation, which can make abdominal entry and visualization difficult.
- Previous upper abdominal operations such as laparoscopic cholecystectomy may make liver retraction difficult and require mobilization of adhesions to expose the hiatus.

Anesthesia and Patient Positioning

- General anesthesia with orogastric tube placement for gastric decompression (if not performing intraoperative upper endoscopy) and Foley catheter. Arterial lines are generally not needed.
- Foot pads should be placed at the end of the bed to allow for steep reverse Trendelenburg positioning.
- Robotic-assisted
  - Both arms tucked to allow clearance of the robotic arms and placement of a liver retractor port
- Laparoscopic
  - Left arm tucked with right arm extended to allow for placement of a liver retractor port
- Laparotomy
  - Left arm tucked with right arm extended to allow for placement of a Bookwalter retractor

Instruments and Equipment

Robotic

- Hassan port (8 mm), direct optical, or Veress needle for entry
- 30°, 8-mm robotic camera
- Four 8-mm robotic ports, 5-mm liver retractor port, 8-mm assistant port
- Robotic vessel sealer and long bipolar electrocautery for tissue dissection
- Large needle driver and large suture cut needle driver
- 5-mm laparoscopic liver retractor: snake or Nathanson
- Bougie dilators

Laparoscopic

- Hassan port (12 mm) or Veress needle for entry
- 30°, 10-mm laparoscopic camera
- Two 5-mm laparoscopic ports, one 10-mm port, 5-mm disposable liver retractor port
- Atraumatic laparoscopic graspers
- Laparoscopic harmonic scalpel for tissue division
- Endo Stitch device (Medtronic, Minneapolis, MN) or laparoscopic needle driver
- Bougie dilators

Technique

Port Placement, Robotic

- Entry to the abdomen is obtained to the left of the midline approximately 16 cm from the xyphoid process to avoid the falciform ligament using a Hassan or Veress technique (Figure 30.1).

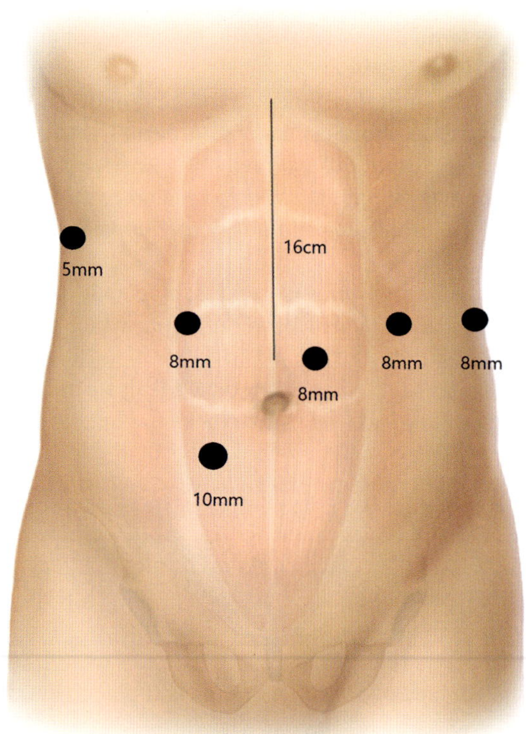

FIGURE 30.1 ▮ Robotic port placement positions. (Modified from Chapman WC Jr, Mutch MG. Total Abdominal Colectomy: Laparoscopic Technique. In: Hawn MT. *Operative Techniques in Surgery*. 2nd ed. Wolters Kluwer; 2023:1030-1042. Figure 4.25.2.)

- If direct optical entry is used, this is typically performed in the left midclavicular line with care taken to avoid the inferior epigastric vessels. Insufflation pressure of 5 mm Hg CO_2 should be applied to the optical port during entry.
- Two additional left-sided 8-mm ports are placed one hand breadth away from each other (9-10 cm) and 2 to 3 cm superior to the camera port to minimize collisions between the arms. The lateral most port is used for retraction during dissection.

- An 8-mm right upper quadrant port is placed and is used as the surgeon's left hand.
- The liver retractor port is placed as far lateral as possible in the right upper quadrant. Care should be taken during placement to avoid injury to the ascending colon.
- A 10-mm assistant port is placed in the right lower quadrant. This port must be large enough to allow for suture passage by the assistant. (Note: One may choose to avoid an assistant port and pass sutures via a working robotic port; however, this requires removing an instrument each time.)

Port Placement, Laparoscopic

- Hassan entry into the abdomen at approximately 10 to 12 cm from the xyphoid to the left of midline (Figure 30.2)

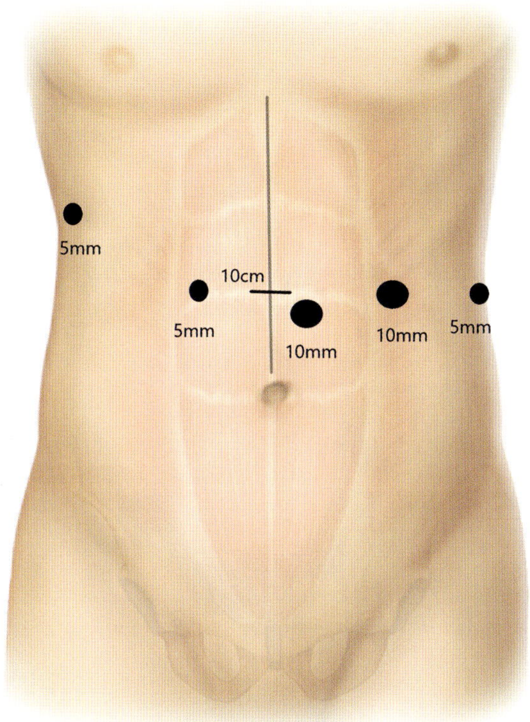

FIGURE 30.2 ‖ Laparoscopic port positions. (Modified from Chapman WC Jr, Mutch MG. Total Abdominal Colectomy: Laparoscopic Technique. In: Hawn MT. *Operative Techniques in Surgery*. 2nd ed. Wolters Kluwer; 2023:1030-1042. Figure 4.25.2.)

- Two additional left-sided ports are placed one hand breadth away from each other at the level of the camera port; the surgeon's right hand port is a 10-mm port to allow for passage of a suture or use of an Endo Stitch device (Ethicon).
- Right upper quadrant 8-mm port placed for the left hand
- Far right upper quadrant 5-mm liver retractor port (identical as described for robotic port placement)

Laparotomy

- Upper midline laparotomy, which may require extension above the xyphoid process if hiatal hernia repair is required
- Use of the Bookwalter retractor is recommended to optimize exposure of the hiatus.

Surgical Approach: Nissen Fundoplication (360° wrap)

- The hiatus is examined for the presence of a hernia requiring repair.
- The short gastric arteries are identified and divided to the level of the left crus. The lessor sac is entered during this dissection. There will often be adhesions between the gastric cardia and the left crus of the diaphragm, which will need to be divided prior to fundoplication (Figure 30.3).

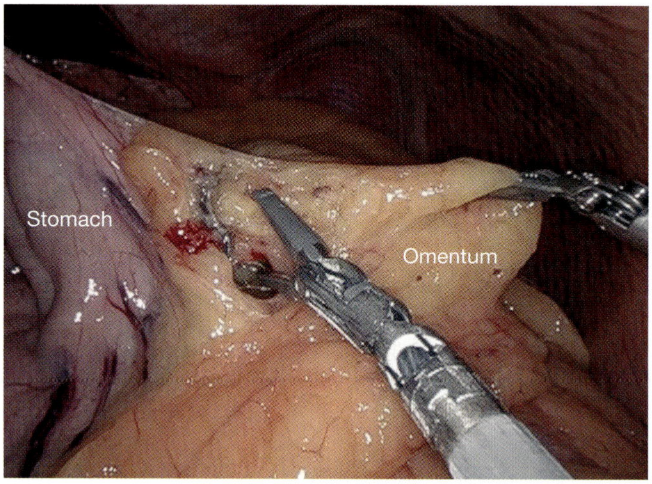

FIGURE 30.3 ▮ Division of the short gastric arteries proceeding along the greater curve of the stomach.

TIPS

In the setting of a hiatal hernia, the short gastric arteries are often tethered and may be easily injured at the level of the left crus of the diaphragm. Similarly, excessive traction on the short gastric arteries and the gastrosplenic ligament can cause injury to the spleen. Proceed with caution in this area.

- The gastrohepatic ligament is then divided with exposure of the right crus.

TIPS

A Penrose drain (Figure 30.4) is passed from the right to the left side of the esophagus at the level of the hiatus, allowing for manipulation of the esophagus. This will also allow for atraumatic manipulation of the esophagus if a hiatal hernia repair is required.

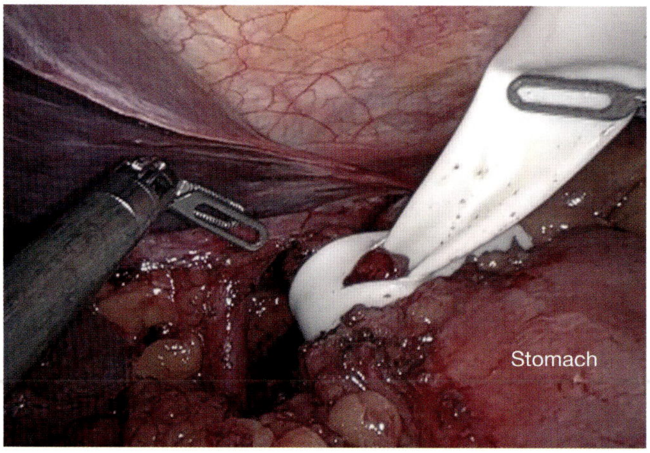

FIGURE 30.4 ▮ A Penrose drain is used to encircle the esophagus.

- The phrenoesophageal fat pad is mobilized to expose the gastroesophageal (GE) junction (Figure 30.5).
- A bougie ranging from 48 to 54 French is passed through the GE junction.

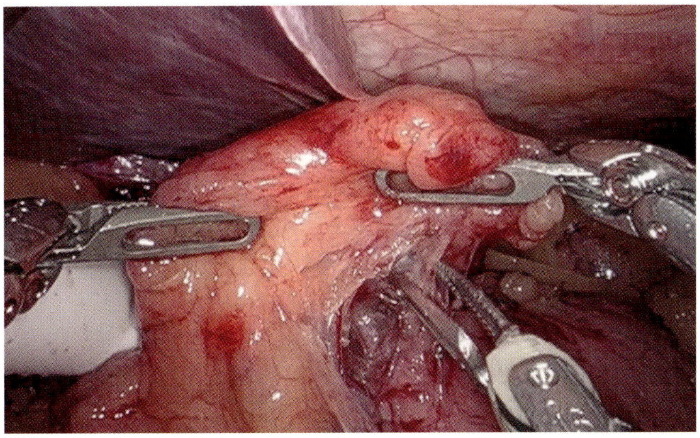

FIGURE 30.5 ▌ The phrenoesophageal fat pad is mobilized carefully off the gastroesophageal junction. Care is taken to avoid injury to the anterior vagus nerve during this step.

- The fundus of the stomach is brought posterior to the esophagus and grasped with the left hand, the right hand picks up the fundus to the left of the esophagus, and it is brought to the midline. A "shoeshine" maneuver is performed to ensure free movement of the wrap posteriorly (Figure 30.6).

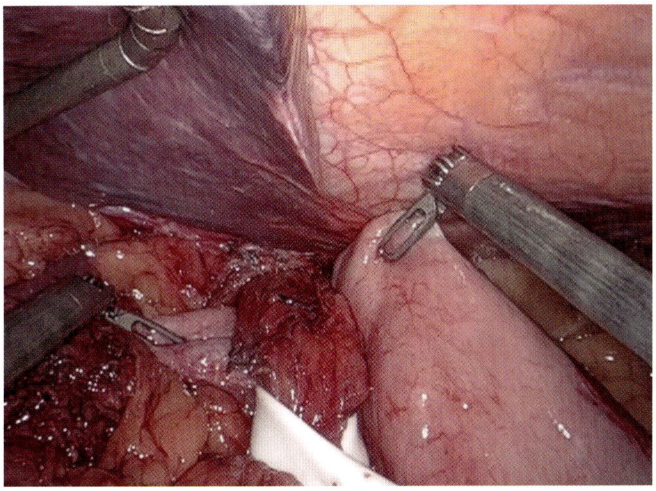

FIGURE 30.6 ▌ Performance of the "shoeshine" maneuver.

TIPS

Avoid performing the fundoplication using the body of the stomach as this is a cause of late wrap failure.

- An initial stitch is placed at the superior aspect of the wrap and the suture ends are left long to allow for manipulation and placement of the wrap at the GE junction.
- Additional stitches between the ends of the fundoplication should incorporate a bite of the esophageal wall to prevent slippage of the wrap.
- The length of the wrap should be 1.5 to 2.5 cm in length to avoid dysphagia (Figure 30.7).

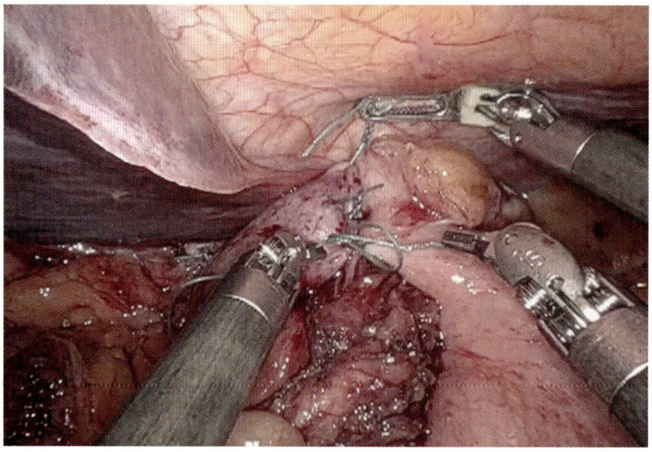

FIGURE 30.7 ▌ Completion of the Nissen fundoplication with tying of the final stitch. Note the use of the suture ends from the initial stitch being used for retraction.

Dor Fundoplication (180° Anterior Wrap)

- The short gastric arteries are divided. (Note: The short gastric arteries do not necessarily need to be divided to perform a Dor; however, this will decrease the tension on the wrap.)
- The angle of His is recreated with a stitch between the fundus and the left side of the esophagus (Figure 30.8).

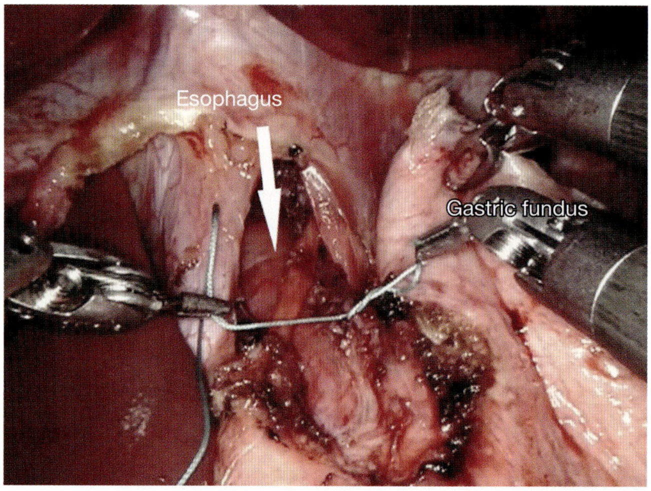

FIGURE 30.8 ▌ Recreation of the angle of His.

- Two to three additional stitches are placed between the fundus and the left crus of the diaphragm (Figure 30.9).

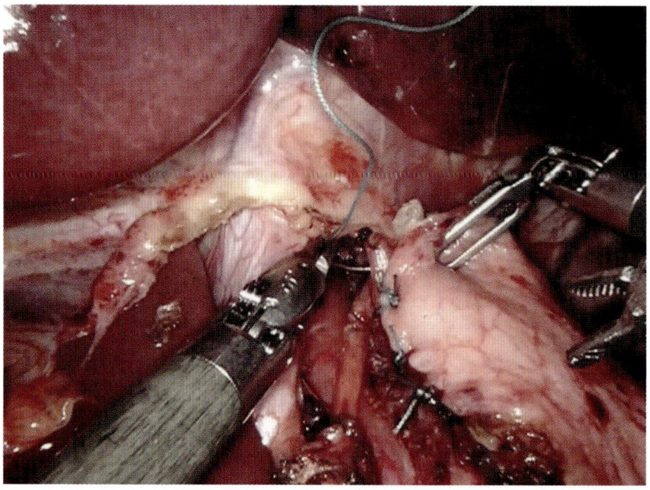

FIGURE 30.9 ▌ Stitches placed between the esophagus, left crus of the diaphragm, and the gastric fundus.

- The fundus is then grasped and brought 180° anterior to the esophagus.
- Sutures are placed between the fundus and the right crus of the diaphragm (Figure 30.10).

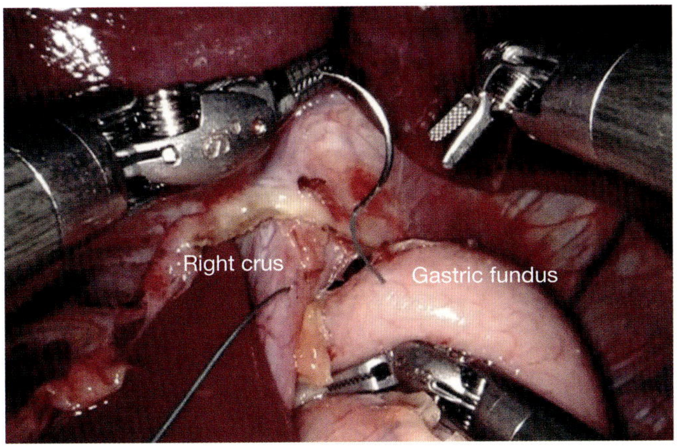

FIGURE 30.10 ▮ Stitches placed between the right crus, the esophagus, and the gastric fundus.

- An apical stitch is placed between the fundus and the apex of the hiatus (Figure 30.11).

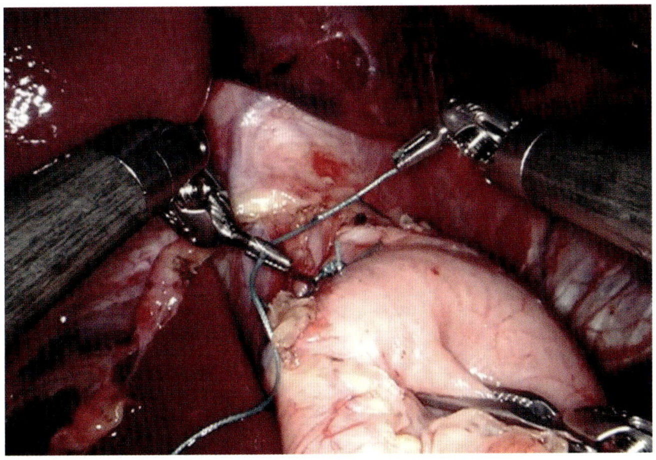

FIGURE 30.11 ▮ Apical hiatus stitch performed completing the wrap.

Toupet Fundoplication (180-270° Posterior wrap)

- After division of the short gastric arteries, the fundus is brought posterior to the esophagus and sutured to the right side of the esophageal wall.
- Three interrupted sutures are typically placed between the wrap and the right side of the esophageal wall.
- To complete the wrap, the fundus is grasped and sutured to the left side of the esophagus leaving a 90° gap between the ends of the wrap creating a 270° wrap (Figure 30.12).

Postoperative Care

- Nasogastric tubes are not routinely placed following fundoplication.
- The patient is advanced to clear liquids the day following surgery and can be discharged on full liquids.
- The diet is advanced slowly over the course of several weeks following surgery.
- A swallow study can be useful if there is concern for mucosal injury; alternatively, an endoscopy can be performed at the end of the procedure to assess for mucosal injury.

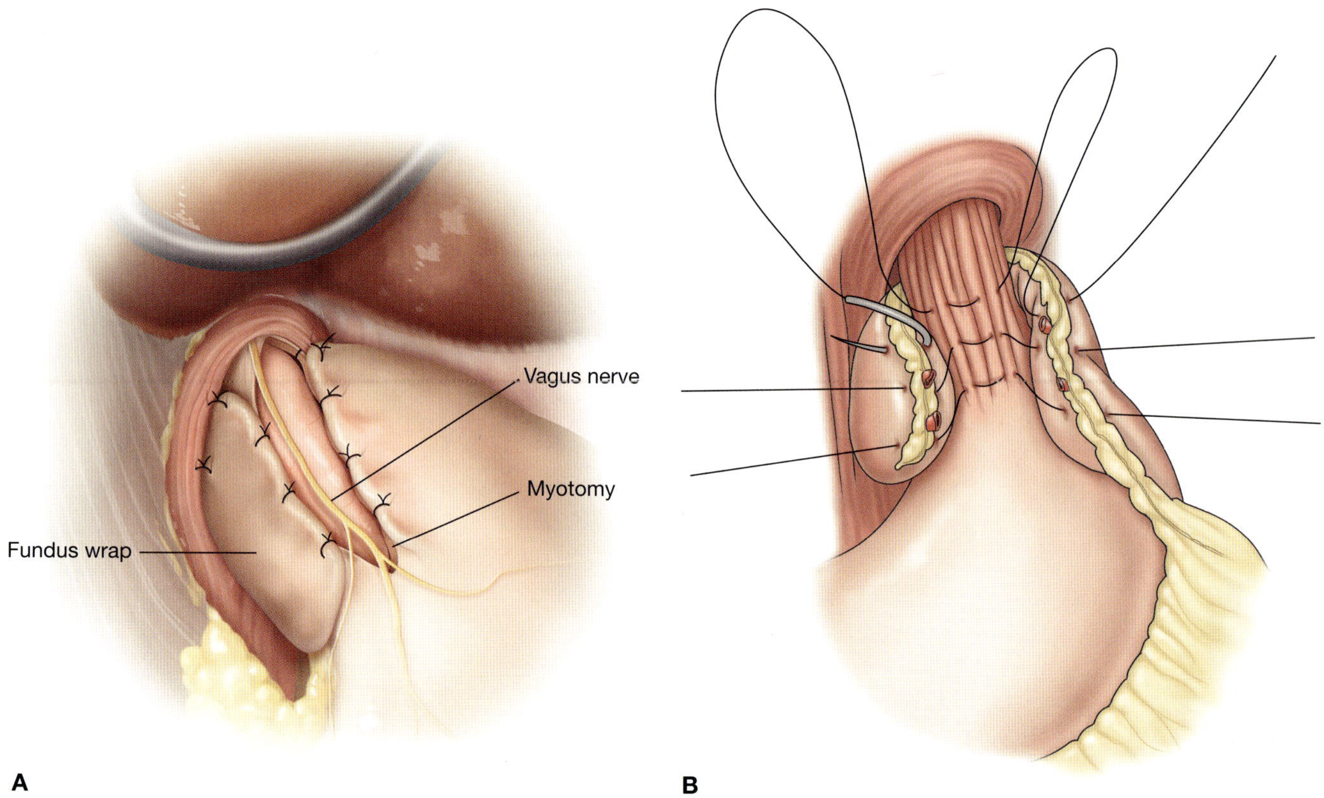

FIGURE 30.12 ▌Toupet fundoplication **(A)** performed in conjunction with a Heller myotomy **(B)**. (**A.** From Shah RD, Hoppo T, Jobe BA. *Laparoscopic Heller myotomy and fundoplication for achalasia*. In: *Master Techniques in Surgery: Esophageal Surgery*. Wolters Kluwer; 2015:161-171. Figure 14.6C.)

PEARLS AND PITFALLS

- Patients should be carefully selected and the fundoplication choice should be tailored to the patient's symptoms, the performance of additional procedures, and the presence of esophageal dysmotility to ensure acceptable clinical outcomes.
- During laparoscopic or robotic dissection, careful grasping of the stomach should be used to prevent serosal injury to the stomach.
- During division of the short gastric arteries, care should be taken to avoid injury to tethered arteries near the left crus of the diaphragm.
- Careful attention to proper positioning of the fundoplication and avoidance of placing the wrap around the stomach will avoid postoperative dysphagia and "slipped fundoplication" phenomenon.
- Careful identification and preservation of the vagus nerve fibers will prevent delayed gastric emptying following fundoplication.

Suggested Readings

1. Ellis FH. The Nissen fundoplication. *Ann Thorac Surg*. 1992;54(6):1231-1235.
2. Spechler SJ, Hunter JG, Jones KM, et al. Randomized trial of medical versus surgical treatment for refractory heartburn. *N Engl J Med*. 2019;381(16):1513-1523.
3. Watson DI, Jamieson GG, Lally C, et al. Multicenter, prospective, double-blind, randomized trial of laparoscopic Nissen vs anterior 90 degrees partial fundoplication. *Arch Surg*. 2004;139(11):1160-1167.
4. Hakanson BS, Lundell L, Bylund A, Thorell A. Comparison of laparoscopic 270° posterior partial fundoplication vs total fundoplication for the treatment of gastroesophageal reflux disease: a randomized clinical trial. *JAMA Surg*. 2019;154(6):479-486.
5. Morino M, Pellegrino L, Giaccone C, Garrone C, Rebecchi F. Randomized clinical trial of robot-assisted versus laparoscopic Nissen fundoplication. *Br J Surg*. 2006;93(5):553-558.

Chapter 31

Paraesophageal Hernia Repair: Robotic-Assisted Laparoscopic Approach/ Transthoracic Approach

BRETT L. BROUSSARD
ELBERT KUO

ROBOTIC-ASSISTED LAPAROSCOPIC APPROACH

Perioperative Considerations

- Minimally invasive approaches to paraesophageal hernia (PEH) repair have become the standard approach given improved morbidity/mortality, decreased blood loss, and decreased length of stay despite increasing comorbidities in the patient population.
- Robotic-assisted laparoscopic repair adds improved stable high-definition 3-D optics, wristed instruments, tremor filtering, and ability to self-first assist as just a few enhancements to this approach. These improvements have allowed surgeons to dissect higher in the mediastinum almost eliminating the need for an esophageal lengthening procedure and repairing primary hiatal hernias from a chest approach.

Indications

- Surgical repair is warranted in the presence of moderate to large PEH/hiatal hernias with symptoms that are related to hiatal/PEH anatomy. Symptoms may include heartburn, regurgitation of food, sour taste in mouth in morning, dysphagia, chest pain/pressure, postprandial bloating, and shortness of breath (if lung volume loss due to compression).
- Caution should be used when a small hiatal hernia is found (<3 cm) in the setting of intense symptomology despite compliance with proton-pump inhibitor therapy as further evaluation may be needed including esophageal manometry and 24-hour pH impedance/BRAVO testing to confirm that acid reflux is causing symptoms.
- Relative contraindications to repair include severe cardiopulmonary dysfunction leading to inability to tolerate general anesthesia. Age of the patient, size of hernia, and previous abdominal surgeries are not contraindications, but a history of extensive prior abdominal surgeries may change the surgeon's approach (see transthoracic approach below).

Preoperative Testing

- Basic laboratory testing including complete blood cell count, chemistry panel with albumin to assess nutritional status. Liver function panel, coagulation studies may be indicated given other medical history.
- Barium esophagram/upper gastrointestinal (UGI) is the radiographic standard and should be completed on all patients. Computed tomography (CT) can be used as a substitute if esophagram is

unable to be performed or may be complementary to esophagram/UGI to further evaluate anatomy, especially in a redo operation. Chest radiograph should be performed if chest CT is not done to rule out other pulmonary pathology.

- Upper endoscopy should be performed preoperatively or intraoperatively. Attention should be paid to:
  - esophageal tortuosity
  - esophageal length
  - hiatal pinch
  - the presence of Cameron ulcers
  - if it is possible to get to the duodenum
  - if the pylorus is tight
- Pulmonary function testing is not routinely required, but if a patient's symptomology centers around shortness of breath or recurrent pneumonias, it should be obtained.
- The need for physiologic esophageal testing in the setting of moderate to large PEH is debatable. We typically try to obtain esophageal manometry, which can be helpful in determining the type of fundoplication and rule out achalasia.
- pH studies are not routinely performed in moderate to large hiatal hernias as this does not change our surgical management.
- Nuclear medicine gastric emptying study should be performed in all settings of redo foregut surgery and selectively used in first time operations where a component of slow emptying or gastroparesis is suspected.

Instruments and Equipment

- We currently use a Da Vinci Xi robot surgery platform (Intuitive Surgical).
- Robotic instruments used:
  - 30° endoscope plus
  - SynchroSeal (alternative is to use Long Bipolar Grasper & Vessel Sealer Extend)
  - Cadiere forceps (×2)
  - Large SutureCut needle driver
  - 8-mm cannula (×5) with bladeless optical obturator (We used one metal 8-mm cannula for the assist port since it is more cost effective than a disposable 8-mm trocar and the needles slide better down the metal trochar)
  - 5-mm trocar (liver retractor)
- Liver retractor of choice
  - We used a 5-mm Pretzel Liver Retractor (Artisan Medical Devices, Medford, NJ) via a right upper quadrant 5-mm trocar. A Nathanson liver retractor is also acceptable, and when placed appropriately, it should avoid collision with the robotic arms, but this should be considered when positioning.
- 1-cm Penrose drain cut to 4 in
- Kittner roll gauze sponge (Carefree Surgical, New Castle, CA)
- Optional: Cor-Knot Device, 5-mm diameter, 31 cm length shaft (LSI Solutions, Victor, NY)
- Optional: GORE Bio-A mesh, 7 × 10 cm (W. L. Gore and Associates, Flagstaff, AZ)
- A Wayne pneumothorax catheter set, 14F, should be available in the room in case the pleural space is entered and the patient becomes hemodynamically unstable (Cook Medical, Bloomington, IN).

Positioning

- General anesthesia is used with a single-lumen endotracheal tube.
- Complete paralysis is ideal for appropriate relaxation of the patient tissues.
- Two large bore peripheral intravenous (IV) lines are typically adequate. If insufficient access, a central venous line can be placed.
- We routinely use radial arterial line catheters given the shifts in blood pressure seen with reverse Trendelenburg positioning and the possibility of entering the pleural space.
- Foley catheter is also placed.
- The lower chest and abdomen are prepped and draped from just below the nipples to the pubic symphysis and as far laterally as feasible.

- The patient is supine in the center of the operating room table with arms out at a 90° angle and secured to the arm board.
- Special care should be made to pad and protect all pressure points of the patient including IV tubing and electrocardiogram leads.
- A foot board is used on the end of the bed so that steep reverse Trendelenburg position can be safely tolerated.
- Upper endoscopy is performed at the beginning of the case if the patient has not previously been scoped by the surgeon. If this is performed at the beginning of the case, we prefer to use carbon dioxide (CO_2) insufflation versus air and are very judicious about how much insufflation we use.
- An orogastric (OG) tube should be placed by anesthesia; however, if it doesn't go easy, it may need to be advanced after the hernia is reduced.

TIPS

- *It is essential to address risk factors for increased intra-abdominal pressure (body mass index >35, heavy lifting, constipation, and future pregnancy) prior to offering hiatal hernia surgery or the risk of recurrence will be high.*
- *If the presenting symptom involves chest pain, a thorough cardiac evaluation may be warranted prior to undergoing surgical repair.*
- *Close evaluation of preoperative imaging should be performed as other conditions such as thoracic scoliosis or conditions of the descending aorta can distort normal hiatal anatomy.*
- *The long bipolar grasper and vessel sealer can be exchanged for a single SynchroSeal instrument.*
- *The extraperitoneal hernia sac is best entered at the 12-o'clock position.*
- *Arm 4 should provide constant counter tension on the hernia sac.*
- *Anterior and posterior vagal nerves should be identified and preserved.*

Technique

Port Placement

- The midline is marked from the xiphoid to the umbilicus and then divided into thirds. The camera port (8-mm robotic port) is placed approximately 2 to 3 cm to the patient's left of midline near the lower third mark. Access to the abdomen can be obtained in numerous methods, but we employ a Veress needle technique and use 15 mm Hg CO_2 pneumoperitoneum. This is followed by optical insertion of the robotic 8-mm cannula with a 5-mm 0° laparoscope (Figure 31.1).
- The remainder of the robotically docked ports (8-mm robotic port) will be in the same horizontal line all 8 cm apart. Two more ports will be placed to the patient's left and one port on the patient's right of midline. The port on the patient's right can be spaced 10 cm apart to give more room for the assistant.
- A 5-mm port will be placed in the right upper quadrant as high in the abdomen and low toward the table as possible for the liver retractor if a pretzel is used. If the Nathanson is used, the 5 mm port is used to make a hole in the peritoneum midline.

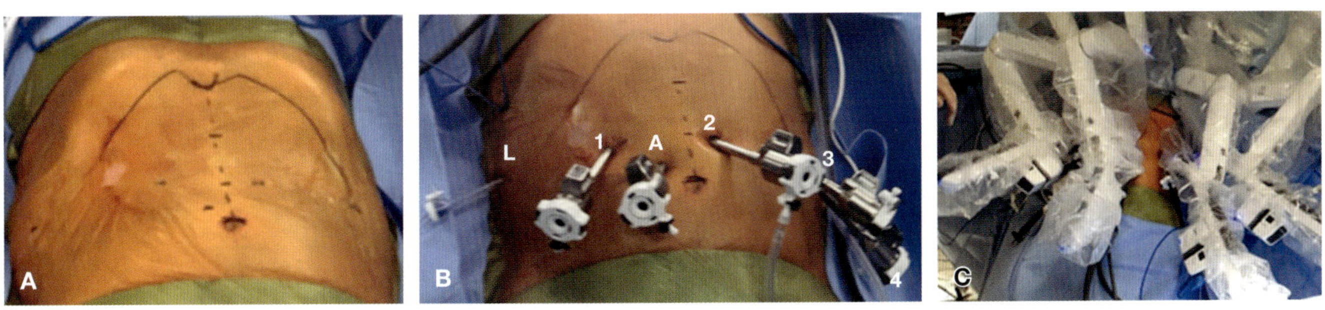

FIGURE 31.1 | The patient is in reverse Trendelenburg with a foot board in place. Five 8-mm robotic ports are used. **A.** The first port placed is the camera port 2 cm to the patient's left of midline and two-thirds the distance from the xiphoid to the umbilicus. The other working ports are placed in the same horizontal plane all 8 cm apart. **B.** The ports are labeled based on which robotic arm will be docked. Port "A" is the assistant port, and port "L" is the liver retractor port. **C.** This is the view once the robot is docked and instruments are in place.

- An assistant port (8-mm robotic port) will be placed on the patient's right side in the periumbilical area. This can be triangulated with the camera port and the right-sided robotic port. This should be above the umbilicus to allow the assistant to reach the hiatus.
- The robotic instruments are docked (for a right-handed surgeon) with the surgeon's "right hand"/ arm 3 as the long bipolar grasper, and "left hand"/arm 1 and "retracting hand"/arm 4 are both Cadiere forceps. The camera is in arm 2.

Hernia Sac Dissection and Reduction of the Sac/Stomach

- The patient is placed in reverse Trendelenburg position.
- This positioning allows gravity reduction of hernia contents such as omentum and bowel, which leads to better hiatal visualization (Figure 31.2).
- Dissection begins with using arm 4 and arm 1 Cadiere forceps to reduce the hiatal hernia contents back to the abdomen. Then the arm 4 Cadiere forcep is used to retract the lesser curve of the stomach to screen right and inferior. This presents the avascular gastrohepatic ligament, which is entered sharply with the bipolar. This plane is dissected toward the top of the right crus and toward the arch of the hiatus. This allows visualization of the right crus.
- Once at the 12-o'clock position, the arm 4 retracting Cadiere is used to evert the hernia sac while arms 1 and 3 are used to open the hernia sac at the phrenoesophageal ligament and peritoneal reflection. This allows access into the posterior mediastinum where the pericardial plane is at the surgeon's cephalad position. This space has characteristic "wispy" areolar tissue and is mostly avascular.
- Blunt and sharp dissection are then used to divide these areolar attachments and identify the posterior mediastinal borders and structures. Special care should be made to visualize the pleural boundaries, esophagus, vertebrae, aorta, and anterior/posterior vagal nerves. As more of the hernia sac is dissected, counter traction on the hernia sac is provided by arm 4. Direct retraction of the stomach should be avoided.
- Once the majority of the hernia sac has been delivered from the mediastinum, the sac must be dissected off of the crura bilaterally. Special care must be taken to avoid removing the peritoneal lining of the crura.
- The bipolar is then used to enter the lesser sac approximately midway down the greater curve of the stomach. The bipolar is then exchanged for the vessel sealer, which is used to divide the short gastric vessels along the greater curve. If the SynchroSeal is used, no instrument exchange is needed. This is taken to the base of the left crus where previous hiatal dissection was performed.
- A Penrose drain is then placed around the distal esophagus and used as a retractor. Prior to sinching down the Penrose drain, the surgeon should ensure an OG tube has traversed the gastroesophageal junction (GEJ) and is in the stomach. This adds rigidity to the Penrose retraction and avoids traction injury to the esophagus (Figure 31.3).

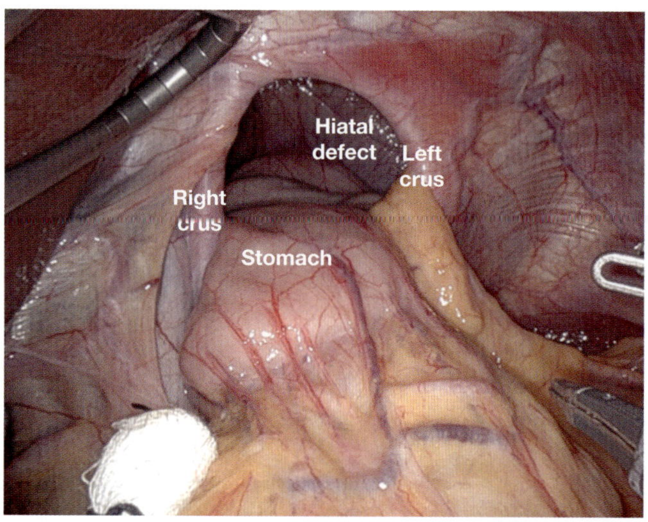

FIGURE 31.2 ▌ The stomach is noted to be in the mediastinum. A large hiatal defect is noted with left and right crus identified.

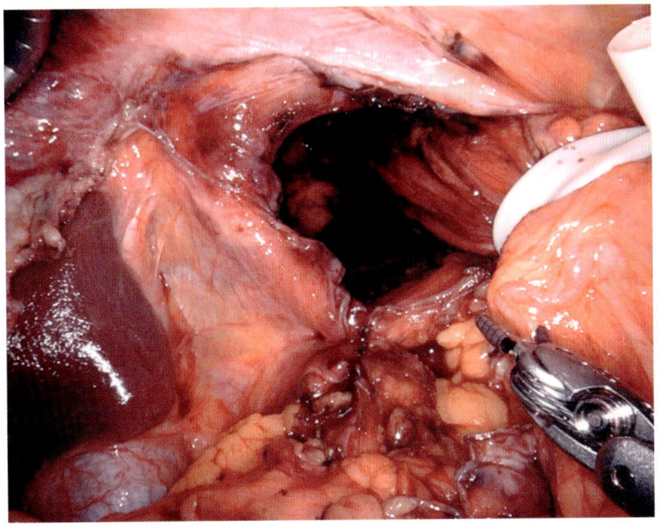

FIGURE 31.3 ▌ Circumferential hiatal dissection with reduction of stomach and hernia sac from the mediastinum. The Penrose drain is used for retraction.

Intra-Abdominal Esophageal Length

- Arm 4 is then used to grab the Penrose and expose the mediastinal esophagus, allowing for circumferential mediastinal mobilization of the esophagus. It is here that special attention is made to avoid vagal nerve injury. This maneuver also provides intra-abdominal esophageal length, which is key for decreasing the risk of recurrence.
- The hernia sac and gastric fat pad are then mobilized off the stomach and distal esophagus to fully visualize the GEJ.
- There should be at least 2.5 cm of intra-abdominal esophageal length to successfully perform a tension-free repair.
- If this is not achieved, more mediastinal dissection may be needed. If length is still not adequate, Collis gastroplasty may be required (please see separate chapter on Collis gastroplasty).

Hiatal Repair

- Crural closure is initiated by placing interrupted 0-polyester permanent braided suture. These are placed in a caudal to cephalad direction bringing the base of both crura together.
- If the hiatal defect is large or tension appears to be an issue, further sutures can be placed at the top of the left and right crus, respectively, to the arch of the crus to form a chevron-type closure. This allows for better distribution of tension across the repair.
- These stitches can be secured with robotic instrument tying or using the Cor-Knot device closure (Figure 31.4).
- The use of biosynthetic mesh can be considered at this point to reinforce crural closure. This is typically cut in a letter "U" shape and placed retroesophageal. This is secured in place with 2-0 absorbable suture such that the mesh is not in contact with the posterior portion of the esophagus (Figure 31.5).

Antireflux Procedure

- The decision to perform a fundoplication and the type of fundoplication varies by surgeon and patient characteristics. Patient age, preoperative symptoms, and manometry (if performed) may help guide the surgeon's decision.
- We find that most patients can tolerate a Toupet partial fundoplication. This is typically done over a 54-French bougie and is further described in a previous chapter (Figure 31.6).

Postoperative Care

- Postoperatively, the patient is kept nothing by mouth and maintained with IV fluids. The Foley catheter is removed at midnight following the procedure as long as adequate output has been recorded.
- We follow an enhanced recovery pathway that minimizes narcotic use in the postoperative setting. This is aided by the routine use of transversus abdominis plane block by our anesthesia colleagues.

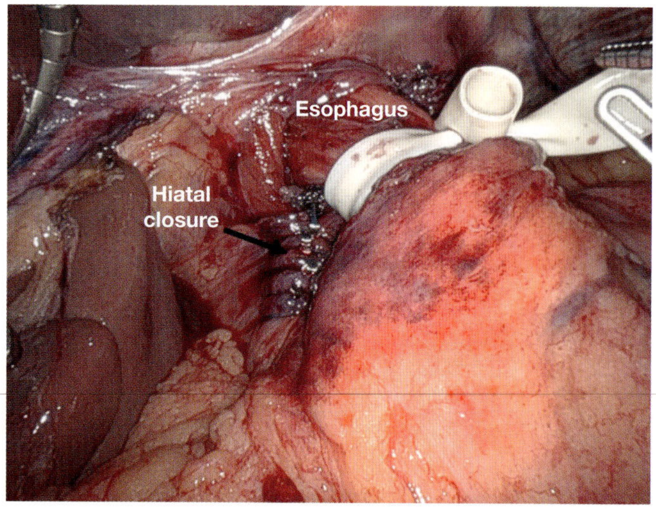

FIGURE 31.4 ▮ The hiatus has been closed with interrupted 0-polyester permanent braided suture using a Cor-Knot device. These are placed in a caudal to cephalad direction bringing the base of both crura together.

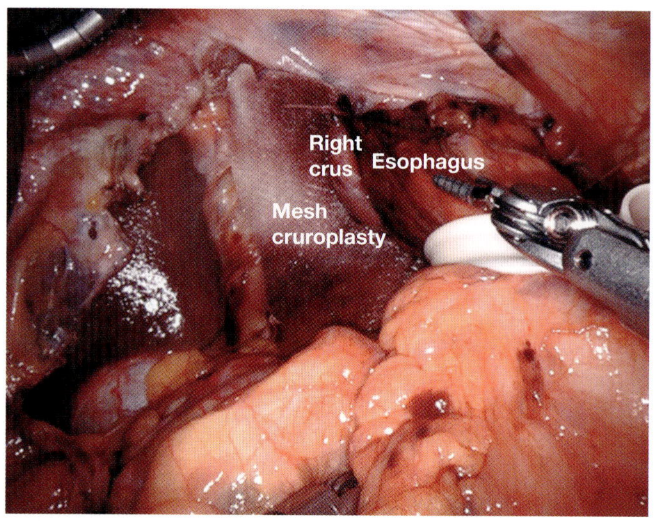

FIGURE 31.5 ▮ Mesh cruroplasty can be performed to reinforce the primary crural repair. The mesh is configured in a "U" shape below the esophagus. The posterior esophagus should not rub against the mesh.

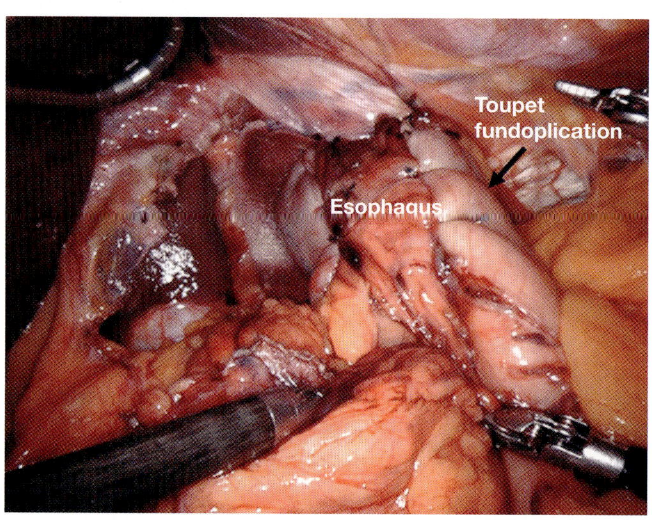

FIGURE 31.6 ▮ Toupet fundoplication is performed at the end of the hiatal hernia repair. Interrupted 2-0 polyester permanent braided suture using a Cor-Knot device is used to secure the fundoplication in place.

- We routinely get postoperative UGI tract radiography (UGI/esophagram) the following morning. This evaluates for the absence of esophageal or gastric leak, subdiaphragmatic positioning of the fundoplication, flow of contrast through the GEJ, and transit into the small intestine.
- The patient is then trialed on a clear liquid diet and then expeditiously advanced to full liquids if tolerating liquids.
- The patient will be discharged home with 2 weeks on a full liquid diet followed by 1 week of soft diet. At 3 weeks postoperatively, the patient is encouraged to slowly advance to a regular diet with special precaution to take small bites, eat slowly, and avoid hard/dry solid foods such as dry bread/chicken for at least 6 weeks.

PEARLS AND PITFALLS

Robotic-Assisted Laparoscopic Approach

- Establishing the correct plane between the hernia sac and the mediastinum is key to complete hernia sac reduction and avoiding injury to mediastinal structures. If the patient is not a redo, this plane should be virgin and easily dissected. If it is not easy, you are usually in the wrong plane. Much of this dissection can be done bluntly with a sponge.
- On the left crural dissection, at the base stay on top of the aortic plane and sweep the esophagus up and to the patients right. Do the opposite on the right crus side. If you can connect the right and left dissection above the aorta and below the esophagus, this will allow easy passage of the Penrose drain.
- When dissecting the short gastrics off the greater curve, the key maneuver is arm 1's retraction of the stomach. We find that if you grab the underside of the stomach and pull down and to the left, this exposes the short gastrics to allow you to take multiple bites with the SynchroSeal before having to adjust your retraction again making you more efficient.
- Adequate intra-abdominal esophageal length of at least 2.5 cm is required for tension-free repair and reduce risk of recurrence.
- Crural closure should close the defect, and chevron closure may be needed to adequately distribute points of tension across the repair.
- If you are using the tie knot device, make sure the assistant port is above the level of the umbilicus so that instrument can reach the hiatus.
- Biosynthetic mesh may or may not be used to reinforce the repair.
- Antireflux procedures should be performed while taking into account the patient's age, symptoms, and esophageal manometry.
- The most common areas of recurrence are posterior and along the left crura. We will often tack our wrap with permanent 2-0 suture in these areas to prevent recurrence.

LAPAROSCOPIC APPROACH

- The perioperative considerations and postoperative care for hiatal hernia repair are not different for laparoscopic versus robotic approaches. Indications and preoperative testing are the same.
- Equipment differences include five standard laparoscopic ports. These include three 5-mm ports and two 12-mm ports. A standard, preferably high definition, 30° laparoscope is needed. Two atraumatic bowel graspers will be needed for retraction and tissue manipulation. A laparoscopic harmonic energy device will be needed for tissue dissection (Ethicon, Bridgewater, NJ). The suture device recommended for hiatal closure and fundoplication suture is the EndoStitch Suturing Device (Medtronic, Minneapolis, MN).
- Positioning of the patient is identical as the robotic approach with the arms out and footboard used to facilitate reverse Trendelenburg position. A split leg position can be considered depending on the surgeon preference.
- Port placement is identical to the robotic approach with the two 12-mm ports serving as the two most medial ports (of the four working ports). The assistant's left hand drives the camera in the 12-mm port and right hand uses a grasper to retract and assist the surgeon. The surgeon's right hand uses the other 12-mm port for the harmonic dissection and EndoStitch when called for. If the patient is noted to have a longer torso, all ports can be elevated a few centimeters to facilitate mediastinal dissection.

- The hiatal and hernia dissection in the laparoscopic approach is identical to the robotic approach with the obvious exception that the assistant drives the camera and provides the traction/counter-traction needed to assist the surgeon. The principle and goals are otherwise the same.
- The EndoStitch device is then used on the surgeon's right hand (12-mm port) to close the hiatus. Nonabsorbable polyester suture material is recommended as in the robotic repair.
- At the end of the procedure, the anterior fascia should be closed on the two 12-mm ports. This can be done primarily or via a suture pass device.

TRANSTHORACIC APPROACH

Perioperative Considerations

- Factors that may influence a surgeon's decision to consider transthoracic repair over other approaches include:
  - History of extensive previous abdominal surgery
  - Morbid obesity
  - Shortened esophagus
  - Giant PEHs
  - Concurrent esophageal pathology such as motility disorders or esophageal diverticulum
  - Perforation of the stomach or esophagus
- Indications and preoperative testing are the same, no matter the approach (see above). The surgeon should have a lower threshold for CT of the thorax if considering a transthoracic approach. Pulmonary function testing should be performed to assess lung function and reserve considering the approach and need for single-lung ventilation.

Instruments and Equipment

- Standard thoracotomy tray should be utilized and will vary by institution.

Positioning

- General anesthesia is used with a double-lumen endotracheal tube or bronchial blocker to allow single-lung ventilation.
- The patient is positioned in the right lateral decubitus position. Pressure points are padded well, and the table is gently flexed at the midpoint to optimize intercostal spaces.
- The left chest is widely prepared and draped with special care to include the left upper quadrant of the abdomen in the field.

TIPS

- *With the improved manual dexterity and improved visualization offered by robotic surgery, the need for a transthoracic approach has become limited.*
- *A good place to identify the esophagus is near the left inferior pulmonary vein as this is usually above the hernia.*
- *A 0-silk suture can be placed on the diaphragm and pulled caudally to assist in visualization of the hiatus.*
- *The right crus is typically deep and may be hard to define. Understanding the caudate lobe of the liver is deep to it, and inferior vena cava posterior is helpful to avoid injury to these structures.*

Technique

Incision

- A standard left posterolateral thoracotomy is performed. This includes dividing the latissimus dorsi muscle but preserving the serratus anterior.

- The chest is entered in the sixth intercostal space. The seventh space can be considered, but the diaphragm may obstruct the surgeon's view. The seventh rib can be shingled or partially resected to improve exposure.
- The left lung is deflated, and the inferior pulmonary ligament is divided up to the level of the inferior pulmonary vein. The lung can then be packed superiorly and anteriorly.

Hernia Dissection

- The esophagus is located anterior to the descending aorta near the inferior pulmonary vein, and the mediastinal pleura is opened over it. Special care is made to identify and protect both vagus nerves.
- The esophagus is encircled, and a Penrose drain or umbilical tape is used as a retractor (Figure 31.7).
- The esophagus is mobilized proximally to the aortic arch and inferiorly to the level of the hernia sac.
- The esophagus and hernia sac are then completely mobilized from the mediastinum. This can be done with sharp and blunt dissection. This is carried out circumferentially, including the pericardial and right pleural planes, down to the hiatus.
- The hernia sac is then opened anteriorly and divided circumferentially. At the level of the hiatus, a 2-cm margin should be kept on the crura to maintain peritoneum on the crura.
- The hernia sac is then dissected free from the esophagus and stomach circumferentially. Special care is again made at this step to avoid injury to the vagus nerves.
- The GE fat pad is then removed. This begins anterior to the right vagus nerve and continues across to the left vagus.

Hiatal Repair

- The GEJ should be clearly identified with the lower half of the intrathoracic esophagus fully mobilized. The diaphragmatic hiatus should be clearly exposed.
- The stomach is reduced into the abdomen, and a decision on esophageal length should be made. As in abdominal approaches, 2 to 3 cm of esophageal length should be in the abdomen without tension. Collis gastroplasty can be considered from the chest and is technically identical to abdominal approaches. This is discussed in another chapter.
- Crural sutures are then placed. A Babcock clamp can be used to grasp and elevate each crural pillar. Interrupted 0-polyester permanent braided sutures are then placed 0.5 cm apart beginning in the caudal direction. Anterior sutures may be placed if the hiatus is very large to avoid angulation of the esophagus as it passes through the hiatus. These sutures are tagged and left untied until the fundoplication is completed (Figure 31.8).

Belsey Mark IV Fundoplication

- A 54- or 56-French Maloney dilator or bougie is then passed through the esophagus.

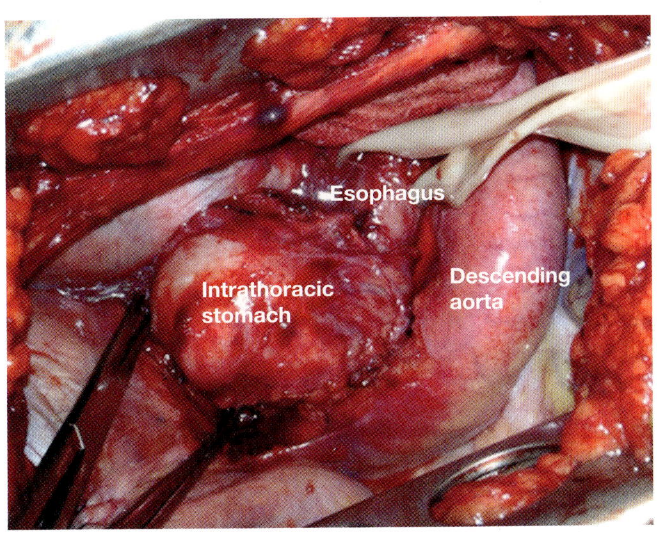

FIGURE 31.7 ▌ The proximal esophagus has been circumferentially dissected, and Penrose drain is placed around it. The intrathoracic stomach has been dissected, and Babcock clamps are placed on the left and right crus. (Courtesy of Douglas J. Minnich, MD.)

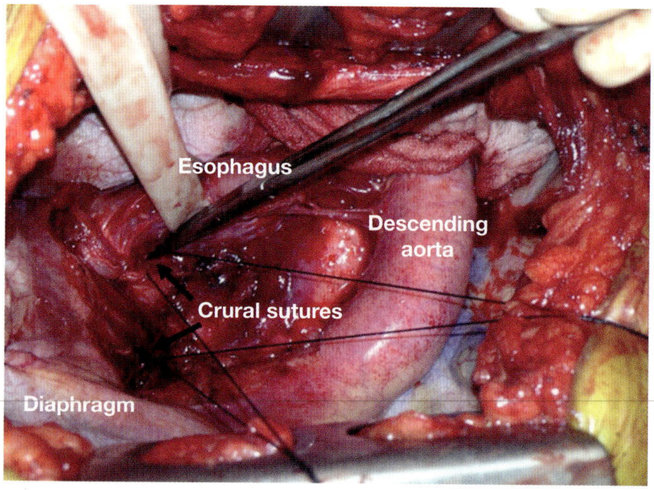

FIGURE 31.8 | Heavy silk sutures are placed for the crural closure but not tied. These are clamped and will be tied after the fundoplication. (Courtesy of Douglas J. Minnich, MD.)

- A double-armed 2-0 silk suture should be used with an atraumatic needle.
- The first suture is placed longitudinally in the esophageal muscle for a distance of 0.5 cm and begun 1.5 cm above the GEJ. This should be located just anterior to the mobilized right vagus nerve posteriorly. It is then passed through the seromuscular layer of the fundus 1.5 cm distal to the GEJ. The second arm of the suture is then placed in a similar fashion 0.5 cm away from the first.
- The second suture is placed in a similar fashion at the midline of the esophagus approximately 135° from the first.
- The third suture is once again placed like the previous two but 135° further from the second suture (Figure 31.9).
- The first three sutures are then tied down in sequence. It is important to have consistent spacing of the fundal stitches to avoid bunching of the fundus as it rolls up.
- A second tier of sutures are then placed in a similar fashion starting 1.5 cm above the previous esophageal sutures. After passing the needle through the fundus, the needles should be kept on the suture.
- A malleable or spoon is then used to protect the abdominal viscera, and the suture is passed through the diaphragmatic hiatus from the abdominal side to the chest side. The stomach is gently reduced into the abdomen, and the sutures are then tied sequentially (Figure 31.10).
- The crural closure sutures are then tied (Figure 31.11).
- An index finger of space should be noted between the last crural stitch and the third Belsey fundoplication stitch.
- A pleural drain is then placed, the left lung is reinflated, and the chest is closed in the standard fashion. We do not routinely use a nasogastric tube.

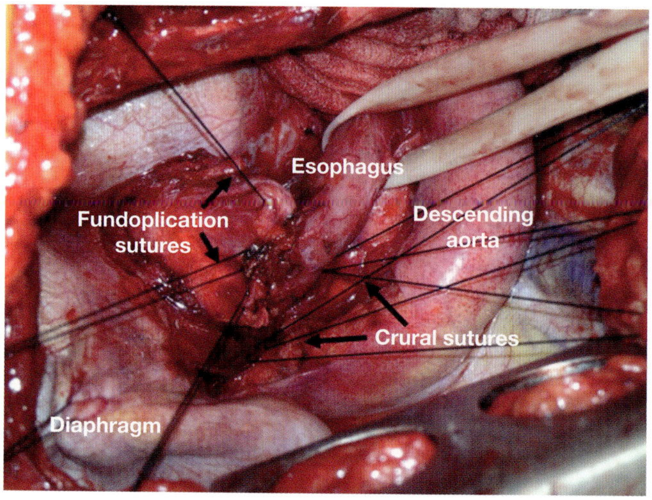

FIGURE 31.9 | A double-armed 2-0 silk suture is then used to start the Belsey fundoplication. The sutures are placed longitudinally 1.5 cm above the gastroesophageal junction (GEJ) through the esophagus and then the fundus of the stomach, 1.5 cm distal to the GEJ and approximately 0.5 cm apart in parallel. These are tied down sequentially after three total sutures are placed 135° apart. (Courtesy of Douglas J. Minnich, MD.)

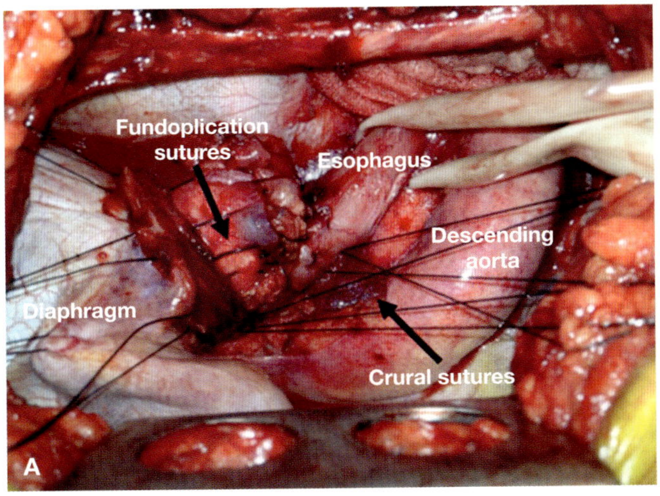

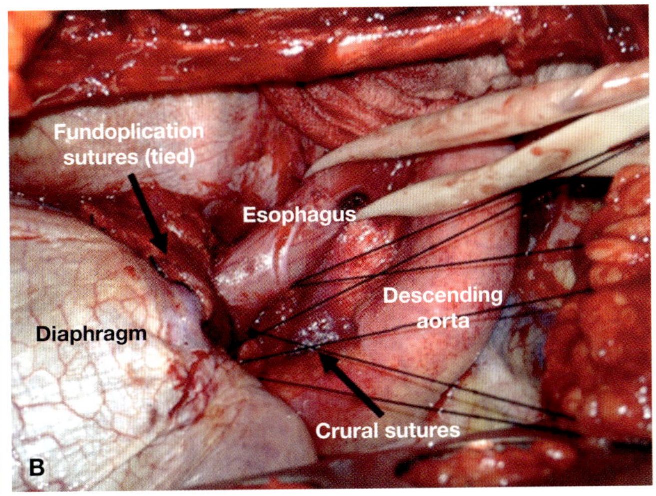

FIGURE 31.10 ‖ **A.** Another row of double-armed 2-0 silk suture are placed in a similar fashion, 1.5 cm above the previous layer. These are also passed through the stomach and then through the crus of the diaphragm. A malleable or spoon can be used through the hiatus to ensure no damage to intra-abdominal structures. **B.** These are then tied down sequentially. (Courtesy of Douglas J. Minnich, MD.)

Postoperative Care

- The initial postoperative course is identical to transabdominal approaches (see above).
- The exception is postoperative pain control. An erector spinae nerve block is performed in the operating room by our anesthesia colleagues. The patient is also given IV pain medicine via patient-controlled analgesia overnight while the patient is NPO.
- If the UGI on the morning of postoperative day 1 is satisfactory, the patient is advanced to clears followed by full liquids as described above.
- The patient is transitioned to oral pain medicine as soon as possible. As this is usually the rate-limiting factor to hospital discharge.

PEARLS AND PITFALLS

Transthoracic Approach

- When dissecting the esophagus off the aortic plane, there can sometimes be large perforators. If one of these is dislodged, the bleeding can be profuse. Special care should be made to ligate these as they are found.
- If the hernia and GEJ are not reduced below the diaphragm with minimal tension, then esophageal lengthening (Collis) can be completed from the chest.

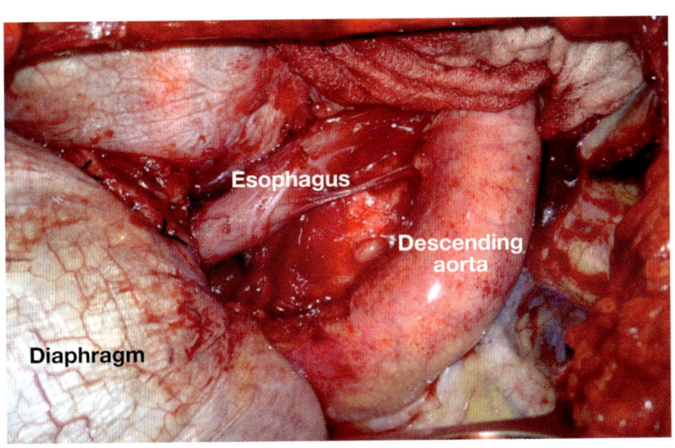

FIGURE 31.11 ‖ The hiatal sutures are then tied. The stomach should be completely reduced. The hiatus should be loose enough to slide a finger periesophageal without too much tension. (Courtesy of Douglas J. Minnich, MD.)

Suggested Readings

1. Allen MS. Belsey procedure—how I teach it. *Ann Thorac Surg*. 2016;102:4-6.
2. Karush J, Sarkaria IS. Robotic-assisted giant paraesophageal hernia repair and Nissen fundoplication. *Oper Tech Thorac Cardiovasc Surg*. 2013;18(3):204-214.
3. Skinner DB, Belsey RH. Surgical management of esophageal reflux and hiatus hernia: long-term results with 1,030 patients. *J Thorac Cardiovasc Surg*. 1967;53:33-54.
4. Laan DV, Agzarina J, Harmsen WS, et al. A comparison between Belsey Mark IV and laparoscopic Nissen fundoplication in patients with large paraesophageal hernia. *J Thorac Cardiovasc Surg*. 2018;156:418-428.
5. Luketich JD, Nason KS, Christie NA, et al. Outcomes after a decade of laparoscopic giant paraesophageal hernia repair. *J Thorac Cardiovasc Surg*. 2010;139:395-404.
6. Sarkaria IS, Laftif MJ, Bianco VJ, et al. Early operative outcomes and learning curve of robotic assisted giant paraesophageal hernia repair. *Int J Med Robot*. 2017;13(1):e1730.

Chapter 32

Collis Gastroplasty

S. ANSLEY SMITH
JESSICA L. MASCH
MATTHEW P. FOX

Perioperative Considerations

- Gastroplasty is usually performed in conjunction with a fundoplication procedure in patients with a shortened esophagus.
- Esophageal lengthening is usually needed if the gastroesophageal (GE) junction is at or above the hiatus after the mediastinal esophagus is fully mobilized.
  - Long-standing history of gastroesophageal reflux disease (GERD) with or without a failed antireflux operation or evidence of dysmotility or a shortened esophagus on manometry should increase suspicion of a shortened esophagus and possible need for Collis gastroplasty.

Anesthesia and Patient Positioning

- General endotracheal anesthesia with chemical paralysis and an orogastric tube
- Supine positioning with arms tucked in steep reverse Trendelenburg position to improve visualization of the GE junction
  - Alternately, low lithotomy with the surgeon standing between the patient's legs

Instruments and Equipment

- 5- to 10-mm 30° laparoscope
- Self-retaining liver retractor
- Two 5-mm atraumatic bowel graspers
- 5-mm vessel-sealing device
- 45-mm articulating linear endoscopic stapler with blue loads

Technique

Port Placement

- Demonstrated in Figure 32.1A-E
- Place the camera port 12 to 15 cm below the xiphoid process slightly to the patient's right (Figure 32.1C)
- A 5-mm subxiphoid self-retaining liver retractor to retract the left lobe of the liver anterolaterally (Figure 32.1B)
- A 5-mm port in the right subcostal margin for the surgeon's left hand (Figure 32.1A)
- A 12-mm working port in the left midclavicular line for the stapler (Figure 32.1D)
- A 5-mm assistant port in the left subcostal margin for retraction on the stomach (Figure 32.1E)

Surgical Approaches

- Can be performed transthoracic via a left thoracotomy, transabdominally via open or laparoscopic techniques, or through a combined transthoracic/transabdominal approach
  - Transabdominal approach usually as part of a Nissen fundoplication or other antireflux procedure

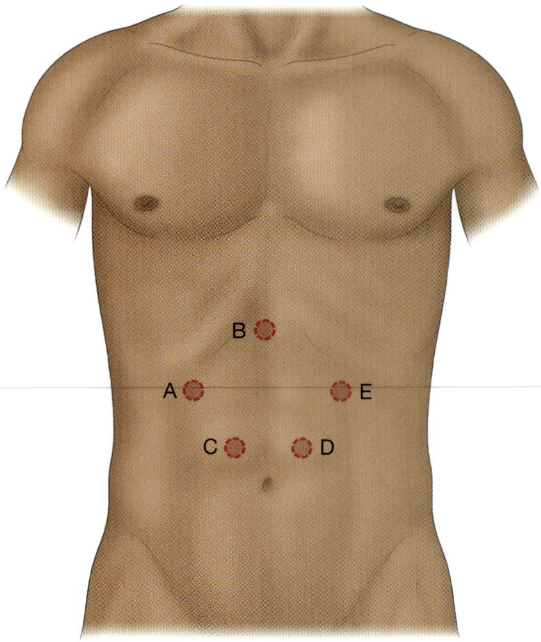

FIGURE 32.1 ▮ Trocar placement. **A.** 5-mm port for left hand. **B.** 5-mm port for self-retaining liver retractor. **C.** 5- to 10-mm port for camera. **D.** 12-mm working port for stapler. **E.** 5-mm assistant port.

Historical Approaches

- Original Collis gastroplasty—vertical suture line parallel to the esophagus performed through a right-sided thoracoabdominal incision
  - Lesser curvature suture line forms the "connecting tube" or neoesophagus
  - Fundal suture line placed below the diaphragm
- **Thoracoscopic/laparoscopic**—stapler introduced through a port site in the right chest and placed parallel to and above the abdominal esophagus flush against the dilator
- **Laparoscopic circular**—circular stapler creates a sealed gastric window through which a linear stapler is fired vertically adjacent to the dilator

Laparoscopic Transabdominal

- After mobilization of the esophagus and removal of the epiphrenic fat pad, perform gastroplasty if the intra-abdominal length is less than or equal to 3 cm or if the GE junction is not below the hiatus.
  - Place a 48-French bougie along the lesser curvature of the stomach.
  - Identify and mark the stomach 2.5 to 5 cm below the angle of His at the location of the new GE junction (Figure 32.2).
    - This marks the inferior edge of the vertical staple line.
    - This provides enough length to perform a short, floppy fundoplication around the neoesophagus.
  - Introduce the stapler through the 12-mm working port at the left midclavicular line (Figure 32.3).
    - Angle the stapler maximally to the patient's right perpendicular to the bougie toward the target of the new GE junction.
    - Grasp the stomach at the angle of His with the left hand while the assistant grasps along the greater curvature and retracts inferiorly.
  - An additional staple load is typically needed to reach the target.
  - Fire a single vertical staple load parallel to the bougie (Figure 32.4).
  - Inspect the staple lines and remove the gastric wedge.
  - Perform a fundoplication if indicated.

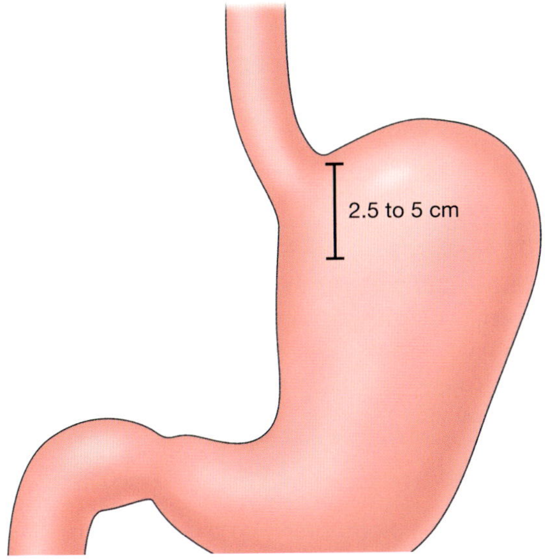

FIGURE 32.2 ▮ Location of the new gastroesophageal junction.

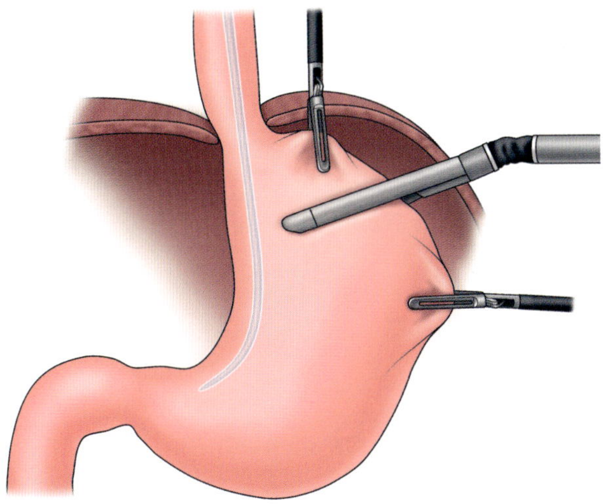

FIGURE 32.3 ▮ Angle the stapler perpendicular to the bougie toward the target of the new gastroesophageal junction.

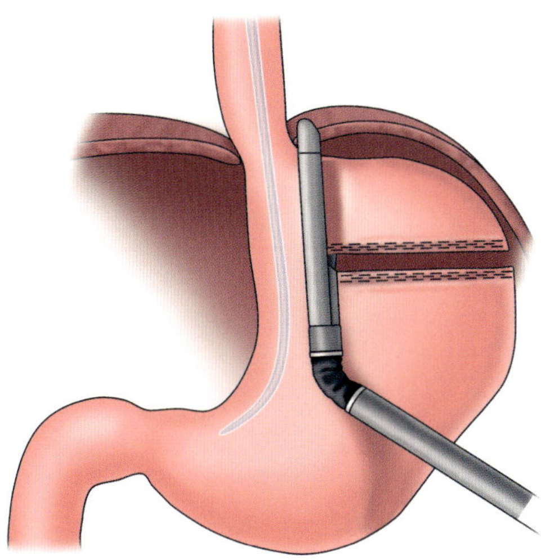

FIGURE 32.4 ▮ Single vertical staple load parallel to the bougie to complete the formation of the new neoesophagus.

TIPS

Make sure to push the bougie out of the stapler to prevent a redundant gastric tube.

Postoperative Care

- Patients remain nothing by mouth until postoperative day 1.
- Gastric decompression is typically not needed in the postoperative period.
- Perform contrast esophagram on postoperative day 1 to assess for leak.
- Advance to clear liquids if no leak on esophagram and slowly to full liquids/soft foods thereafter.
- Patients are usually ready for discharge on postoperative day 1 after tolerating clear liquids.

Possible Complications and Functional Issues

- Leak from staple lines, necrosis if the blood supply to the neoesophagus is compromised, or early dysphagia if the neoesophagus is too tight.
- GERD symptoms may not completely resolve after surgery due to the presence of functioning gastric mucosa in the neoesophagus.

PEARLS AND PITFALLS

- Trocar placement 12 to 15 mm from xiphoid process is key.
    - Placement at the umbilicus may prevent adequate mobilization of the esophagus in the mediastinum.
- If fundoplication is performed, make sure that the first bite is on the native esophagus and not on the neoesophagus to avoid a slipped fundoplication.

Suggested Readings

1. Collis JL. An operation for hiatus hernia with short oesophagus. *Thorax*. 1957;12(3):181-188.
2. Horvath KD, Swanstrom LL, Jobe BA. The short esophagus: pathophysiology, incidence, presentation, and treatment in the era of laparoscopic antireflux surgery. *Ann Surg*. 2000;232(5):630-640.
3. Johnson AB, Oddsdottir M, Hunter JG. Laparoscopic Collis gastroplasty and Nissen fundoplication. A new technique for the management of esophageal foreshortening. *Surg Endosc*. 1998;12(8):1055-1060.
4. Swanstrom LL, Marcus DR, Galloway GQ. Laparoscopic Collis gastroplasty is the treatment of choice for the shortened esophagus. *Am J Surg*. 1996;171(5):477-481.

Chapter 33

Reoperative Antireflux Surgery: Minimally Invasive Surgery/Thoracotomy

NIKHIL PANDA
PAUL W. FURLOW
CHRISTOPHER R. MORSE

Perioperative Considerations

- Minimally invasive techniques (ie, laparoscopic- and robotic-assisted) are the gold standard operative approaches for antireflux surgery.
- Fundoplication failure rates range from 20% to 30% with 3% to 6% of patients undergoing revisional, or "redo," operations.
- Prior to reoperation, evaluation includes:
  - Comprehensive history and physical exam focusing on symptom complex (eg, gastroesophageal reflux disease, dysphagia, pain) and health-related quality of life assessment
  - Review of all prior operative reports (eg, operative anatomy, use of mesh, type of fundoplication)
  - Preoperative testing with contrast esophagography, pH testing, manometry, esophagogastroduodenoscopy, and gastric emptying studies. Computed tomography of the chest, abdomen, and pelvis is valuable.
  - Cardiopulmonary assessment including pulmonary function testing, especially among patients for whom open transthoracic approaches are planned.
- The goals of reoperative antireflux surgery is to:
  - restore "normal" anatomy with complete takedown of prior sutures/fundoplication/repair,
  - restoration of intra-abdominal gastroesophageal junction,
  - esophageal mobilization with adequate intra-abdominal esophageal length,
  - crural repair, and
  - often an antireflux operation, typically a partial fundoplication.

Instruments and Equipment

Minimally Invasive Approach

- Ports (Figure 33.1): Optical entry (5-mm) versus Hasson (12-mm camera), liver retractor (5-mm), surgeon grasper (5-mm), surgeon dissector/suture (12-mm), assistant grasper (5-mm)
- 10-mm 30° laparoscopic
- Flexible articulating laparoscopic liver retractor
- Two atraumatic bowel graspers
- Energy device (eg, laparoscopic harmonic scalpel)
- Endoscopic suturing device
- Endoscopic stapling device
- Endoscope for esophagogastroduodenoscopy
- Esophageal bougies (eg, Maloney tapered bougies)

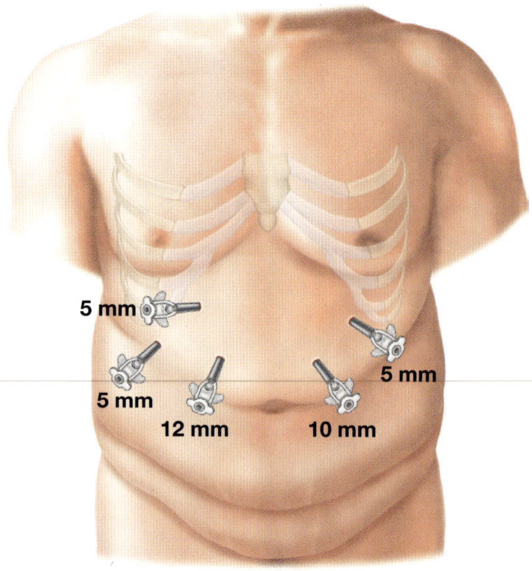

FIGURE 33.1 ▌ Laparoscopic port placement for minimally invasive antireflux surgery. (From Smith BR, Nguyen NT. Gastric bypass. In: Luketich J, ed. *Master Techniques in Surgery: Esophageal Surgery*. Wolters Kluwer; 2015:97-107. Figure 9.1.)

Open Approach

- Double-lumen endotracheal tube with pediatric flexible bronchoscopy
- Standard thoracotomy/laparotomy instruments
- Fixed retractor system (eg, Thompson or Omni-Tract)
- Endoscope for esophagogastroduodenoscopy
- Esophageal bougies (eg, Maloney tapered bougies)

Patient Positioning

- Minimally invasive approach:
  - Supine position
  - Arms abducted at 90° with padding on hands, joints, intravenous catheters, and monitoring devices
  - Adjustable foot board
  - Laparoscopic monitors placed above arm boards at eye level

Open Approach

- Right lateral decubitus position, hips and arms secured, padding on hands, joints, intravenous catheter, and monitoring devices
- Operating table flexed

TIPS

- *Coordination with an experienced anesthesiologist and use of rapid sequence intubation is encouraged.*
- *Use of an arterial line including in MIS approaches can be helpful for monitoring hemodynamics during insufflation and inadvertent capnothorax.*
- *For reoperative laparoscopic entry, place the first laparoscopic port away from prior incisions to avoid injury to intra-abdominal structures.*
- *If capnothorax occurs with hemodynamic compromise, a 12-French pigtail catheter is placed on the affected side and placed to suction during the remainder of the case.*
- *In the crural repair, endoscopy can be used to evaluate if there is a concern of tight crural closure with diaphragmatic or crural indentation.*
- *Use of endoluminal functional lumen imaging probe (EndoFLIP) preoperatively or intraoperatively as an adjunct during crural repair/fundoplication can provide objective measures of gastroesophageal junction morphology.*
- *For open cases, we employ thoracoabdominal approach, balancing the added pain of a thoracotomy with the unparalleled exposure of the esophagus, gastroesophageal junction, and abdomen.*

Techniques

Minimally Invasive Approach

- Anesthetic and monitoring: single-lumen endotracheal tube, two large-bore peripheral intravenous catheters, arterial line for hemodynamic monitoring, nasogastric tube
- Endoscopic evaluation: assessment of mucosal pathology (eg, Barrett esophagus), location and integrity of prior repair/wrap, mechanism of failure (eg, twisted or herniated wrap), esophageal length
- Incisions and exposure
  - Open technique for initial port placement
  - If adhesions prevent standard port placement as described above, an additional 5-mm port in the right or left lower quadrant is placed for lysis of adhesions before converting to standard ports (Figure 33.1).
  - Position the patient in reverse Trendelenburg to displace mobile intestine and omentum into the pelvis.

Esophagogastric Dissection

- Meticulous dissection with lysis of adhesions
- Typically work clockwise beginning between esophagogastric junction and liver and dissecting anteriorly, left laterally, and then posteriorly (Figure 33.2)

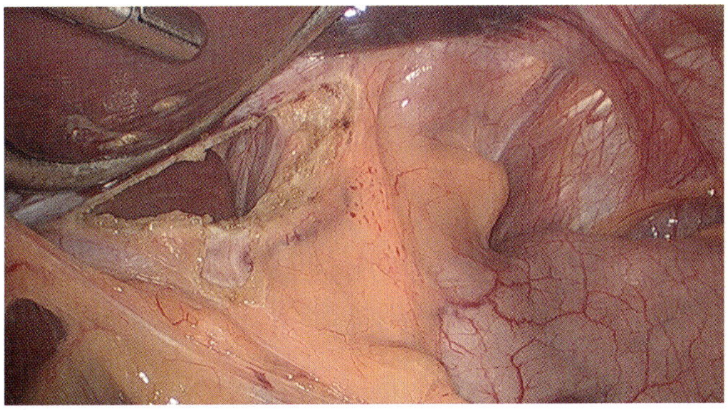

FIGURE 33.2 ▮ Laparoscopic esophagogastric dissection. (From Mittal SK. Laparoscopic Nissen fundoplication. In: Luketich J, ed. *Master Techniques in Surgery: Esophageal Surgery*. Wolters Kluwer; 2015:1-13. Figure 1.4.)

- The goal is to complete the dissection circumferentially, but in a reoperative field, the surgeon may need to regularly move to a different location if not making progress.
- All prior sutures and complete takedown of the fundoplication must be performed to identify anatomy and allow subsequent esophageal mobilization.

Esophageal Mobilization ± Lengthening

- The intra-abdominal and intrathoracic esophagus is mobilized circumferentially to allow 3 cm of intra-abdominal length (Figure 33.3).

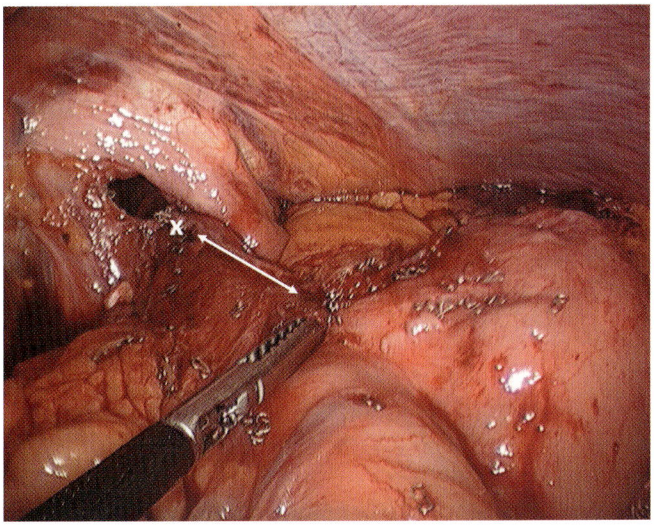

FIGURE 33.3 ▮ Esophagogastric junction dissection and esophageal mobilization demonstrating adequate length (3 cm) of intra-abdominal esophagus. (From Antonoff MB, Andrade RS, Maddaus MA. Laparoscopic Collis gastroplasty. In: Luketich J, ed. *Master Techniques in Surgery: Esophageal Surgery*. Wolters Kluwer; 2015:65-74. Figure 6.10.).

- The gastroesophageal junction fat pad, if present, is resected.
- If the esophagus is shortened, an esophageal lengthening procedure with a wedge fundectomy (eg, laparoscopic Collis gastroplasty) is performed (Figure 33.4):

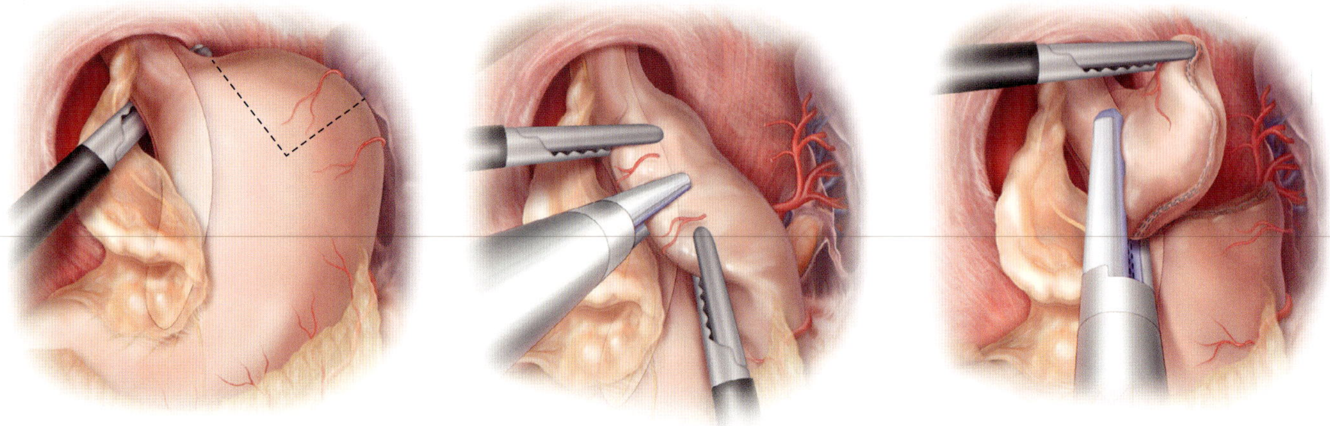

FIGURE 33.4 ▌ Technique of laparoscopic Collis gastroplasty (ie, wedge fundectomy) for purposes of esophageal lengthening. (From Nason KS, Luketich JD. Laparoscopic paraesophageal hernia repair. In: Luketich J, ed. *Master Techniques in Surgery: Esophageal Surgery*. Wolters Kluwer; 2015:121-135. Figure 11.7.)

- A 54- to 56-French Maloney tapered bougie is placed across the esophagogastric junction toward the incisura angularis along the lesser curvature of the stomach.
- Atraumatic graspers proximally and distally splay out the fundus of the stomach toward the spleen to visualize the position of the bougie, angle of His, and fundus without any folds or twists.
- An endoscopic stapler is then used to place a first staple fire from the greater curvature toward the lateral edge of the esophageal bougie.
- Additional staple fires are placed along the esophageal bougie to complete the gastric wedge resection.

Crural Repair

- A posterior crural repair is performed with a series of simple, interrupted, permanent sutures.
- The crura are approximated such that the distance of a single finger breadth between the esophagus and crura remain (Figure 33.5).

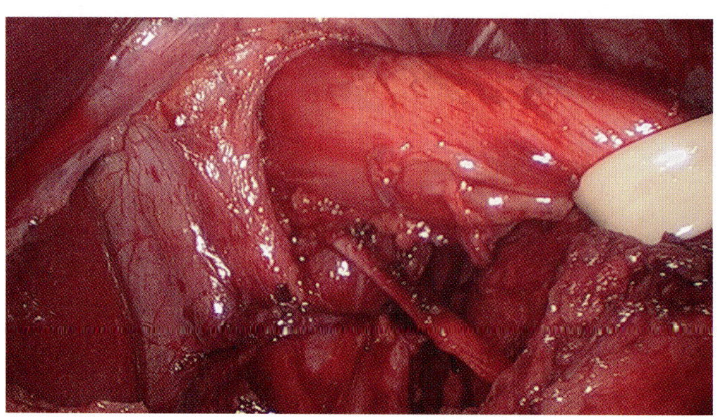

FIGURE 33.5 ▌ Posterior suture approximation of crura. (From Mittal SK. Laparoscopic Nissen fundoplication. In: Luketich J, ed. *Master Techniques in Surgery: Esophageal Surgery*. Wolters Kluwer; 2015:1-13. Figure 1.10.)

- If the crura cannot be approximated in a tension-free manner, a relaxing incision is made in the diaphragm; the incision is typically 2 cm away and parallel to the right crus or anteriorly/radially along the diaphragm (Figure 33.6).
- Following crural closure, the diaphragmatic defect from the relaxing incision is closed (Figure 33.6). When mesh is needed, we favor biologic porcine mesh.

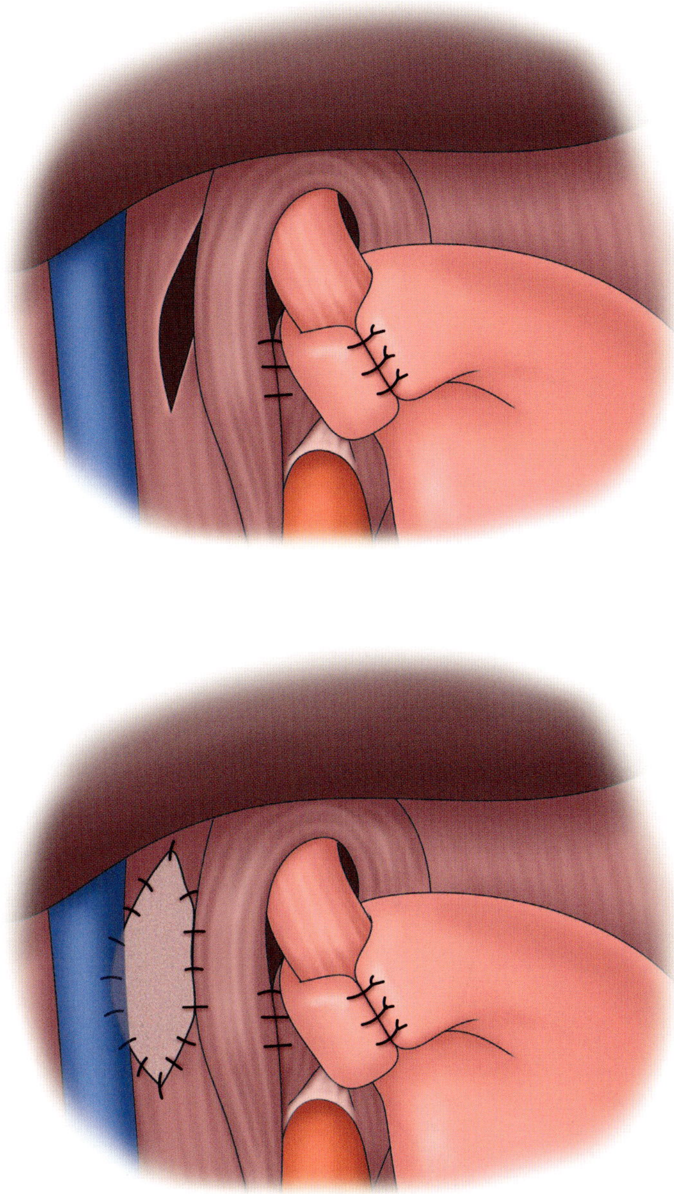

FIGURE 33.6 | Relaxing incision adjacent to right crus for a large hiatus with overlying mesh, separated from crural repair.

Fundoplication

- We typically perform a partial Toupet or complete 360° Nissen fundoplication, informed by preoperative manometry and assessment of esophageal motility. For the partial Toupet fundoplication:
  - The mobilized fundus is delivered behind the esophagus (Figure 33.7).

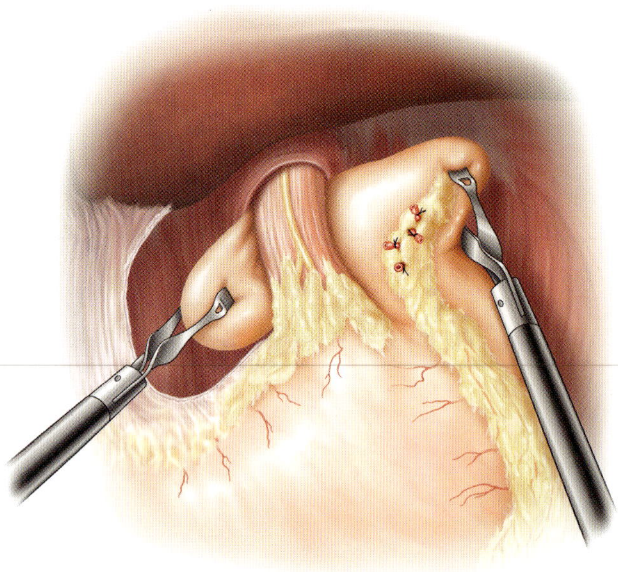

FIGURE 33.7 ■ Delivery of fundus posteriorly to the mobilized esophagus to assess position of subsequent fundoplication. (From Kastenmeier AS, Swanstrom LL. Laparoscopic partial fundoplications. In: Luketich J, ed. *Master Techniques in Surgery: Esophageal Surgery*. Wolters Kluwer; 2015:15-28. Figure 2.6.)

- Simple, interrupted, permanent sutures are placed between the delivered fundus and the right crus with additional sutures placed between the fundus and the esophagus (Figure 33.8).

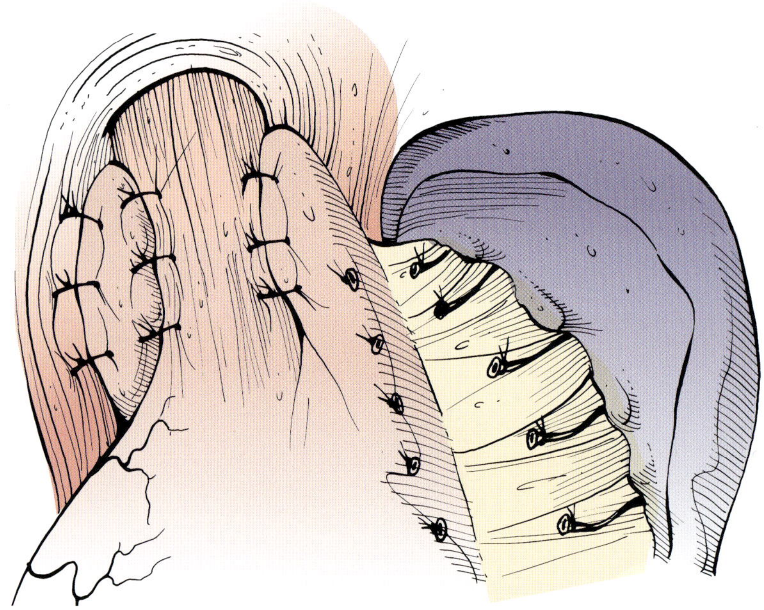

FIGURE 33.8 ■ Toupet fundoplication demonstrating sutures between fundus and esophagus with additional anchoring sutures between fundus and crura. (From Soper, Hungness ES. Laparoscopic antireflux surgery. In: Fischer JE, ed. *Fischer's Mastery of Surgery*. 7th ed. Wolters Kluwer; 2019:945-961. Figure 74.6.)

- Similar sutures are placed left of the esophagus between the fundus and left crus, as well as the fundus and esophagus.
- Completion endoscopy can be performed if desired. The nasogastric tube is removed prior to closing and extubation.

Open Approach

- Anesthetic and monitoring: thoracic epidural anesthesia, double-lumen endotracheal tube, two large-bore peripheral intravenous catheters, arterial line for hemodynamic monitoring, nasogastric tube, Foley catheter

- Endoscopic evaluation as described above
- A left curvilinear thoracoabdominal incision is made beginning below the scapular angle, crossing the left costal margin, and oriented toward a location halfway between the xiphoid and umbilicus (Figure 33.9). The left chest is entered in the seventh interspace.

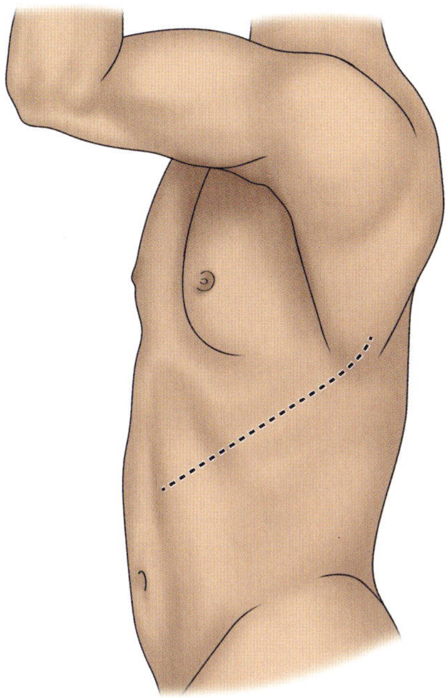

FIGURE 33.9 ‖ Incision for thoracoabdominal approach to the esophagogastric junction. A line is drawn from the scapular angle across the costal margin to half way between the xiphoid and umbilicus.

- Like the laparoscopic approach, the conduct of the operation includes careful dissection of the esophagogastric junction (Figure 33.10), takedown of the prior repair, esophageal mobilization with potential esophageal lengthening, crural approximation, and fundoplication.

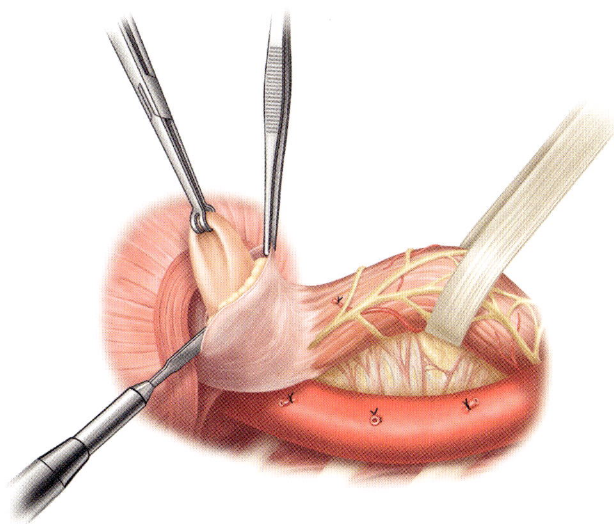

FIGURE 33.10 ‖ Transthoracic esophagogastric and hiatal dissection. (From Darling G, Griffith FP. Open paraesophageal hernia: transthoracic approach. In: Luketich J, ed. *Master Techniques in Surgery: Esophageal Surgery*. Wolters Kluwer; 2015:137-146. Figure 12.1.)

- In specific cases, the left thoracoabdominal approach also allows for creation of a Roux-en-Y gastrojejunostomy (eg, severe gastric dysmotility and reflux) or esophagogastrectomy. Typically, this need arises when the lower esophageal sphincter is not reconstructable following multiple previous procedures. The conduct of these operations is discussed elsewhere in this text.
- Prior to closure of the chest, a 28-French chest tube and 19-French Blake drain are placed into the left pleural space.
- Completion endoscopy is performed and a nasogastric tube is placed prior to closing and extubation.

Postoperative Care

Minimally Invasive Approach

- **Postoperative Day 0:** Patients are transported to the postoperative anesthesia care unit, and postoperative chest radiograph to evaluate for capnothorax is obtained. Strict nil per os diet with nasogastric tube continuous suction.
- **Postoperative Day 1:** Gastrografin and dilute barium swallow study is obtained with initiation of limited clear liquid diet and hospital discharge.
- **Postoperative Day 2 to 14:** Slow advancement from limited clear liquids, to full liquids, to soft solid diet.
- **Postoperative Day 14:** Surgical follow-up appointment and first health-related quality of life assessment.

Open Approach

- **Postoperative Day 0:** Patients are transported to the surgical intensive care unit, where an immediate postoperative chest radiograph is obtained. Strict nil per os diet with nasogastric tube to continuous suction.
- **Postoperative Day 1 to 3:** Patients are transferred to the postoperative recovery ward. The epidural catheter and nasogastric tube remain, the chest tube is discontinued, and patients are kept nil per os.
- **Postoperative Day 4:** Gastrografin and dilute barium swallow study is obtained with subsequent nasogastric tube removal and initiation of limited clear liquid diet. Epidural, Foley, and Blake drain are removed.
- **Postoperative Day 5:** Discharge on limited clear liquid diet.
- **Postoperative Day 14:** Surgical follow-up appointment and first health-related quality of life assessment.

PEARLS AND PITFALLS

- All efforts should be made to avoid inadvertent esophageal entry or gastrotomy during gastroesophageal junction dissection and esophageal mobilization. There is a tendency to err toward the stomach/wrap to avoid esophageal or vagal nerve injury; however, multiple gastrotomies and repairs limit subsequent fundoplication options.
- It is critical to completely takedown the prior repair and fundoplication to restore "normal" anatomy. It may be tempting to only partially takedown or remove sutures to avoid damage to nearby structures. This approach leads to a higher rate of failure of the revision.
- When considering an open approach, a transabdominal approach can be considered. However, our experience is that the transthoracic approach provides superior exposure, fewer adhesions, and greater versatility in revisional operations.

Suggested Readings

1. Awais O, Luketich JD, Schuchert MJ, et al. Reoperative antireflux surgery for failed fundoplication: an analysis of outcomes in 275 patients. *Ann Thorac Surg*. 2011;92(3):1083-1090.
2. Morse CR, Broussard BL. Laparoscopic techniques in reoperation for failed antireflux repair. In: Darling GE, Baumgartner WA, Jacobs JP, eds. *Pearson's General Thoracic Surgery. STS Cardiothoracic Surgery E-Book*. 2020; Society of Thoracic Surgeons.
3. Su B, Attaar M, Wong H, et al. Using a standardized intra-operative endoflip protocol during fundoplication to identify factors that affect distensibility. *Surg Endosc*. 2021;35(10):5717-5723.

Chapter 34

Achalasia

AARON DINERMAN
LEONIDAS TAPIAS

Perioperative Considerations

General

- It is an absolute necessity to rule out malignancy, mass lesions, or other causes of pseudoachalasia.
- Previous upper gastrointestinal surgeries, especially history of fundoplication or hiatal hernia repair, can lead to sequelae of symptoms mimicking achalasia.
- Esophageal manometry is key in the diagnosis. Findings consist of aperistalsis of the esophagus and impaired relaxation of the lower esophageal sphincter (LES) with occasional elevated LES pressures.
- Computed tomography of the chest and abdomen is optional but can be useful to rule out pseudoachalasia.
- It is very important to establish if the patient has undergone any other treatment for achalasia. Botox injections and balloon or Savary dilations can make the myotomy more tedious.
- There are three types of achalasia: Type I (classic) involves little or no contractility in the majority length of the esophagus, type II involves oscillatory periods of esophageal contraction, and type III (spastic) involves spastic contractions of the distal esophagus.
- Type II achalasia has optimal response to treatment, followed by type I. Type III achalasia has very poor treatment response.

Preoperative Instruction

- It is imperative to discuss with the patient the possibility of future interventions and to manage expectations.
- The patient should follow a liquid diet prior to surgery to help clear the esophagus and prevent having food debris in the esophageal lumen.

Technical Considerations

Transthoracic

Anesthesia and Positioning

- Preoperative placement of an epidural catheter for postoperative pain control
- Double-lumen endotracheal tube to allow single-lung ventilation of the right lung during left thoracotomy
- Patient is placed in the right lateral decubitus, standard thoracotomy position with slight tilting of the hips back in the remote case that the incision needs to be extended to the abdomen.

Instruments and Equipment

- Esophagogastroduodenoscope (EGD)
- Penrose drain
- Energy device (harmonic scalpel and electrocautery)
- Esophageal bougie (54-French)

- Sutures for fundoplication (2-0 nonabsorbable)
- Kittners for blunt dissection

Technique

- EGD is done at the beginning of the case to assess for retention of food debris and the integrity of the esophageal mucosa.
- Left thoracotomy is performed in the seventh intercostal space.
- Retraction of the lung anteriorly and superiorly. The inferior pulmonary ligament is transected to help expose the distal esophagus.
- Mediastinal pleura is opened, and the esophagus is dissected circumferentially. A Penrose drain can be placed around the esophagus to help with retraction and exposure.
- Myotomy is performed with a combination of forceps and Kittners. In some instances when anatomy permits, myotomy can be done with the harmonic scalpel using the cold arm of the instrument to dissect the muscle and the hot arm to transect. It is important to avoid sharp dissection or heat when in close proximity to the submucosa.
- The length of the myotomy can vary but usually involves the proximal 5 to 7 cm and about 1 cm into the stomach, to the level of the submucosal gastric veins.
- Placing an esophageal bougie can help stretch the mucosa, thereby avoiding folds and making the myotomy easier and safer.
- A fundoplication should be performed in the setting of a hiatal hernia or when a longer myotomy is needed in the stomach.
- A 28-French chest tube is placed under direct visualization and the left thoracotomy is closed in layers.

Laparoscopic

Anesthesia and Positioning

- Single-lumen endotracheal tube
- Supine with arms out and footboard in preparation for steep reverse Trendelenburg position

Instruments and Equipment

- EGD
- Laparoscopic ports: two 12-mm ports, two 5-mm ports
- Liver retractor (ie, Nathanson retractor)
- Energy device (harmonic scalpel and electrocautery)
- Esophageal bougie (54-French)
- Endoscopic Kittners for blunt dissection

Technique

- Start with EGD. It is very important to minimize insufflation to prevent bowel distention that might interfere with laparoscopic visualization.
- An open technique is used to place the first port. A 1-cm incision is performed two-third of the distance from the xiphoid to the umbilicus on the left paramedian side to place the first 12-mm port. The second port is placed a hand breath to the right. The two 5-mm ports are placed on each flank. A small incision is made in the subxiphoid area to place the Nathanson retractor.
- Start by dividing the gastrohepatic ligament. This dissection is carried anteriorly toward the left crus. It is important to maintain the peritoneal covering of the crura (Figure 34.1)

TIPS

At this point, it is very helpful to start dividing the short gastric vessels and retract the stomach to the patient's right side. This allows a better dissection of the hiatus and helps identifying higher and more posterior short gastric vessels (Figures 34.2 and 34.3).

- Define the gastroesophageal junction. Separate the longitudinal fibers with the help of two graspers.

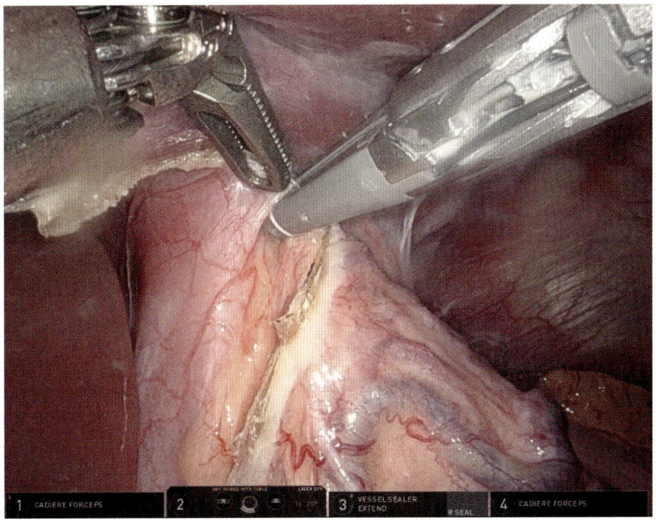

FIGURE 34.1 | The phrenoesophageal membrane is incised along the right crus, taking care to minimize violation of the crura peritoneum.

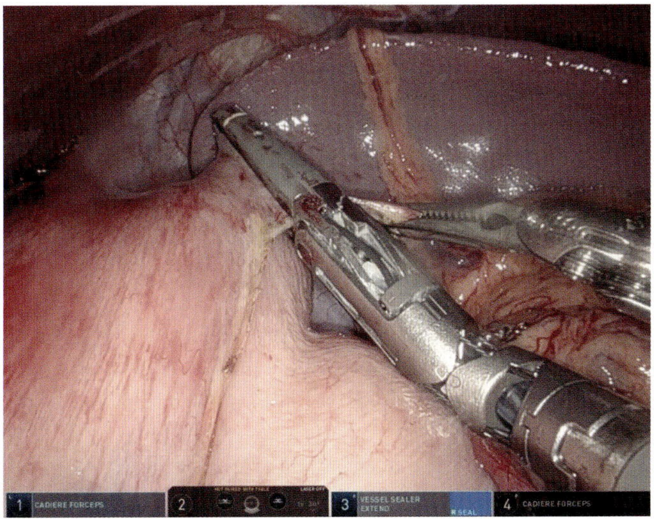

FIGURE 34.2 | Intraoperative view of robotic Heller myotomy demonstrating division of the short gastrics within the gastrosplenic ligament utilizing energy device (robotic vessel sealer).

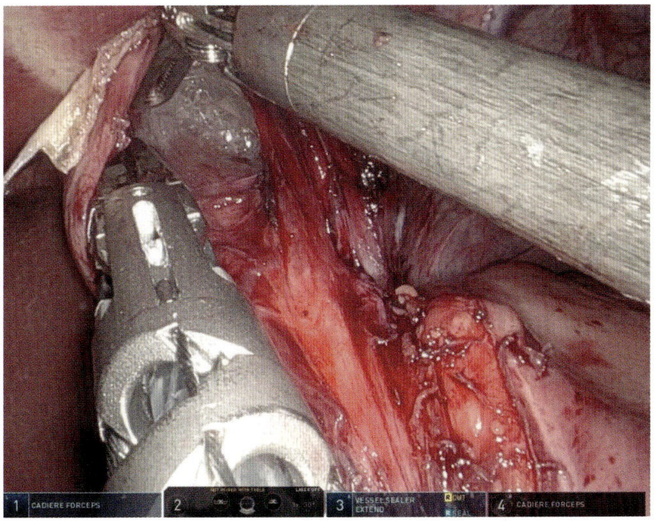

FIGURE 34.3 | Ample mediastinal dissection is imperative to accommodate enough esophageal length for the myotomy.

TIPS

During this part of the operation, it is helpful to insert a bougie. The bougie distends the mucosa, preventing folding which can cause accidental injuries (Figure 34.4).

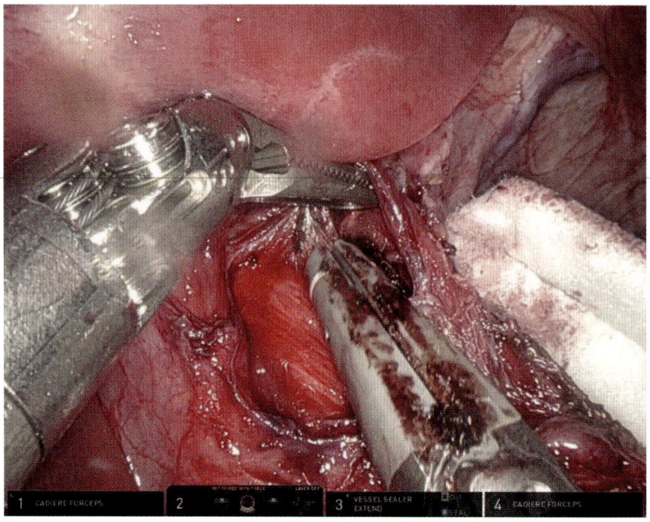

FIGURE 34.4 | Separation of the adventitia reveals the longitudinal muscle fibers as the myotomy is initiated with energy device (robotic vessel sealer).

- Circular fibers are identified and separated from the submucosa. The extension of the myotomy is usually 5 cm proximal and 2 to 3 cm distal. Some use impedance planimetry (ie, EndoFLIP) to assess the myotomy and the need for a longer extension.
- Once there is a good mucosal bulging, an EGD can help visualize the distal esophagus and assess for any mucosal injury.
- The hiatus is repaired, and a partial fundoplication is performed (ie, Dor vs Toupet). The advantage of a Dor fundoplication is the ability to "buttress" the myotomy site (Figure 34.5).

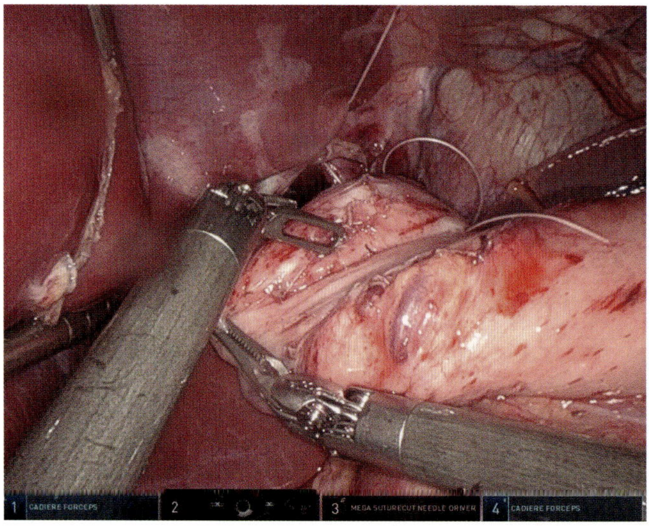

FIGURE 34.5 | An anterior fundoplication taking care to avoid serosal injury to the fundus.

Endoscopic

Anesthesia and Positioning

- General anesthesia with a single-lumen endotracheal tube
- Supine position

Instruments and Equipment

- Standard forward-viewing diagnostic gastroscope, preferably with large working channel (3.2 mm)
- Transparent distal tapered hood
- Triangle-tip knife
- Coagulation forceps
- CO_2 insufflation
- Methylene blue dye
- 25 G injection needle

General Technical Points

- Submucosal injection of methylene blue dye, approximately 10 mL to create a satisfactory dissection place for clear distinction of the mucosa and submucosa for proper visualization of the muscular layers of the esophagus
- Consistent verification of the integrity of the submucosal flap to ease in dissection and avoid unnecessary nonanatomical tunneling
- Reinjection of dye may be necessary at several points during the dissection of the submucosal flap to create an optimal visualization.
- Mucosotomy—Longitudinal 2-cm incision to facilitate enough space for entrance of endoscope at 2-o' clock position
- Using electrocautery, triangle-tip knife, create a submucosal tunnel.
- Identification of the gastroesophageal junction is based on the length of the endoscope, narrowing of the submucosal tunnel, visualization of palisade vessels, and abrupt widening of the submucosal tunnel.

TIPS

If there is difficulty creating a dissection plane, restarting a new tunnel 90° from the original dissection is helpful.

- Create the myotomy incision 2-cm distal to the submucosal tunnel entrance and it should not be carried beyond 10-cm proximal to gastroesophageal junction.
- Take every effort to incise both the longitudinal and circular muscle layers of the muscular layer of the esophagus; however, only a circular muscle myotomy can be potentially done with this technique.
- Myotomy incision can be extended to a greater extent in peroral endoscopic myotomy due to lack of mediastinal and abdominal cavity dissection required for myotomy.
- In the event of a perforation, endoclips can be used. Evidence of pneumoperitoneum is the best way to ascertain the gravity of the perforation. Have a low threshold to convert to an open or laparoscopic procedure to help with diagnosis or to intervene.
- Closure of the mucosotomy is done with hemostatic endoclips at approximately 5-mm integrals.

Postoperative Considerations

General

- No placement of any esophageal tubes in the postoperative period unless done under direct endoscopic guidance
- Nausea and vomiting needs to be treated actively. If persistent or sustained tachycardia, the patient must return to the operating theater for endoscopic evaluation.
- A postoperative day 1 esophagram is obtained to assess myotomy, rule out leak, and assess esophageal/gastric emptying.
- Once evidence of a good myotomy and no leak is confirmed, diet can be advanced progressively.

Transthoracic

- Chest tube can usually be removed as early as postoperative day 1.

Endoscopic

- Evaluation of the myotomy and integrity of the mucosal flap is done on postoperative day 1 with an esophagram. If there are any doubts as to the status of the repair or myotomy, the patient should undergo a repeat upper endoscopy.

PEARLS AND PITFALLS

- Always rule out other causes of pseudoachalasia, such as malignancy, and obtain esophageal manometry to make a diagnosis.
- Creating a sufficiently long myotomy is crucial, while also ensuring not to cause mucosal damage.
- Patient selection is crucial. Identify the patient's comorbidities and surgical history to choose the appropriate approach for myotomy (open, video-assisted, or endoscopic).

Suggested Readings

1. Schlottmann F, Neto RML, Herbella FAM, Patti MG. Esophageal achalasia: pathophysiology, clinical presentation, and diagnostic evaluation. *Am Surg*. 2018;84(4):467-472. PMID: 29712590.
2. Gaissert HA, Lin N, Wain JC, Fankhauser G, Wright CD, Mathisen DJ. Transthoracic Heller myotomy for esophageal achalasia: analysis of long-term results. *Ann Thorac Surg*. 2006;81(6):2044-2049. PMID: 16731127.
3. Werner YB, Rösch T, Reddy DN. Endoscopic or surgical myotomy in achalasia. Reply. *N Engl J Med*. 2020;382(14): 1377-1378. PMID: 32242373.
4. Rawlings A, Soper NJ, Oelschlager B, et al. Laparoscopic Dor versus Toupet fundoplication following Heller myotomy for achalasia: results of a multicenter, prospective, randomized-controlled trial. *Surg Endosc*. 2012;26(1):18-26.
5. Schaheen LW, Sanchez MV, Luketich JD. Peroral endoscopic myotomy for achalasia. *Thorac Surg Clin*. 2018;28(4): 499-506. PMID: 30268295.
6. Schlottmann et al., 2018 Schlottmann F, Luckett DJ, Fine J, Shaheen NJ, Patti MG. Laparoscopic Heller myotomy versus peroral endoscopic myotomy (POEM) for achalasia: a systematic review and meta-analysis. *Ann Surg*. 2018;267(3): 451-460. PMID: 28549006.

Chapter 35

Zenker Diverticulum

LUCY NAM
CHRISTOPHER R. MORSE

Perioperative Considerations

- A barium swallow and upper gastrointestinal esophagoscopy, often performed at the time of procedure, should be performed in patients suspected of having a Zenker diverticulum after history and physical exam.
- A barium swallow typically reveals a cervical midline protrusion at the level of the posterior hypopharyngeal wall between the inferior constrictor muscle and the cricopharyngeus muscle (Killian triangle) (Figure 35.1).

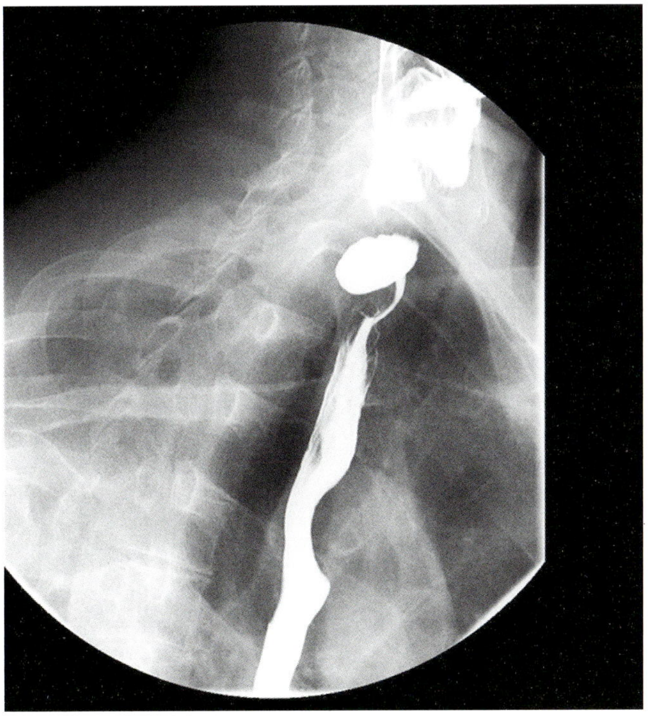

FIGURE 35.1 ❙ Barium swallow demonstrating a Zenker diverticulum.

- Surgical options include both transcervical open approaches (diverticulectomy/diverticulopexy and cricopharyngeal myotomy) and transoral, endoscopic approaches. The endoscopic approach is gaining popularity and avoids the need for a left neck incision (Figure 35.2).
- When considering a transoral stapled endoscopic approach, the diverticulum should be at least 2.5 to 3 cm in size to allow for entrance of the stapler and a complete cricopharyngeal myotomy with division of the common septum. Patients should be evaluated for limited mouth opening, fragile dentition, and inability to extend the neck, which makes placement of the Weerda laryngoscope difficult.

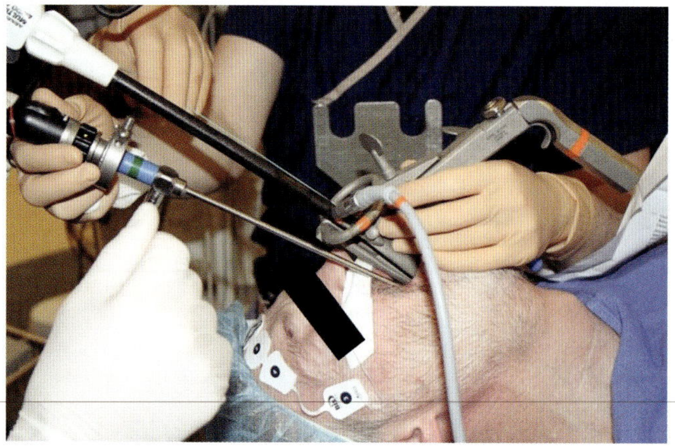

FIGURE 35.2 ▮ Transoral stapling of a Zenker diverticulum.

Instruments and Equipment

- Open transcervical diverticulectomy/diverticulopexy and cricopharyngeal myotomy:
  - 48-French Maloney bougie placed in the esophagus prior to stapling of the diverticulum
  - TA-30 stapler for resection of the diverticulum
- Transoral endoscopic diverticulectomy:
  - Weerda scope laryngoscope (Karl Storz, Tuttlingen, Germany)
  - Endo GIA stapler (Medtronic, Minneapolis, MN)
  - 5-mm 30° laparoscope to assist with visualization
  - Endo Stitch device (Medtronic, Minneapolis, MN)
  - 0-Ethibond suture (48 cm length)

Patient Positioning

- Open transcervical diverticulectomy/diverticulopexy and cricopharyngeal myotomy:
  - Placed supine
  - Arms tucked
  - Padding beneath shoulders to gently flex the neck
  - Head turned to right to expose left neck
  - Back of the bed raised to a slight "chair" position
- Transoral endoscopic diverticulectomy using rigid endoscopy:
  - Placed supine
  - Arms tucked
  - Head at top of the operating table
  - Gentle padding beneath the head to achieve "sniffing position"

Technique

- Open transcervical diverticulectomy or diverticulopexy with cricopharyngeal myotomy.
- Initial flexible esophagoscopy to assess the size of the diverticulum and remove any retained material from the diverticulum.
- After prep and drape of left neck, incision along anterior border of left sternocleidomastoid muscle. Divide platysma muscle.
- Reflect carotid sheath laterally and larynx medially.
- If necessary, divide the omohyoid muscle for visualization.
- Continue dissection toward prevertebral fascia and once identified, move medially to identify the esophagus.
- Dissect out the posterior and lateral esophagus and identify the diverticulum extending posteriorly and inferiorly.
- Elevate the diverticulum, often with the assistance of a clamp, and dissect circumferentially to the base of the diverticulum. Remove all connective tissue surrounding the diverticulum at its origin between the inferior constrictors of the pharynx and cricopharyngeal muscle below. This should define a clear plane between the mucosa of the diverticulum and esophageal muscle (Figure 35.3).

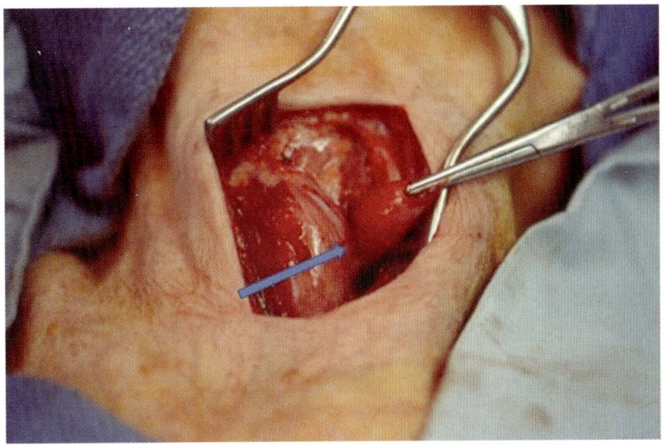

FIGURE 35.3 ❙ Open, transcervical approach to a Zenker diverticulum with the diverticulum elevated with a clamp and the blue arrow indicting the base of the diverticulum.

- Create a myotomy extending 5 to 6 cm distally from the inferior base of the diverticulum, completely through the cricopharyngeus. This should allow "pouting" of the mucosa.
  - We extend the myotomy directly from the base of the diverticulum, careful to divide all cricopharyngeal fibers.
- For a diverticulectomy:
  - Place a 48-French Maloney bougie into the esophagus. Place under direct vision across the esophageal myotomy.
  - Staple the base of the diverticulum with a TA-30 stapler.
    - If the diverticulum is resected sharply, perform a two-layer technique with absorbable suture for the inner layer. In this situation, the myotomy should be made lateral to the diverticulectomy and the muscle closed over the mucosa as a second layer.
- For a diverticulopexy:
  - Suspend the dissected diverticulum with four or five silk stitches superiorly to the prevertebral fascia in this region.
  - Esophageal myotomy in this circumstance should be made lateral the diverticulopexy.

Transoral Endoscopic Diverticulectomy

- Perform flexible esophagoscopy to assess size of the diverticulum and remove retained material from the diverticulum.
  - As mentioned, the diverticulum needs to be 3 cm in size to allow for an adequate cricopharyngeal myotomy.
- We use a small endotracheal tube (6.0) taped to the lateral mouth opening.
- Rigid esophagoscopy using Weerda laryngoscope (Karl Storz, Tuttlingen, Germany)

TIPS

Occasionally, it is helpful to advance the flexible endoscope through the Weeda scope to assist in positioning the rigid laryngoscope.

- Place one jaw of the laryngoscope in the true lumen of the esophagus (anterior) and the other in the diverticulum (posterior). This should allow for good visualization of the diverticular septum (Figure 35.4).
- Continue to expand the jaws to allow clear visualization of the diverticulum and the common septum.
- Use a 5-mm 30° laparoscope inside/alongside the Weerda laryngoscope to enable further visualization.
- Place a traction suture (0 Ethibond) in the common septum using an Endo Stitch device (uncut suture) (Figure 35.5).
  - Using the Endo GIA stapler, one jaw in the esophagus and one in the diverticulum (across the septum) and fire stapler

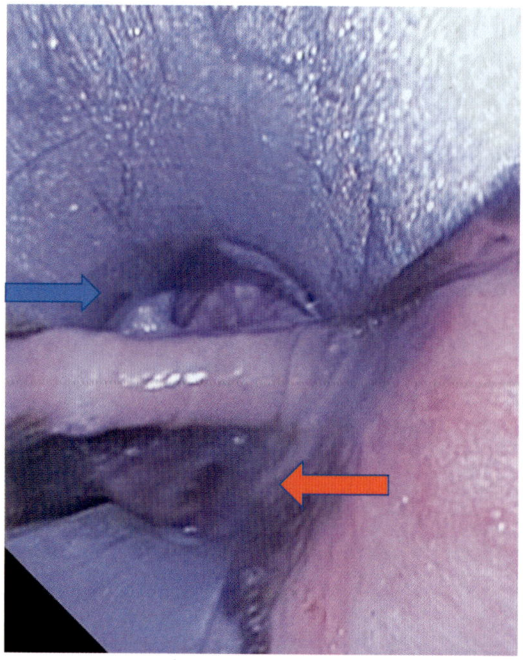

FIGURE 35.4 ▮ View of Weeda laryngoscope in position with good visualization of diverticular septum. Blue arrow indicates the esophagus and the red arrow demonstrates the diverticulum.

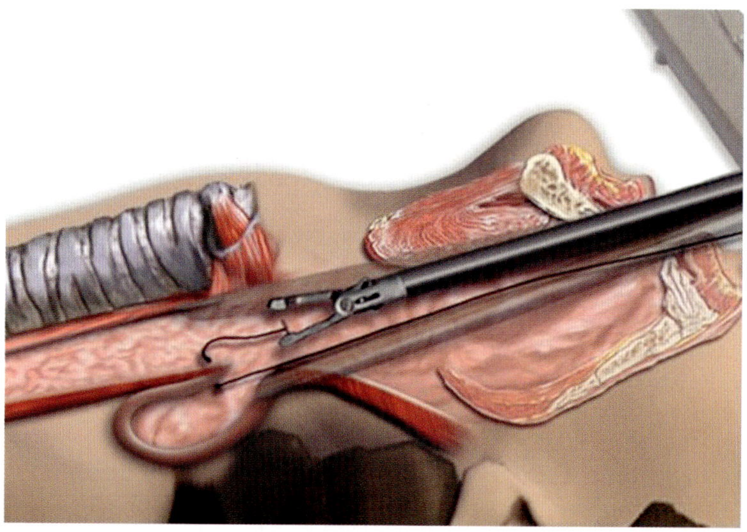

FIGURE 35.5 ▮ Placement of an Endo Stitch through the septum to facilitate stapling of common wall.

TIPS

It is helpful to provide gentle traction on stitch to pull the septum of the diverticulum into the stapler.

- Fire as many staple loads (often 2) as needed to ensure the common septum is divided completely to the base of the diverticulum.
- Replace the stitch as necessary after firing to further expose the septum. When the stitch is replaced, we attempt to place the new stitch at the base of the previous staple line to further draw the septum into the stapler.

Postoperative Care

- With an open approach, a 15-French Blake drain is left adjacent to the repair. On postoperative day 1, a barium swallow is obtained to confirm the absence of any leak and the patient is placed on a clear liquid diet. The drain is removed after the barium swallow and the patient is discharged home on the same day. Occasionally, we will challenge the patients with "grape juice" and follow drain output in lieu of a barium swallow.

- The postoperative care for a transoral endoscopic approach is similar, except there is no drain placed. On a follow-up barium swallow, a small residual spur is often noted at the inferior aspect of the divided cricopharyngeus, which is thought to be of minimal clinical significance (Figure 35.6).
- We employ a standard weekly advancement of diet from liquids to more solid foods over the course of several weeks.

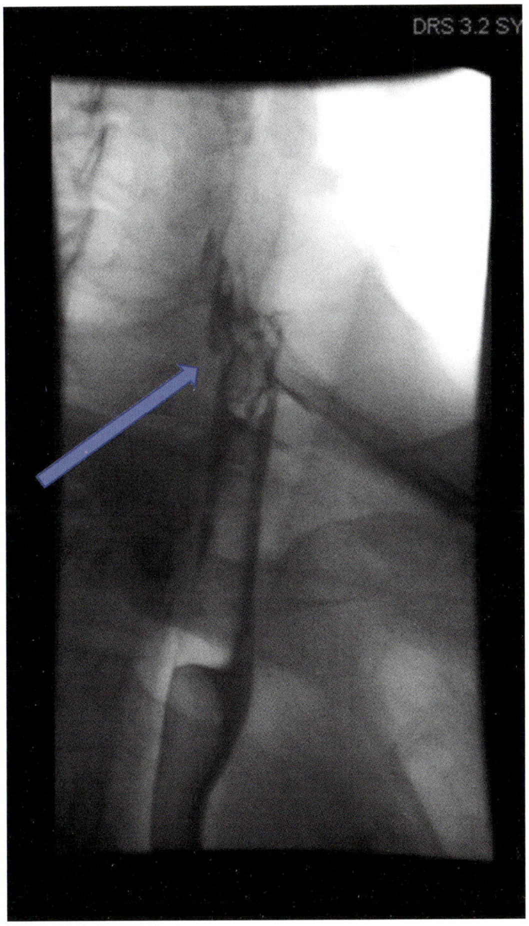

FIGURE 35.6 ‖ Postoperative swallow after a transoral stapling of a Zenker diverticulum. Note the slight residual "spur" as highlighted by the blue arrow.

PEARLS AND PITFALLS

Open transcervical procedure:

- A left-sided incision is commonly used as the cervical esophagus is positioned slightly off midline toward the left, behind the trachea.
- Careful traction and dissection on the larynx/esophagus to avoid injury to the recurrent laryngeal nerve.
- When performing an open diverticulectomy, take care not to narrow the esophageal lumen when coming across with the stapler to divide the diverticulum. We typically use a 48-French bougie in the esophagus when stapling to avoid this problem.
- Cricopharyngeal myotomy alone can treat small, early pouches (typically <1 cm) as the diverticulum will "disappear" as the mucosa pouts within the myotomy. These small diverticulum should not be treated with a transoral, endoscopic approach as there is not enough "length" in the divided septum to allow for an adequate cricopharyngeal myotomy.
- Consider the various advantages of each procedure: diverticulopexy leads to decreased risk of a postoperative leak as there is no violation of the hypopharyngeal mucosa. An advantage of diverticulectomy is the elimination of the pouch completely, thus reducing the very small risk of diverticular carcinoma.

Transoral endoscopic stapled approach:

- Deep paralysis with anesthesia and placing the patient in a subtle "sniffing" position will assist with the placement of the Weeda laryngoscope.
- Dental injury from placement of the laryngoscope can occur and is the most commonly described complication of the transoral approach. Descending mediastinitis can also occur causing significant morbidity, though this is a very rare issue.
- The traction suture helps to expose the septum and facilitate a complete cricopharyngeal myotomy.
- There are a number of flexible endoscopic options as well. They can be performed without need for neck flexion. Techniques used to divide the common septum include electrocautery using needle knife with techniques similar to POEM (peroral endoscopic myotomy) for achalasia. This approach does not address the Zenker diverticulum.

TIPS

If it is difficult to see the diverticulum, it may be helpful to advance the flexible scope through the Weeda laryngoscope to determine distance to the diverticulum.

Suggested Readings

1. Chang C, Payyapilli R, Scher R. Endoscopic staple diverticulostomy for Zenker's diverticulum: review of literature and experience in 159 consecutive cases. *Laryngoscope*. 2003;113(6):957-965.
2. Dohlman G, Mattsson O. The endoscopic operation for hypopharyngeal diverticula: a roentgencinematographic study. *AMA Arch Otolaryngol*. 1960;71:744-752.
3. Gutschow CA, Hamoir M, Rombaux P, Otte JB, Goncette L, Collard JM. Management of pharyngoesophageal (Zenker's) diverticulum: which technique? *Ann Thorac Surg*. 2002;74(5):1677-1683.
4. Lerut T, van Raemdonck D, Guelinckx P, Dom R, Geboes K. Zenker's diverticulum: is a myotomy of the cricopharyngeus useful? How long should it be? *Hepato-Gastroenterology*. 1992;39(2):127-131.
5. Yuan Y, Zhao YF, Hu Y, et al. Surgical treatment of Zenker's diverticulum. *Dig Surg*. 2013;30:214-225.

Chapter 36

Epiphrenic Diverticulum Repair

LUIS F. TAPIAS

Perioperative Considerations

Preoperative Evaluation

- Workup of an epiphrenic diverticulum includes:
  - Contrast esophagram to determine the size and location of the diverticulum
  - Esophagoscopy to rule out mucosal abnormalities within the diverticulum (eg, rare cases of squamous cell carcinomas secondary to food stasis) or concomitant distal esophageal pathology
  - Esophageal manometry is used selectively, as the majority of epiphrenic diverticula are associated with an esophageal motility disorder. In addition, there are technical limitations related to probe placement that might limit the results of this study.
  - Computed tomography of the chest/abdomen might be useful in select cases to better understand the relationships of the diverticulum to surrounding structures.
  - A complete blood count can help establish the possibility of concomitant pulmonary infections secondary to aspiration and iron deficiency anemia secondary to blood loss. Chemistries to establish nutritional status are helpful.
- Workup to establish medical candidacy for surgery includes:
  - Cardiovascular evaluation
  - Pulmonary function testing if a transthoracic approach is planned

Preoperative Instructions

- Ask patients to follow a liquid diet for 2 to 3 days before surgery. This will help clear the esophageal lumen and diverticulum of food debris, to avoid interference on the day of surgery.

TIPS

- *Rarely, patients can present with two or more epiphrenic diverticula. Carefully review all preoperative studies, as all diverticula need to be addressed in some form during the operation. If small, additional diverticula can be dealt with by performing a myotomy only or by imbrication. Alternatively, small diverticula can be left alone in select cases.*
- *Epiphrenic diverticula can present acutely. Rare case reports have described perforation of the diverticulum or upper gastrointestinal bleeding from mucosal ulceration.*
- *The majority of true epiphrenic diverticula project toward the right chest. However, this should not push you to attempt a surgical approach from the right chest, which is not recommended routinely. Typically, if a transthoracic approach is planned, it should be a left-sided approach, as it allows better access to the gastroesophageal junction and facilitates performing a myotomy, or access to the gastric fundus in cases where a partial fundoplication is planned.*

Technique

Left Thoracotomy Approach

Anesthesia

- Placement of a preoperative epidural catheter is recommended for postoperative pain management.
- General anesthesia with a double-lumen endotracheal tube (left-sided for easier placement).
- Peripheral vascular access is adequate.
- Foley catheter

Instruments and Equipment

- On-table esophagogastroduodenoscopy (EGD) in all cases
- Standard thoracotomy tray
- Electrocautery and/or energy device (eg, harmonic scalpel)
- Penrose drain (for esophageal retraction)
- Esophageal bougie (50-56 French)
- Mechanical staplers with thin or medium tissue thickness loads

Positioning

- Right lateral decubitus with bed flexion (standard thoracotomy position)

Technique

- Start the procedure by performing an EGD. Rule out malignant disease in the diverticulum or the rest of the esophagus. Look for retention of food debris and clear this from the epiphrenic diverticulum, if possible.
- Perform a standard left posterolateral thoracotomy through the seventh or eighth intercostal space.
- It is strongly recommended to harvest the intercostal muscle as a posteriorly based pedicled flap at the planned thoracotomy intercostal space for later use.
  - Develop the subperiosteal plane on the rib above and below using a Matson-Alexander rib elevator and bluntly separate the intercostal muscle and its neurovascular bundle away from the ribs.
  - Dissect the intercostal muscle as anteriorly as possible and divide it sharply with scissors, while ligating the cut end on the anterior chest wall.
  - Protect the intercostal muscle flap with a moist gauze during the procedure.
- Take down the left inferior pulmonary ligament and retract the left lung anteriorly and superiorly to expose the esophageal bed in the posterior mediastinum.
- Open the mediastinal pleura in front of the aorta to dissect the esophagus. Encircle the esophagus and pass a Penrose drain, either superiorly or inferiorly. The Penrose drain provides improved retraction and exposure for further dissection and mobilization of the esophagus.
- The esophagus and diverticulum (usually projecting to the right chest) are dissected progressively from the contralateral pleura and surrounding mediastinal structures.

TIPS

There can be significant inflammation and adhesions around the diverticulum. Patiently work layer by layer to avoid injuries to surrounding structures.

- Once fully mobilized, the esophagus and diverticulum are rotated into the left chest. The diverticulum is directly grasped, and the neck of the diverticulum is dissected to identify the defect in the muscle fibers and to isolate the true mucosal neck of the epiphrenic diverticulum (Figure 36.1).

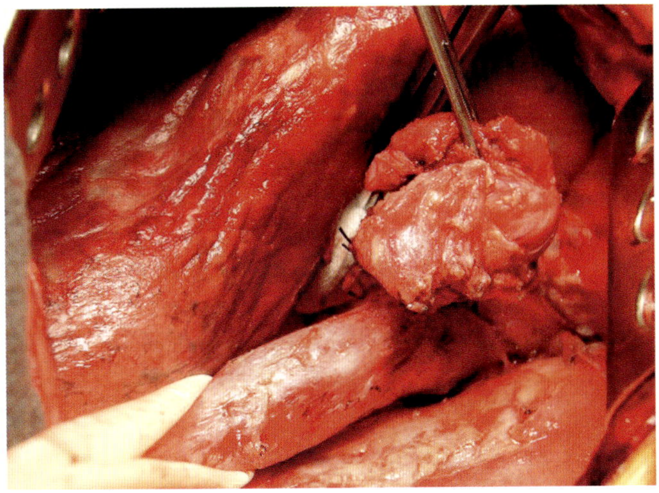

FIGURE 36.1 ▮ Left thoracotomy approach. Completely dissected epiphrenic diverticulum grasped with a clamp. A Penrose drain is seen around the more distal esophagus to assist with retraction.

- A large esophageal bougie is placed (50-56 French) before resection of the diverticulum. This prevents narrowing the esophageal lumen when completing a diverticulectomy.
- The diverticulum is resected by firing a mechanical stapler with a medium tissue thickness load across its neck (Figure 36.2).

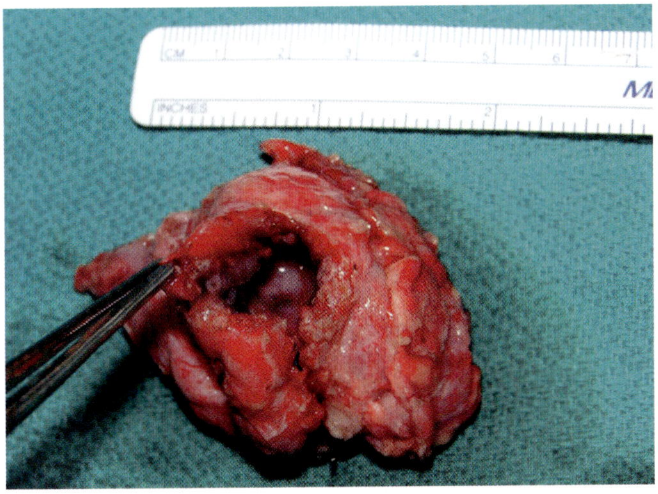

FIGURE 36.2 ▮ Diverticulectomy specimen.

TIPS

If there is significant food retention inside the diverticulum identified during the initial EGD, then consider opening the diverticulum in a controlled fashion to evacuate the retained food debris. Otherwise, this can get caught in the staple line during diverticulectomy and, potentially, predispose to a leak.

- Depending on the location of the diverticulum, the diverticulectomy site can be part of the esophageal myotomy. If inadequate, then the esophageal muscular layer is closed over the diverticulectomy site. This is done by placing multiple simple interrupted 4-0 silk sutures to reapproximate the muscular edges (Figure 36.3).

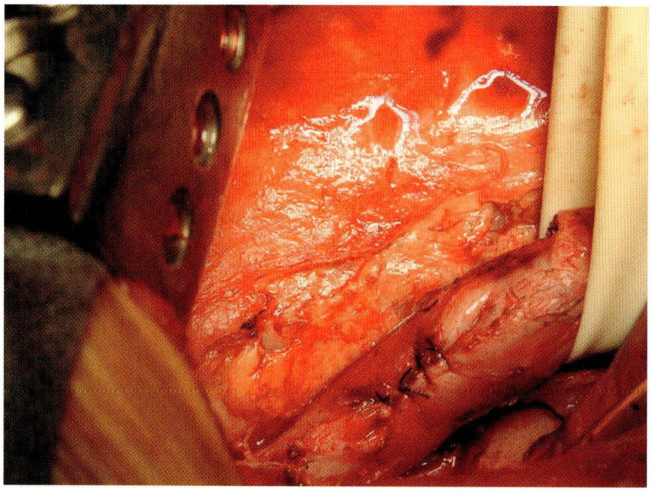

FIGURE 36.3 ▌ Left thoracotomy approach. After diverticulectomy, the muscular layer of the esophagus can be re-approximated to cover the mucosal diverticulectomy site.

- Following diverticulectomy, the esophagus can fall into its natural position in preparation for the esophageal myotomy.
- The esophageal myotomy must extend from the upper border of the diverticulum to 1 cm into the gastric cardia (Ellis technique), which causes minimal disruption of the gastroesophageal junction and can enable the omission of a concomitant antireflux procedure.

TIPS

Esophageal epiphrenic diverticula are pulsion in nature. They are a direct reflection of a functional distal obstruction of the esophagus due to an esophageal motility disorder. This needs to be addressed as part of the operation by performing a long esophageal myotomy, without exceptions.

- The myotomy is done sharply to avoid thermal injury of the esophageal mucosa. Stay sutures on the muscular edges of the esophageal myotomy can assist with retraction and exposure to extend the myotomy to the desired length (Figure 36.4).

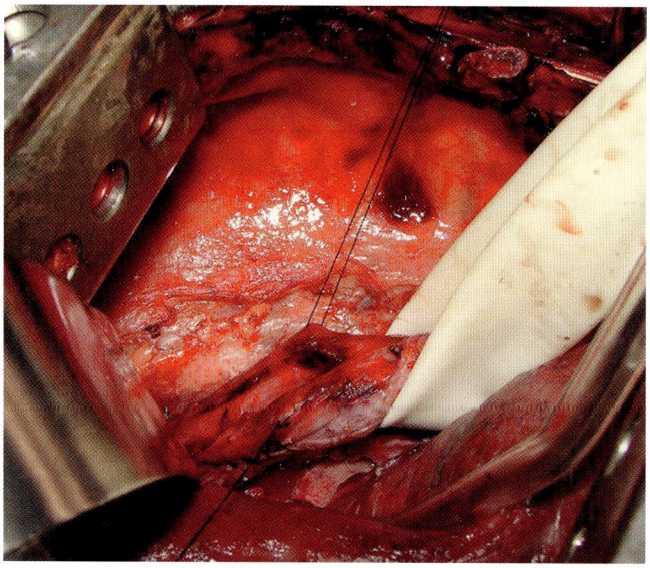

FIGURE 36.4 ▌ Left thoracotomy approach. A thoracic esophageal myotomy must always be performed. Stay sutures on the edges of the myotomy assist with retraction and exposure, thus facilitating extension of the myotomy.

- If a fundoplication is planned, then the operation continues with this step. Through a left thoracotomy approach, a Belsey fundoplication (anterior 240° wrap) can be constructed.

- Finally, the intercostal muscle flap is used to buttress the diverticulectomy and/or myotomy site. It is secured with simple or horizontal mattress sutures using 4-0 silk. If covering the myotomy site, it should be anchored to the muscular edges of the myotomy. This helps keeping the myotomy open (Figure 36.5).

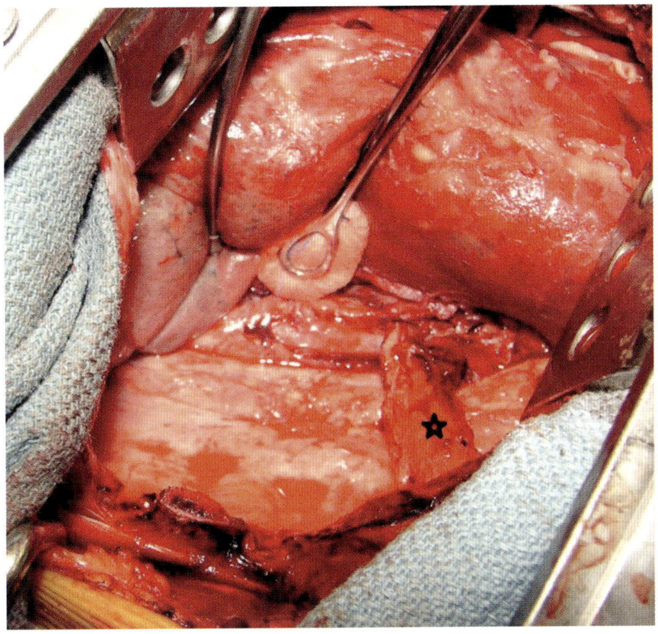

FIGURE 36.5 | Left thoracotomy approach. An intercostal muscle flap (star) can be used to cover the diverticulectomy or esophageal myotomy sites. This provides reinforcement to these areas, minimizing the risk of leaks.

- A large-bore (28-French) chest tube is placed and directed toward the apex to manage fluid and air (in case there is an air leak secondary to lung manipulation). A soft small-bore chest tube is placed in the posterior mediastinum to help control a potential esophageal leak.
- The left thoracotomy is closed in layers in the standard fashion.

Minimally Invasive Approach

Considerations

- Laparoscopy:
  - It can be used to approach very distal esophageal epiphrenic diverticula in a transhiatal fashion.
  - It allows for a familiar approach to perform an esophageal myotomy that extends into the cardia of the stomach.
  - It also provides an easy and familiar approach to perform a hiatal hernia repair and/or fundoplication.
  - Point of caution—With a "normally sized" esophageal hiatus, it may be difficult to perform a safe mediastinal dissection and consideration should be made to enlarging the hiatus to allow for the dissection of the epiphrenic diverticulum
- Video-assisted thoracic surgery (VATS):
  - VATS can be used alone or in combination with laparoscopy.
  - It can be used for the resection of diverticula higher up in the chest.
  - It allows for a more proximal extension of the esophageal myotomy.
  - It can prove useful in cases of redo operations after failed laparoscopic procedures.
  - The major disadvantage of VATS is the difficulty in performing a hiatal hernia repair and/or fundoplication.

Anesthesia

- Laparoscopy:
  - General anesthesia with single-lumen endotracheal tube
  - Complete neuromuscular paralysis is needed for adequate abdominal insufflation with CO_2.

- VATS:
  - General anesthesia with double-lumen endotracheal tube

Instruments and Equipment

- On-table EGD in all cases
- Laparoscopy:
  - Hasson port (12 mm)
  - Three 5-mm ports
  - One 12-mm port
  - Liver retractor
  - Atraumatic graspers
  - Energy device for dissection (eg, harmonic scalpel)
- VATS:
  - Standard VATS tray
  - Atraumatic graspers
  - Energy device for dissection (eg, Harmonic scalpel)
- For all approaches:
  - Bougie (50-56 French)
  - Mechanical staplers with medium thickness loads

Positioning

- Laparoscopy:
  - Supine with arms out
  - A footboard is placed to allow for a steep reverse Trendelenburg position intraoperatively.
- VATS:
  - Lateral decubitus position with bed flexion (standard thoracotomy/VATS position)

Technique

- Start the procedure by performing an EGD. Rule out malignant disease in the diverticulum or the rest of the esophagus. Look for retention of food debris and clear this from the epiphrenic diverticulum, if possible.
- Laparoscopy:
  - Divide the pars flaccida of the gastrohepatic omentum and carry the dissection toward the right crus of the diaphragm.
  - Mobilize the phrenoesophageal membrane and bluntly dissect the esophagus away from the right crus of the diaphragm.
  - Divide the short gastric vessels and retract the stomach toward the right side to expose the left crus of the diaphragm. Dissect the esophagus away from it.
  - Dissect the inferior aspect of the esophagus, find the junction between the right and left diaphragmatic crura, and encircle the esophagus.
  - Dissect the esophagus into the mediastinum circumferentially.
  - Identify the diverticulum in the lower esophagus and dissect it free to define its neck (Figure 36.6).

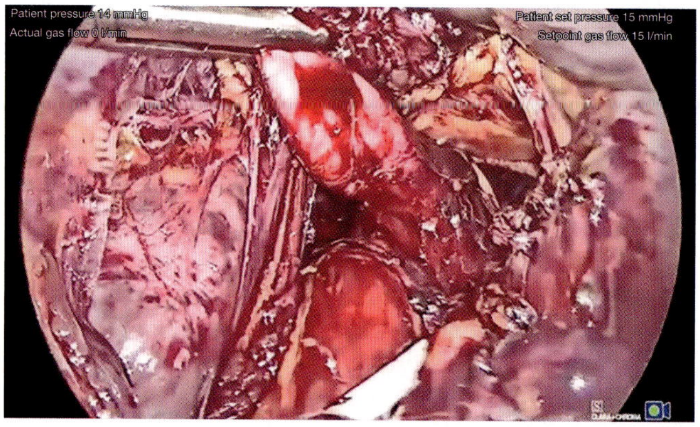

FIGURE 36.6 Laparoscopic transhiatal approach. A low epiphrenic diverticulum can be identified and dissected while working through the esophageal hiatus.

  - Pass an esophageal bougie.
  - Perform a diverticulectomy by transecting the diverticulum at its neck with a mechanical stapler with a medium thickness load (Figure 36.7).

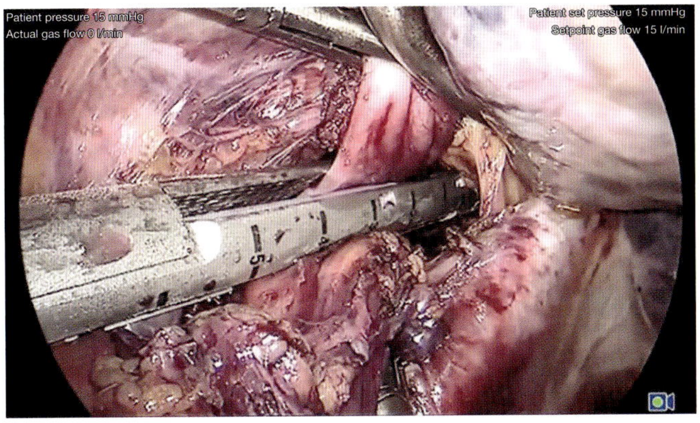

FIGURE 36.7 | Laparoscopic transhiatal approach. A diverticulectomy is performed using a mechanical stapler while having an esophageal bougie in place.

  - Perform an esophageal myotomy in the standard fashion (Heller technique, described elsewhere in this book).
  - Perform a repair of the diaphragmatic hiatus and a partial fundoplication.
- Left VATS:
  - Divide the inferior pulmonary ligament.
  - Open the mediastinal pleura just anterior to the aorta to gain access to the esophagus.
  - Dissect the esophagus and encircle it with a Penrose drain to improve retraction and exposure.
  - The esophagus and diverticulum are dissected progressively from the contralateral pleura and surrounding mediastinal structures. The diverticulum is dissected to define its neck (Figure 36.8).

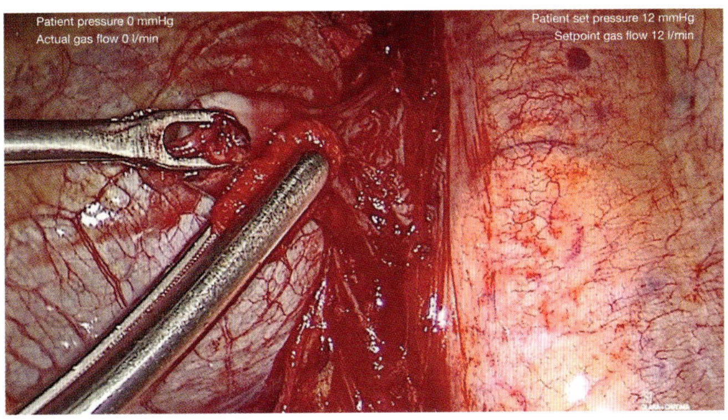

FIGURE 36.8 | Left video-assisted thoracic surgery approach. The diverticulum is dissected from the surrounding tissues to define its neck before resection.

  - Pass an esophageal bougie.
  - A diverticulectomy is performed by transecting the diverticulum at its neck with a mechanical stapler with a medium thickness load (Figure 36.9).

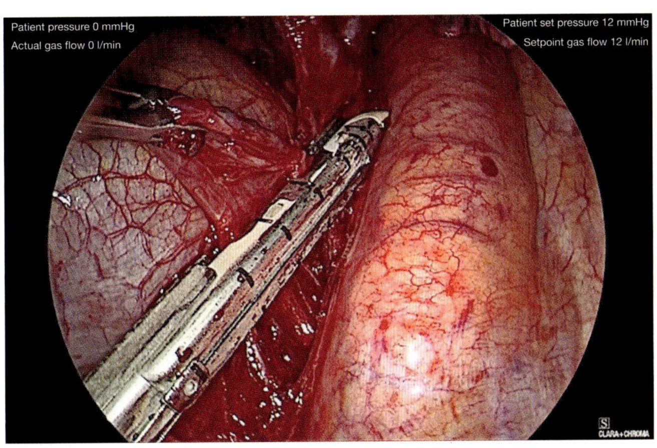

FIGURE 36.9 | Left video-assisted thoracic surgery approach. A diverticulectomy is performed using a mechanical stapler while having an esophageal bougie in place.

- A long esophageal myotomy can be performed next. Stay sutures on the edges of the myotomy assist with exposure and extension of the myotomy (Figure 36.10).

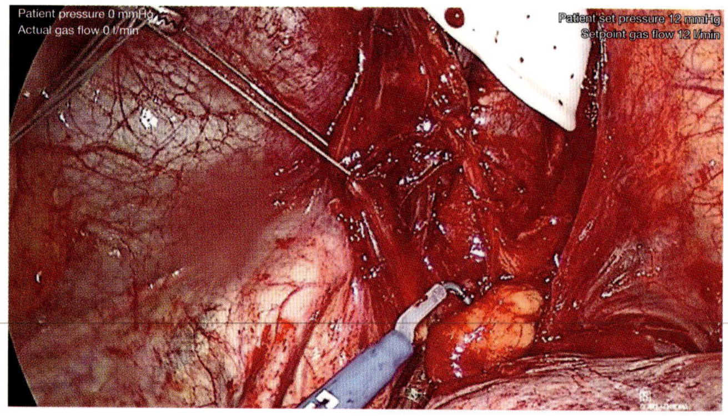

FIGURE 36.10 ▌ Left video-assisted thoracic surgery approach. A long esophageal myotomy is performed. Stay sutures on the muscular layer of the esophagus assist with retraction.

- Combined laparoscopy and VATS:
  - Combined approaches can be useful in certain situations, such as the presence of multiple diverticula or diverticula located higher up in the chest.
  - VATS can be used to perform a diverticulectomy and provide a more proximal extension of the esophageal myotomy.
  - Laparoscopy can be used to perform a Heller myotomy and partial fundoplication.

Postoperative Care

- A large-bore chest tube can be removed on postoperative day (POD) 1 if there is no air leak.
- A small-bore soft chest tube in the posterior mediastinum is left in place until a contrast esophagram is obtained. This can be used to control a potential esophageal leak.
- A contrast esophagram is obtained approximately on POD 4 to 5 to assess the integrity of the repair and rule out active esophageal leaks. If negative, diet can start.
- In addition, measuring drain fluid amylase levels can increase the sensitivity at detecting esophageal leaks.
- Diet is advanced progressively. A recommended sequence is 5 days of clears liquids, 5 days of full liquids, and 5 days of soft food.
- The patient is discharged from the hospital on POD 5 to 6.

PEARLS AND PITFALLS

- Favor an open posterolateral thoracotomy approach unless extremely experienced and comfortable with minimally invasive techniques. Epiphrenic diverticula are rare and, therefore, it is difficult to accumulate large experiences.
- When an open transthoracic approach is planned, an epiphrenic diverticulum should be approached through the left chest, even if it projects toward the right chest. A left chest approach provides better access to the gastroesophageal junction to complete all the steps of the operation.
- All patients undergoing surgical treatment of an epiphrenic diverticulum should have an esophageal myotomy.
- Failure to perform a myotomy results in high leak rates from the diverticulectomy staple line and increases the risk of late recurrence of the diverticulum.
- If a transthoracic approach is used, the myotomy can be fashioned in a way to prevent too much disruption of the gastroesophageal junction, thus avoiding a fundoplication.
- If a laparoscopic transhiatal approach is used, reconstruction of the esophageal hiatus and a partial fundoplication must be done to avoid development of a hiatal hernia or significant postoperative reflux.

Suggested Readings

1. Tapias LF, Morse CR, Mathisen DJ, et al. Surgical management of esophageal epiphrenic diverticula: a transthoracic approach over four decades. *Ann Thorac Surg*. 2017;104(4):1123-1130.
2. Benacci JC, Deschamps C, Trastek VF, Allen MS, Daly RC, Pairolero PC. Epiphrenic diverticulum: results of surgical treatment. *Ann Thorac Surg*. 1993;55(5):1109-1114.
3. Macke RA, Luketich JD, Pennathur A, et al. Thoracic esophageal diverticula: a 15-year experience of minimally invasive surgical management. *Ann Thorac Surg*. 2015;100(5):1795-1802.
4. Sudarshan M, Fort MW, Barlow JM, et al. Management of epiphrenic diverticula and short-term outcomes. *Semin Thorac Cardiovasc Surg*. 2021;33(1):242-246.
5. Allen TH, Clagett OT. Changing concepts in the surgical treatment of pulsion diverticula of the lower esophagus. *J Thorac Cardiovasc Surg*. 1965;50(4):455-462.

Chapter 37

Transhiatal Esophagectomy

DANNY WANG
CHRISTOPHER R. MORSE
PHILICIA MOONSAMY

Transhiatal esophagectomy remains an important procedure in the armamentarium of a thoracic surgeon. Since a thoracotomy is avoided, the transhiatal approach offers less morbidity for the patient. Additionally, a cervical anastomosis minimizes the potential for mediastinitis in the setting of anastomotic leak. Performing a cervical anastomosis comes with associated risks such as recurrent laryngeal nerve injury and potentially a higher incidence of anastomotic leak, but this may be justified in a select group of patients who would benefit from avoiding a transthoracic approach.

Indications

- Tumors involving the upper to midesophagus (less than 25 cm from the incisors) where it may be difficult to get a negative margin with an intrathoracic approach/anastomosis.
- Long segment Barrett's esophagus less than 20 cm from the incisors.
- Patient with significant pulmonary comorbidities or prior right thoracotomy where it is particularly advantageous to avoid a transthoracic approach.
- Benign disease/end-stage motility disorders/chemical injury to the esophagus necessitating near total esophagectomy.
- Surgeon preference.

Preoperative Considerations

- Age and performance status: Patients with significant comorbidities or advanced age are at a higher risk of postoperative complications.
- Nutritional status, particularly if the patient received neoadjuvant chemoradiotherapy.
- Cardiopulmonary reserve.
- Patient with a history of coronary artery disease and or significant risk factors should undergo preoperative cardiology assessment.
- Pulmonary function tests.
- For patients with more proximal disease, it may be advantageous to perform a bronchoscopy to eliminate the potential of airway involvement.
- Ideally, esophageal resection is performed within 4 to 6 weeks of completion of neoadjuvant therapy, although some patients may be too weak and dehydrated to undergo a major procedure and careful risk assessment must be performed.

Surgical Technique

Anesthetic Considerations

- An arterial catheter should be placed to closely monitor blood pressure throughout the procedure, particularly with compression of the heart and mediastinal structures during blunt dissection through the posterior mediastinum.

- Transhiatal esophagectomy requires close cooperation between the anesthesia team and surgeon to avoid prolonged hypotension.
- A transhiatal esophagectomy can typically be performed with a single-lumen endotracheal tube. A double-lumen endotracheal tube is rarely used and may lead to increased airway injuries during esophageal blunt dissection due to its large size.

Surgical Considerations

- Every transhiatal esophagectomy begins with an endoscopy and possible bronchoscopy to survey the extent of disease and any airway involvement (if this has not already been accounted for).
- The arms are carefully padded and placed at the patient's side, and the skin of the neck, chest, and abdomen is prepped and draped from the pubis to the mandible and to the midaxillary lines.

Abdominal Phase

- Following a supraumbilical incision, the left lobe of the liver is retracted to the left upper quadrant and the abdomen is inspected for any evidence of metastatic disease.
- Beginning along the greater curve of the stomach, the greater omentum is freed from the stomach by entering the lesser sac in an avascular portion of the omentum. The right gastroepiploic artery is fully preserved, and the short gastric vessels are ligated typically with an energy device (Harmonic scalpel).

TIPS

- *Avoid thermal injury to the gastroepiploic along the greater curve of the stomach. Staying a centimeter off the vessel with the energy device is typically adequate.*
- *Due to concerns with injuring the gastroepiploic artery, surgeons often dissect too far caudally into the greater omentum when dissecting along the greater curve of the stomach. This results in a large amount of residual omentum remaining attached to the gastric conduit. The goal is indeed to preserve the gastroepiploic, but bringing a large amount of omental fat into the mediastinum with the conduit can make it more difficult to position and bring it up to the neck.*

- Retroantral and retrofundal attachments of the stomach in the lesser sac are taken down with the cautery device.
- The gastrohepatic omentum is opened, and the left gastric artery and vein are isolated with all nodal tissue swept up with the specimen and the vessels are divided with a linear stapler (vascular load).
- This dissection is then carried up along the right crus and circumferentially at the esophageal hiatus.
- With the stomach mobilized, a generous Kocher maneuver is performed to allow the pylorus to be lifted into the mediastinum if necessary.
- We do not typically perform a gastric emptying procedure.
- The esophagus is then retracted toward the abdominal cavity with a Penrose drain around the esophagus, and the aortic esophageal branches are divided under vision.
- The esophageal hiatus may need to be widened slightly by dividing one of the diaphragm crura to allow entrance of the hand into the posterior mediastinum.
- When performing blunt dissection of the esophagus in the mediastinum, care is taken to preserve the integrity of the membranous wall of the airway.

Cervical Phase

- A 7-cm incision is made along the anterior border of the left sternocleidomastoid (SCM) muscle from the angle of the mandible to the sternal notch.
- The SCM and the carotid sheath are retracted laterally. We avoid placing a self-retaining retractor between the SCM and larynx to prevent recurrent laryngeal nerve injuries.
- A finger or peanut is used to retract the larynx medially, and dissection is carried down toward the prevertebral fascia. Once the prevertebral fascia is identified, the esophagus typically lies medial and under the airway.

- The esophagus is then dissected bluntly using the fingers into the superior mediastinum, and the cervical esophagus is encircled with a Penrose drain.
- With some gentle upward traction on the Penrose drain, dissection of the upper thoracic esophagus continues. Vessels were taken with an energy device if they could be seen with retraction. Care is again taken not to injure the membranous wall of the airway.

Mediastinal Phase

- With a hand placed through the esophageal hiatus via the abdomen and blunt dissection performed through the cervical incision (hand/sponge stick), progress is made superiorly and inferiorly until there is a connection of the two dissection planes in the posterior mediastinum.
- In performing the dissection through the cervical esophagus, traction is placed on the Penrose drain to elevate the cervical esophagus to allow for more precise division of vessels and vagus nerve branches. With a hand placed through the esophageal hiatus, blunt dissection is used to take down small vessels and vagal branches.
- Close communication with the anesthesia team to address hypotension is important during the mediastinal dissection.
- Hypotension is addressed by stopping dissection or administering additional fluid/pressor agents.
- The esophagus is then divided in the neck with a stapling device (Figure 37.1), and the specimen is retracted down through the hiatus.

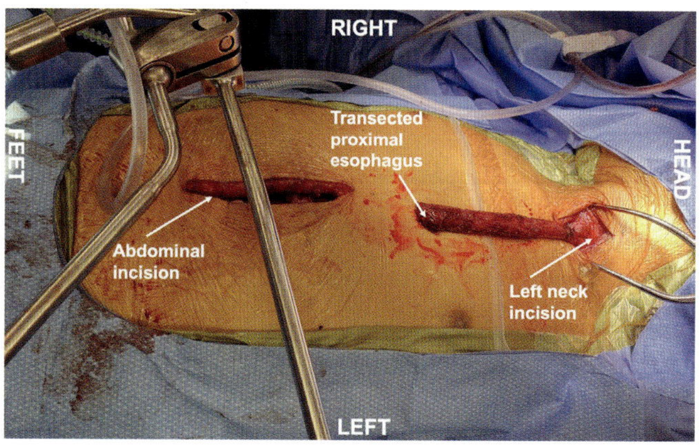

FIGURE 37.1 ▮ The esophagus is transected and removed from the mediastinum via the neck incision.

- Any bleeding within the mediastinum is tamponaded with lap sponges as needed.
- The gastric conduit is created using successive fires of a linear stapler to exclude the lesser curve of the stomach. The staple fires should be aligned parallel to the greater curve, and the final conduit should have a width of approximately 5 to 6 cm.
- We use a three-step process to transport the gastric conduit to the neck:
- An Argyle chest tube is delivered from the neck to the abdomen via the mediastinum. The tip of the chest tube secured to the end of a Foley catheter using a stitch, and the tip of the Foley is then inserted into a sterile plastic bag (with the balloon blown up). This tip of the Foley is secured to the bag using a tied suture just proximal to the balloon.
- The chest tube is pulled up through the neck, delivering the Foley catheter into the posterior mediastinum where the conduit will eventually lie. The sterile bag should still be down in the abdomen with the Foley balloon at this juncture. The chest tube is freed from the Foley catheter in the neck (Figure 37.2).
- The gastric conduit is placed into a sterile plastic bag, maintaining its proper orientation. Suction is applied to the end of the Foley catheter, and the catheter is pulled up through the neck, drawing plastic bag containing the conduit cephalad and depositing the conduit into the posterior mediastinum. This allows for atraumatic positioning of the conduit (Figure 37.3).

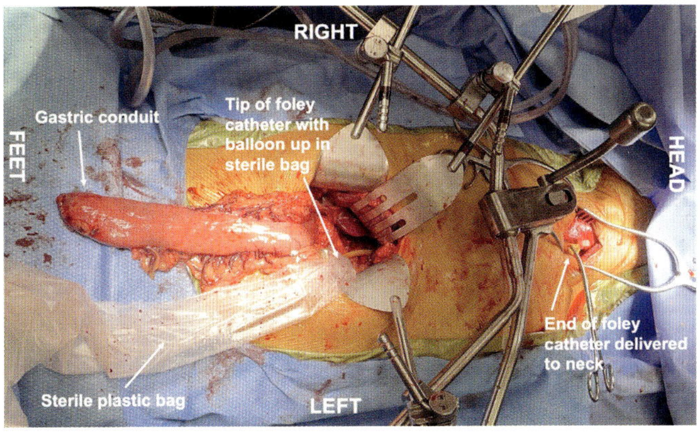

FIGURE 37.2 | A chest tube (not pictured) has been used to draw a Foley catheter up to the neck through the posterior mediastinum. This figure shows the balloon of the Foley catheter inserted into a sterile bag and inflated. The distal end of the Foley catheter exits in the neck (secured here with a Kelly clamp). The gastric conduit is inserted into the plastic bag in the correct orientation, suction is applied to the end of the Foley at the neck, and conduit is drawn up to the neck whilst in the plastic bag. The assistant pulls the Foley out through the neck while the surgeon guides the conduit and plastic bag up through the posterior mediastinum to make sure the correct orientation is maintained.

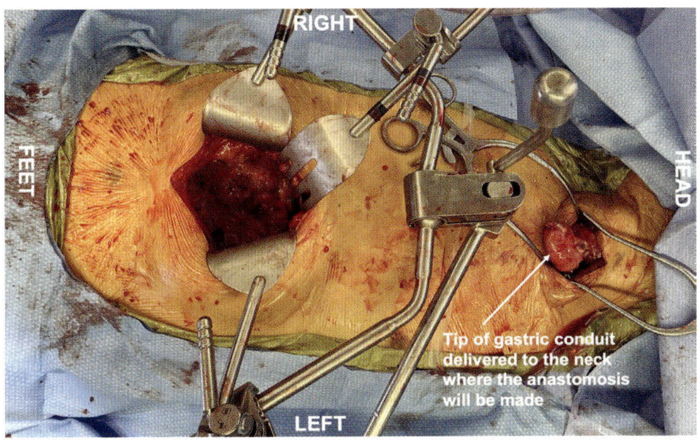

FIGURE 37.3 | The conduit has been delivered to the neck, and the plastic bag and Foley has been removed.

TIPS

- *When making the gastric conduit, it is important to note that length for the conduit comes from creating a staple line starting at the top of the fundus rather than the gastroesophageal junction. Placing the stomach on stretch will demonstrate this and allow for a longer, more perfused conduit.*
- *The conduit must remain in the proper orientation when it is delivered to the neck. We have found the most reproducible method of orientation is keeping the gastric conduit staple line facing the right chest. Any "twisting" of the conduit can lead to vascular compromise and conduit dysfunction.*

Anastomotic Phase

- We use a circular end-to-end anastomosis (EEA) 25 mm stapler to perform most of our cervical anastomoses.
- With the proximal esophageal open, the anvil is placed and secured with several purse-string sutures.
- The tip of the gastric conduit is then opened along the distal end of the staple line, and the stapler was inserted and brought out along the greater curve where it is connected to the anvil. Two complete tissue donuts must be created after the stapler is fired.
- The gastrotomy is then closed with one to two applications of a linear Endo GIA stapler.
- Gentle traction is applied to the gastric conduit from the abdomen to pull the anastomosis from the neck to lie in the esophageal bed.
- The gastric conduit is then secured with circumferential silk sutures at the esophageal hiatus.
- A nasogastric tube is placed and secured with its tip just above the esophageal hiatus.

Postoperative Care

- The patient is extubated in the operating room and typically will spend one night in a monitored bed.
- The patient should be ambulatory the end of the day of surgery or on postoperative day 1.
- Tube feedings are started via the jejunostomy on postoperative day 2 and advanced after return of bowel function.
- The nasogastric tube is typically left in for 5 days when a barium swallow is obtained.
- On the barium swallow, we are looking for an intact anastomosis and emptying of the gastric conduit.
- The patient goes home taking by mouth (orally) and advances their diet over several weeks.
- We do not typically leave a neck drain near the surgical anastomosis.
- If there is concern of an anastomotic leak, the neck wound can be opened, drained, and packed to expedite healing.

Management of Complications

- Anastomotic leak is manifested by redness and drainage from the cervical incision, which should be then opened and packed. Jejunostomy feeds are instituted as well as antibiotic coverage and either nothing per mouth or sips of water.
- Postoperative pneumothoraces can occur and can be managed with a chest tube depending on the size of the pneumothorax. Similarly, pleural effusions identified at any point postoperatively may also require chest tube drainage.
- Recurrent laryngeal nerve injuries are managed initially with injection of the vocal cords and medialization. Traction injuries may resolve on their own but ultimately may require a more permanent medialization procedure.
- Early recognition and intervention are essential to maintain good pulmonary toilet.

PEARLS AND PITFALLS

- Most bleeding in the mediastinum can be controlled with packing and patience.
- If an EEA circular anastomosis is not feasible, an end-to-end double layer handsewn anastomosis is a viable alternative.
- The delivery of the stomach through the mediastinum is accomplished with the sterile plastic bag as described and with gentle pressure and support of the gastric conduit through the esophageal hiatus by the operating surgeon via the abdomen as the assistant draws the catheter up through the cervical incision with suction applied to the bag.
- It is essential to be certain that the conduit is not twisted in the mediastinum after it is delivered to the neck.
- A jejunostomy is often placed prior to closing the cervical incision and the abdominal incision.

Suggested Readings

1. Lin J, Iannettoni MD. Transhiatal esophagectomy. *Surg Clin North Am*. 2005;85(3):593-610.
2. Orringer MB. Transhiatal esophagectomy: how I teach it. *Ann Thorac Surg*. 2016;102(5):1432-1437.
3. Parry K, Ruurda JP, van der Sluis PC, van Hillegersberg R. Current status of laparoscopic transhiatal esophagectomy for esophageal cancer patients: a systematic review of the literature. *Dis Esophagus*. 2017;30(1):1-7.
4. Scipione CN, Chang AC, Pickens A, Lau CL, Orringer MB. Transhiatal esophagectomy in the profoundly obese: implications and experience. *Ann Thorac Surg*. 2007;84(2):376-383.
5. Orringer MB, Marshall B, Iannettoni MD. Transhiatal esophagectomy: clinical experience and refinements. *Ann Surg*. 1999;230(3):392-403.

Chapter 38

Left Thoracoabdominal Esophagectomy

PIERRE DE DELVA
CORBIN CLEARY

- Left thoracoabdominal esophagectomy was popularized by Edward Churchill and Richard Sweet and for many years was considered a standard technique.
- In current practice, other approaches, including minimally invasive techniques, are favored by most surgeons and the role of thoracoabdominal esophagectomy is more limited.
- The distal esophagus and gastroesophageal junction (GEJ) can be difficult to expose in obese patients and in the setting of advanced malignancy or reoperative surgery.
    - The thoracoabdominal approach provides excellent access to the GEJ in both benign and malignant conditions, including perforation, trauma, esophageal cancer, or difficult hiatal hernia and antireflux surgery.
- It is in the setting of a challenging operation focused at GEJ that the thoracoabdominal approach is ideal, as it provides unparalleled exposure and concurrent access to the abdominal and thoracic cavities.
- Every thoracic surgeon managing complex GEJ pathology should be familiar with this approach.

Perioperative Considerations

- Patients considered for this approach should be evaluated for adequate pulmonary reserve as the combination of a thoracotomy, laparotomy, and diaphragmatic incision can lead to higher pulmonary morbidity in marginal patients.
- Nutritional status should be optimized for any patient requiring esophagectomy to promote appropriate anastomotic healing and postoperative recovery.
- The stomach is the preferred conduit, even in the setting of multiple previous operations. However, in complex cases benefiting from the thoracoabdominal approach, surgeons should be prepared to use alternative conduits.

TIPS

Preoperative angiography can be helpful in evaluating the integrity of the blood supply of the stomach and colon.

- Esophagoscopy or esophagogastroduodenoscopy should be performed by the surgeon to confirm the diagnosis and extent of pathology.

Instruments and Equipment

- Standard thoracotomy and laparotomy instruments
- Abdominal and chest wall retractors
- Vessel sealing devices provide for rapid hemostatic dissection and mobilization
- Surgical staplers for conduit creation and anastomosis

Anesthesia Considerations

- Given the extent of the incision and dissection, all patients should be considered for neuraxial blockade.
- Single-lung ventilation is essential to optimize the exposure for the procedure and can be obtained either by dual-lumen endotracheal tube or bronchial blocker.

Patient Positioning

- The patient should be placed in right lateral decubitus position with the left hip slightly rotated posteriorly to enhance access to the abdominal cavity (Figure 38.1).

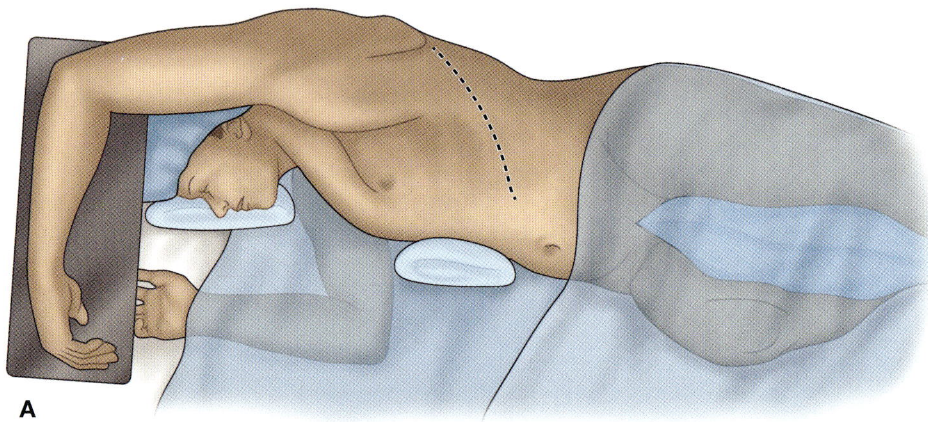

A

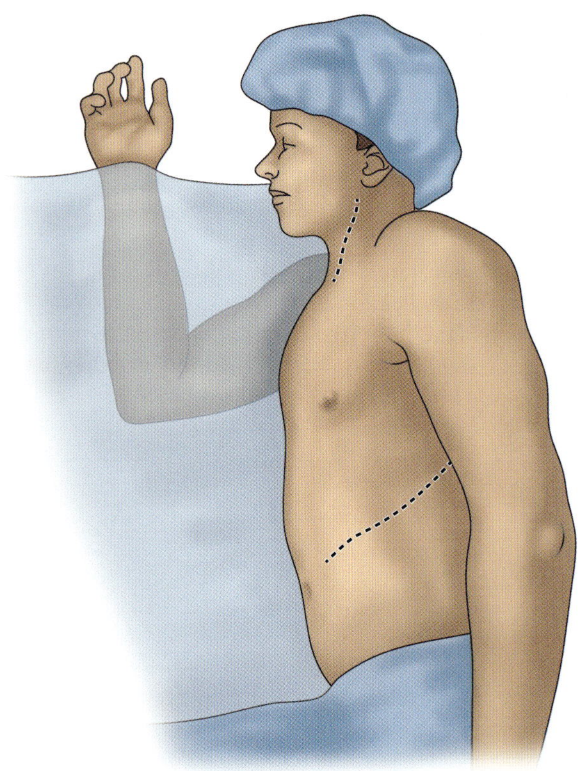

B

FIGURE 38.1 ▮ A and B. Patient positioning and incision for thoracoabdominal esophagectomy. Proper positioning provides concurrent exposure to the chest and abdomen. The incision extends from the tip of the scapula, across the costal cartilage and into the abdomen.

- Flexion should be created at the costal margin.
- The left arm should be draped across the patient's body.
  - If a cervical incision is planned for a high anastomosis, the arm can be included in the operative field so that it can be positioned for access to the left neck.
- A single sterile preparation can be utilized; if a neck anastomosis is planned, this should be included within the field.

Technique

- Incision and division of the diaphragm:
  - The incision can start either in the abdomen or the thorax.
    - If there is concern for resectability in cases of malignancy, an abdominal incision can be performed first to evaluate for metastatic disease prior to committing to the entire incision and division of the costal cartilage and diaphragm.
  - The standard thoracoabdominal incision for esophageal surgery extends from the tip of the scapula to a point in the upper abdomen, typically halfway between the xiphoid and umbilicus (Figure 38.1).
    - A sixth intercostal space incision is ideal for creation of the anastomosis just below the aortic arch.
  - If the anastomosis needs to be created above the aortic arch, the skin incision is extended cephalad between the posterior edge of the scapula and the spine.
    - A fourth or fifth intercostal incision provides optimal exposure for a high intrathoracic anastomosis, but access to the abdominal cavity may be limited.
  - The costal cartilage is divided, and the diaphragm is incised to gain exposure to the abdominal cavity (Figure 38.2A).
    - The diaphragm can be divided either circumferentially or radially.
      - We prefer a circumferential incision because it preserves phrenic function while providing good exposure to the hiatus (Figure 38.2B).
      - Radial incision creates the most direct and unobstructed view of the GEJ but divides lateral branches of the phrenic nerve.
    - A 2-cm margin of diaphragm should be left attached to the chest wall to ease closure.
      - everal stay/marking sutures are placed along the diaphragmatic incision to realign the closure.

Thoracic Portion

- The inferior pulmonary ligament is divided. The posterior pleura is opened, and the lower esophagus is freed with appropriate caution given to division of the aortoesophageal branches.
- A Penrose drain can be used to encircle the esophagus to provide gentle traction.
- The dissection continues proximally to the subcarinal space.
  - En bloc lymphadenectomy is performed in malignant disease; otherwise, the dissection is maintained on the esophagus to minimize trauma to adjacent structures.
  - If further cephalad dissection is needed, careful blunt dissection should be utilized to minimize trauma to the airway and the recurrent laryngeal nerve.

The Abdominal Portion

- The greater omentum is divided off the stomach, ensuring protection of the right gastroepiploic artery (Figure 38.3A).
  - If desired by the surgeon, a variable amount of the omentum may be harvested with the stomach to serve as a buttress flap.
- Division of gastrosplenic ligament and division of the short gastric arteries is then performed.
- The gastrohepatic ligament is divided with care, observing for the presence of replaced or accessory hepatic vessels.
- The left gastric artery is divided as close to its origin as possible, allowing for appropriate lymphadenectomy when necessary (Figure 38.3B).
  - This may be best approached by rotating the greater curvature of the stomach toward the patient's right.

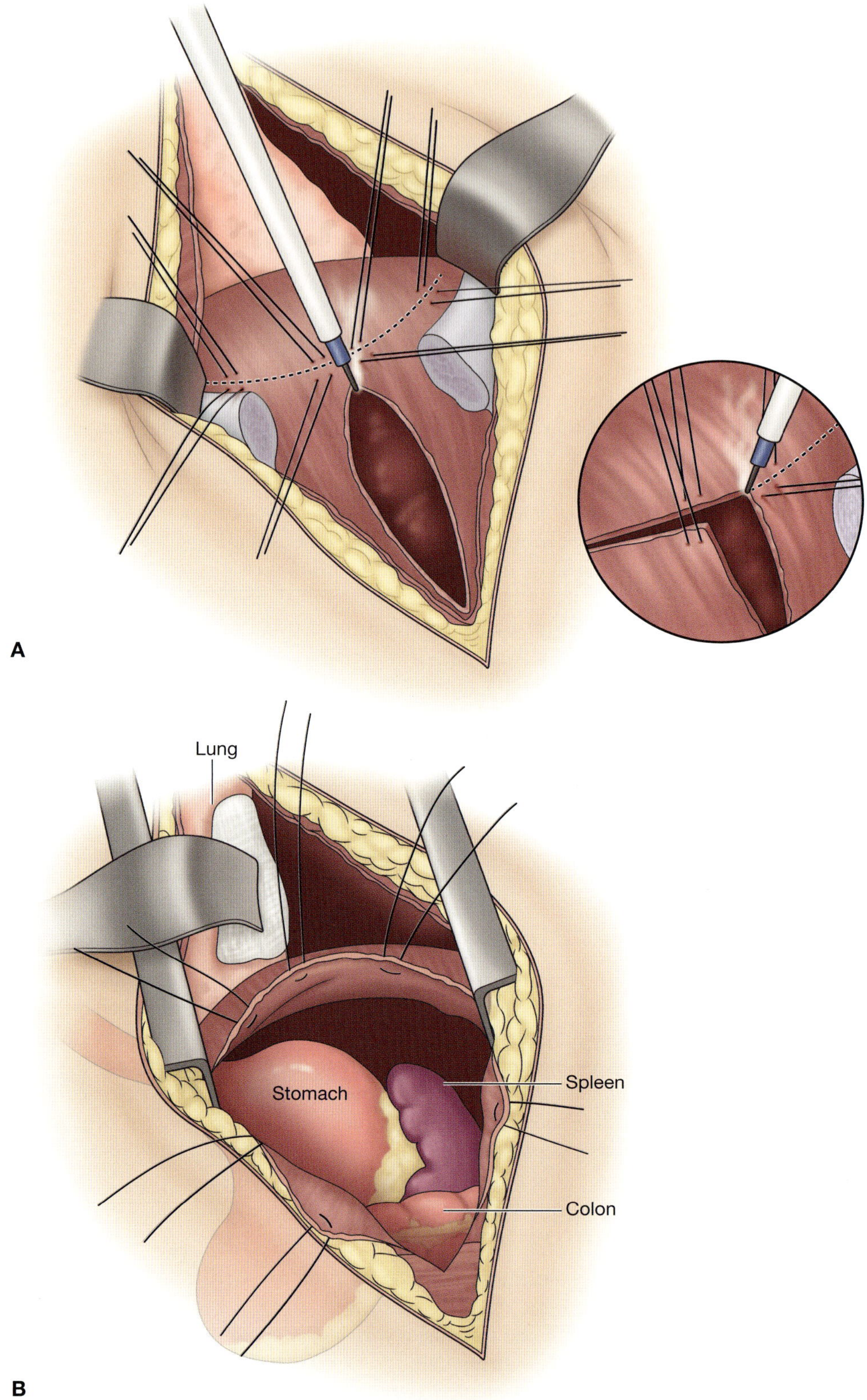

FIGURE 38.2 ▮ **A.** Circumferential diaphragm incision with alignment stay sutures. Incision is perpendicular to the abdominal muscular incision. **B.** Exposure of the gastroesophageal junction.

- A Kocher maneuver can be performed to medialize the duodenum and enhance the cephalad mobility of the conduit.
- The stomach is divided with sequential stapler firings.
    - A tubularized or whole stomach conduit can be fashioned, with the former having the advantage of more length and potentially better emptying.

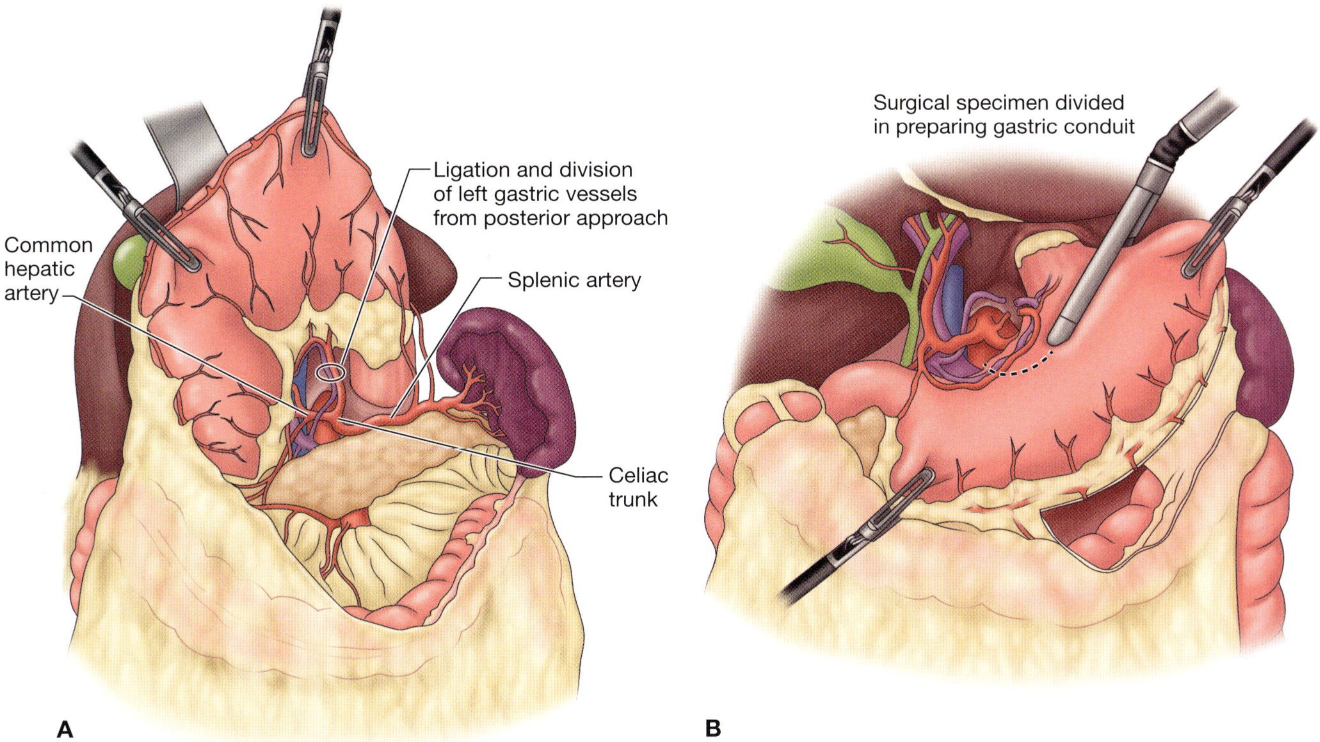

FIGURE 38.3 | A. Mobilization of the stomach in preparation for conduit formation. **B.** Ligation of the left gastric artery through the gastrocolic ligament with the stomach retracted to the right.

- The gastric conduit is then delivered into the chest, ensuring appropriate orientation.
  - The thoracoabdominal approach facilitates proper alignment and positioning of the gastric or alternatives conduit, such as short-segment colonic or jejunal interposition.
- A jejunostomy is created for postoperative enteral access if needed.

The Anastomosis

- After delivery of the stomach into the chest, the pathological portion of the esophagus and stomach is resected, balancing between optimal proximal and distal margins, the length of well-vascularized conduit, and tension.
- Care should be taken to ensure the anastomosis is created close to the end of the right gastroepiploic arcade.
- The anastomosis is routinely placed below the aortic arch; however, supra-aortic or cervical anastomotic sites may be selected depending on the extent of pathology, desired margin, or surgeon preference.
- A variety of techniques exist to create an adequate anastomosis, including stapled, hand-sewn, and combined approaches.
  - Stapled anastomoses can be performed through a variety of techniques, including end-to-end, end-to-side, side-to-side (Orringer approach).
  - Hand-sewn methods can also be utilized and preferred by many surgeons.
    - The two-layer, hand-sewn Sweet anastomosis is well described and has demonstrated low leak rates and excellent functional results.

Closure and Drainage

- Pleural drains are placed and at least one of the drains should be targeted to control potential anastomotic leaks.
- A nasogastric tube is placed with surgeon guidance though the chest.
- The diaphragm and abdominal musculature are closed with interrupted sutures, using the stay sutures to aid in alignment (Figure 38.4A).
  - Diaphragm is closed with nonabsorbable sutures.

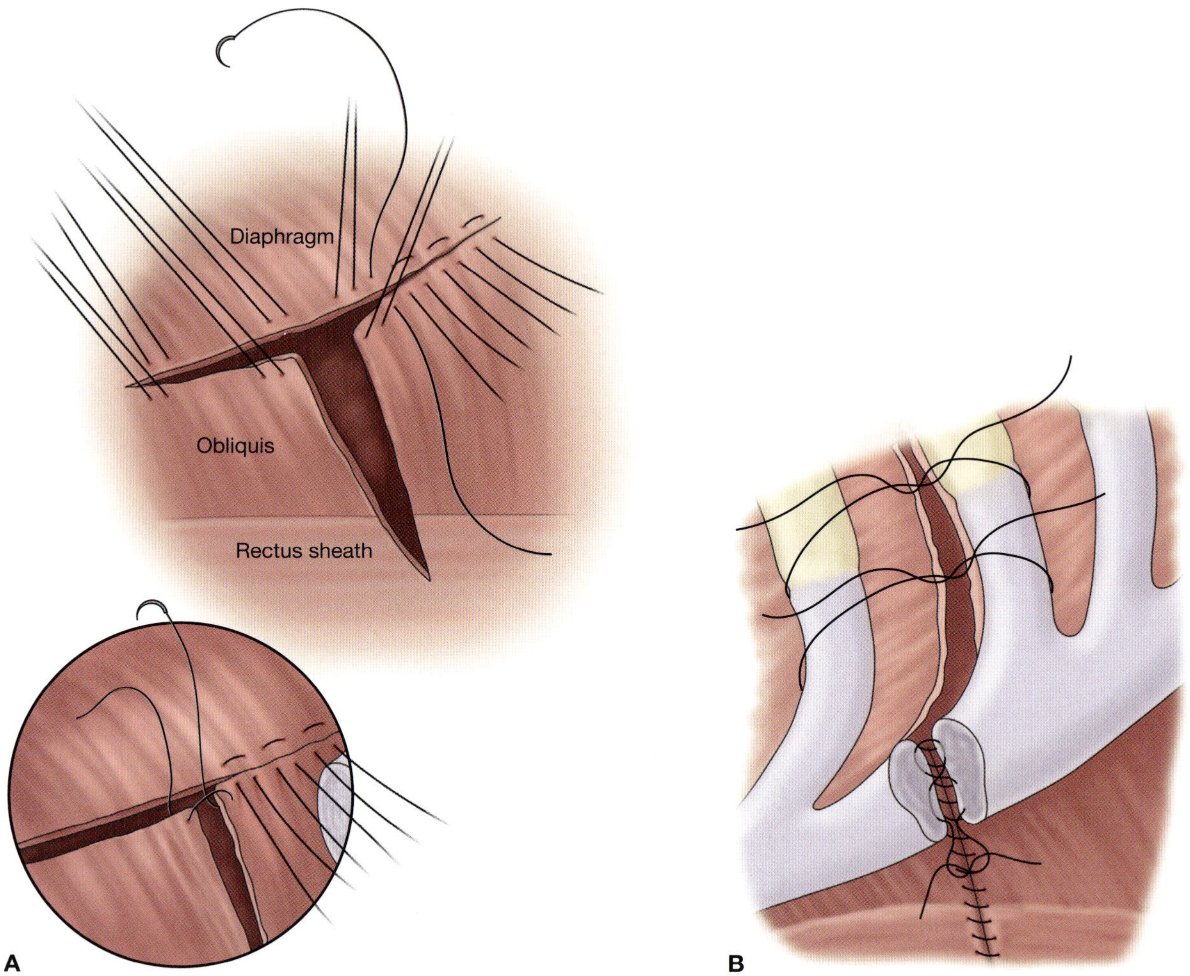

FIGURE 38.4 ▌ A. Closure of the circumferential diaphragmatic incision, using the stay sutures for alignments. **B.** Closure of the chest incisions and approximation of the costal cartilage.

- The ribs are reapproximated with standard pericostal sutures, and the costal margin can be reapproximated with sutures, wires, or plates (Figure 38.4B).
- If a neck incision is used, the dermis and platysma are closed in separate layers and a drain may be placed through the incision into the mediastinum.

Postoperative Care

- Patients typically spend their first postoperative day in the intensive care unit.
- Meticulous attention to volume status and oxygen delivery is crucial for conduit perfusion and anastomotic healing.
- The nasogastric tube is placed on low intermittent suction and flushed appropriately to prevent conduit distention.
- Neuraxial analgesia should provide adequate pain control; regimens of standing ketorolac, acetaminophen, and gabapentin provide for additional pain control in appropriate patients.
- An esophagogram may be performed to evaluate for evidence of anastomotic leaks, assess gastric emptying, and rule out aspiration.
- Chest tubes and drains are removed as the drainage decreases and no signs of infection, chyle leak, or bleeding.
- Esophagectomy is prone to complications and a high index of suspicion, and meticulous patient care and rapid recognition and rescue are crucial to prevent significant morbidity and mortality.

PEARLS AND PITFALLS

- The thoracoabdominal approach is ideal for distal pathology and contraindicated in conditions involving the upper thoracic esophagus, as exposure is hindered by the aorta and great vessels and would be best approached via the right thoracic cavity.
- Postoperative outcomes start with appropriate preoperative planning.
- Wide exposure is fundamental to this approach, and division of the costal cartilage and diaphragm provides better exposure than counter abdominal and thoracic incisions or a thoracic-only incision with transdiaphragmatic access to the abdomen.
- Incisional morbidity can be minimized with proper opening and closure of the incision.
- A well-vascularized and tension-free anastomosis is paramount to the success of the operation.
- Intraoperative assessment of gastric conduit perfusion with fluorescent indocyanine green imaging can assist in determining an ideal anastomotic site.

Suggested Readings

1. Churchill ED, Sweet RH. Transthoracic resection of tumors of the esophagus and stomach. *Ann Surg*. 1942;115(6):897-920. PMID: 17858052; PMCID: PMC1543875.
2. Gillies RS, Simpkin A, Sgromo B, Marshall RE, Maynard ND. Left thoracoabdominal esophagectomy: results from a single specialist center. *Dis Esophagus*. 2011;24(3):138-144. PMID: 20819097.
3. Li B, Guo Q, Yang H, et al. Left thoracoabdominal approach in surgical treatment of adenocarcinoma of the esophagogastric junction in the Northern Henan Province of China. *Dig Surg*. 2011;28(1):2-8. PMID: 21293125.
4. Morse CR, Mathisen DJ. Left thoracoabdominal approach. In: Sugarbaker DJ, Bueno R, Colson Y, Jaklitsch M, Krasna M, Mentzer S, eds. *Adult Chest Surgery*. 2015:183-195.
5. Murthy S. Left Thoracoabdominal expsosure for esophagectomy and complex hiatus pathology. In: Luketich JD, ed. *Master Techniques in Surgery: Esophageal Surgery*. 2014:263-272.
6. Sweet RH. *Operations of the Esophagus*. W. B. Saunders Company; 1954.

Chapter 39

McKeown (3-Hole) Esophagectomy

SMITA SIHAG
DANIELA MOLENA

McKeown esophagectomy, also known as 3-hole esophagectomy, is the preferred surgical technique for resection of midesophageal malignancies. It allows for a three-field lymph node dissection with a cervical neck anastomosis. However, because of the significant morbidity that can result from the extensive nature of this operation, minimally invasive techniques have evolved to mitigate some of these effects. Ivor Lewis esophagectomy with intrathoracic anastomosis is often preferred for distal esophageal malignancies, whereby neck dissection and related complications, such as recurrent laryngeal nerve injury, may be avoided. In the current era of esophageal surgery, however, surgeons are able to select the appropriate operation or approach on the basis of the extent of disease, and McKeown esophagectomy remains an important and necessary technique in a surgeon's armamentarium.

Indications

- Tumors involving the upper to midesophagus (<30 cm from incisors) especially if there is concern for either a positive or an inadequate margin (<3 cm) using an Ivor Lewis approach.
- Tumors with nodal involvement above the level of the carina (ie, paratracheal or supraclavicular lymph nodes) necessitating a three-field lymph node dissection.
- Extension of long-segment Barrett metaplasia/dysplasia <25 cm from incisors.
- Need for upfront intrathoracic exploration to evaluate surgical resectability, ie, concern for tumor invasion into airway or pericardium.
- Benign diseases affecting the entire esophagus, ie, end-stage motility disorders or chemical injury.
- Surgeon preference or patient factors favoring cervical versus intrathoracic anastomosis.
- Prior radiation to the upper thoracic esophagus or mediastinum.

Perioperative Considerations

- **Age and performance status:** Octagenarians and patients with an Eastern Cooperative Oncology Group score ≥2 are at higher risk of postoperative complications.
- **Nutritional and metabolic status:** Laboratory studies including albumin and prealbumin and serial weights should be assessed. Preoperative feeding tube placement (jejeunostomy or gastrostomy) is reasonable to optimize malnourished patients with severe dysphagia or radiation esophagitis. Insertion of a feeding tube is preferred over an expandable stent given increased operative difficulty after prolonged stent placement.
- **Cardiopulmonary reserve:** Nearly all patients should undergo a comprehensive cardiopulmonary evaluation with a stress echocardiogram and pulmonary function tests.
- **Surgical planning:** In addition to appropriate staging studies, bronchoscopy, upper endoscopy, and/or diagnostic laparoscopy should be considered prior to resection to rule out airway involvement,

assess the adequacy of the conduit, map the location of distal margin, and rule out metastatic disease in the abdomen.

Technique

Regardless of whether an open or minimally invasive technique is used, the steps of the operation are nearly identical. A minimally invasive laparoscopic/thoracoscopic approach is described in depth below, with additional tips and tricks to improve exposure and efficiency. These steps can also be easily translated to open or robotic cases.

Thoracic Component

- Following induction of general anesthesia, the patient is intubated with a double-lumen endotracheal tube following flexible bronchoscopy and endoscopy to rule out invasion of the airway and to assess the extent of disease in the esophagus.
- The operation begins with the patient in the left lateral decubitus position, with slight rotation anteriorly. Thoracoscopic ports are placed as shown in Figure 39.1. There are two ports for the primary surgeon anteriorly and one for the assistant posteriorly, along with one port for either a 5- or 10-mm 45° camera.

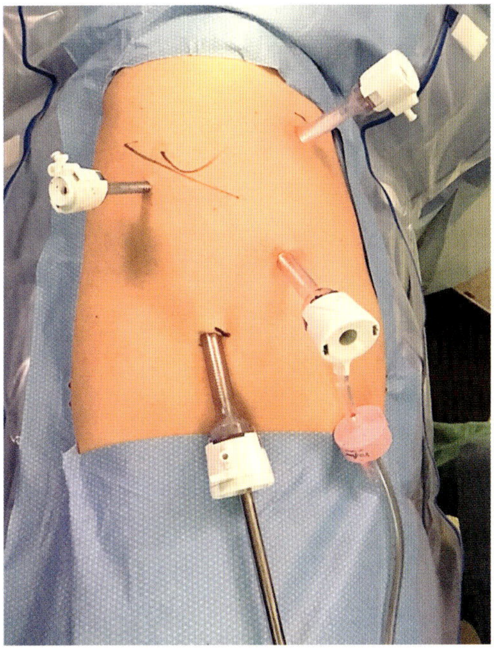

FIGURE 39.1 ▮ Thoracoscopic port placement.

TIPS

Either carbon dioxide insufflation to 8 mm Hg or a retraction figure-of-eight stitch in the central tendon of the diaphragm is used to help improve visualization of the thoracic sulcus.

- After the posterior mediastinal pleura is incised using a vessel-sealing device, such as either the Harmonic scalpel (Ethicon) or LigaSure (Medtronic), the azygous vein is divided with a linear Endo GIA stapler (Medtronic) (Figure 39.2).

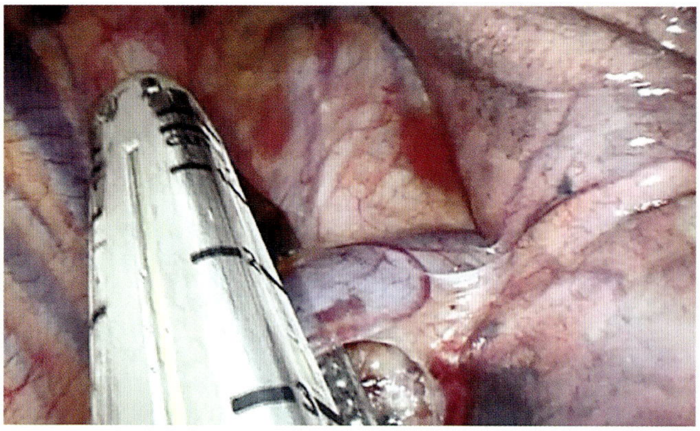

FIGURE 39.2 ▌ Division of the azygous vein using a linear Endo GIA stapler.

TIPS

Care must be taken to avoid thermal injury to the airway when using the Harmonic scalpel.

- The esophagus is mobilized from the hiatus to the thoracic inlet. A circumferential quarter-inch Penrose drain is placed around the esophagus, secured with hemoclips, to facilitate retraction (Figure 39.3).

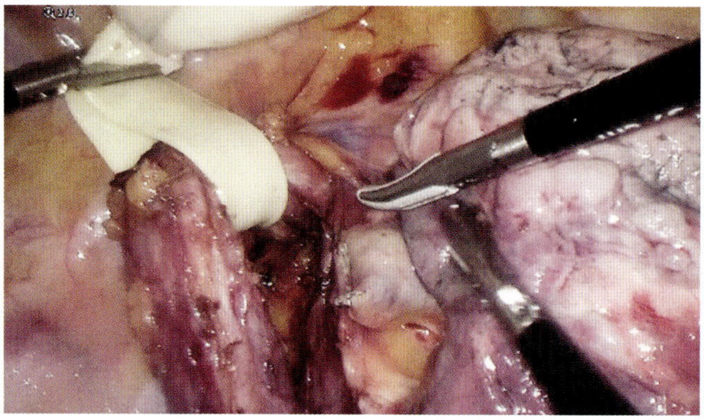

FIGURE 39.3 ▌ Retraction of the esophagus using a Penrose drain while dissecting along the periesophageal plane from the diaphragm to thoracic inlet.

TIPS

Stay in the periesophageal plane during the dissection, primarily to avoid left mainstem injury.

TIPS

The thoracic duct should be prophylactically ligated if it is visualized during the procedure; however, routine ligation is not generally necessary or recommended.

- Paraesophageal lymph nodes are removed en bloc with the esophagus, while a complete lymphadenectomy of the subcarinal (Figure 39.4) and right paratracheal nodal packets is performed separately after esophageal mobilization.
- A Penrose drain is left in place in the thoracic inlet to help identify the esophagus from the cervical dissection.

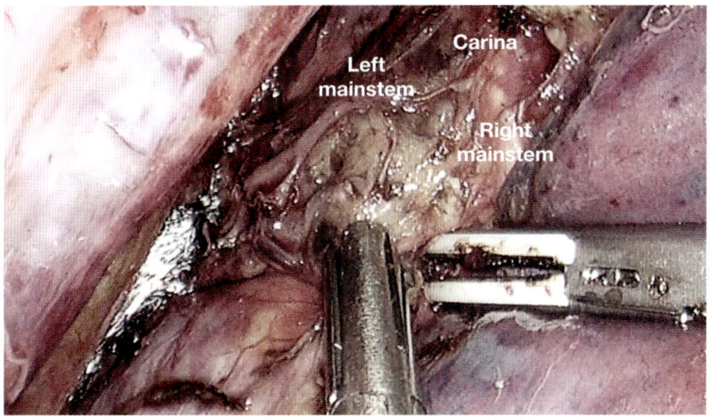

FIGURE 39.4 ▮ Subcarinal lymphadenectomy.

TIPS

Take extra care to protect the recurrent laryngeal nerves as the dissection of the esophagus is continued into the thoracic inlet.

- A second Penrose drain is placed in the diaphragmatic hiatus inferiorly to assist with retraction and easy identification of the esophagus during the abdominal phase of the operation.
- Once dissection is complete, a 28-French chest tube is placed through the most inferior port and positioned posteriorly and apically. An intercostal nerve block is then performed using bupivacaine. Epidural catheters were routinely placed for thoracotomy but not for minimally invasive procedures.

Abdominal Component

- The patient is repositioned supine and secured with a foot board with arms tucked. A shoulder roll is placed with the head directed toward the right to expose the left neck. A midline port is placed below the falciform and above the umbilicus for a 45° camera, followed by 5- and 12-mm ports for the primary surgeon in the right upper quadrant and 5- and 12-mm ports for the assistant in the left upper quadrant (Figure 39.5). This configuration is optimal if both a first and second assistant are available. An additional 5-mm subxiphoid port is used for the Nathanson Liver Retractor (Cook Medical).

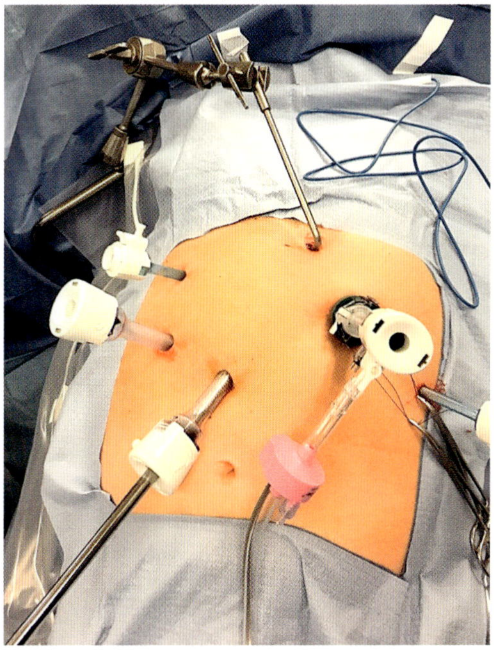

FIGURE 39.5 ▮ Abdominal port placement.

- Once the patient is placed in steep reverse Trendelenburg position, dissection begins at the lesser curve, and the gastrohepatic ligament is divided up to the hiatus.

TIPS

Beware of a replaced left hepatic artery. Celiac axis lymphadenectomy is then performed, removing all lymph nodes along the hepatic artery and the left gastric artery (Figure 39.6A).

- The left gastric artery is skeletonized and divided with a linear Endo GIA stapler (Figure 39.6B).

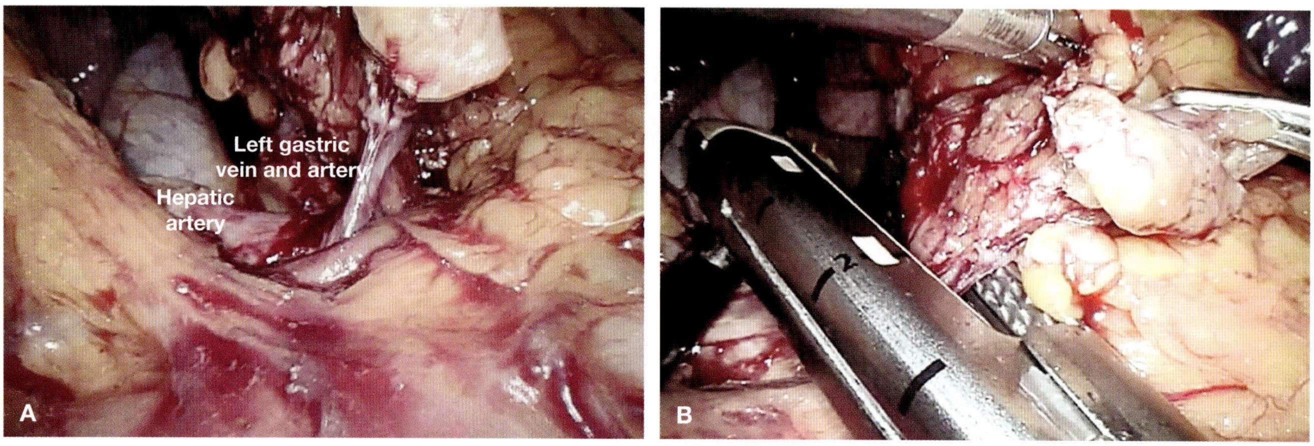

FIGURE 39.6 ❙ A. Dissection of hepatic artery and celiac plexus lymph nodes with skeletonization of the left gastric vessels. **B.** Division of the left gastric artery and vein using a linear Endo GIA stapler.

- The gastroepiploic arcade is then identified visually along the greater curve, and the lesser sac is entered through the gastrocolic ligament (Figure 39.7A). The dissection is continued along the greater curve toward the left crus, ensuring that the short gastric artery branches are well cauterized (Figure 39.7B).

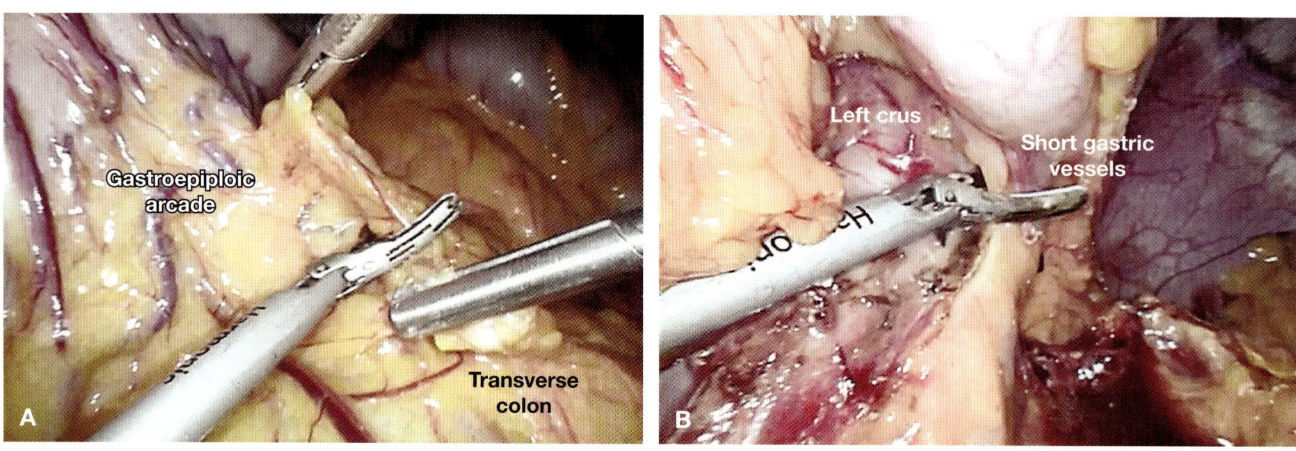

FIGURE 39.7 ❙ A. Entry into the lesser sac while carefully preserving the gastroepiploic arcade. **B.** Division of the short gastric vessels along the stomach all the way to the left crus.

- The dissection is then continued toward the duodenum, separating the stomach from the transverse mesocolon. The authors do not perform a pyloric drainage procedure routinely. In addition, the authors do not perform a full Kocher maneuver, as fully releasing the peritoneal reflection along the gastroepiploic pedicle to the first portion of the duodenum is usually sufficient to allow the gastric conduit to reach the neck (Figure 39.8).

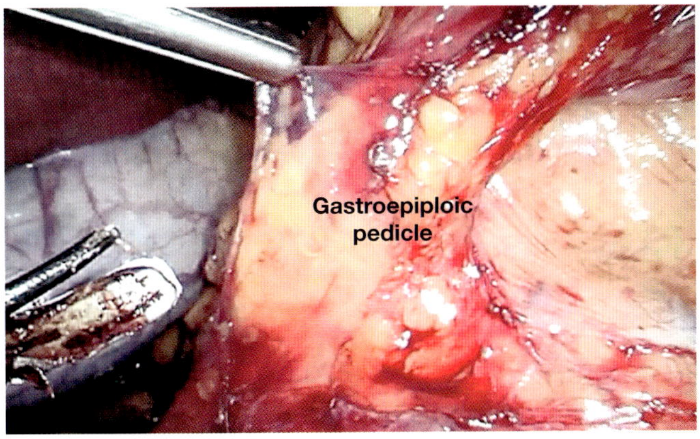

FIGURE 39.8 | Division of the peritoneal reflection over the gastroepiploic pedicle to the first portion of the duodenum to allow full mobilization of the stomach allowing the pylorus to easily reach the right crus. A complete Kocher maneuver is not necessary.

- Next, the phrenoesophageal ligament is divided, and the esophagus is circumferentially mobilized at the hiatus extending into the mediastinum. Continuity with the chest dissection is established by identifying the Penrose drain in the diaphragmatic sulcus (Figure 39.9).

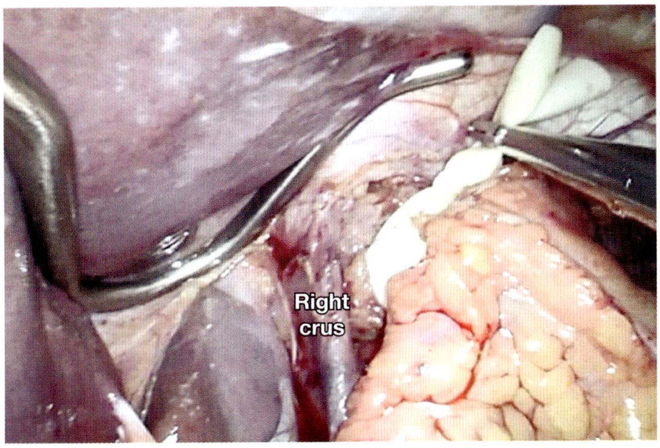

FIGURE 39.9 | Using the Penrose drain to establish continuity between the thoracic and abdominal dissection at the hiatus.

- With full mobilization of the stomach complete, the gastric conduit is fashioned with serial firings of a linear Endo GIA stapler from the incisura to the tip of the fundus (Figure 39.10A). A conduit diameter of 3 to 5 cm is preferred, and the conduit is completely detached from the specimen.
- PINPOINT (Stryker) laparoscopic fluorescence imaging technology may be used to assess the perfusion of the conduit to the tip of the fundus following intravenous bolus of indocyanine green (Figure 39.10B).

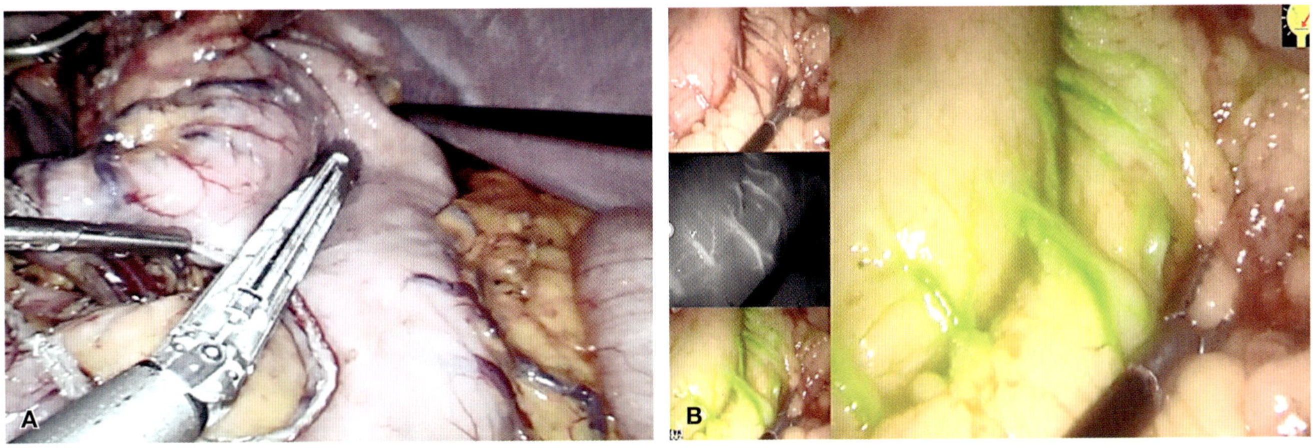

FIGURE 39.10 | **A.** Construction of the gastric conduit, typically 3 to 5 cm in width. **B.** Indocyanine green perfusion of the gastric conduit demonstrates that the gastroepiploic arcade is intact and patent.

- Last, a jejunostomy tube (J-tube) is placed. Once the omentum and transverse colon are retracted superiorly, the ligament of Treitz is identified, and a segment of jejunum 30 to 40 cm distal to the ligament is used to insert the J-tube.
- The Endo Stitch device (Medtronic) with a 2-0 polysorb suture is used to place sutures in four quadrants to tack the jejunum to the abdominal wall. The J-tube is inserted using the Seldinger technique, and an antitorsion stitch is placed once the tube is secured to the abdominal wall.

Cervical Component

- A left neck incision along the anterior sternocleidomastoid muscle is made. The carotid sheath is retracted laterally, the thyroid is retracted medially, and the tracheoesophageal groove is identified (Figure 39.11). The dissection is continued toward the thoracic inlet, and continuity is established with the previous chest dissection, where the Penrose drain was retained.

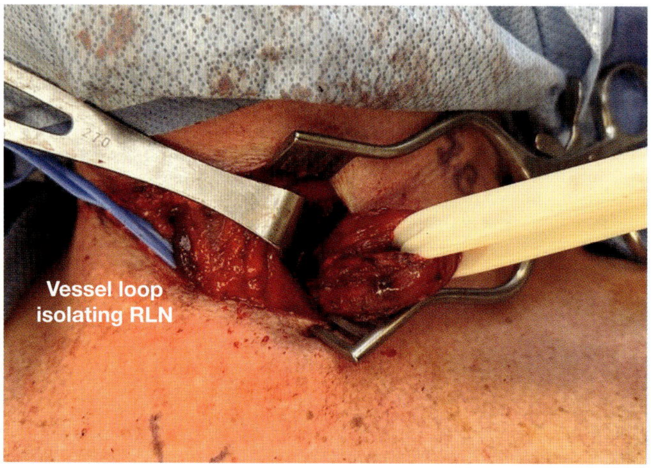

FIGURE 39.11 ▌ Left neck incision with mobilization of the cervical esophagus using the Penrose drain. Blue vessel loop is isolating the recurrent laryngeal nerve (RLN).

TIPS

As in the chest, the dissection is limited to the plane immediately adjacent to the esophagus, and blunt techniques are used once the space is opened to avoid recurrent laryngeal nerve injury.

- The specimen is pulled out carefully through the neck while the assistant feeds the distal end through the hiatus and mediastinum laparoscopically. The proximal esophagus is divided sharply with a knife, and the specimen is sent to pathology for frozen section analysis of the proximal and distal margins.
- To facilitate delivery of the conduit to the neck, a large Foley catheter or 28-French chest tube is passed through the neck incision and posterior mediastinum and into the abdomen. The tip is secured to the gastric conduit using the Endo Stich device with a 2-0 Surgidac suture, and the conduit is brought up into the neck, again, with laparoscopic assistance in carefully feeding it through the hiatus in the correct orientation.

TIPS

A less traumatic method for transposition of the gastric conduit to the neck involves placing the gastric conduit into a plastic ultrasound probe bag with a Foley catheter with an inflated balloon secured to both the bag and the conduit (Figure 39.12A and B). This greatly facilitates passage of the conduit through the posterior mediastinum or substernally.

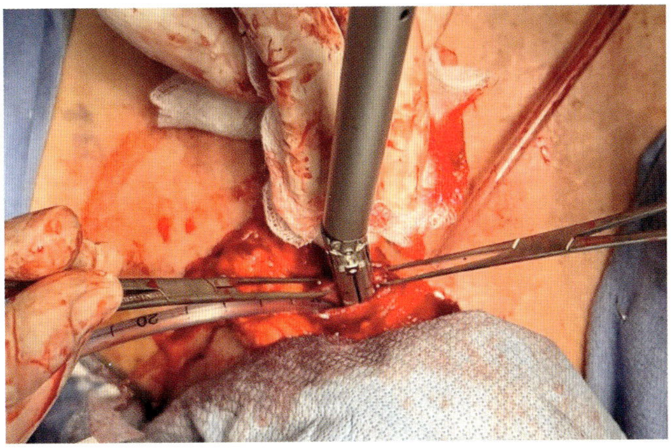

FIGURE 39.13 | Technique for stapled cervical anastomosis using a linear Endo GIA stapler.

- The anastomosis is constructed with either a linear Endo GIA or EEA stapler (Medtronic) (Figure 39.13). A nasogastric tube (NGT) is passed through the anastomosis and secured at 45 cm from the nares. A Jackson-Pratt (JP) drain is positioned beside the anastomosis, and the wounds are closed.

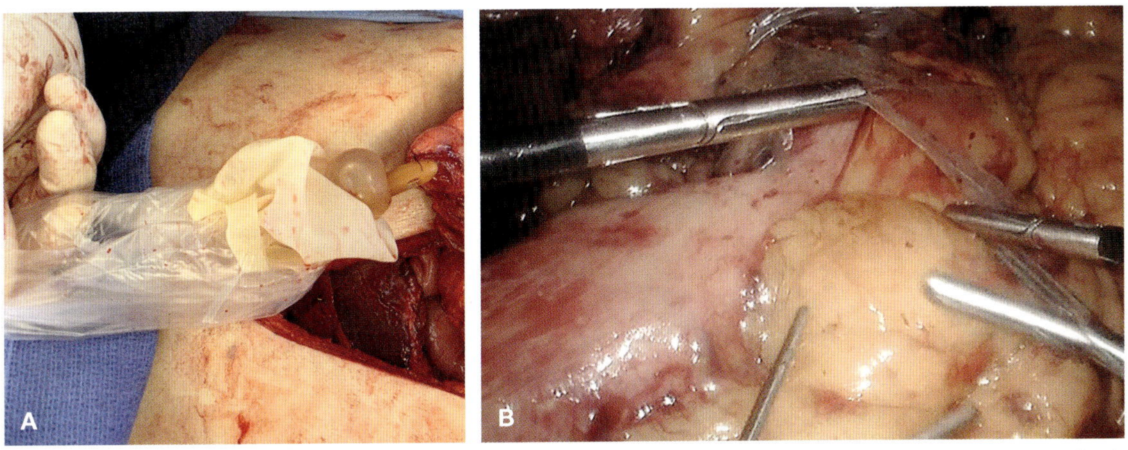

FIGURE 39.12 | **A.** The Foley catheter and ultrasound bag sutured to the conduit. **B.** Insertion of the gastric conduit into a sterile ultrasound probe bag laparoscopically to facilitate atraumatic transposition to the neck. Applying suction to the Foley catheter as the conduit is delivered to the neck via the posterior mediastinum.

TIPS

Any redundancy of the conduit may be reduced by gently pulling the conduit back into the abdomen laparoscopically. In addition, a large hiatal opening can be repaired if there is concern for future paraconduit hernia formation.

Postoperative Care

Enhanced recovery protocols after surgery have been successfully implemented for both open and minimally invasive McKeown esophagectomy patients at low to moderate risk of postoperative complications with good results. Modifications should be considered for patients at high risk of postoperative complications or who deviate from a routine postoperative course.

- **Pain control:** A patient-controlled analgesia pump is sufficient for patients undergoing minimally invasive procedures, while a thoracic epidural is still preferred for patients undergoing thoracotomy and/or laparotomy. Patients are transitioned to liquid analgesics via jejeunostomy tube once they are tolerating goal tube feeds.

- **Nutrition:** Tube feedings are initiated on day 2 via jejeunostomy tube at 30 mL/h and advanced slowly by 10 mL/h every 6 hours as bowel function resumes. Once the goal feeding rate is well tolerated, tube feeds are then cycled for 8 to 10 hours overnight. Oral intake begins with clear liquids by day 5 or 6 if there are no apparent complications, such as anastomotic leak or recurrent laryngeal nerve injury. Patients are transitioned to full liquids around day 10 and soft foods by day 14.
- **Chest tube:** A 28-French chest tube is managed on water seal postoperatively. Once a chyle leak is ruled out by day 3, the chest tube is removed by day 4 or 5 when the drainage is less than 300 mL/24 h period.
- **NGT:** The NGT is kept to low wall suction until bowel function resumes and the output is less than 300 mL over a 24-hour period. Usually by day 5, the NGT is removed and sips of liquids are initiated.
- **Neck drain:** A JP drain near the anastomosis is maintained either on or off suction per surgeon preference. This drain remains in place until the patient is tolerating liquids without evidence of anastomotic leak. If there is evidence of anastomotic leak, the drain is kept in place until it is fully healed. The neck wound may also be partially opened and packed if needed to allow for better drainage or management of wound infection.

Management of Common Complications

- **Anastomotic leak:** Patients are at higher risk of anastomotic leak following McKeown esophagectomy in comparison to Ivor Lewis approach. However, leaks are much more easily managed with intravenous antibiotics, adequate drainage, and nothing by mouth or sips of water only.
- **Recurrent laryngeal nerve injury:** This complication occurs in 10% to 15% of patients following McKeown esophagectomy. If this is suspected, a laryngologist should be consulted for laryngoscopy. Early vocal cord medialization is recommended if indicated to prevent aspiration and facilitate effective pulmonary toilet.
- **Chyle leak:** If a chyle leak is observed postoperatively, outputs should be monitored carefully. For low output leaks, elemental tube feedings may allow it to resolve. For high output leaks, lymphangiography with ablation is effective if an experienced interventionalist is available to perform the procedure. If not, surgical thoracic duct ligation may be necessary.

PEARLS AND PITFALLS

- If following the thoracic dissection, there is concern that postoperative radiotherapy may be needed for residual disease or close margins, consider substernal reconstruction.
- If the gastric conduit appears inadequate for any reason at the time of reconstruction, esophageal diversion with cervical esophagostomy followed by delayed substernal reconstruction using a colon interposition is usually a safe option to consider.
- If the conduit barely reaches the neck, partial resection of the manubrium may facilitate a tension-free anastomosis for a substernal conduit.
- An end-to-end double layer hand sewn anastomosis is an alternative if a stapled anastomosis is not technically feasible.

Suggested Readings

1. Deng J, Su Q, Ren Z, et al. Comparison of short-term outcomes between minimally invasive McKeown and Ivor Lewis esophagectomy for esophageal or junctional cancer: a systematic review and meta-analysis. *OncoTargets Ther*. 2018;11:6057-6069.
2. Kernstine KH, DeArmond DT, Shamoun DM, Campos JH. The first series of completely robotic esophagectomies with three-field lymphadenectomy: initial experience. *Surg Endosc*. 2007;21(12):2285-2292.
3. Korst RJ, Sukumar M, Burt ME. Atraumatic gastric transposition after transhiatal esophagectomy. *Ann Thorac Surg*. 1997;64(3):867-869.
4. Luketich JD, Pennathur A, Awais O, et al. Outcomes after minimally invasive esophagectomy: review of over 1000 patients. *Ann Surg*. 2012;256(1):95-103.
5. McKeown KC. Total three-stage oesophagectomy for cancer of the oesophagus. *Br J Surg*. 1976;63(4):259-262.

6. Mu JW, Gao SG, Xue Q, et al. Updated experiences with minimally invasive McKeown esophagectomy for esophageal cancer. *World J Gastroenterol*. 2015;21(45):12873-12881.
7. Patel S, Petrov R, Abbas A, Bakhos C. Robotic-assisted McKeown esophagectomy. *J Vis Surg*. 2019;5:43.
8. Swanson SJ, Batirel HF, Bueno R, et al. Transthoracic esophagectomy with radical mediastinal and abdominal lymph node dissection and cervical esophagogastrostomy for esophageal carcinoma. *Ann Thorac Surg*. 2001;72(6):1918-1925. discussion 1924-1925.
9. Taguchi S, Osugi H, Higashino M, et al. Comparison of three-field esophagectomy for esophageal cancer incorporating open or thoracoscopic thoracotomy. *Surg Endosc*. 2003;17(9):1445-1450.
10. van der Sluis PC, van der Horst S, May AM, et al. Robot-assisted minimally invasive thoracolaparoscopic esophagectomy versus open transthoracic esophagectomy for resectable esophageal cancer: a randomized controlled trial. *Ann Surg*. 2019;269(4):621-630. .
11. van Workum F, Bouwense SA, Luyer MD, et al. Intrathoracic versus cervical anastomosis after minimally invasive esophagectomy for esophageal cancer: study protocol of the ICAN randomized controlled trial. *Trials*. 2016;17(1):505.
12. Wang C, Pan C, Mao W, Chen Q, Liu J, Hu J. Thoracolaparoscopic McKeown esophagectomy. *J Thorac Dis*. 2019;11(6):2564-2566.
13. Yang Y, Zhang X, Li B, et al. Short- and mid-term outcomes of robotic versus thoraco-laparoscopic McKeown esophagectomy for squamous cell esophageal cancer: a propensity score-matched study. *Dis Esophagus*. 2020;33(6):doz080.

Chapter 40

Ivor Lewis (Robotic-Assisted Minimally Invasive/Open) Esophagectomy

NATHANIEL R. EVANS III
UZMA RAHMAN

Perioperative Consideration

- The majority of esophageal cancer patients have received preoperative chemotherapy ± radiation therapy. We endeavor to operate on these patient 6 to 8 weeks after completion of therapy.
- Nutrition status should be optimized preoperatively. Most patients' ability to tolerate oral diet improves during preoperative treatment. Esophageal stents or jejunostomy tubes may be used as adjuncts when oral intake is not adequate during preoperative therapy.
- Jejunostomy tubes may be placed at the time of esophagectomy. Centers with low anastomotic leak rates and early (<5 days) oral feeding routines can safely avoid jejunostomy.
- Pyloric drainage, if desired, can be performed via pyloroplasty, pyloromyotomy, or pyloric injection of botulinum during laparoscopy or endoscopy.
- When available, stomach is the most reliable conduit. Colon and jejunum are alternatives when the stomach is not a viable option.
- When incising the gastrohepatic ligament or skeletonizing the left gastric (LG) pedicle, it is important to ensure that there is no replaced left hepatic artery (LHA) originating from the LG artery.
  - If this anatomic variant is present, the LG pedicle should be divided distal to the takeoff of the LHA.
- The right gastroepiploic artery is the sole blood supply to the gastric conduit. Therefore, mobilization of the greater curvature of the stomach should be performed cautiously to avoid compromising this vessel.

TIPS

- *Regional anesthesia can be placed preoperatively to optimize multimodal pain control and improve postoperative mobilization. We routinely use erector spinae pain catheters with ropivacaine infusion as they avoid the potential vasoplegia associated with epidurals.*
- *Dissecting at the hiatus and mobilization of the lower esophageal sphincter from the abdomen can facilitate completion of the thoracic mobilization.*

Anesthesia and Patient Positioning

- General anesthesia with left-sided double-lumen endotracheal tube
- Flexible bronchoscopy to confirm appropriate positioning of the endotracheal tube and rule out any endobronchial lesions

- Esophagogastroscopy to visualize mucosal abnormalities. Pyloric injection can be performed during this procedure.
- Patient positioned supine, secured with footboard and straps for the abdominal portion of the case
  - For an open case, both arms are out.
  - For minimally invasive surgery (MIS), both arms are tucked. The patient is placed in steep reverse Trendelenburg position before docking the robot.
- After the abdominal portion, patient is positioned in left lateral decubitus for the thoracic portion of the case.

Instruments and Equipment

Laparoscopic

- Hasson port (12-mm diameter)
- 8-mm 30° angled laparoscope
- Three 8-mm operating ports
- Triangular articulating liver retractor
- Advanced energy device
- Robotic vascular stapler to divide the LG pedicle
- Robotic 45-mm stapler to create the gastric conduit

Thoracoscopic

- Four robotic ports and one assistant port
- Advanced energy device
- Robotic vascular stapler to divide the azygos vein
- 29-mm end-to-end anastomosis (EEA) stapler
- 18-French nasogastric tube (NGT) and bridle
- Robotic green load stapler
- 28-French chest tube
- 24-French Blake drain

ABDOMINAL PORTION

Port Placement for Laparoscopic surgery

- Four robotic ports and a liver retractor (Figure 40.1)

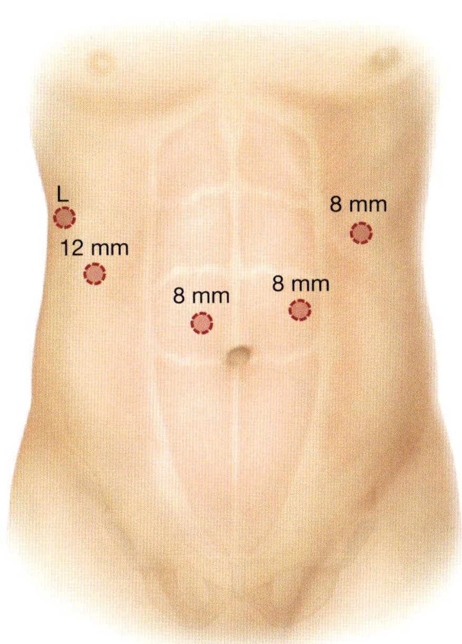

FIGURE 40.1 | Abdomen port placement. (Modified from Morris AM. Sigmoid colectomy: laparoscopic technique. In: Hawn MT, ed. *Operative Techniques in Surgery*. 2nd ed. Wolters Kluwer; 2023:984-991. Figure 4.20.7.)

- 12-mm port placed via open technique in the right upper quadrant
- Three 8-mm ports to the left of that
- Liver retractor port placed far lateral on the right side
- An additional 12-mm port may be placed for a bedside assistant

Technique

- For MIS cases, elevate the left lateral edge of the liver with the liver retractor to expose the gastrohepatic ligament.
  - For open cases, enter the abdomen via a midline laparotomy from the xiphoid to the umbilicus.
  - Divide the falciform ligament and diaphragmatic attachments of the left lobe of the liver. This will facilitate its rightward retraction and exposure of the hiatus.
- Examine the liver and surrounding structures for any metastatic disease. Any suspicious lesions should be biopsied and sent for frozen section analysis.
- Divide the gastrohepatic ligament to the level of the right crus.
- Continue to dissect at the hiatus to expose the right crus (Figure 40.2) and skeletonize the LG pedicle (Figure 40.3A).

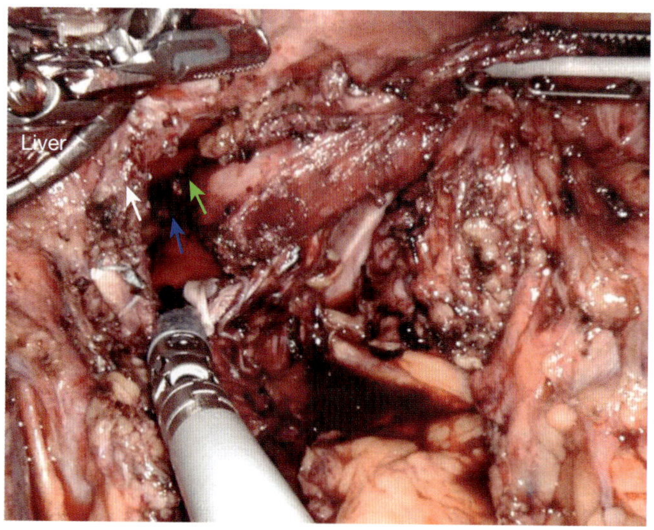

FIGURE 40.2 | Dissecting at the right crus (white arrow: right crus, blue arrow: esophageal hiatus, green arrow: pericardium).

- Dissection is carried toward the left crus, dividing the phrenoesophageal ligament, such that the hiatus is circumferentially free of attachments.
- Divide the gastrosplenic ligament and short gastric vessels up to the left crus.
- Using the robotic vascular stapler, divide the LG pedicle (Figure 40.3B).

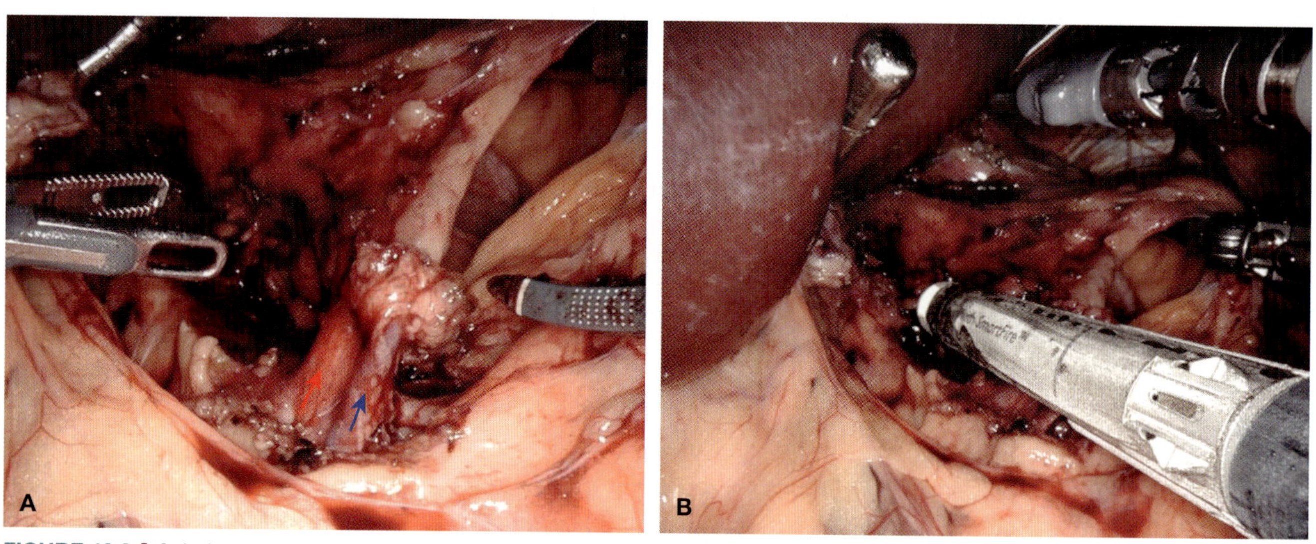

FIGURE 40.3 | A. Left gastric pedicle skeletonized (red arrow is artery, blue arrow is vein). **B.** Left gastric pedicle divided.

- For open cases, use a vascular load stapler, or clamp and ligate the LG pedicle.
- Divide the gastrocolic ligament, posterior short gastric vessels, and any attachments of the stomach to the omentum and retroperitoneum (Figure 40.4). At this point, the stomach should be circumferentially free.

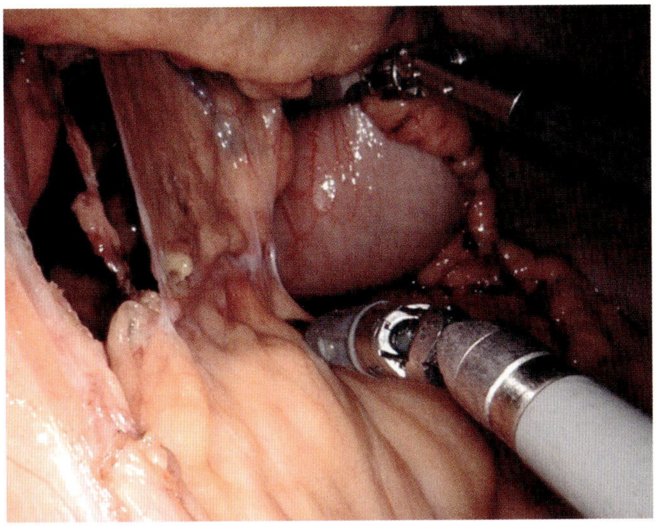

FIGURE 40.4 ▌ Dividing the posterior attachments of the stomach.

- Pylorus can be injected at this point, using 1 to 2 mL of botulinum toxin at different locations for a total of 10 mL.
- Intravenous indocyanine green (ICG) can be used to visualize and ensure preservation of the right gastroepiploic vessels (Figure 40.5). We use 10 mg of intravenous ICG.

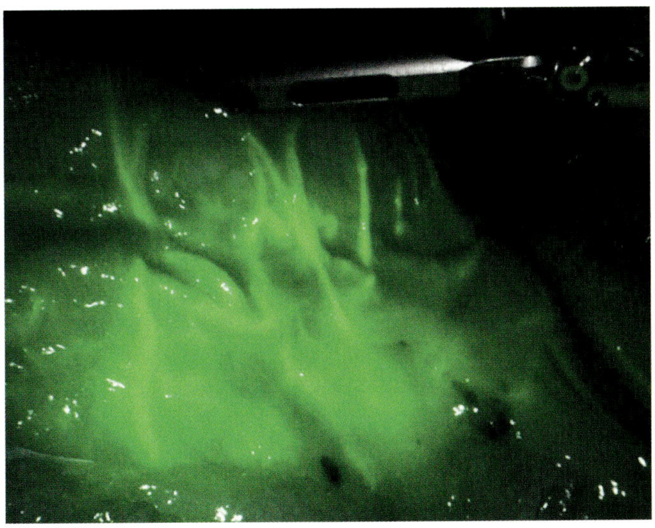

FIGURE 40.5 ▌ Indocyanine green injection showing robust perfusion to future gastric conduit via right gastroepiploic artery.

- Using the robotic 45-mm green stapler, create a 4-cm gastric conduit along the greater curvature of the stomach (Figure 40.6).
    - For open cases, use serial firings of a GIA stapler.
- This completes the abdominal portion. The robot is undocked, and fascia and skin incisions closed. Patient is repositioned for the thoracic portion of the case.

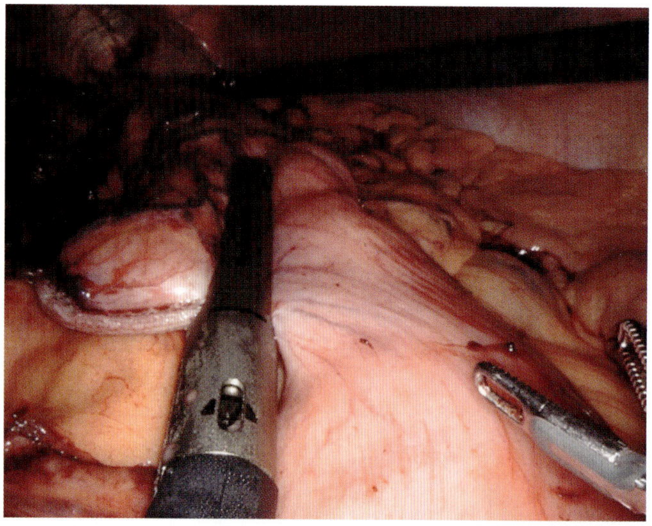

FIGURE 40.6 ▌ Creating gastric conduit.

THORACIC PORTION

Port Placement for Thoracoscopic portion

- Four robotic ports and an assistant port as shown in (Figure 40.7).

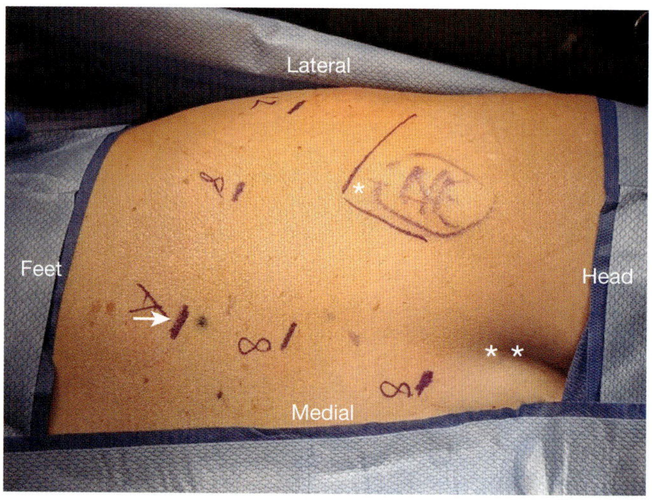

FIGURE 40.7 ▌ Right thorax port placements (* = tip of the scapula, ** = posterior axillary line, arrow = assistant port).

- 12-mm, 8-mm, and assistant ports are along eighth intercostal space.

Technique

- For an open case, a standard right posterolateral thoracotomy incision is made through the sixth intercostal space and rib retractors are placed.
- We start by dividing the inferior pulmonary ligament until the inferior pulmonary vein (Figure 40.8).

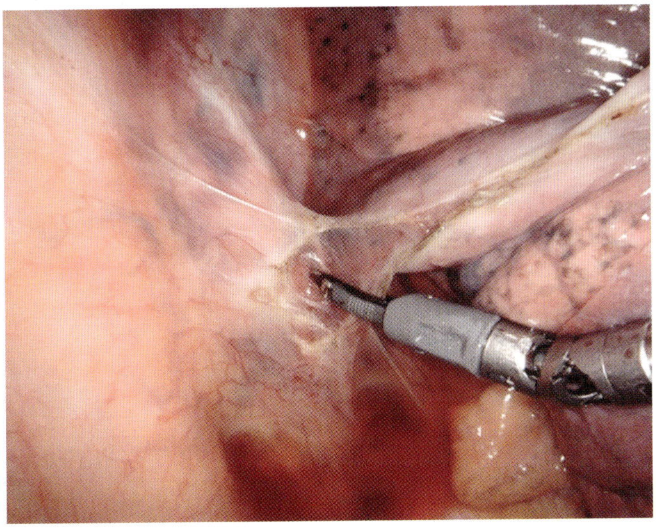

FIGURE 40.8 ▮ Dividing the right inferior pulmonary ligament.

- Continue the dissection by incising the pleura posterior to the lung leading up to the azygos vein (Figure 40.9). Any bronchial artery branches encountered during this dissection are divided using the vessel sealer.

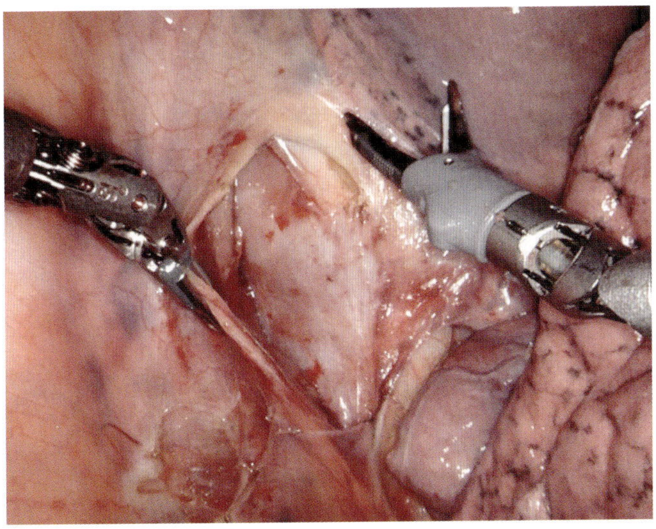

FIGURE 40.9 ▮ Dividing the posterior pleura.

- Divide the vagus nerve with the vessel sealer (Fig. 40.10).

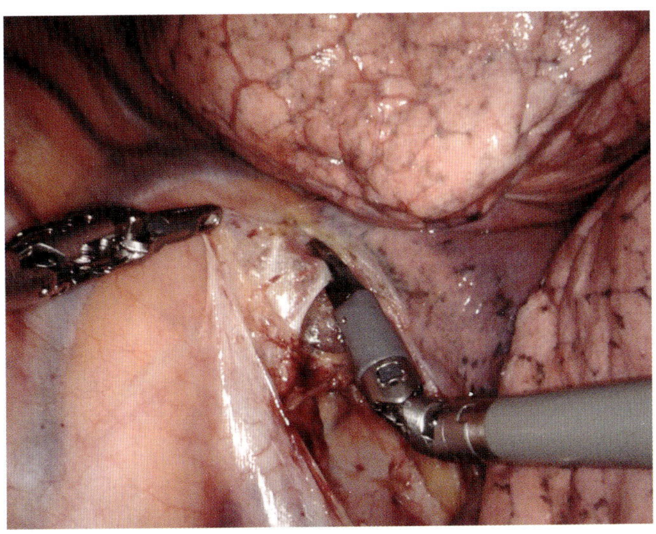

FIGURE 40.10 ▮ Dividing the vagus nerve.

- Dissect and create a window circumferentially around the azygos vein (Fig. 40.11A) and divide it using a vascular stapler (Fig. 40.11B).

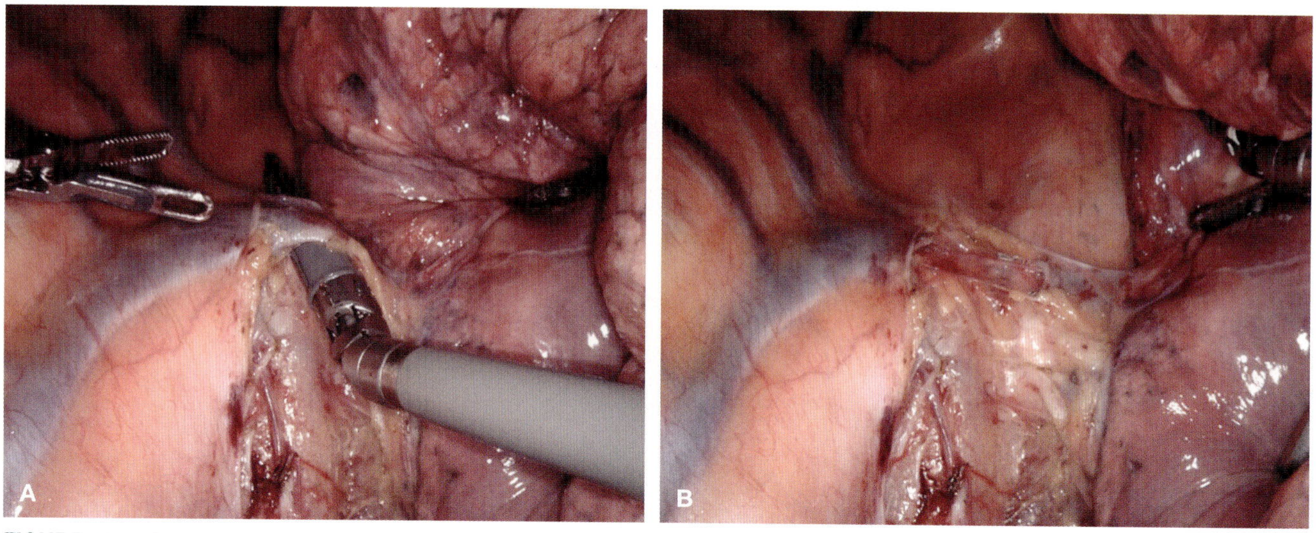

FIGURE 40.11 ‖ **A.** Creating a window around the azygos. **B.** Azygos vein divided.

- At the level of the carina, divide the vagus nerve using the vessel sealer.
- Subcarinal lymph nodes are excised at this point (Fig. 40.12).

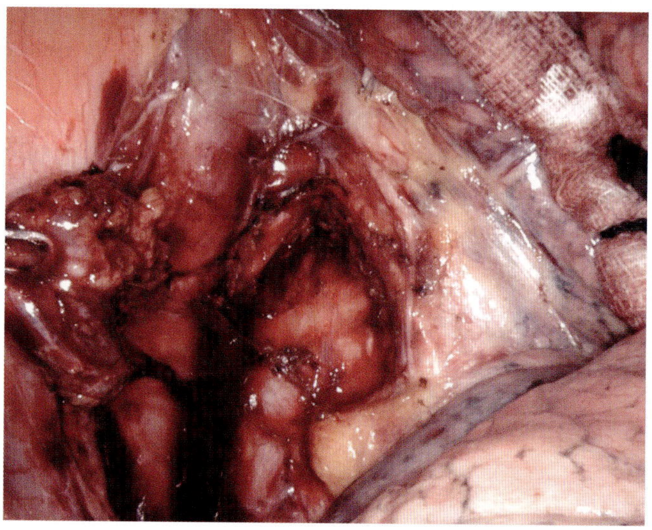

FIGURE 40.12 ‖ Excising the subcarinal lymph nodes.

- Incise the pleura posterior to the esophagus, staying in the avascular plane between the periaortic and periesophageal fat.
- Any blood vessels in this plane are divided with the vessel sealer until the esophagus is completely free inferiorly. At this point, the specimen is withdrawn into the chest and separated from the conduit (Fig. 40.13).
- Free the esophagus superiorly and transect it just above the azygos vein. The specimen includes most of the thoracic esophagus, proximal stomach, and lymph nodes.
- Place a circumferential row of suture in the proximal esophagus using full-thickness bites.
- Enlarge the 12-mm port and place a wound protector (Fig. 40.14). Deliver the pathologic specimen and introduce the anvil via this incision.
- Insert the 28-mm EEA anvil into the proximal esophagus. Cinch and secure by tying the sutures previously placed.
- Place a second row of sutures circumferentially, staying in the muscle layer only, and tie to secure the anvil in place.

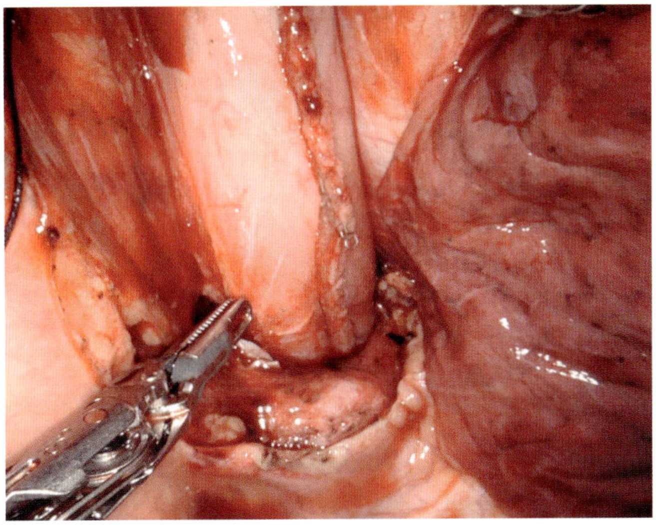

FIGURE 40.13 ■ Retracting the gastric conduit into the chest.

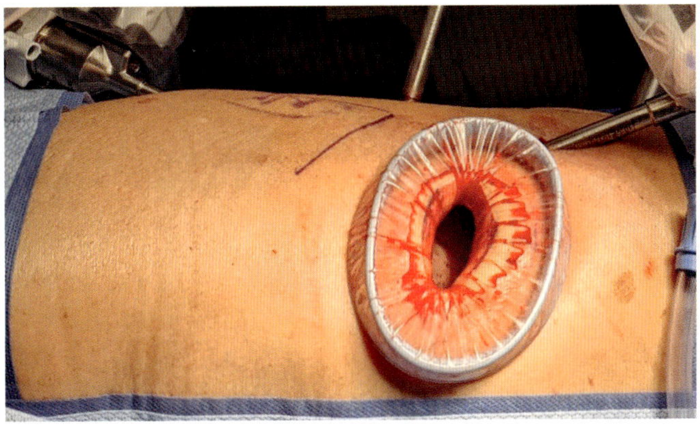

FIGURE 40.14 ■ A 12-mm port enlarged and wound protector in place to deliver the pathologic specimen.

- Make a gastrostomy at the tip of the conduit and insert the EEA stapler.
- Advance the spike through the greater curve side of the conduit and align with the anvil.
- Close the anvil and fire the EEA stapler. Examine the specimen on the stapler to ensure that there are two intact donuts of tissue.
- Close the gastrotomy in the conduit using a stapler.
- Suture the neo-esophagus to the diaphragm using a permanent suture.
- Communicate with anesthesia to advance the nasogastric tube to the level of the diaphragm.
- After undocking the robot, place a straight 28-French chest tube posteriorly, irrigate the right chest, and reinflate the right lung under direct visualization.
- We also place a 24-French Blake drain along the diaphragm to drain fluid and monitor for chylous output postoperatively.

Postoperative Care

- Patients are routinely extubated in the operating room. If the patient needs to remain intubated, the double-lumen endotracheal tube is replaced with a standard single lumen tube.
- Patient remains strict NPO until an esophagram is obtained on postoperative day (POD) 5.
- We place our esophagectomy patients on intravenous diltiazem or resume home beta-blocker for atrial fibrillation prophylaxis.
- Patient is monitored in the surgical intensive care unit at least until POD 1.
- Hemodynamics are followed closely to ensure that the patient is well-resuscitated but not hypervolemic.
- Early mobility and aggressive pulmonary toilet are key to optimal postesophagectomy recovery.
- Daily CXRs are obtained with special attention paid to NGT position and dilation of the conduit.

- Patient remains strict NPO until a fluoroscopic study is obtained on POD 5 and NGT is removed.
- If fluoroscopic study is negative for an anastomotic leak and stenosis, chest tube is removed, and patient is given a liquid diet.
- Patients are typically discharged on POD 6 to 7.

PEARLS AND PITFALLS

- The presence of accessory hepatic arteries may necessitate more distal dissection along the LG artery.
- During the laparoscopic portion, avoid getting into the pleura when dissecting around the hiatus as it will create capnothorax.
- The right gastroepiploic artery is the only blood supply to the gastric conduit. While mobilizing the greater curvature of the stomach and dividing its attachments to the omentum, the right gastroepiploic artery should be identified and preserved.
- When dividing the gastrosplenic ligament, be mindful that aggressive tension in this region can cause splenic injury.
- When creating the gastric conduit, care must be taken to staple parallel to the greater curve of the stomach. Avoid "spiral" staple lines.
- Use of a 45-mm staple allows for a staple line that mimics the natural curve of the stomach.
- As much as possible, avoid dissecting lymph nodes individually. Sweeping the lymph nodes toward the specimen is more efficient as it allows for lymphadenectomy with the pathologic specimen.
- When dissecting the subcarinal lymph nodes and the mid-esophagus, care must be taken to avoid the left mainstem bronchus. When a double lumen endotracheal tube is used, the left mainstem is distended and particularly prone to injury.
- Identifying the avascular plane between the periesophageal fat and the periaortic fat helps prevent inadvertent injury to the thoracic duct.
- We prefer to transect the proximal esophagus in two layers. First, incise the muscle layer circumferentially, then divide the mucosal layer 1 to 2 mm more distal to avoid retraction of the mucosa.
- When placing the initial row of sutures to secure the anvil in the esophagus, using full-thickness bites also prevents the mucosal layer from retracting within the muscle layer. We typically use 15 cm of 2-0 PDS sutures for this.
- Make sure to communicate with anesthetist that there is no tube in the esophagus when creating the gastric conduit, transecting the esophagus, or creating the anastomosis.

Suggested Readings

1. Bakshi A, Sugarbaker DJ, Burt BM. Alternative conduits for esophageal replacement. *Ann Cardiothorac Surg*. 2017;6(2):137-143.
2. Fransen LFC, Luyer MDP. Effects of improving outcomes after esophagectomy on the short- and long-term: a review of literature. *J Thorac Dis*. 2019;11(suppl 5):S845-S850.
3. Fenton JR, Bergeron EJ, Coello M, Welsh RJ, Chmielewski GW. Feeding jejunostomy tubes placed during esophagectomy: are they necessary? *Ann Thorac Surg*. 2011;92(2):504-512.
4. Antonoff MB, Puri V, Meyers BF, et al. Comparison of pyloric intervention strategies at the time of esophagectomy: is more better? *Ann Thorac Surg* 2014;97(6):1950-1658.
5. Noussios G, Dimitriou I, Chatzis I, Katsourakis A. The main anatomic variations of the hepatic artery and their importance in surgical practice: review of the literature. *J Clin Med Res*. 2017;9(4):248-252.
6. Okusanya OT, Hess NR, Luketich JD, Sarkaria IS. Technique of robotic assisted minimally invasive esophagectomy (RAMIE). *J Vis Surg*. 2017;3:116.

Chapter 41

Colon Interposition

HENNING A. GAISSERT
MARIA LUCIA L. MADARIAGA

Choice of Esophageal Substitution

Colon is selected for esophageal replacement because of its reliable blood supply, the straight course, and a lumen comparable to the esophagus. These qualities specifically apply to the left colon, and conduits based on the ascending branch of the left colic artery are therefore superior to right-sided colon. Replacing esophagus with colon, however, remains a complex operation requiring three intestinal anastomoses; stomach is therefore preferred for its simplicity and lower risk after esophageal resection.

Perioperative Considerations

Colon may serve to replace long and short segments of esophagus; in this chapter, the technique of long-segment interposition is described.

- The operation follows a sequence of colonic mobilization, test clamping of arteries and veins prior to division, preparation of a substernal tunnel, creation and placement of the interposition conduit, and sequential completion of the three anastomoses.
- This operation consists of multiple steps with narrow margins for error, places an important segment of intestine at risk of ischemia, and requires excellent patient selection and preparation for a disease requiring complex reconstruction.
- Substitution of the esophagus with colon is often conducted after previous operations and within a scarred field. To limit time-consuming intraoperative assessment, preoperative angiography should have confirmed the following information, particularly in elderly patients with comorbid conditions:
  - The inferior mesenteric artery (IMA) has no flow-limiting stenosis. An example of an IMA stenosis is shown in Figure 41.1.
  - The middle colic artery has either a single or two branches communicating with each other to provide continuous arterial supply to the hepatic flexure (Figure 41.2).
  - The territories of middle colic and inferior mesenteric arteries communicate by either Drummond artery or the arc of Riolan or both (Figure 41.3).
- Angiography may be deferred in young patients without vascular disease. Where angiography is not available, colon interposition may be performed but more time must be devoted during operation confirming vascular supply and condition. A study of vascular anatomy is appended as Suggested Readings. To understand a contrary opinion to mesenteric angiography, we also suggest a study from interventional radiologists that argues that mesenteric angiography before esophageal reconstruction did not improve outcomes; however, no surgeon was involved in data acquisition or drawing of conclusions, and a comparison to patients without angiography, as stated in their conclusion, did not occur.
- Colon interposition in anyone above the age of 40 years or with risk factors for cancer or inflammatory bowel disease should be preceded by colonoscopy.

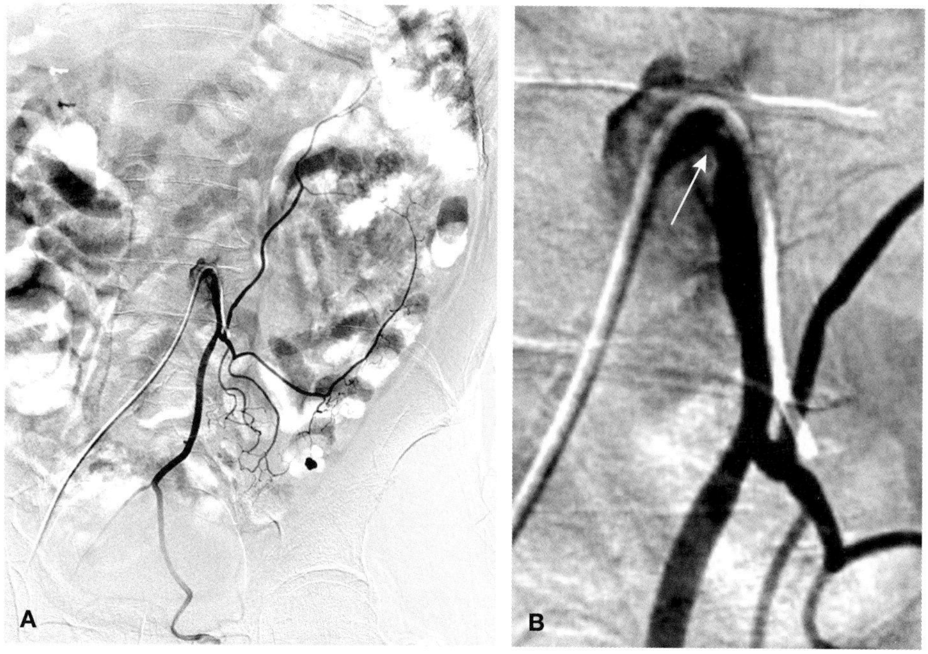

FIGURE 41.1 ▌ **A and B.** Angiographic injection of the inferior mesenteric artery demonstrates a stenosis at its origin (arrow) precluding the use of the left colon.

Instruments and Equipment

An upper hand retractor, a relic by now in many operating rooms, elevates the xiphoid and exposes the subxiphoid region; if unavailable, an internal mammary retractor will do. Soft vascular bulldog clamps are required for trial clamping. Standard endoscopic stapling devices are used to divide the intestine. The conduit is placed for transfer through the mediastinum in a laparoscopy camera bag.

Positioning

The patient is placed in supine position. Arms are padded and placed alongside the body; knees are relaxed on one pillow. When a long operative time is anticipated or the patient has a low body mass index, intraoperative warming equipment using forced hot air is applied underneath in addition to covering the lower body.

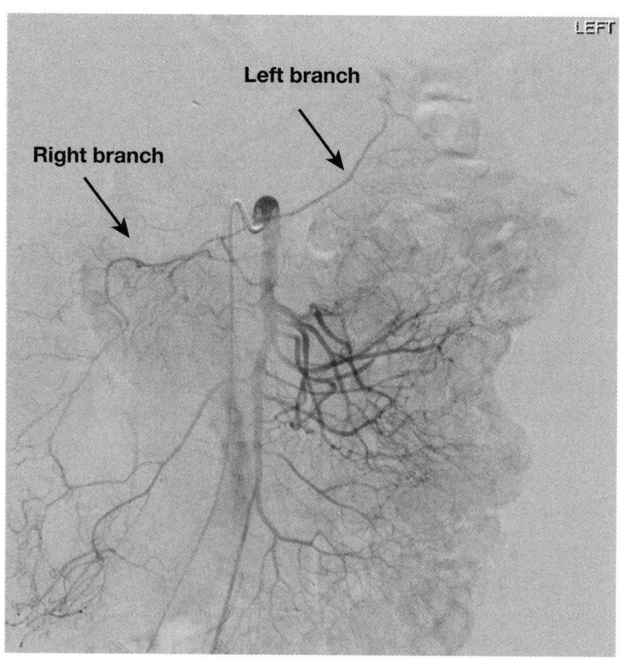

FIGURE 41.2 ▌ Angiogram of the superior mesenteric artery demonstrates a patent, long middle colic artery (MCA). Competitive flow from the left limits opacification of the MCA at the splenic flexure. This finding is not unexpected.

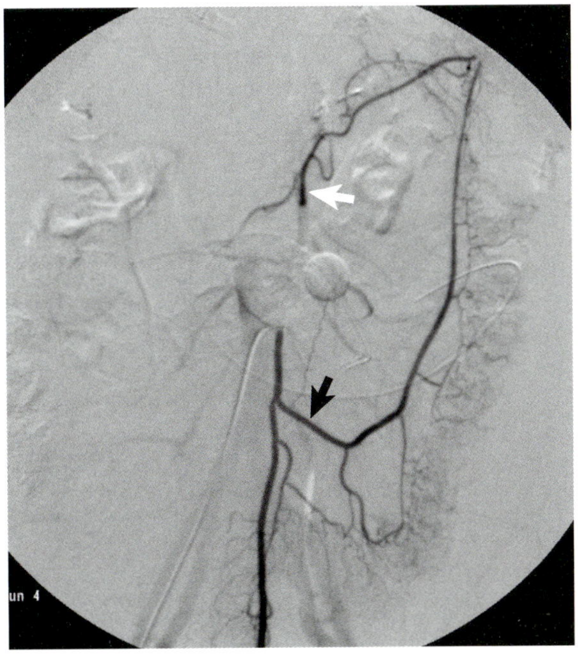

FIGURE 41.3 | Angiogram of the inferior mesenteric artery (IMA) demonstrates a well-developed ascending left colic artery branch (black arrow) in continuity with the middle colic artery (MCA, white arrow). The MCA forms a single trunk from which both left and right branches arise. The image suggests absence of vascular disease and communication between IMA and MCA.

Technique

Colon interposition via laparotomy is presented here in the belief that the gain of manual control during critical operative steps, specifically for judging tension at the pedicle, preserving a closed pleura for the length of the substernal tunnel, and passing the vascular pedicle and colon into the neck, dwarfs the disadvantage of a long incision. While this assumption may be proven wrong over time, the functional outcome of the esophageal substitute depends, independent of the approach, on several relevant details:

- The substernal colonic segment must be perfectly straight and contained within the mediastinal pleura; a loop of colon displaced into the pleural space may be expected to enlarge due to the forces of respiration and obstruct over time with delay of orogastric transit.
- In planning conduit length, consider the *effective length* as limited by the reach of the pedicle and commit only to division of the transverse colon when tension-free reach to the neck is certain because that is where the anastomosis is commonly performed. Conduit length may then be adjusted to achieve a straight course of the remaining esophagus and colon.
- For best emptying of the substernal or posterior mediastinal substitute, the cologastric anastomosis should be placed within posterior gastric wall. Small stomach remnants after prior gastrectomy obstruct easily, while Roux-en-Y colojejunostomy maintains excellent long-term emptying characteristics, at the price of lifelong vitamin B_{12} substitution.
- The technique selected for intestinal anastomosis must reliably achieve absence of leak and patency as close to 100% as possible. We find this goal is best accomplished with hand-sewn anastomoses.
- The arterial anatomy of the conduit requires close attention and preoperative angiographic study.
- A colon conduit with reversed peristalsis, based on the middle colic or ileocolic artery, for example, in a patient with IMA occlusion, is to be avoided. While prograde peristalsis is not observed in colon conduits, reversal of peristalsis results in luminal obstruction and oral regurgitation.

Figure 41.4 shows common sites of late conduit obstruction.

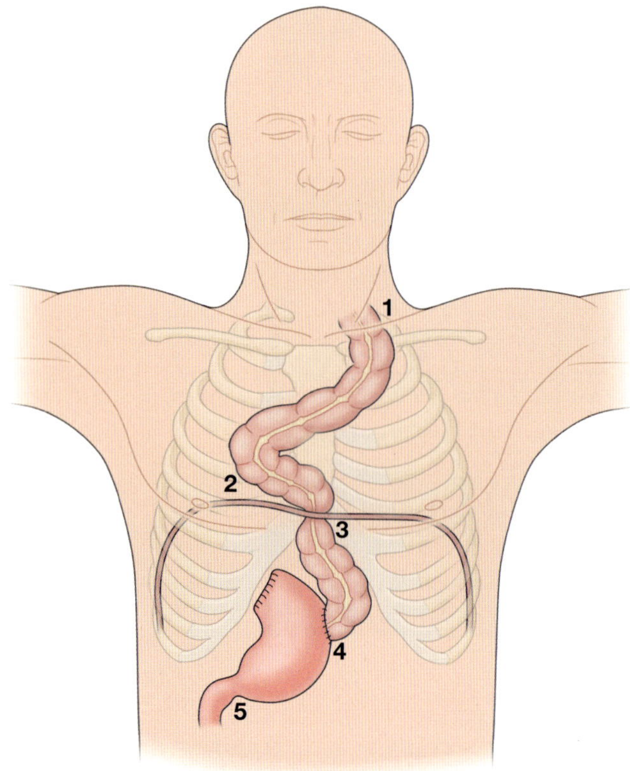

FIGURE 41.4 ▮ Sites of potential obstruction late after colon interposition. 1—thoracic inlet narrowed by sternoclavicular joint, 2—herniation of redundant colon from anterior mediastinum into pleural space, 3—narrowed diaphragmatic hiatus (posterior mediastinal conduit), 4—narrowed cologastric anastomosis, 5—obstructed pylorus.

TIPS

- *Avoiding long-term complications during colon interposition:*

Complication	Cause	Prevention
Conduit obstruction—pleural space	Angulation	Neck: avoid excessive conduit length
	Exposure to respiratory forces	Substernal: preserve mediastinal pleura
Conduit obstruction—stomach	Cologastric anastomosis	Wide cologastric anastomosis, large gastric pouch
	Gastric outlet	Pyloroplasty
Acid or bile reflux	Stomach within pleural space	Long (>5 cm) abdominal conduit segment
	Colon within pleural space	Avoid intrapleural conduit

Mobilizing Transverse and Descending Colon

- Following midline incision from xiphoid to below the umbilicus, the transverse and descending colon and their mesentery are separated from stomach and retroperitoneum to expose the full length of the inferior mesenteric pedicle and the origin of the middle colic artery. The hepatic and splenic flexures are completely mobilized.
- The proposed levels of colonic division are marked with preliminary sutures. While vascular supply must not be skeletonized, the anticipated sites of eventual ligation are exposed, dissected, and clamped with soft bulldog clamps, ie, sigmoid branches that constrain the ascending branch of the left colic artery from rising toward the hiatus, the vessels close to the colonic wall at the lower and upper end of colonic division, and the origin of the middle colic artery. Conversely, arterial duplications supplying the left colon and an arc of Riolan coexisting with Drummond artery are preserved.
- Substantial arterial or venous tributaries to the hepatic flexure must not be overlooked during trial clamping, since otherwise conduit ischemia is unmasked only after completed arterial and intestinal isolation. Note the branch variations of the middle colic artery as these determine where the vessels are clamped and later divided; the surgeon should ascertain a continuously patent middle colic

artery connecting the two sides of the transverse colon and recognize opportunities to reconstruct a very proximal separation of two middle colic arteries. Once bulldog clamps are applied and complete isolation of the proposed conduit on its left colic pedicle is confirmed, the conduit passage to the neck is created.

Conduit Position

A left colon conduit may reach as high as the base of the skull whether its course is the posterior mediastinum, the retrosternal space, or either pleural space. Among these alternatives, the pleural route is the least desirable because it is the most diverting. The pleural space further leaves the intestinal lumen exposed to respiratory forces that dilate a conduit over time, creating redundancy and obstruction. The substernal position with preserved mediastinal pleura is the optimal location and will therefore be described here. After previous sternotomy with opened pericardium, a pleural route may have to be accepted.

Preparation of the Mediastinal Passage

- In the abdomen, the retroxiphoid region is exposed. The plane anterior to the pericardium is opened by taking down the diaphragmatic attachments at the sternum and for about 5 cm on each side of the sternum. Lifting the sternum with narrow retractors, first from below and then from above, a midline passage is developed without haste separating pericardium from sternal surface and then enlarging this opening toward the mediastinal pleura. Dissection is slowly carried out with tonsil sponge-tipped ring forceps to gradually widen the passage while avoiding large tears in the pleura. Pleural openings permit colon to gradually drift into the pleural space, resulting in conduit redundancy and obstruction as shown in Figure 41.5. Depending on anatomy, the inserted surgeon's hand may gently enlarge the dissected tunnel.
- The neck is exposed on the side of the cervical esophageal stoma, selecting either a low one-sided collar incision or one along the anterior contour of the sternocleidomastoid muscle. The sternoclavicular joint and the clavicular head are resected to enlarge the thoracic inlet and prevent swallowing obstruction as shown in Figure 41.6.

Preparation of Esophagus and Conduit

- At the time of prior esophagectomy, the esophagus extracted at the neck should be left long without any tailoring or shortening. Benign disease is permitted to be present at the cutaneous stoma, and ischemic discoloration or inflammatory strictures are tolerated. A long esophageal segment is most

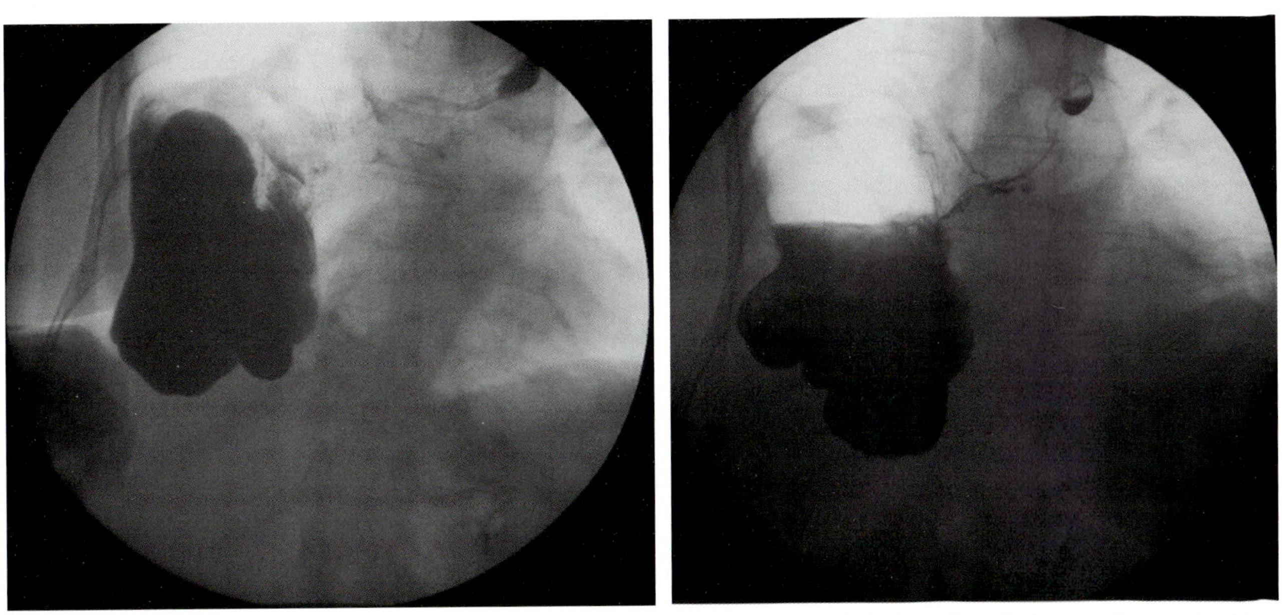

FIGURE 41.5 ▌ Late displacement of substernal colon into the right pleural space with clinical obstruction. The images show contrast in distended conduit overlying lung in the right pleural space. The patient underwent a box resection of the redundant colon segment while preserving Drummond artery and mesentery by sternotomy. The operation relieved the obstruction.

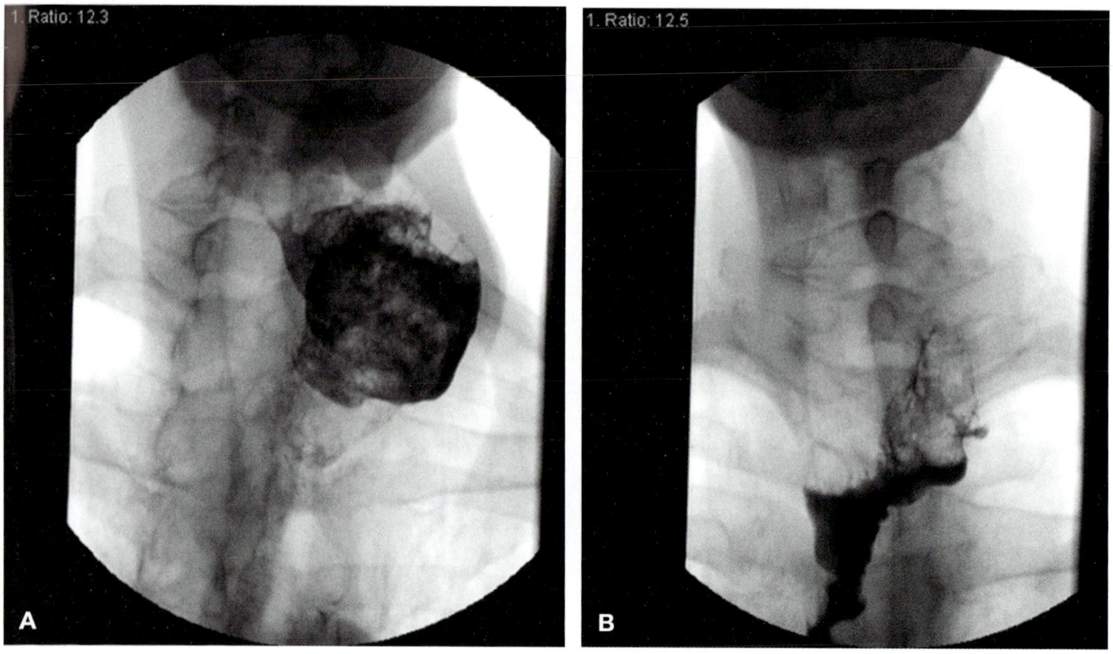

FIGURE 41.6 ▮ Leaving the manubrium and clavicle intact during substernal colon interposition often causes obstruction, particularly when the anastomosis remains located in the neck, as shown in a 56-year-old man who underwent the operation as an infant and presents with long-standing regurgitation. **A.** The early barium bolus. **B.** Delayed emptying.

desirable, while a segment as short as 1 or 2 cm may be accepted for anastomosis. In lye strictures with obliteration of the esophageal lumen and scarring of the pyriform sinus, the anastomotic site may be to the lateral or the posterior hypopharyngeal wall at or above the level of the arytenoid.

- The cutaneous esophageal stoma is circumscribed, and the esophagus is separated from its pectoral position over the entire length. If the esophagus is located behind the sternocleidomastoid muscle, muscular attachments are taken down from manubrium and clavicle and are now separated from the esophagus. Positioning the esophagocolic anastomosis below the thoracic inlet within a constraining environment is preferred, though anastomosis to even a very short esophagus above the thoracic inlet is possible.
- While preparing the substernal tunnel, the surgeon has repeatedly checked perfusion and color of the conduit. The left colic artery and the middle colic artery distal to the clamp should maintain a palpable pulse, while the veins show no engorgement. The lower conduit is prepared first to recognize the cephalad reach of the vascular pedicle. The point of the colon in direct extension of the ascending arterial branch is gently extended toward the xiphoid and marked with a suture; the level of reach is also marked on the skin. The distance measured from the subxiphoid skin to the proposed level of the anastomosis is generously transposed to the colon at the hepatic flexure with a second stitch. DeMeester's method of measuring conduit length is described under Suggested Readings and in Figure 41.7.
- The descending colon is divided from the sigmoid to achieve an eventual conduit length between gastric anastomosis and diaphragm between 10 and 15 cm. The clamped sigmoid and middle colic vessels are ligated; the leaves of the mesentery may be incised along intestinal vessels for mobilization, but the vessels are not exposed. The proximal colon at the hepatic flexure is divided last with particular attention to vascularity and adequate conduit length.
- Trimming conduit length in the neck is easy, working with a short conduit is not. If the conduit is discovered to be short in the neck but long enough to reach the esophagus, a sternotomy is performed. Tension on the vascular pedicle or the conduit must be avoided, while conduit redundancy is kept to a minimum.

Conduit Transposition to the Neck

The conduit is lifted to orient the vascular pedicle without torsion. The pedicle is placed posterior to the stomach, and the cologastric anastomosis is performed to the posterior gastric wall. A tubelike plastic bag made for sterile enclosure of surgical endoscopes (MTI, Tucson, AZ) is moistened with sterile saline and passed over the conduit to provide a low-friction transfer vehicle through the mediastinum.

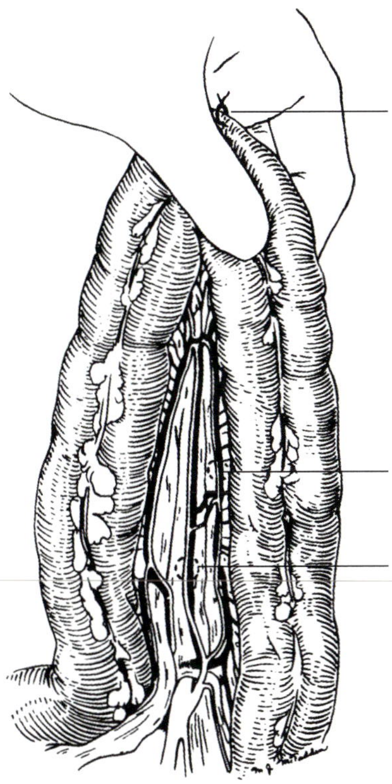

FIGURE 41.7 ▮ Method determining the length of the conduit according to DeMeester (see Suggested Readings). The left colon is lifted opposite to where the ascending branch of the left colic artery tethers the colon. This point is marked as shown with a suture and typically reaches the xiphoid level. The distance of the xiphoid to the anticipated level of anastomosis in the neck is measured from this suture to an equidistant point proximal on the transverse colon or the hepatic flexure that is marked with a second suture. (Reprinted with permission from DeMeester TR, Johansson KE, Franze I, et al. Indications, surgical technique, and long-term functional results of colon interposition or bypass. *Ann Surg*. 1988;208:460-74.)

A long vascular clamp is inserted into the mediastinal tunnel from the neck under direct vision and passed to the diaphragm where the bag is grasped. Alternatively, an umbilical tape passed through the mediastinum may be secured to the top of the bag. Filling the mediastinum with warm saline, the bag is passed to the neck with gentle pull from above and guidance from below. No effort is made to overcome resistance to upward movement; in this event, the conduit is returned to the abdomen, and the tunnel is inspected for enlargement. One may place lap sponges into the plastic tube to gently enlarge the substernal passage while avoiding tension or tearing of the conduit.

Sequence of Anastomoses

- The esophagocolic anastomosis is performed first. The esophagus is trimmed sufficiently to expose all layers. The conduit is positioned well into the cervical wound to facilitate the anastomosis, above its final location, and shortened so that its later course will be straight and not redundant. We use a manual, double-layer anastomosis for all three anastomoses because of its highly reliable outcome. From habit, the outer layer consists of obliquely placed, interrupted 4-0 silk sutures and the inner layer of interrupted 4-0 Vicryl, with knots tied on the luminal side, though many variations of this technique exist. Should a long segment of cervical esophagus be trimmed to permit a neck anastomosis? We prefer gentle delivery of additional conduit into the neck, with downward transposition of the completed anastomosis into the mediastinum.
- Following completion, the anastomosis is gently guided into the mediastinum if esophageal length permits. A nasocolonic sump drain is left in the upper colon to prevent regurgitation of colon contents and removed after 2 to 3 days. A closed suction drain (10 mm × 20 cm, Cardinal Health, Dublin, OH) is placed into the neck wound without contact to the anastomosis. Colon is attached to the diaphragm with interrupted sutures to reduce the risk of intestinal herniation.
- A cologastric anastomosis of wide diameter is performed next so as not to pose any obstruction. A pyloroplasty is often added because vagal dysfunction after nerve transection commonly impairs gastric emptying. If the gastric remnant is small, completion gastrectomy and drainage of the conduit into a Roux-en-Y segment of sufficient length (≥40 cm) is preferred to avoid bile reflux.
- For colo-colostomy, the two ends are united below the small bowel mesentery and over the terminal ileum, attaching colon mesentery to retroperitoneum and ileum with interrupted sutures to avoid the risk of internal herniation.

Feeding Tube

We perform jejunostomy to secure enteral nutrition while the patient accommodates to the esophageal substitute.

Postoperative Care

- The patient is usually extubated in the operating room. The patient is mobilized toward ambulation on the first or second postoperative day. The nasocolonic drain is removed after 2 or 3 days; sips of water are begun thereafter. Enteral nutrition is begun on the second or third day with low continuous tube feedings; starting feedings at 20 mL/h and advancing the rate by 20 mL/h each day is tolerated by most patients.
- A thin barium contrast study is obtained 6 or 7 days after the operation, and contrast is observed until passed into the small bowel. A modified barium swallow under the direction of a speech and swallowing therapist is preferred when the cervical anastomosis is created at the pharynx in patients with lye stricture.
- Diet advancement occurs gradually from clear liquids to full liquids. Soft solids are often started when the patient has already left the hospital. Before discharge, the patient and their family are instructed in the use of jejunal drip feedings, to enable troubleshooting the feeding pump. The jejunostomy is finally removed when the patient tolerates at least a soft solid diet.

PEARLS AND PITFALLS

- The angiographic study determining the substitute choice is best reviewed in advance of the operation with a radiologist to ensure correct interpretation of its findings.
- While the separation of tasks, such as colon preparation to general surgeon and esophageal connection to thoracic surgeon, offers superficial attraction, a unifying planning, sequencing of operative steps, and deliberate control over each seemingly unimportant detail in one surgeon offer important advantages.
- The surgeon should prepare for more than one substitute choice in advance, although the preference for left colon due to its vascular and conduit properties is abandoned only for good reasons.

Suggested Readings

1. Boukerrouche A. Left colonic graft in esophageal reconstruction for caustic stricture: mortality and morbidity. *Dis Esophagus*. 2013;26(8):788-793.
2. Chirica M, Veyrie N, Munoz-Bongrand N, et al. Late morbidity after colon interposition for corrosive esophageal injury: risk factors, management, and outcome. A 20-years experience. *Ann Surg*. 2010;252(2):271-280.
   Chirica et al and Boukerrouche describe reconstruction after lye ingestion, a difficult entity because confluent scarring from the pharynx to the stomach present in many cases raises challenging issues during and after operation. The pharyngeal anastomosis to colon requires particular attention, and the authors share their valuable experience.
3. de Delva PE, Morse CR, Austen WG Jr, et al. Surgical management of failed colon interposition. *Eur J Cardio Thorac Surg*. 2008;34(2):432-437.
   This manuscript is valuable for its description of long-term obstructive complications. Because these are sometimes preordained at the time of operation, a dedicated "box tip" is included above.
4. DeMeester TR, Johansson KE, Franze I, et al. Indications, surgical technique, and long-term functional results of colon interposition or bypass. *Ann Surg*. 1988;208(4):460-474.
   Having aged very well, this report summarizes not only the results of one of the most experienced surgical groups but also provides detailed advice on surgical technique.
5. McDermott S, Deipolyi A, Walker T, Ganguli S, Wicky S, Oklu R. Role of preoperative angiography in colon interposition surgery. *Diagn Interv Radiol*. 2012;18(3):314-318.
   The MGH interventional radiologists report here mesenteric angiography as performed for esophageal reconstruction. While their correlation with surgical outcome occurred without our participation, the manuscript is of interest; however, contrary to what their conclusions suggest, there was no comparison to interposition without preoperative angiography.
6. Peters JH, Kronson JW, Katz M, DeMeester TR. Arterial anatomic considerations in colon interposition for esophageal replacement. *Arch Surg*. 1995;130(8):858-863.
   The effects of anatomic variations and vascular disease are of great importance to the outcome of the operation. As noted in the discussion, whether angiography is obligatory and what precise criteria are applied to guide conduit use are still controversial. Since the existing practice climate tolerates only success and angiography is a safe test, the surgeon has little reason not to obtain this information in advance.
7. Wain JC, Wright CD, Kuo EY, et al. Long-segment colon interposition for acquired esophageal disease. *Ann Thorac Surg*. 1999;67(2):313-318.
   As we present Massachusetts General Hospital techniques and tips, the authors wish to acknowledge this reference as their source of teaching and learning; there are no tricks.

Chapter 42

Repair of Esophageal Perforation

CHASE C. MARSO
JARROD D. PREDINA
UMA M. SACHDEVA

Perioperative Considerations

General

- Esophageal perforation is associated with significant morbidity and mortality.
- Suspicion for esophageal perforation should be high to facilitate early recognition and treatment.
- Treatment consists of intravenous antibiotics and NPO (nothing by mouth) status and may include endoscopic or surgical intervention.
- The most frequent cause of esophageal perforation is iatrogenic injury following esophagogastroduodenoscopy with or without additional endoscopic procedures. Foreign body ingestion, trauma, malignancy, and increased luminal pressure from emesis (Boerhaave syndrome) or obstruction are also common causes of perforation.
- Patient presentation is subject to the extent and duration of perforation, location of esophageal injury (cervical, thoracic, or gastroesophageal [GE] junction), and communication with the mediastinum, pleura, or peritoneum. Patients may present with acute onset of neck, chest, or abdominal pain; fevers; chills; dyspnea; or odynophagia. When patients present more than 24 hours after the initial injury, hemodynamic instability, respiratory failure, and altered mental status may be present.

Diagnosis

- Chest X-ray (CXR): pleural effusion, pneumothorax, pneumomediastinum, pneumoperitoneum, subcutaneous emphysema, mediastinal widening, and anterior displacement of trachea in lateral views
- **Contrast esophagram:**
  - Fluoroscopic swallow study
    - Begin with Gastrografin if low aspiration risk. Proceed to thin barium if negative.
    - Assess for contrast extravasation into mediastinum or pleural space.
    - Identify location and laterality of perforation (Figure 42.1).
  - Computed tomography with intravenous (IV) and oral Gastrografin.
    - Beneficial for assessing mediastinal collections, pleural spaces, and lung fields as well as contrast extravasation.
    - May be less sensitive than swallow study.
- **Endoscopy**
  - Identify location and size of injury and assess extent of full-thickness perforation. It can be difficult to identify the exact location of an acute perforation endoscopically.
  - Assess for associated pathology including malignancy, stricture, diverticulum, or esophagitis.
  - Insufflate conservatively. May place chest tube prior to endoscopy if concern for the development of tension pneumothorax resulting from insufflation (Figure 42.2).

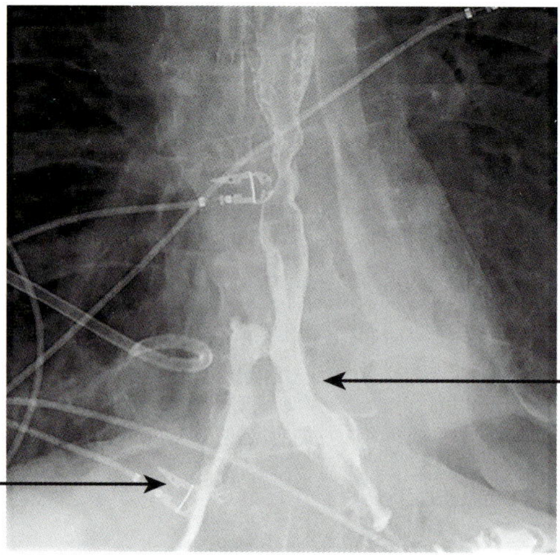

FIGURE 42.1 ▮ Contrast esophagram with iodine-based dye (Gastrografin) from patient with distal esophageal perforation. Right pigtail catheter had been placed in right pleural space prior to the esophagram.

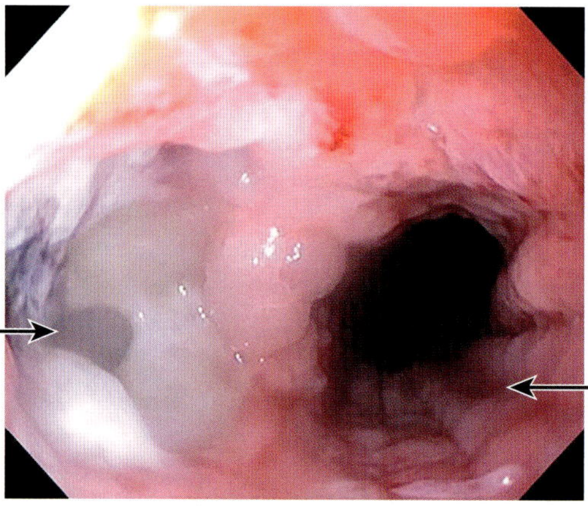

FIGURE 42.2 ▮ Endoscopic visualization of distal esophageal perforation.

Initial Management

- Admit to intensive care unit.
- Support hemodynamics.
- Blood cultures to evaluate for sepsis.
- Prompt initiation of medical therapy: NPO, IV fluids, broad spectrum antibiotics including antifungal therapy (common regimens include vancomycin/cefepime/metronidazole/fluconazole or piperacillin-tazobactam/fluconazole).
- May consider medical management as above if patient is stable and perforation is small and contained on imaging.
  - For a perforation to be contained, contrast must exit and then re-enter the esophagus with no free-flowing contrast into the mediastinum or pleural spaces.

Indications for Intervention

- Free extravasation of contrast into mediastinum or pleural space.
- Hemodynamic instability.
- Large perforation.

Interventions for Management

- Video-assisted thoracoscopic surgery (VATS) washout and wide drainage of pleural space or mediastinum, potentially in conjunction with esophageal stenting.
- Endoscopic stenting.
- Open repair via thoracotomy.

- Esophagectomy: reserved for perforations associated with malignancies (techniques are discussed in Chapters 37-40).
- Cervical washout and wide drainage.

Choice of Intervention

- All operations should begin with endoscopic evaluation of the entire length of the esophagus and perforation site, noting perforation location, size, and any associated pathologies.
- Endoscopic stenting has become the procedure of choice at most centers for small to moderate-sized esophageal perforations located within the thoracic esophagus but not involving the GE junction. This procedure may be used for either clinically stable patients or patients who are critically ill and would not tolerate a large open operation. Stenting may be used in the setting of acute esophageal perforation, such as iatrogenic perforation or Boerhaave syndrome, or in the setting of subacute perforation (perforations presenting after 48 hours). If the pleural space is contaminated, stenting should be combined with VATS washout and drainage of the pleural space.
- Open repair is the gold standard operation for relatively healthy patients presenting with acute esophageal perforation (<48 hours old), who are not yet critically ill. Open repair includes thoracotomy on the side of the perforation, as indicated by preoperative radiographic studies and intraoperative endoscopic evaluation, followed by chest washout and debridement, identification of the perforation site with debridement to healthy tissue, and open suture repair in two layers with placement of intercostal muscle flap to buttress the repair. Open repair may also be used for cervical esophageal perforations, though these can often be treated with cervical exploration and wide drainage without formal repair of the perforation site.
- VATS washout, decortication, and drainage can be utilized alone for very sick patients who are unable to tolerate open repair and whose perforations are not amenable to endoscopic stenting or can be used in combination with endoscopic stent placement if there is pleural soilage.

Anesthesia and Positioning

- General endotracheal anesthesia with paralysis.
- Radial arterial line.
- Central venous access.
- Single-lumen endotracheal tube and supine position for initial endoscopy, stenting, and cervical exploration.
- May place a nasogastric tube in the stomach beyond the perforation site with position confirmed endoscopically.
- If VATS decortication or open repair are planned, exchange single lumen for double-lumen endotracheal tube and place patient in lateral decubitus position with operative side facing up.
- Common Exposures:
  - Left neck exposed with head turned to the right for cervical esophageal injuries.
  - Left lateral decubitus for midesophageal injuries.
  - Right lateral decubitus for distal one-third or GE junction injuries.

VIDEO-ASSISTED THORACOSCOPIC WASHOUT AND DRAINAGE

Perioperative Considerations

Indications

- Perforation of unknown duration (>48 hours).
- Pleural soilage.
- Loculated pleural or mediastinal collections.

Instruments and Equipment

- Diagnostic gastroscope.
- 18-French nasogastric tube.

- 5- or 10-mm thoracoscopic camera.
- Two or three 10-mm plastic or metal thoracoscopic ports.
- Ring forceps or preferred instrument for lung manipulation.
- Yankauer and VATS suction tips.
- 5-mm endoscopic Kittner and metal pediatric suction for decortication.
- One to three chest drains: combination of 28-French chest tubes and 19-round Blake drains often used. Drains are usually placed to the apex, along the posterior mediastinum, and at the diaphragm.

TIPS

- *Principles of operation: Washout of soiled pleural space, pulmonary decortication as needed, and wide drainage of chest cavity.*
- *Consider performing in combination with esophageal stenting and placement of jejunal feeding access.*

Technique

- Confirm lung isolation.
- Place 2 or 3 standard VATS ports.
- Obtain pleural fluid for gram stain and culture.
- Evacuate all fluids in pleural space, paying special attention to loculated collections abutting the mediastinum, at the costophrenic angle, and within the fissures.
- Decorticate lung if needed by holding rind with ring forceps and gently teasing lung parenchyma off the rind using endoscopic Kittner or pediatric suction.
- Continue decortication until all parenchyma cells are free.
- Irrigate chest with 1 g vancomycin in 1 L warm normal saline solution.
- **Leave drains:** 28-French anteriorly to apex, 28-French posteriorly adjacent to esophagus, and 19-round Blake at diaphragm.
- Close incisions in layers as per standard closure techniques.

ENDOSCOPIC STENT PLACEMENT

Perioperative Considerations

Indications

- Patient with localized perforation of any age (acute or subacute or unknown age >48 hours).
- Poor candidates for open repair.
- Perforation located >3 to 4 cm from the cricopharyngeus or the EG junction to allow for sufficient stent landing zone and to minimize chance of distal migration.

Instruments and Equipment

- Gastroscope.
- Fluoroscopy including C-arm, certified radiation technologist, and appropriate lead shielding.
- Jagwire.
- Three paperclips.
- Surgical tape.
- Ruler.
- Covered esophageal stent (eg, EndoMAXX stent).
  - These come in several diameters and lengths. 23 mm diameter with 10, 12, or 15 cm length stents are most commonly used.
  - Covered esophageal stents may be secured via endoscopic suture placement to prevent migration.

TIPS

- *Stent should fully cover the perforation, with 2 to 5 cm proximal and distal coverage to prevent leakage around stent.*
- *To prevent migration:*
  - *It can be useful to upsize the stent radial diameter (23 mm) to help achieve fixation.*
  - *Covered stents may also be secured proximally by placing one to two endoscopic sutures.*
- *Stents are most effective for mid- or mid-distal esophageal perforations.*
- *If stent crosses GE junction, it is more prone to distal migration and patients will have increasing reflux symptoms.*
- *With stenting in the upper third of esophagus, the proximal end of the stent must be below the cricopharyngeus.*
- *All team members in the operating room at the time of fluoroscopy should have lead shielding, including a thyroid shield. It is the surgeon's responsibility to confirm appropriate shielding of all team members prior to initiating fluoroscopy.*

Technique (Video 42.1)

- After perforation is identified by initial endoscopy, Jagwire is placed into working channel of gastroscope.
- Position the tip of the gastroscope at the location of the perforation. Under fluoroscopic guidance, the site of perforation is marked at the skin level by affixing an unfolded paper clip to the skin using surgical tape.
- At the level of the skin, measure half of the length of the chosen stent and secure a second paperclip at this distance cephalad to the first paperclip. Repeat with a third paperclip caudal to the original paperclip.
- The gastroscope is removed from the mouth, leaving the Jagwire in place. Load the stent deployment device on the tip of the Jagwire.
- Under fluoroscopic guidance, the stent is threaded over the Jagwire into the esophagus and positioned using the paper clip-marked sites.
- The stent is deployed by pulling back the tabs at the end of the deployment device sequentially. Watch the stent deploy under continuous fluoroscopy.
- Remove the stent deployment device and Jagwire from the mouth and reinsert the gastroscope to evaluate stent position.
- If necessary, the stent can be repositioned more proximally using the stent retrieval forceps by grasping the proximal loop of the stent cage. This should be done under fluoroscopic guidance until the stent is positioned between the externally marked proximal and distal sites.
- It is better to err distally in deployment rather than proximally, as it is easier to reposition the stent proximally. If distal repositioning is required, consider removing the stent and deploying a new stent, deploying a longer stent, or placing a second "kissing stent" at the distal site.
- Perform CXR postoperatively to define initial stent placement. This allows for monitoring stent migration (Figures 42.3-42.6).

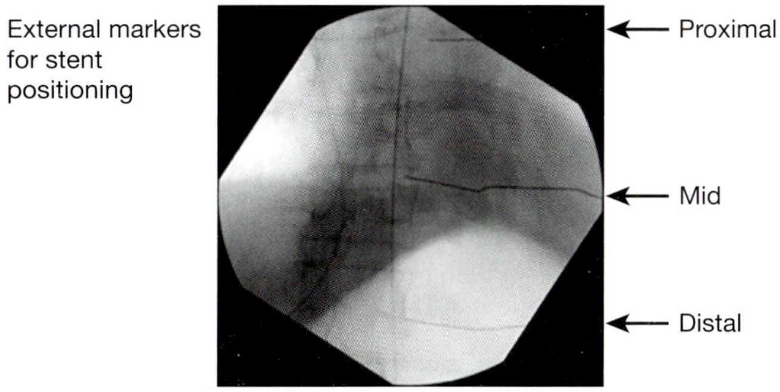

FIGURE 42.3 | Preparing to deploy the stent using fluoroscopic guidance. A guidewire has been inserted into the esophagus. Radiopaque objects (paperclips) placed at skin level are used to mark the location of the perforation (middle), proximal target for the stent (superior), and distal target for the stent position (inferior).

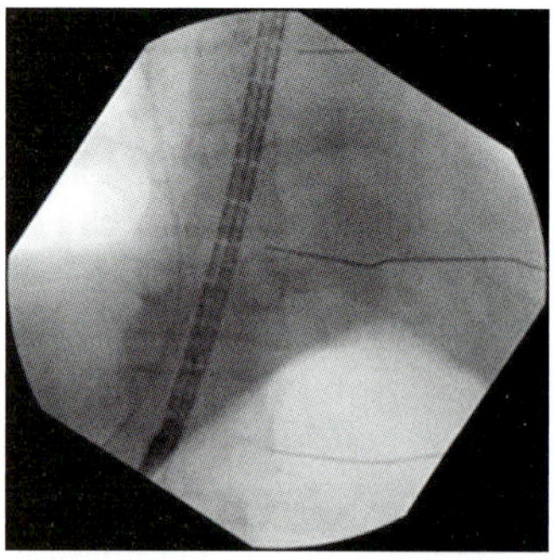

FIGURE 42.4 | The stent deployment device is inserted over the guidewire and appropriately positioned based on external marks.

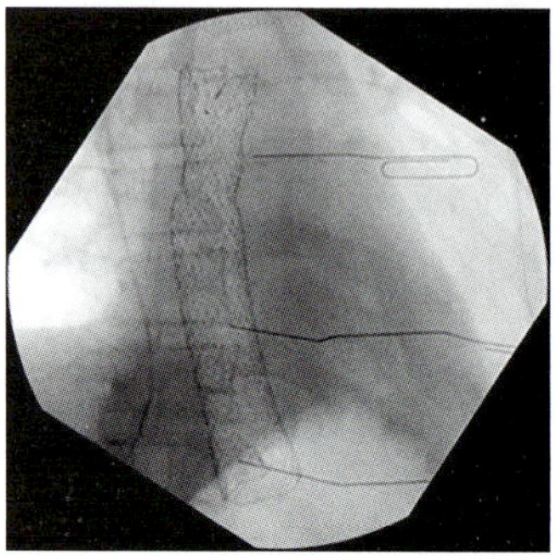

FIGURE 42.5 | The stent is deployed, and the guidewire is withdrawn.

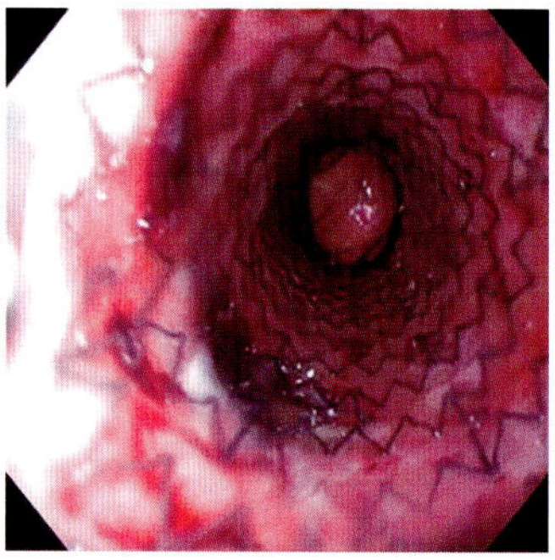

FIGURE 42.6 | Postoperative endoscopic visualization of esophageal stent.

OPEN REPAIR VIA THORACOTOMY

Perioperative Considerations

Indications

- Perforation of known duration, best if <24 to 48 hours.
- Relatively well patient, able to tolerate thoracotomy and heal subsequent repair.

Instruments and Equipment

- Thoracotomy tray.
- 4-0 polydioxanone (PDS) or 4-0 Vicryl sutures.
- 4-0 silk sutures.
- Chest drains as above, may use one or two 19-round Blake drains.

TIPS

- *Determine side of perforation through preoperative imaging and endoscopy to inform laterality of thoracotomy.*
- *Best outcomes if patient is volume resuscitated and hemodynamically stable at the time of repair (should continue resuscitation intraoperatively).*
- *Repair may be buttressed with intercostal muscle flap, pericardium, pleura, or omentum.*

Technique (Video 42.2)

- Exposure:
  - Right-sided approach common for upper 2/3 thoracic esophagus. Pleural entry at fifth or sixth intercostal space.
  - Left-sided approach common for distal 1/3 thoracic esophagus. Pleural entry at seventh or eighth intercostal space.
- Harvest intercostal muscle flap prior to pleural entry.
- Clean pleural space and decorticate lung, as described for VATS washout.
- Divide inferior pulmonary ligament to retract lung anteriorly and cephalad.
- Open mediastinal pleura along anterior and posterior esophagus.
- Identify perforation site and repair with two-layer closure.
  - Often need to extend myotomy to expose the extent of mucosal injury.
  - Ensure NG tube placement distal to perforation site prior to closure of mucosal layer.
  - Repair mucosa with running 4-0 PDS suture or interrupted 4-0 Vicryl sutures with knots traditionally placed on the inside (luminal surface) of esophagus.
  - Repair muscular layer with interrupted 4-0 silk sutures with knots on the outside (Figures 42.7 and 42.8A-C).

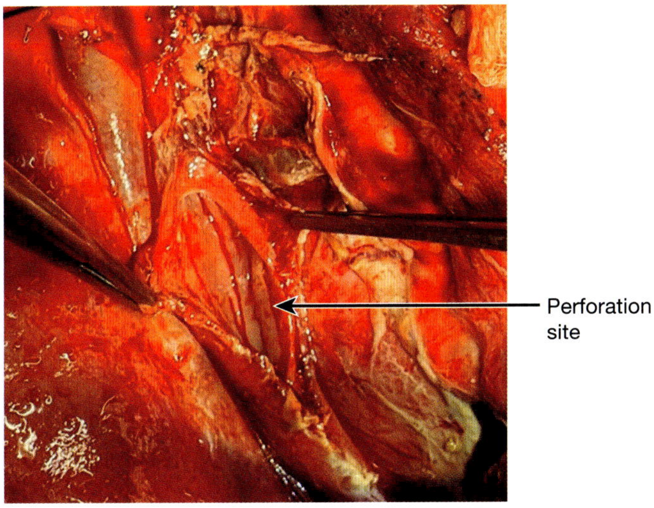

FIGURE 42.7 | Esophageal perforation site prior to open repair.

- Place intercostal muscle flap over repair and secure circumferentially using mattressed 4-0 silk sutures.
- Place drains, including one 19-round Blake drain adjacent to repair.
- Place jejunostomy tube for enteral feeding by either open or laparoscopic approach.

ESOPHAGECTOMY

Perioperative Considerations

Indications

- Malignancy.
- Distal esophageal obstruction due to high-grade stricture or long-standing severe achalasia.

TIPS

- *Foregut reconstruction is often delayed in unstable patients. Instead, may create cervical esophagostomy with transthoracic closure of hiatus.*
- *Longer remnant of proximal esophagus facilitates later reconstruction.*

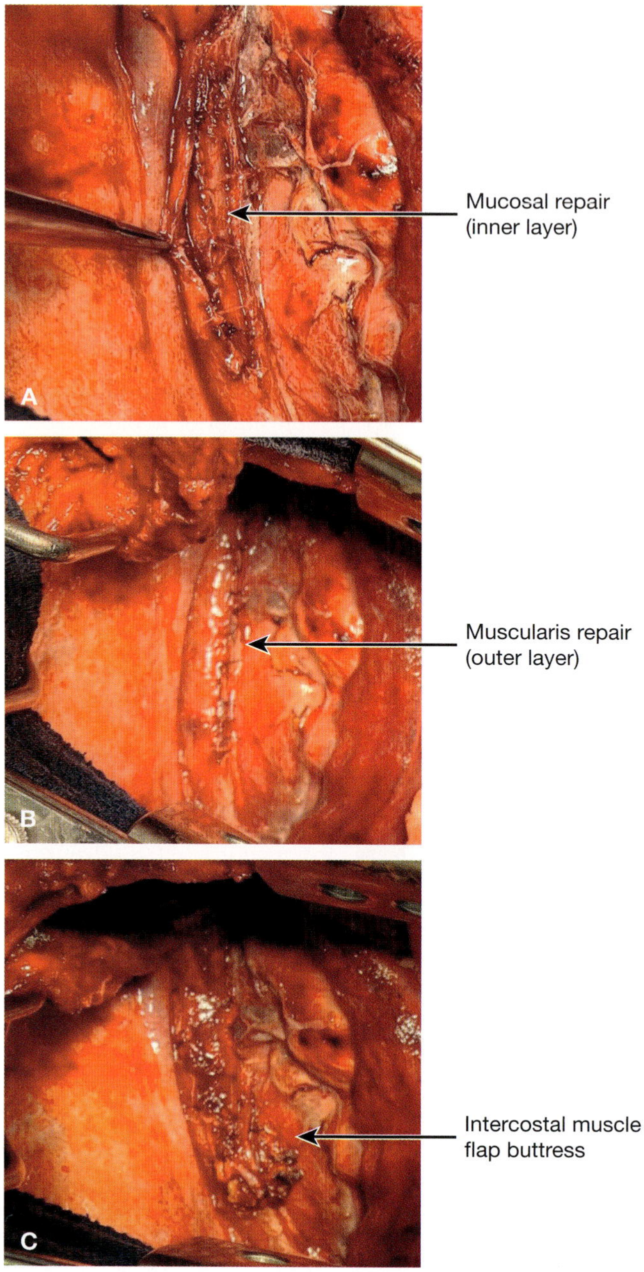

FIGURE 42.8 ▮ A-C. Suture repair of perforation in two layers. The inner layer constitutes the mucosal repair with interrupted Vicryl sutures, with knots placed on the inside. The outer layer constitutes the muscularis repair with interrupted silk sutures. The final layer is the intercostal muscle flap buttress overlying the primary repair site.

- May consider performing esophageal exclusion/diversion rather than esophagectomy in sick patients who would not tolerate esophagectomy. Exclusion/diversion techniques include:
- Distal exclusion at GE junction with stapler and placement of pharyngostomy tube for proximal esophageal drainage.
- End cervical esophagostomy, with or without plan for delayed reconstruction.
- Esophageal T-tube or side-cervical esophagostomy are less commonly performed but can provide proximal drainage in very sick patients with large irreparable perforations. Esophageal T-tube is slowly withdrawn over the course of months as perforation site heals by secondary intention.
- Feeding jejunostomy tube must be placed with any esophageal diversion or exclusion procedure.

CERVICAL WASHOUT AND WIDE DRAINAGE

Perioperative Considerations

Indications

- Cervical esophageal perforation with fluid collection, evidence of neck infection, or contrast extravasation on esophagram.

Technique

- Exposure:
  - Left cervical incision, anterior to sternocleidomastoid muscle, from sternal notch to cricoid cartilage.
- Ligate middle thyroid vein, divide omohyoid muscle, retract carotid sheath laterally, and retract trachea/thyroid medially.
- Irrigate thoroughly with antibiotic-infused saline.
- Leave drains adjacent to esophagus.
- May leave neck open with packing or close loosely with interrupted nylon sutures to allow for drainage.

POSTOPERATIVE CARE

- Patients with pre-existing esophageal pathology (achalasia and strictures) or distal obstruction are at high risk of repair failure.
- Strict NPO and surgical feeding (G or J tube, total parenteral nutrition) for nutrition.
- Consider performing contrast study 48 hours after stenting to ensure adequate stent coverage (Figure 42.9A and B).

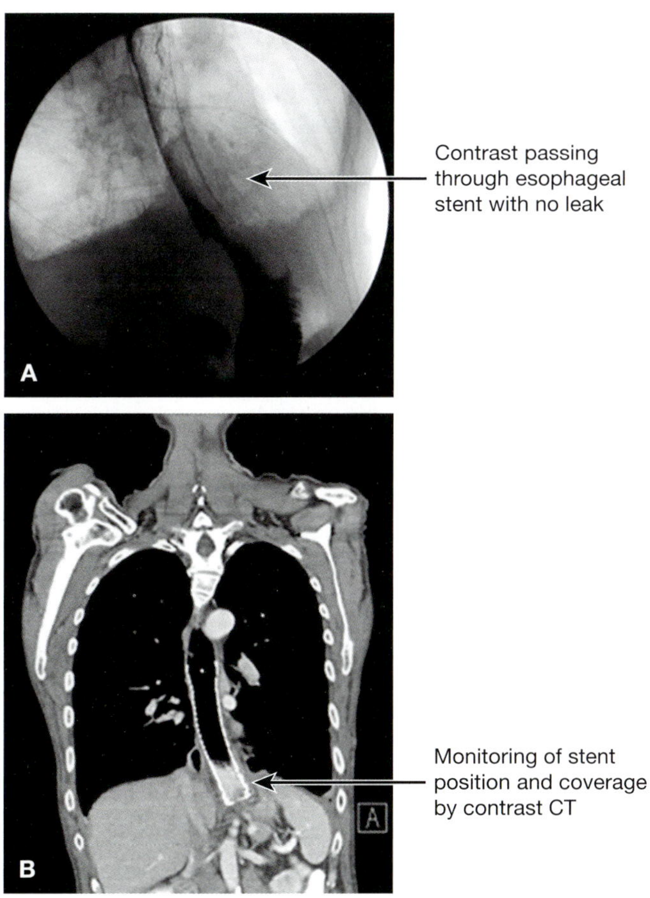

FIGURE 42.9 | A. Contrast esophagram 48 hours after stent placement demonstrating adequate stent placement and coverage of esophageal perforation site, with no contrast extravasation. **B.** Computed tomography esophagram on postoperative day 7 after stent placement. The stent remains in position and has not migrated. Contrast is seen flowing through the stent and reaching the stomach, with no contrast extravasation or leakage around stent.

- Obtain contrast study to evaluate for persistent leak at 5 to 7 days postoperatively following open repair or wide drainage.
- If no evidence of ongoing leak, plan for slow diet advancement over weeks, beginning with only clear liquids.
- If esophageal stent placed, plan for stent removal and re-revaluation with contrast esophagram in 3 to 6 weeks.

PEARLS AND PITFALLS

- Early diagnosis and management are critical to reduce morbidity and mortality.
- When performing open repair, closure should be buttressed with intercostal muscle flap or other healthy tissue (pericardium or pleura).
- Regardless of approach and technique to address esophageal perforation, morbidity and mortality are significant and should be discussed with patients and their families at the time of diagnosis.
- Prompt recognition and intervention can be lifesaving.

Suggested Readings

1. Abbas G, Schuchert MJ, Pettiford BL, et al. Contemporaneous management of esophageal perforation. *Surgery*. 2009;146(4):749-756.
2. Axtell AL, Gaissert HA, Morse CR, et al. Management and outcomes of esophageal perforation. *Dis Esophagus*. 2022;35(1):doab039.
3. Brinster CJ, Singhal S, Lee L, Marshall MB, Kaiser LR, Kucharczuk JC. Evolving options in the management of esophageal perforation. *Ann Thorac Surg*. 2004;77(4):1475-1483.
4. Kaman L, Iqbal J, Kundil B, Kochhar R. Management of esophageal perforation in adults. *Gastroenterology Res*. 2010;3(6):235-244.
5. Krause EM, Carr SR. *Esophageal perforation*. In: *TSRA Clincial Scenarios in Cardiothoracic Surgery*. 2nd ed. TSRA; 2020:166-171.
6. Maxwell R, Reynolds JK. The management of esophageal perforation. In: Camden AM, ed. *Current Surgical Therapy*. 12th ed. Elsevier Saunders; 2017:73-78.
7. Peyre CG, Watson TJ. Esophageal perforation. In: Luketich JD, ed. *Esophageal Surgery*. Wolters Kluwer Health; 2014:413-424.
8. Yang J, Siddiqui A, Kowalski TE, et al. Esophageal stent fixation with endoscopic suturing device improves clinical outcomes and reduces complications in patients with locally advanced esophageal cancer prior to neoadjuvant therapy: a large multicenter experience. *Surg Endosc*. 2017;31:1414-1419.

Chapter 43

Rigid Bronchoscopy and Acute Management of Tracheal Stenosis

ASHOK MUNIAPPAN

Perioperative Considerations

- Severe tracheal stenosis presenting with escalating symptoms is an emergency as mucous or blood can occlude the remaining lumen and lead to anoxia and cardiorespiratory arrest.
- Benign etiologies of tracheal stenosis include postintubation injury (cuff or tracheostomy site), inflammatory disease (idiopathic laryngotracheal stenosis, sarcoidosis, Wegener granulomatosis, relapsing polychondritis), infectious disease (tuberculosis, histoplasmosis), traumatic airway injury, and benign neoplasms (papilloma, amyloid).
- Malignant etiologies of tracheal stenosis include primary tumors (carcinoid, squamous cell, adenoid cystic, and mucoepidermoid carcinomas) and secondary tumors (lung, esophageal, thyroid, and metastatic cancers).
- Benign and neoplastic tracheal obstructions have unique characteristics and require different management.
- Frequently, there is a delay in diagnosis. Supportive care pending intervention includes admission to intensive care unit, airway humidification, supplemental oxygen, heliox therapy, and mild anxiolysis.
- If the patient is not in distress, and the airway is secure, chest computed tomography (CT) is performed to evaluate the tracheal obstruction and concomitant disease.
- Emergent resection of tracheal stenosis or obstruction is almost never necessary.
- The primary goal is to assemble an expert anesthetic and procedural team that can assess and relieve tracheal obstruction.
- A secondary goal is to defer the definitive operation until the assessment is complete (eg, determine length of stenosis, culture airway secretions, stage tumor) and patient's condition is ideal (eg, wean from mechanical ventilation, reduce or eliminate steroids, and treat pneumonia).

Instruments and Equipment

- Flexible bronchoscope (therapeutic, adult diagnostic, and pediatric sizes, ideally with video)
  - Through the scope pneumatic dilators (requires therapeutic bronchoscope)
  - Flexible forceps
- Rigid bronchoscope
  - Jackson rigid bronchoscopes with ventilating side arm (Figure 43.1). Sizes 3.5, 4, 5, 6, 7, 8, and 9 mm.
  - Jackson rigid bronchoscopes have a softer and rounder profile at the tip unlike "spade-like" tips of other models that tend to cut into the stenotic airway.

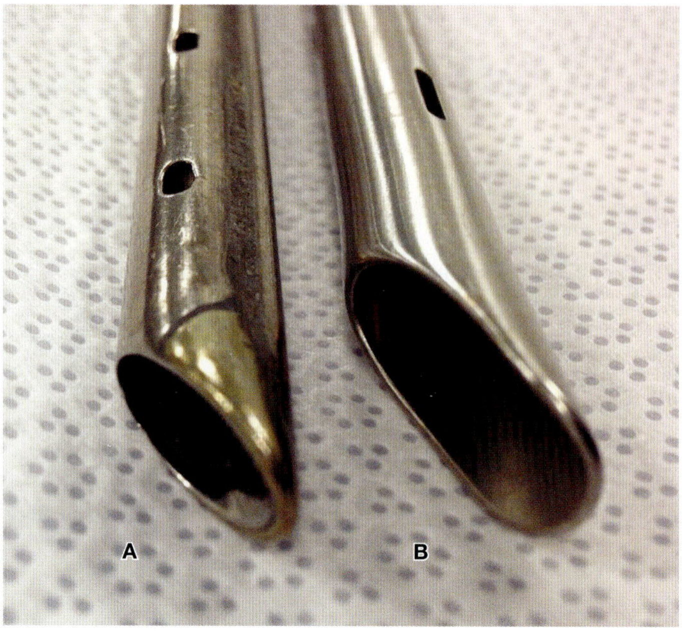

FIGURE 43.1 | Jackson and Storz rigid bronchoscopes. The tip of the Jackson bronchoscope **(A)** is rounder and blunter than that of the Storz bronchoscope **(B)**, which is potentially safer for dilating tracheal stenosis or core-out of tumor. (From Muniappan A. Tracheal dilation. In: Mathisen DJ, Morse C, eds. *Master Techniques in Surgery: Thoracic Surgery—Transplantation, Tracheal Resections, Mediastinal Tumors, Extended Thoracic Resection*. Wolters Kluwer; 2015:321-326. Figure 34.1.)

- Jackson-Pilling esophageal bougies (10-16 French)
- Hopkins rigid telescope
- Wide-bore suction cannula
- Rigid forceps

Anesthesia and Patient Positioning

- General anesthesia is typically induced with an inhalational or intravenous technique; neuromuscular blockade is avoided until it is determined an airway can be easily secured.
- Patient induction through a bag mask or laryngeal mask airway is the best technique.
- The surgeon must be present to assist with emergent intubation or rigid bronchoscopy if the airway is lost or ventilation and oxygenation are inadequate.
- Jet ventilation catheters can be passed through laryngeal mask airway or rigid bronchoscope positioned proximal to stenosis if there is a suitable lumen.
- Rarely, extracorporeal membrane oxygenation can salvage a situation in which tracheal intubation or emergent tracheostomy are not easily performed.
- The patient is positioned supine on an operating room table with a blanket and gel pad beneath the occiput to align the oral, pharyngeal, and laryngeal axes.

Technique

- Flexible bronchoscopy may be used for mild to moderate tracheal stenoses (diameter > 6-7 mm).
  - The location, length of stricture, relationship to cricoid/vocal folds, distance from carina, and presence of concomitant pathology are noted.
  - Biopsy of tumor is performed.
  - Balloon dilation of tracheal strictures is possible, with the caveat that tracheal disruption is possible.
- Rigid bronchoscopy for evaluation and initial treatment of benign tracheal stenosis is the standard technique.
  - After adequate induction of anesthesia, a 7- or 8-mm Jackson rigid bronchoscope is used to examine the larynx, glottis, and subglottis.
    - The bronchoscope must be passed cautiously and in the appropriate orientation to avoid injury to the vocal folds.
    - This bronchoscope is positioned above the stenosis.
    - The side arm of the rigid bronchoscope is used to ventilate and oxygenate the patient.
    - The suction cannula is used to clear secretions.

- The rigid Hopkins telescope is passed through a valved adapter at the end of the rigid bronchoscope and used to examine the stenosis.

- Severe or complex stenoses (<5 mm) are initially dilated with Jackson-Pilling esophageal bougies starting with the smallest size (Figure 43.2).

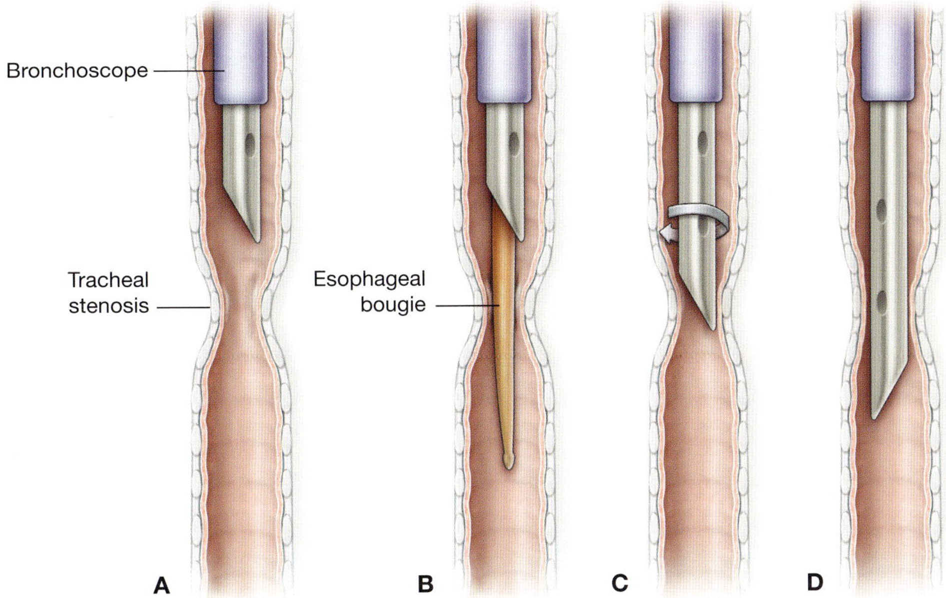

FIGURE 43.2 ▌ Tracheal dilation with rigid bronchoscopy. The rigid bronchoscope remains proximal to the stenosis allowing for examination of the stenosis with a rigid telescope passed distally **(A)**. Very tight stenoses are initially dilated by passing a Jackson-Pilling esophageal bougie (10-16 French) through the stricture **(B)**. The rigid bronchoscope is then used to dilate further by passing distally with a gentle rotatory motion and taking care to remain in the long axis of the trachea **(C)**. Serial dilation with increasing diameter rigid bronchoscopes may be performed **(D)**. (From Muniappan A. Tracheal dilation. In: Mathisen DJ, Morse C, eds. *Master Techniques in Surgery: Thoracic Surgery—Transplantation, Tracheal Resections, Mediastinal Tumors, Extended Thoracic Resection*. Wolters Kluwer; 2015:321-326. Figure 34.3.)

- Bougie dilation of critical stenoses will allow further dilation with the rigid bronchoscope itself.
- Pediatric rigid bronchoscopes, starting with 3.5-mm scopes, are used for severe strictures.
  - Pediatric rigid bronchoscopes (3.5-5 mm) are introduced with a laryngoscope bringing the cords into view.
- The blunt rounded tip of the rigid bronchoscope engages the stenosis, and a gentle "corkscrew" motion is used to navigate and dilate the stricture.
  - Care must be taken to remain in the axis of the airway and not to use excessive force to avoid perforation of the airway.
- Serial dilation with adult bronchoscopes (6-8 mm) is performed. Most benign stenoses will permit at least the 7-mm rigid bronchoscope.
- Dilation may avulse granulation tissue or scar, which are patiently and completely retrieved with suction cannula and biopsy forceps.

TIPS

- *Avoid laser incision of strictures—it could delay definitive care and extend length of stricture.*
- *Use the flexible bronchoscope through the rigid bronchoscope to clear distal secretions and aspirated material.*

- Rigid bronchoscopy and "core-out" of the obstructing tumor can also relieve neoplastic central airway obstruction (Figure 43.3).
  - The core-out technique to remove neoplastic obstruction requires a partial lumen or orifice alongside the tumor.

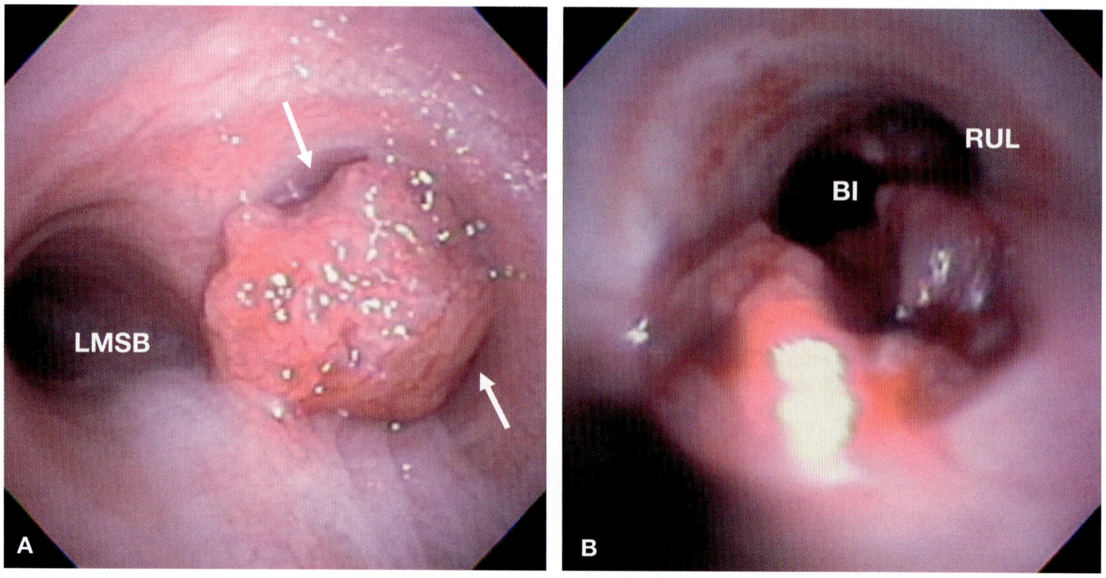

FIGURE 43.3 ▮ Core-out of an obstructing right mainstem endobronchial tumor. A partial orifice or slit (arrows) almost always remains even if a tumor occupies the entire airway lumen **(A)**. The tip of the rigid bronchoscope engages this slit before rotatory motion is performed to core-out the tumor. Tumor fragments are evacuated and the distal bronchus intermedius (BI) and right upper lobe (RUL) bronchial orifice are seen after core-out **(B)**. LMSB, left mainstem bronchus.

- Confirm the tumor is not an arteriovenous malformation or hemangioma, rare lesions that must not be managed with core-out.
- The partial orifice is engaged with the tip of the bronchoscope and a gentle rotatory motion of the scope is used to core-out the tumor.
- Fragments are retrieved with forceps and suction.
- Oozing from the cut surface of the tumor is temporarily tamponaded with the bronchoscope.
- Dilute epinephrine (0.1 mg/mL) may be instilled or applied with soaked pledgets to limit oozing.
- Laser or argon plasma cautery can also be used to debulk and limit oozing of central airway tumors but is rarely required.

Postoperative Care

- After dilation or core-out is completed, an endotracheal tube or laryngeal masked airway is placed to facilitate awakening and return to spontaneous breathing.
- Most patients can be safely extubated in the operating room. If preoperative pulmonary compromise due to pneumonia or significant atelectasis was present, the patient may be weaned from mechanical ventilation in the ICU.
- Antibiotic therapy, empiric or culture directed, is used if there is significant tracheobronchitis or evidence of pneumonia.
- Rigid bronchoscopy can sometimes induce glottic edema. Periprocedural steroids (eg, dexamethasone) are administered if glottic edema is appreciated or anticipated.
- Patients are admitted to a unit or floor with expert respiratory care. Symptoms can recur as the dilation effect may be transient. Patients require excellent pulmonary toilet and other supportive care to regain function and recruit atelectatic lung.
- A postoperative chest x-ray is used to assess for pneumomediastinum or pneumothorax, which are signs of airway disruption. Tube thoracostomy is necessary if a pneumothorax occurs. CT scans, esophagoscopy, and contrast swallow studies are used to diagnose esophageal injuries that could occur if airway disruption occurs in the membranous wall.
- Make plans for definitive treatment of tracheal stenosis or tumor such as tracheal resection and reconstruction, tracheostomy/T-tube placement, radiation, or chemotherapy.

PEARLS AND PITFALLS

- Tracheal dilation or core-out of an obstructing tumor is preferable to urgent tracheal resection. Dilation or core-out of tumor facilitates weaning from the ventilator and steroids, necessary for minimizing potential morbidity of tracheal resection.
- Rigid bronchoscopy and treatment of tracheal stenosis require experienced surgical, anesthetic, and nursing personnel with access to complete and well-maintained equipment and facilities. A spontaneously breathing patient experiencing symptoms of tracheal stenosis must not receive heavy sedation or paralysis until all equipment and personnel are assembled.
- Critical tracheal stenosis (<5 mm) requires initial dilation with a bougie or pediatric size rigid bronchoscope (starting size 3.5 mm) before standard adult rigid bronchoscopes (>6 mm) can traverse the stenosis, to avoid risk of airway perforation.
- Jackson rigid bronchoscopes or models with rounded and blunt tips are preferable for dilation of strictures and core-out as they are less apt to perforate the airway.
- Bleeding after core-out of central airway tumors can almost always be controlled with tamponade by the rigid bronchoscope, obviating the use of laser or cautery. Instillation of dilute epinephrine (0.1 mg/mL) or tranexamic acid (10-20 mg/mL) can also alleviate oozing.
- Rigid bronchoscopy can induce glottic edema or trauma. Experience and careful technique minimize the risk of trauma. Glottic edema can be mitigated by periprocedural steroids (dexamethasone).

Suggested Readings

1. Mathisen DJ, Grillo HC. Endoscopic relief of malignant airway obstruction. *Ann Thorac Surg*. 1989;48(4):469-475.
2. Ost DE, Ernst A, Grosu HB, et al. Complications following therapeutic bronchoscopy for malignant central airway obstruction results of the AQuIRE registry. *Chest*. 2015;148(2):450-471.
3. Sarkiss M. Anesthesia for bronchoscopy and interventional pulmonology: from moderate sedation to jet ventilation. *Curr Opin Pulm Med*. 2011;17(4):274-278.

Chapter 44

Endobronchial Ultrasound and Navigational Bronchoscopy

CAMILLE A. MATHEY-ANDREWS

Perioperative Considerations

- Endobronchial ultrasound (EBUS) is a minimally invasive diagnostic technique used to evaluate structures within the airway wall, lung, and mediastinum.
  - Transbronchial needle aspiration (TBNA) and transbronchial lung biopsy (TBBX) can be performed with EBUS using a convex ultrasound probe (Figure 44.1).
- EBUS may be used to evaluate mediastinal or hilar lymphadenopathy, mediastinal masses, and peribronchial pulmonary nodules.
  - Used to aid in the diagnosis of central lung cancers, lymphoma, and sarcoidosis.
  - Effective approach for non-small-cell lung cancer staging, providing nodal assessment of levels 2, 4, 7, 10, and 11.
  - Capable of providing sufficient samples for tumor genotyping of common mutations, such as epidermal growth factor receptor (EGFR) and anaplastic lymphoma kinase (ALK).
  - Radial (360°) EBUS can be used to provide a detailed assessment of airway involvement by tumors when indicated.
- Navigational bronchoscopy uses imaging-based navigational systems to guide a flexible/ultrathin bronchoscope through the airways, enabling evaluation and biopsy of peripheral pulmonary lesions (PPLs).
- The most common types of navigational bronchoscopy currently in use include:
  - Virtual bronchoscopic navigation (VBN)
  - Electromagnetic navigation bronchoscopy (ENB)
  - Robotic bronchoscopy

Instruments and Equipment

Endobronchial Ultrasound

- Flexible bronchoscope
- EBUS bronchoscope
- EBUS latex probe balloon
- 10 mL of normal saline in a Luer Lock syringe
- Connector tubing with a three-way stopcock
- 19 to 25G EBUS needles (generally 21 or 22G)
- Suction syringe
- Light source and display for bronchoscope and ultrasound images
- Collection slides for rapid on-site evaluation (ROSE) and media for permanent preservation

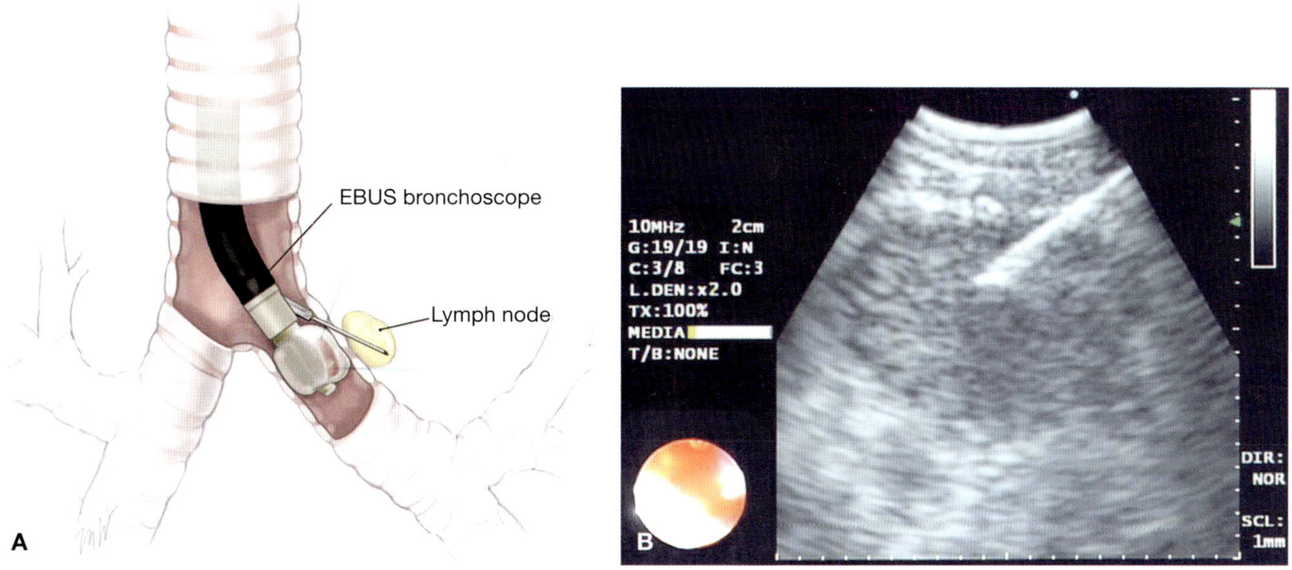

FIGURE 44.1 ▌ A. Endobronchial ultrasound bronchoscope is advanced through the airway, targeted to the area of interest, and its balloon is inflated to maximize the area of contact with the tracheal mucosa. A needle is then advanced through the bronchial wall and into the node of interest as transbronchial needle aspiration is performed. **B.** Ultrasound images demonstrate needle insertion into the target lymph node. (**A.** From Burt BM, Groth SS, Sugarbaker DJ. Pulmonary resection. In: Fischer JE, ed. *Fischer's Mastery of Surgery*. 7th ed. Wolters Kluwer; 2019:799-828. Figure 62.5; **B.** From Lanuti M. Mediastinoscopy and other thoracic staging procedures. In: Kaiser L, Kron IL, Spray TL, eds. *Mastery of Cardiothoracic Surgery*. 3rd ed. Wolters Kluwer; 2014:14-27. Figure 2.17.)

Navigational Bronchoscopy

- Thin slice computed tomography (CT)
- Navigational system with flexible/ultrathin bronchoscope

Anesthesia and Patient Positioning

- Patient is positioned supine.
- Either moderate sedation or general anesthesia may be used.
- Choice of advanced airway
  - Laryngeal mask airway (LMA): may enable better visualization and sampling of level 2R and 2L lymph nodes.
  - Endotracheal intubation: necessary to use size 8.5 endotracheal tube (ETT) or above.
- Topical application of 2% lidocaine to the airways may be helpful to suppress coughing in patients receiving light sedation or in whom neuromuscular blockade is not used.
- No indication for antibiotic prophylaxis.

Technique

EBUS-TBNA: General Principles

- Start with standard white light bronchoscopy to characterize endoluminal anatomy and clear secretions.
- Introduce convex EBUS scope into trachea; position the sheath of the needle and balloon of the probe so that only the tip is visualized by the EBUS bronchoscope.
- Advance the EBUS scope to the area of interest and use gentle flexion to bring the tip of the scope in contact with the endotracheal mucosa.
- Fan the scope clockwise/counterclockwise to identify vascular landmarks and visualize the target lymph node or lesion; visualization may be enhanced by inflation of the probe balloon with normal saline.
- Insert the EBUS needle through the working channel of the EBUS scope, and advance the needle through the bronchial wall into the target lesion using a jabbing motion.

- The needle may push the target lesion out of focus; if this occurs, gently advance the EBUS scope or inflate the balloon to restore visualization.
- Agitate the stylet in and out of the needle several times to dislodge any bronchial wall fragments retained at the tip of the needle and then remove the stylet.
- Apply suction by attaching a syringe to the tip of the needle.
- Under direct visualization, withdraw and introduce the needle from the distal aspect of the lymph node or target lesion to the proximal aspect. Repeat this step 10 to 15 times for each pass.
- Release the needle from suction, and remove the needle from the scope to collect the specimen for permanent evaluation and/or ROSE.
- Perform a minimum of three passes at each target site to maximize yield.

TIPS

EBUS-TBNA

- *The tip of the EBUS scope is distal and posterior to the visual field; therefore, the scope should be flexed slightly forward and anteriorly to effectively pass the scope through the vocal cords when using an LMA.*
- *Access to 4R station can be difficult in some patients if the ETT is too close to the carina as the turn near the right upper lobe orifice as too acute. In these cases, pull back the ETT to just below the cords or consider an LMA airway.*
- *When performing EBUS-TBNA, use a jabbing motion with the EBUS needle to traverse the bronchial wall and enter the target lesion. This is favored over slow needle insertion as it tends to be more effective.*
- *Smaller needle size is generally thought to yield better samples with less blood.*

EBUS-TBNA: Nodal Assessment

- EBUS offers access to all lymph node stations adjacent to the tracheobronchial tree, including levels 2, 4, 7, 10, and 11 (Figure 44.2).

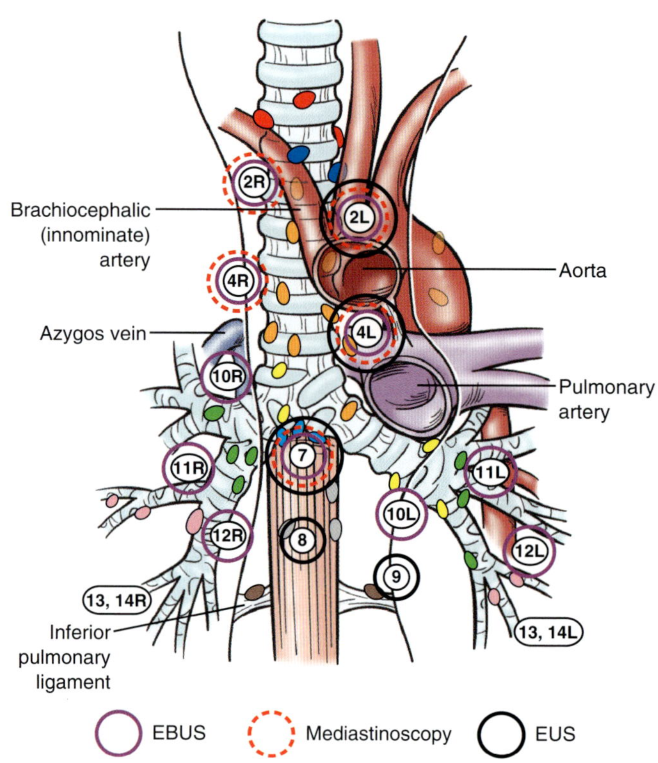

FIGURE 44.2 ▌ Map depicting nodes accessible through various invasive mediastinal staging approaches, with nodes accessible by endobronchial ultrasound circled in purple. (From Lanuti M. Mediastinoscopy and other thoracic staging procedures In: Kaiser L, Kron IL, Spray TL, eds. *Mastery of Cardiothoracic Surgery*. 3rd ed. Wolters Kluwer; 2014:14-27. Figure 2.10a and redrawn after Mountain CF, Dresler CM. Regional lymph node classification for lung cancer staging. *Chest*. 1997;111:1718-1723c.)

- Order of nodal sampling should proceed from "farthest" contralateral station from the tumor to the nearest ipsilateral station (N3 to N1), leaving any positron emission tomography-avid stations last to avoid needle contamination of subsequent nodal stations. If subsequent biopsies are required after a suspicious or positive station has been sampled, the EBUS needle should be sampled and a new needle obtained.
- Assessing left-sided nodal stations:
  - 2L: oppose left tracheal wall above the aortic arch.
  - 4L: oppose left tracheal wall below the aortic arch and above the pulmonary artery (Figurc 44.3).

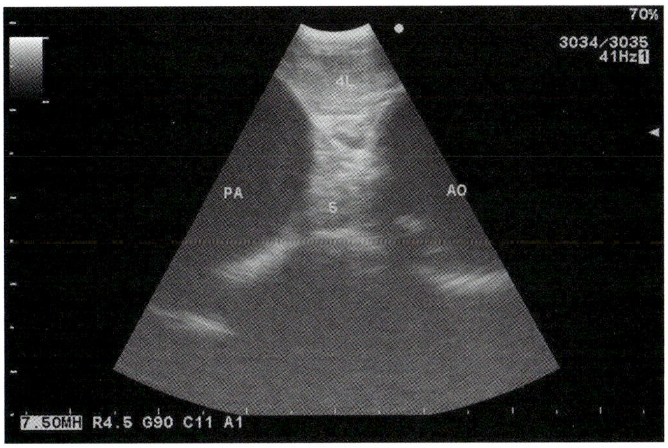

FIGURE 44.3 | Endobronchial ultrasound image of station 4L lymph node, positioned above the pulmonary artery and aorta. (From Kazakov J, Liberman M. Endobronchial and endoscopic ultrasound staging in lung cancer. In: Mathisen DJ, Morse C. ed. *Master Techniques in Surgery: Thoracic Surgery—Lung Resections, Bronchoplasty*, Wolters Kluwer; 2015:19-33. Figure 3.5.)

  - 10L: oppose the lateral aspect of the left mainstem bronchus below the pulmonary artery.
  - 11L: oppose the secondary carina between the left upper and lower lobes.
- Station 7: oppose the left main bronchus or right main bronchus medially below the carina. Look from both sides to identify the best angle and best nodal target.
- Assessing right-sided nodal stations:
  - 2R: oppose right tracheal wall above the intersection of the innominate vein with the superior vena cava.
  - 4R: oppose right tracheal wall above the azygous vein above the right upper lobe take-off.
  - 10R: oppose the lateral aspect of the right mainstem bronchus, below the azygous vein.
  - 11R: oppose the right secondary carina between right upper lobe and bronchus intermedius.

Navigational Bronchoscopy

A more exhaustive review of the techniques used in navigational bronchoscopy is provided by our "Suggested Reading." All modalities can be performed in combination with EBUS-TBNA/TBBX.

- General principles rely upon the use of helical CT to create virtual images that enable navigation through the peripheral airways.
- VBN software (LungPoint, DirectPath) uses high-quality CT images to guide the bronchoscope to a target lesion.
- In ENB (SuperDimension, SPiN), an electromagnetic field is generated around the patient and used in combination with CT-based mapping to correct for respiratory movements during bronchoscope advancement.
- Robotic bronchoscopy (Ion) additionally provides fiber optic shape-sensing technology to guide bronchoscope navigation in combination with CT imaging.
  - Ion software (PlanPoint) generates a 3D airway representation using preprocedure CT.
  - Following endotracheal intubation, the system is docked and live view bronchoscopic images are aligned to the navigation view images at the main carina and at multiple anatomic checkpoints.
  - Once the live and navigation views are synchronized, robotic bronchoscopy is initiated and the operator uses the ion controller to navigate to the biospy target. The ultrathin bronchoscopic catheter can articulate 180° in any direction and reach all 18 segments of the lung.
  - Ion software aids in navigation to the target lesion. Once reached, the catheter is locked in place and Ion's flexion needle is passed through the catheter and into the target location for transbronchial biopsy.

Postoperative Care

- A postoperative chest radiograph should be obtained to evaluate for pneumothorax or bleeding.
- Patients may be discharged from the postanesthesia care unit on the same day.
- Anticoagulation and antiplatelet agents may be resumed immediately.
- Negative biopsies of large or suspicious lymph nodes during lung cancer staging should be evaluated further with direct biopsy via cervical mediastinoscopy or video-assisted thoracic surgery.

PEARLS AND PITFALLS

EBUS-TBNA

- The use of 21- or 22-G needle is recommended, even in cases in which lymphoma or sarcoidosis are suspected.
- The use of suction will increase biopsy yield; however, this may also increase blood contamination.
- A minimum of three passes should be performed each targeted site to optimize yield.
- ROSE aids in ensuring adequate biopsy yield, however, is not required.
- When performing lung cancer staging, start with N3 nodes, then proceed to N2 and N1 to minimize the risk of cross-contamination and false upstaging. Any lymph node with a short axis greater than 5 mm should be sampled.
- Lymph nodes appear hypoechoic and should be differentiated from vascular structures using color Doppler.
- EBUS has a high sensitivity and specificity for detecting malignant involvement of lymph nodes (ie, those that are round, well defined, >1 cm, with heterogeneous echogenicity and absent central hilar structures); however, diagnostic sampling for confirmatory analysis should nevertheless be performed.
- Newer technologies integrated into EBUS, such as elastography and spectral analysis, further aid in distinguishing between benign and malignant tissues.
- In patients undergoing staging for suspected non-small cell lung cancer, additional samples should be obtained for molecular analysis (ie, EGFR, ALK genotyping).

Navigational Bronchoscopy

- Diaphragm motion, atelectasis, and reduced lung volumes with anesthesia can all contribute to CT-to-body-divergence with navigational bronchoscopy, reducing the sensitivity of these platforms.
- Trial data suggest that robotic bronchoscopy provides superior diagnostic yield for small PPLs when compared with ultrathin and ENB.

Suggested Readings

1. Giri M, Dai H, Puri A, Liao J, Guo S. Advancements in navigational bronchoscopy for peripheral pulmonary lesions: a review with special focus on virtual bronchoscopic navigation. *Front Med (Lausanne)*. 2022;9:989184.
2. Hegde P, Goudie E, Liberman M. Endosonographic lymph node staging by combined endobronchial ultrasound (EBUS): technique and technical tricks. *Operat Tech Thorac Cardiovasc Surg*. 2019;23:136-150.
3. Wahidi MM, Herth F, Yasufuku K, et al. Technical aspects of endobronchial ultrasound-guided transbronchial needle aspiration: CHEST guideline and Expert Panel report. *Chest*. 2016;149(3):816-835.
4. Yarmus L, Akulian J, Wahidi M, et al. A prospective randomized comparative study of three guided bronchoscopic approaches for investigating pulmonary nodules: the PRECISION-1 study. *Chest*. 2020;157(3):694-701.
5. Yasufuku K, Chiyo M, Koh E, et al. Endobronchial ultrasound guided transbronchial needle aspiration for staging of lung cancer. *Lung Cancer*. 2005;50(3):347-354.

Chapter 45

Mediastinoscopy and Potential Complications

ZANE T. HAMMOUD

Perioperative Considerations

- Imaging of the mediastinum is mandatory and ideally should reveal target tissue to be biopsied. Beware of aberrant anatomy or heavily calcified lymph nodes and vessels.
- Absence of surgical contraindications, eg, invasion of vessels in the neck and/or mediastinum. Bulky tumors invading critical structures may pose a danger to the procedure.
- Patient must be able to tolerate general anesthesia.
- Patient must be able to extend the neck to allow full visualization of the mediastinum. Lack of neck extension makes mediastinoscopy very challenging if not impossible.
- Presence of large thyroid goiter may make exposure challenging. Careful physical exam and imaging should alert the surgeon to this.
- Previous neck radiation or surgery may result in obliteration of normal tissue planes. These are relative contraindications (but not absolute). If present, consider alternative mediastinal staging modality such as endobronchial ultrasound.
- If performing bronchoscopy (usual), ask anesthetist to intubate with size 7.5 to 8.0 endotracheal tube.
- Indication for mediastinoscopy should dictate a plan for the procedure. For instance, biopsy of mediastinal mass to rule out lymphoma is different than mediastinal staging for lung cancer. Thus, plan should proceed according to indication.

Positioning, Instructions, and Equipment

TIPS

- *Position the patient with arms tucked and shoulder rolled to maximize neck extension (Figure 45.1A and B).*

- Maximal neck extension will draw trachea out of the mediastinum, thus facilitating ability to reach subcarinal space.
- Single-lumen endotracheal intubation with tube directed rightward and downward as much as possible so as not to interfere with the mediastinoscope.
- Entire neck and sternum should be exposed and prepped.
- Arterial line should be placed if patient has evidence of atherosclerotic disease.
- Adjust table height based on surgeon preference (seated vs standing) when performing the procedure.
- Turn table away from anesthetist to create more working space for surgeon.
- If available, video mediastinoscope preferable (Figure 45.2A), as visualization is far superior to the standard scope. However, these are somewhat large, and in thin patients, a standard mediastinoscope may be preferable (Figure 45.2B).

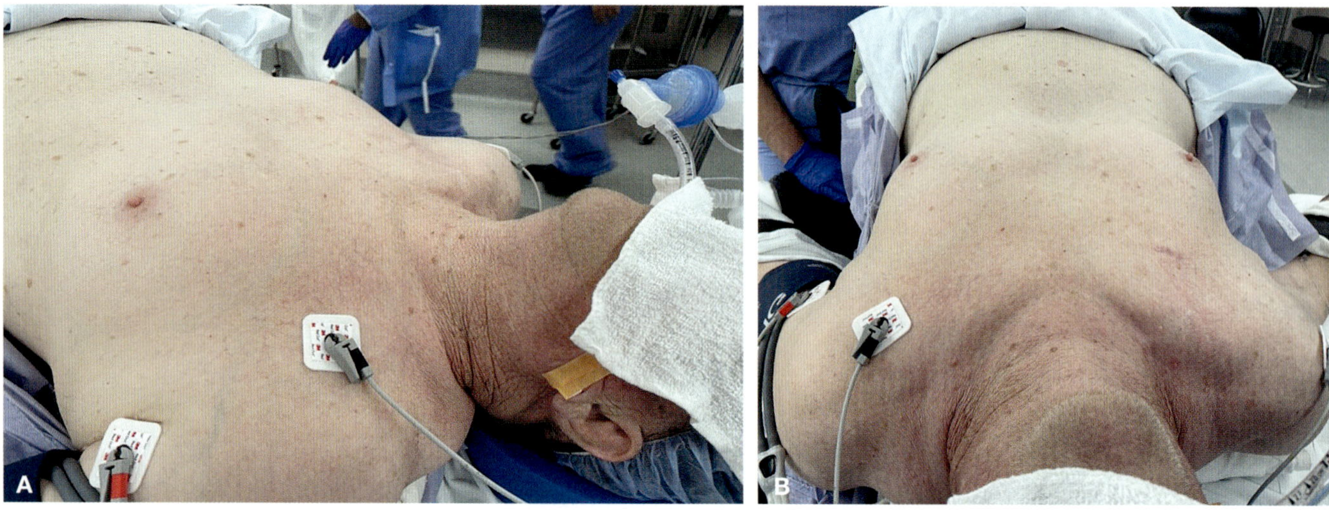

FIGURE 45.1 ▌ A: Preferred position for cervical mediastinoscopy with neck extended and arms at side. **B:** Surgeon's perspective after appropriate positioning for cervical mediastinoscopy with exposure to the neck and chest.

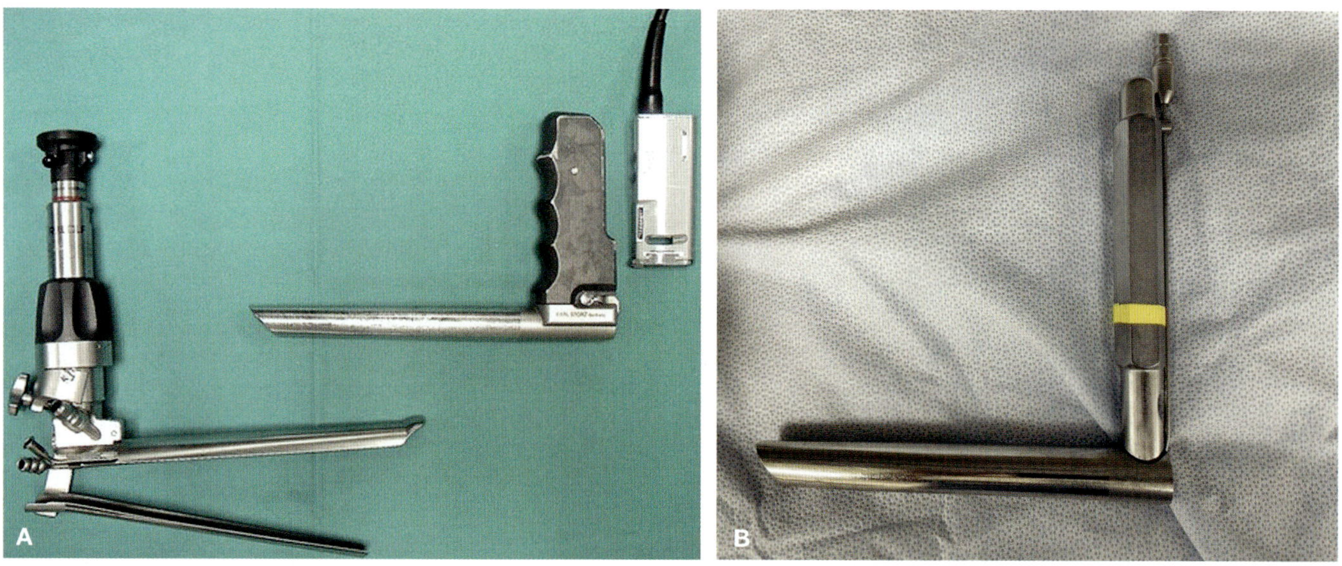

FIGURE 45.2 ▌ A: Video and **(B)** standard mediastinoscopes.

- Have pertinent imaging in the operating room.
- Decide which instruments will be used and make sure they are readily available (Figure 45.3). It is always advisable to review the operative plan with OR personnel to make sure all necessary equipment/instruments are in the room.
- Have a plan regarding biopsy targets based on imaging and clinical situation, eg, if there is suggestion of contralateral nodal disease, this should be biopsied first. If there is contralateral disease, this obviates the need for any further biopsies.
- Communicate with pathologist to give them a "heads up" if frozen section examination is desired. This is especially critical if procedure is being performed to obtain tissue for lymphoma or other mediastinal mass.

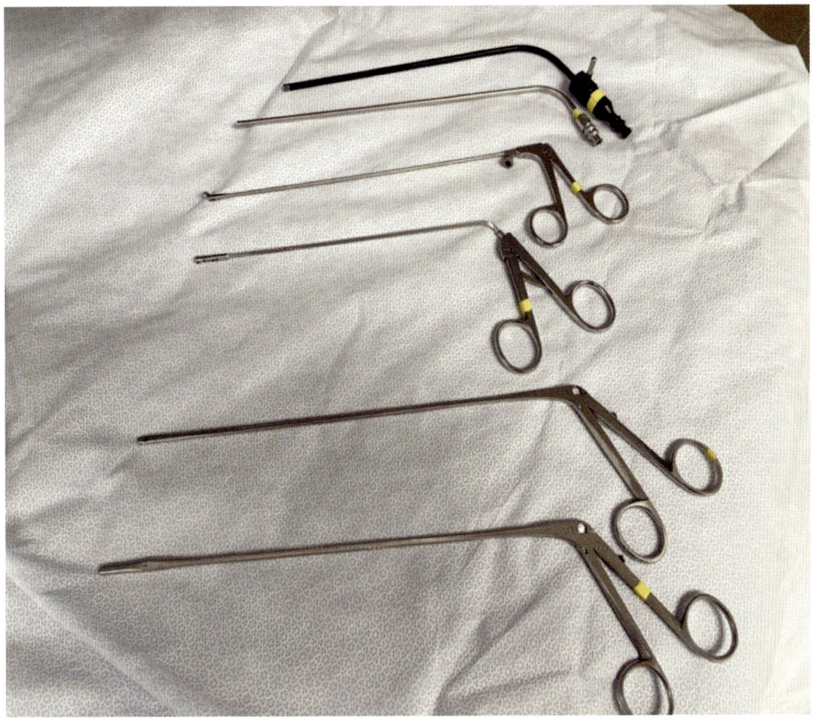

FIGURE 45.3 | Standard instrumentation for cervical mediastinoscopy, including blunt-tipped suction device, long biopsy forceps, and long graspers.

Technique

- Prep and drape the entire neck and chest area (chin to subxiphoid area and nipple to nipple).
- A 2-cm horizontal incision is made approximately 2 cm above the sternal notch and carried through the platysma.
- Divide strap muscles in midline to identify trachea (this should be below the thyroid isthmus, thus obviating need to divide the isthmus). Use digital palpation liberally to feel for the trachea as it may at times be slightly off midline.
- Once trachea is identified, the pretracheal plane is entered sharply with Metzenbaum scissors by lifting the pretracheal fascia, incising it, and gently spreading to create a space in the pretracheal plane.
- Once the pretracheal space has been identified, dissection is carried toward the subcarinal space bluntly and gently with an index finger. (I find it helpful to turn my body such that the palmar side of the index finger is pointing toward the sternum. In this manner, the tip of my index finger can be flexed to feel the innominate artery pulse. This helps to identify the extent of my dissection.)
- After the pretracheal space has been created, the mediastinoscope is gently introduced into the created space and gently advanced into the subcarinal region.
- After exploration of the subcarinal space (station 7), the mediastinoscope is withdrawn slightly and the right and left mainstem bronchi identified.
- After conclusive identification of the mainstem bronchi, the right and left tracheobronchial angles are carefully examined for station 4 lymph nodes.
- Finally, the mediastinoscope is withdrawn further and the tip is tilted upward to search for level 2 lymph nodes.
- After all biopsies have been obtained, inspection is again performed to insure adequate hemostasis.
- Once hemostasis is deemed adequate, the mediastinum is irrigated.
- The strap muscles are reapproximated with interrupted suture and the remainder of the incision is closed in layers.
- Local anesthetic is infiltrated and a dressing is applied.

Postoperative Care

- The patient is monitored in the recovery area for any signs of respiratory distress or instability of vital signs.
- CXR is routinely performed to rule out any evidence of pneumothorax or widening of the mediastinum suggestive of hemorrhage.
- After a minimum of 2 hours of observation, the patient is discharged to home if stable.

PEARLS AND PITFALLS

- Prior to procedure, make sure that the operative team has all necessary instruments and that the mediastinoscope is in good working condition (especially video).
- Some sort of packing material should be readily available in the OR. The packing should be of a size that it can be easily introduced through the neck incision with a long instrument. Once packing is in place, leave a tail protruding through the incision so that the packing can be easily retrieved.
- The entire team, including anesthetist, should be aware of your protocol in the event of massive bleeding. The first hint of bleeding is usually loss of visualization such that one may think that the light on the mediastinoscope has gone out. Even massive bleeding can be controlled with pressure, thus allowing time for the OR staff to get ready for possible sternotomy and to allow anesthesia to obtain proper intravenous access, drugs, blood, etc.
- The most common bleeding is usually minor lymph node bleeding. This can be easily controlled with packing and waiting 5 to 10 minutes before looking again.
- Once the pretracheal plane has been developed, the mediastinoscope can be introduced into the plane with gentle "pushing" to the carina. A blunt-tipped suction device should be used to dissect tissue surrounding lymph nodes so that the lymph node protrudes into the field of view.
- Always keep in mind the indication for the procedure.
- One common mistake (especially if one is inexperienced) is to mistake the right main bronchus for the trachea. Biopsy around the right main bronchus is dangerous. This can be avoided by making sure that one sees both a right and left airway for proper orientation.
- On the right, one must be aware of the proximity of the azygous vein as well as the first pulmonary artery branch. Injury to either of these structures may occur if the surgeon is aggressive with biopsy of structures to the right of the right main bronchus.
- On the left, the recurrent laryngeal nerve crosses the left main bronchus. Aggressive dissection and/or biopsy in this area, particularly on the left of the bronchus, risks injury to the nerve.
- The esophagus is in close proximity to the subcarinal space and may be injured if the surgeon is overly aggressive with deep biopsies in this area. Again, identification of proper anatomy is key.
- If there is any doubt whether or not a structure is a lymph node or a vessel, the structure should be aspirated first prior to any attempt at biopsy.
- Once a lymph node or mass is grasped, a gentle to and fro motion can be used to tease the tissue and to obtain the biopsy. Excessive force is not wise or necessary.
- Extended cervical mediastinoscopy is a procedure with which one should be familiar for historical purposes only. It is the recommendation of this author that this procedure should not be performed as there are other safer procedures that can achieve a similar result.
- Similarly, anterior mediastinotomy (left) is a procedure that traditionally was done to biopsy lymph nodes at stations 5 and 6 for lung cancer. For this indication, video-assisted thoracic surgery is a better alternative. However, every thoracic surgeon should be familiar with this procedure as it may at times be indicated for biopsy of various anterior mediastinal masses.

Suggested Readings

1. Hegde PV, Liberman M. Mediastinal staging: endosonographic ultrasound lymph node biopsy or mediastinoscopy. *Thorac Surg Clin*. 2016;26(3):243-249.
2. Lemaire A, Nikolic I, Petersen T, et al. Nine year single center experience with cervical mediastinoscopy: complications and false negative rates. *Ann Thorac Surg*. 2006;82(4):1185-1189.
3. Wei B, Bryant AS, Minnich DJ, Cerfolio RJ. The safety and efficacy of mediastinoscopy when performed by general thoracic surgeons. *Ann Thorac Surg*. 2014;97(6):1878-1884.

Chapter 46
Esophagogastroduodenoscopy

CHINMAY HARIDAS
CHI-FU JEFFREY YANG

Esophagogastroduodenoscopy (EGD) is the most commonly performed endoscopic procedure. An EGD allows in-depth evaluation of the oropharynx, esophagus, stomach, and proximal duodenum (Figure 46.1).

Perioperative Considerations

- Prepare bite block, check the suction, airflow, and water flow.
- Avoid overinsufflation of air once the scope is in the esophagus and stomach.
- A significant vagal response can be elicited intubation is performed before the patient is adequately anesthetized.
- Suction out any air before removing the scope from the stomach.
- If using general anesthesia, inform the anesthetist before removing the endoscope, as this may dislodge the endotracheal tube.

Indications

Diagnostic

- Persistent upper abdominal symptoms
- New symptoms—nausea, vomiting, etc.
- Refractory gastroesophageal reflux disease
- GI bleeding or screen for esophageal varies
- Biopsy of tissue
- Intraoperative evaluation

Therapeutic

- Evaluate for malignancy in high-risk patients
- Removal of foreign body and polyps
- Dilation of strictures, treatment of bleeding lesions, and intraluminal surgery
- Placement of feeding and draining tubes
- Follow-up after medical, surgical, or endoscopic treatment

Relative Contraindications

- Anatomical limitations that increase the risk of esophageal perforation during intubation
- Congestive heart failure, acute respiratory distress syndrome, and medically unstable patients

Technique

- Place a bite block in the mouth of the patient while in left lateral decubitus position with neck flexed forward. The bite block can either be placed between the teeth or fitted over the instrument shaft.

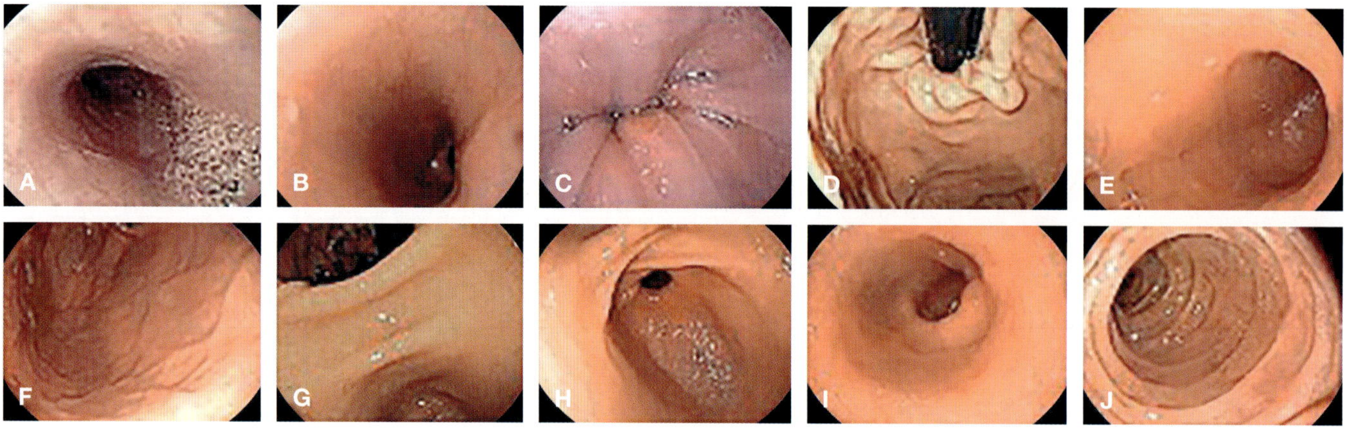

FIGURE 46.1 ▮ Overview of endoscopy: **(A)** Proximal esophagus; **(B)** distal esophagus; **(C)** Z-line and diaphragm indentation; **(D)** cardia and fundus on retroflexed view; **(E)** body (including lesser curvature); **(F)** body on retroflexed view; **(G)** angulus on partial retroflexion; **(H)** antrum; **(I)** duodenal bulb; and **(J)** second part of the duodenum, including the ampulla. (From Marques S, Bispo M, Pimentel-Nunes P, et al. Image documentation in gastrointestinal endoscopy: review of recommendations. *GE Port J Gastroenterol*. 2017;24(6):269-274, Figure 2. Copyright © 2017 Karger Publishers, Basel, Switzerland.)

- Introduce the endoscope into the mouth (either by the blind insertion method or the direct vision insertion method) and to the base of the tongue. Proceed downward to visualize the vocal cords, epiglottis, both piriform sinuses, and the surrounding cartilages (Figure 46.2).

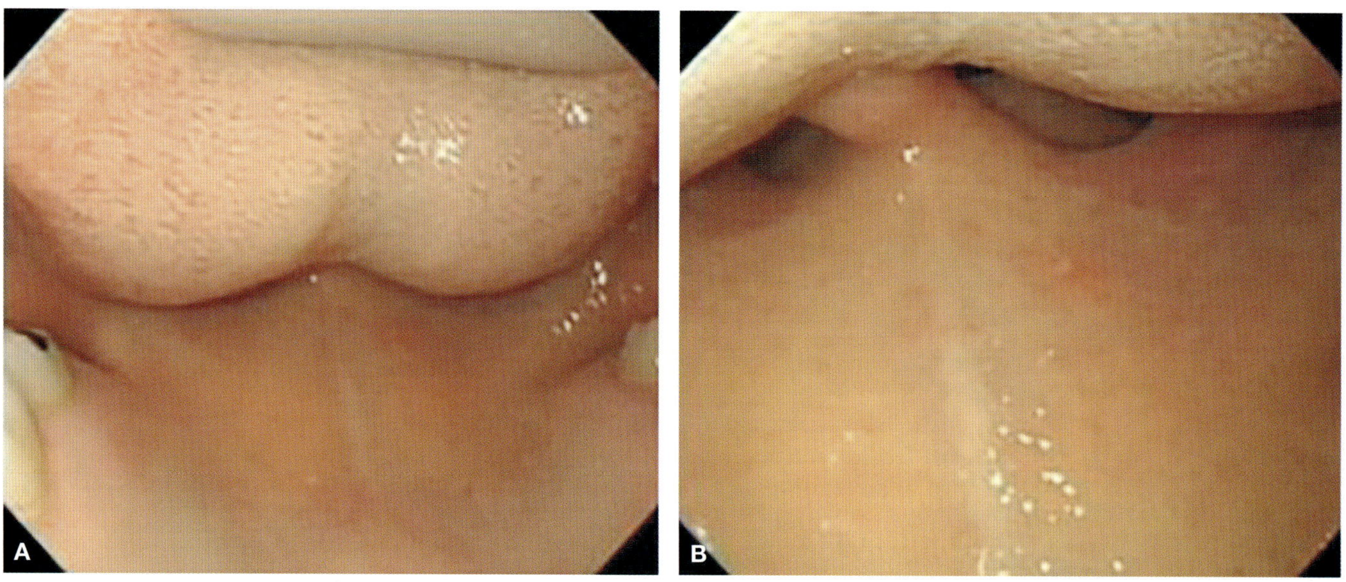

FIGURE 46.2 ▮ Endoscopic images of the **(A)** oral cavity and **(B)** uvula.

- With the help of gentle pressure while insufflating air, pass the scope behind and to the right of the arytenoid cartilage toward the upper esophageal sphincter (UES) (Figure 46.3).

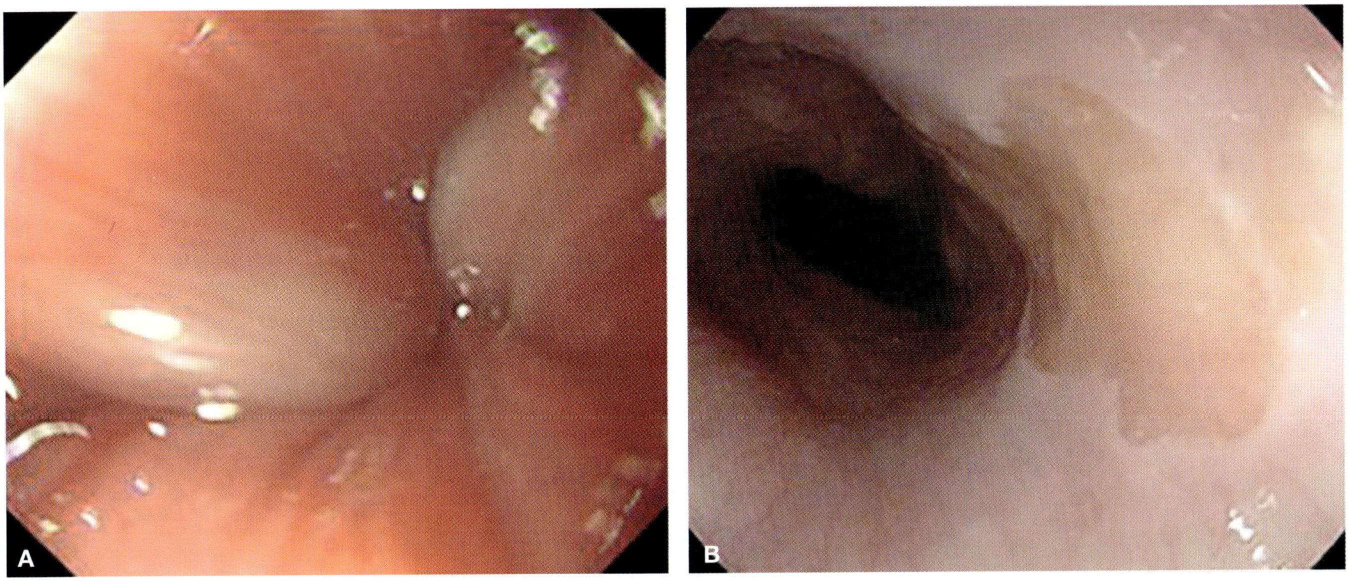

FIGURE 46.3 ▮ Endoscopic image of the cervical esophagus. **A:** Upper esophageal sphincter. **B:** Heterotopic gastric mucosa.

- The esophageal sphincter has a slitlike lumen (hardly visible) through which the endoscope can be passed (Figure 46.4). Examine the gastroesophageal junction and the lower esophageal sphincter (LES) (which can have a typical rosette-like appearance when closed).

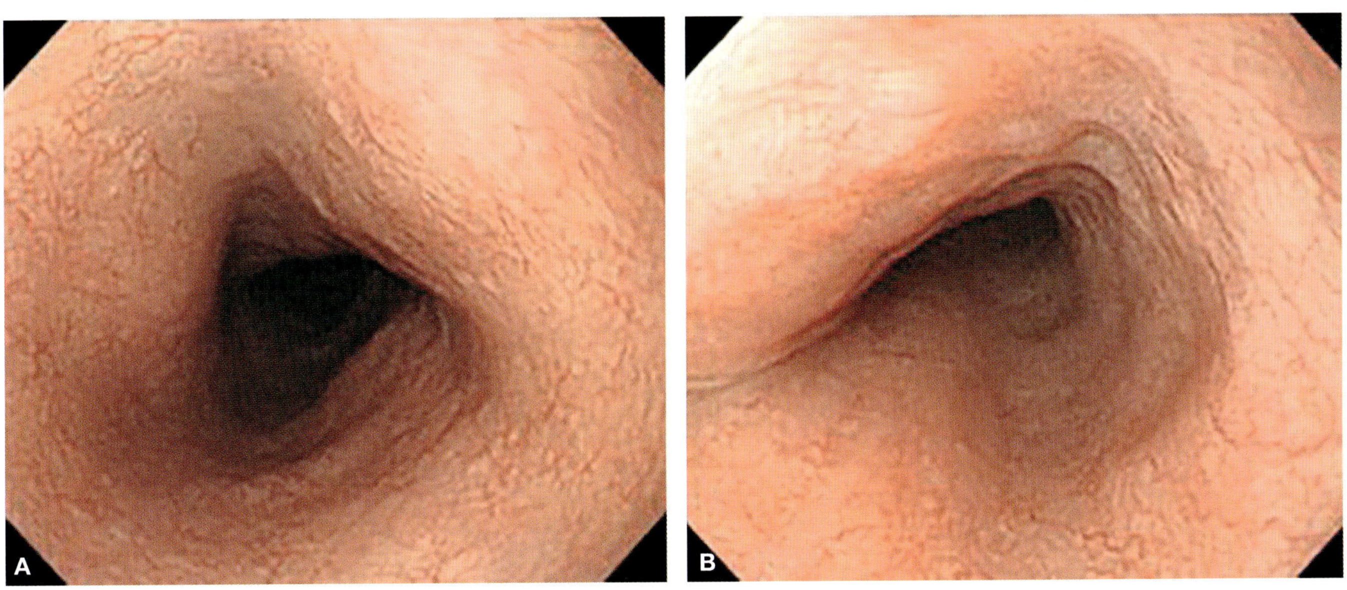

FIGURE 46.4 ▮ Endoscopic image of the thoracic esophagus. **A:** Extrinsic compression from the aortic arch and left main bronchus is observed on the right side of the picture. **B:** Extrinsic compression from the heart, left atrium is seen on the left side of the picture.

- An open sphincter exposes the Z-line and the interior of the stomach (Figure 46.5). The Z-line demarcates the transition between the esophageal and gastric epithelium.

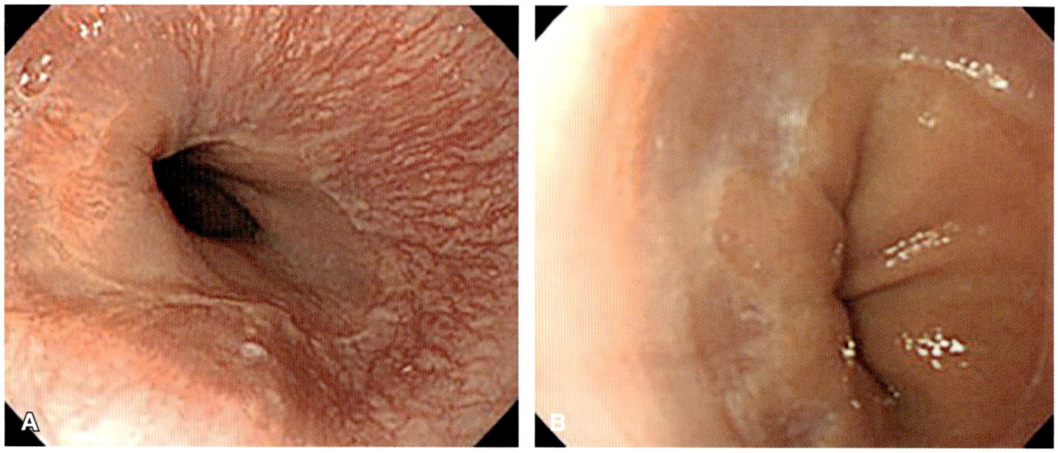

FIGURE 46.5 ❙ **A:** Longitudinal palisade vessels are seen here at the lower esophagus near the stomach. **B:** Gastroesophageal junction.

- Pass down the scope to enter the stomach. In order to improve visualization here and minimize the risk of reflux, the gastric secretions should be suctioned, after which air is insufflated (Figures 46.6-46.8).

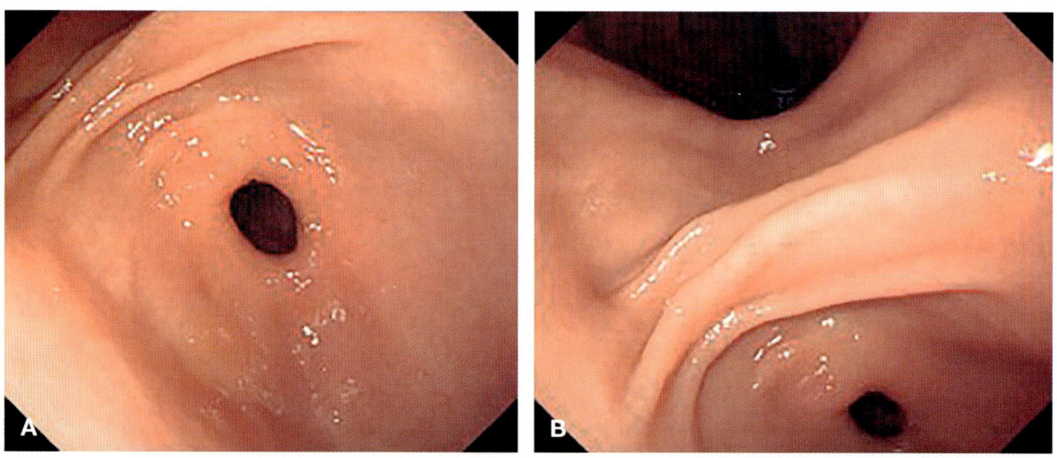

FIGURE 46.6 ❙ **A:** Pyloric channel. **B:** The antral ring is observed below the angle.

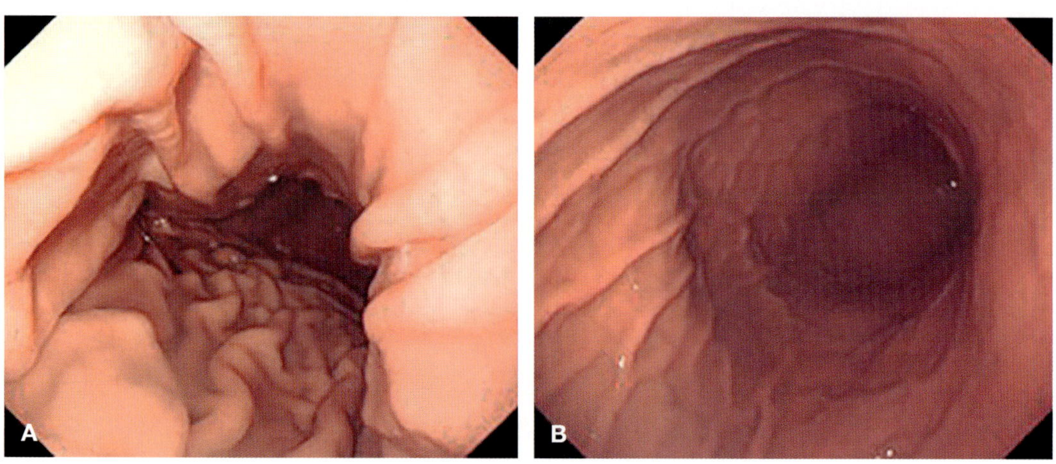

FIGURE 46.7 ❙ **A:** Mucosal folds on the greater curvature of the stomach. **B:** Straightened mucosal folds after insufflation of air.

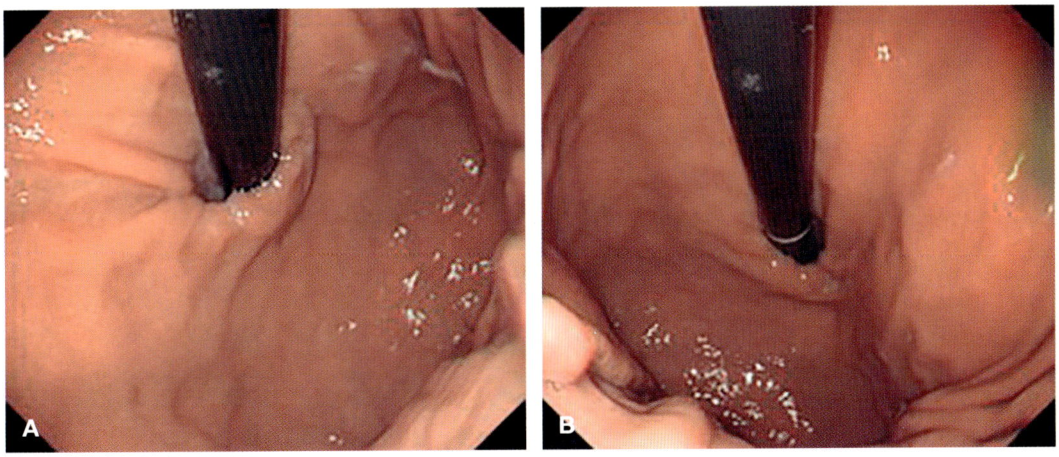

FIGURE 46.8 | A: Retroflexed view of the cardia. **B:** Retroflexed view of the cardia and fundus. (From Kim KO. Normal upper GI findings and normal variants. In: Chun H, Yang SK, Choi MG, eds. *Clinical Gastrointestinal Endoscopy*. Berlin, Heidelberg: Springer; 2014.)

- Enter the duodenal bulb and examine all of its four quadrants. The duodenal bulb has a rounded and oblong appearance.
- If the evaluation of the second and third parts of the duodenum is warranted, then the following maneuvers are performed to advance the scope:
  - Advance the scope into the duodenal bulb and the second part of the duodenum.
  - Rotate the scope and the shaft to the right simultaneously in counterclockwise direction.
  - Advance the scope (Figures 46.9 and 46.10).

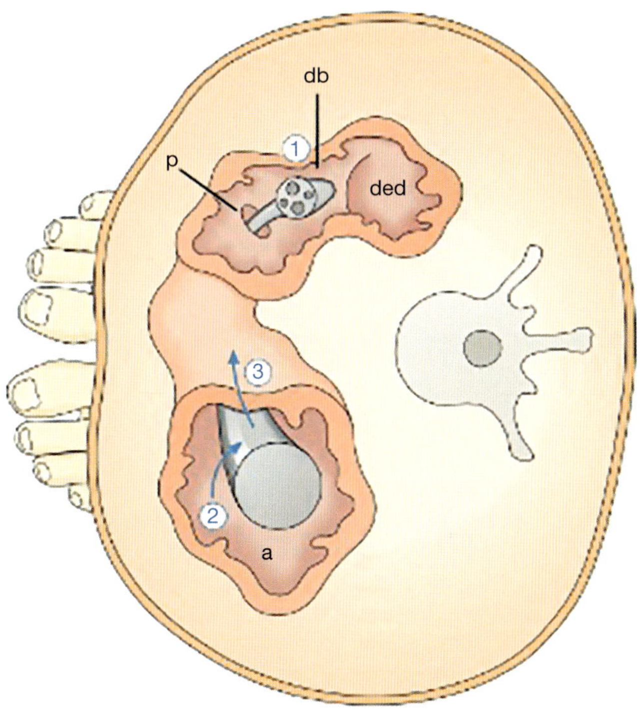

FIGURE 46.9 | To advance the scope into the third part of the duodenum, the endoscopist needs to: (1) first advance the scope into the duodenal bulb and the second part of the duodenum, (2) rotate the scope and the shaft to the right simultaneously in counterclockwise direction, and (3) advance the scope. a, antrum; db, duodenal bulb; ded, descending duodenum; p, pylorus. (Redrawn from Block B, Schachschal G, Schmidt H. *Endoscopy of the Upper GI Tract: A Training Manual*. Stuttgart: Georg Thieme Verlag; 2004.)

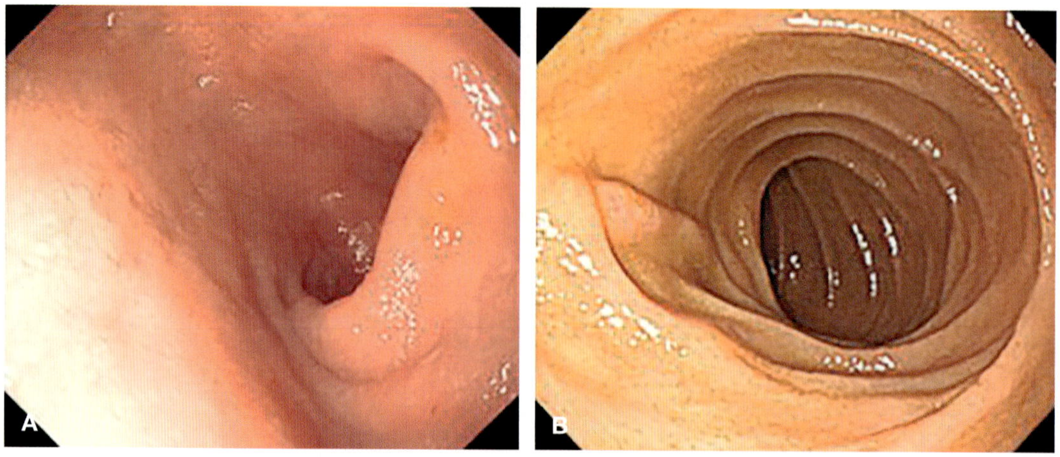

FIGURE 46.10 ▌ **A:** Duodenal bulb and **(B)** duodenal second portion. (From Kim KO. Normal upper GI findings and normal variants. In: Chun H, Yang SK, Choi MG, eds. *Clinical Gastrointestinal Endoscopy*. Berlin, Heidelberg: Springer; 2014.)

ESOPHAGEAL STENT PLACEMENT

Perioperative Considerations

Indications for Stents

- Indications for esophageal stent placement include: (1) esophageal perforation, (2) postsurgical anastomotic leaks, (3) refractory, benign strictures, and (4) tracheoesophageal fistula.
- It is also indicated in patients with malignant esophageal obstruction to manage dysphagia and alleviate symptoms.

Contraindications for Stents

- Esophageal stent placement is contraindicated in patients who are deemed too hemodynamically unstable to undergo upper gastrointestinal endoscopy and in those with uncontrolled coagulopathy and esophageal varices.
- In addition, a stent should not be placed proximally across the UES as this can lead to significant discomfort. A stent across the LES may lead to increased reflux.

Technique

Esophageal stents can be placed with the assistance of an EGD and/or fluoroscopy. There are multiple ways of placing a stent. We show here a common technique (Figure 46.11).

- Identify the proximal and distal aspects of the stricture with the EGD and with fluoroscopy. Place metal clips on the skin to mark the proximal and distal aspects of the stricture. Advance a guidewire through the EGD.
- Keep the wire but withdraw the EGD. Advance the stent over the wire and then deploy a stent across the stricture under fluoroscopic guidance.

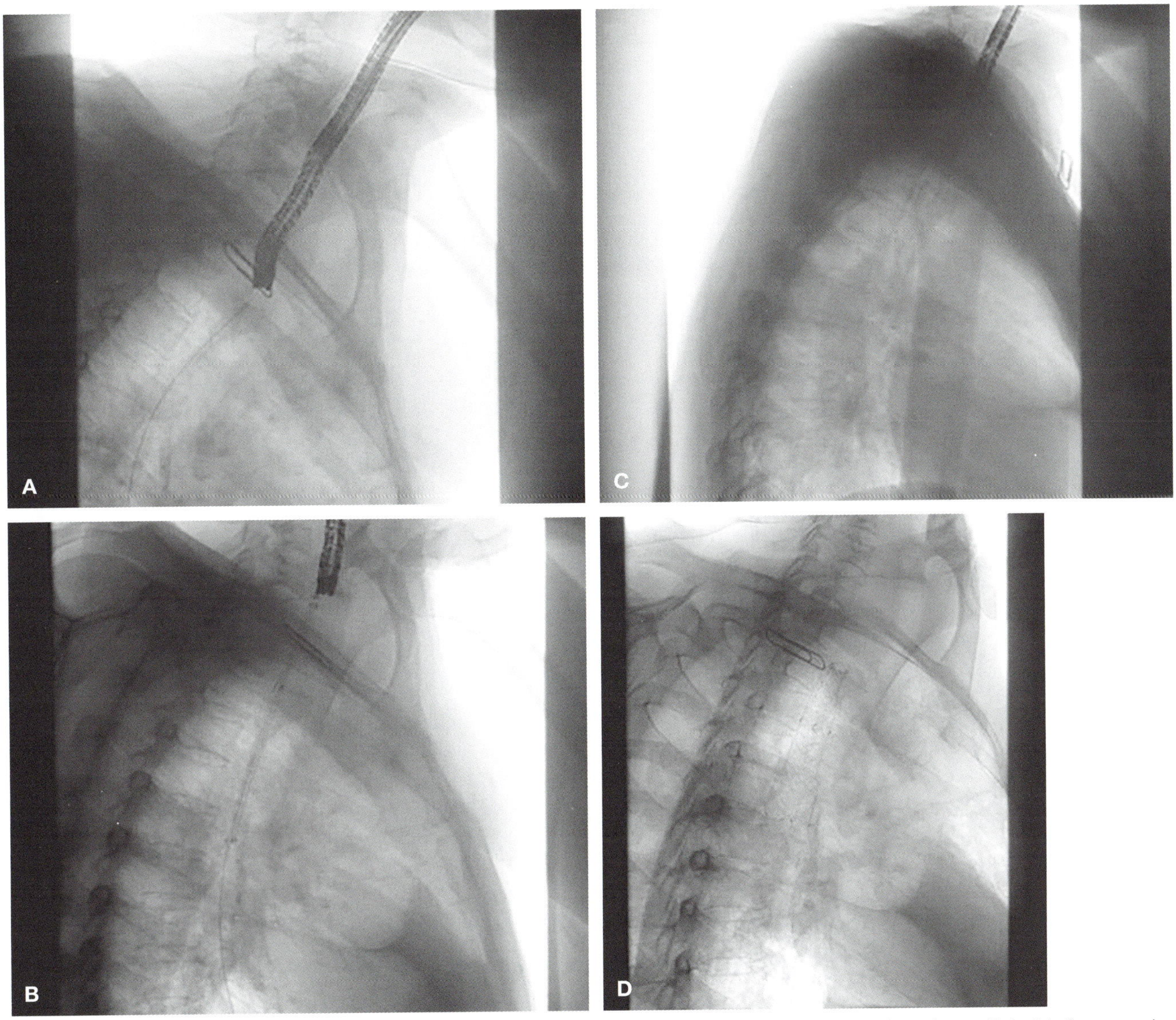

FIGURE 46.11 ▌ **A:** This is a fluoroscopic image showing that the guidewire has been advanced through the stricture. **B:** In this fluoroscopic image, the stent has been placed across the stricture. **C and D:** These fluoroscopic images show the stent after deployment. (From Min BH. Stent placement for malignant esophageal obstruction. In: Chun H, Yang SK, Choi MG, eds. *Therapeutic Gastrointestinal Endoscopy*. Singapore: Springer; 2019.)

PEARLS AND PITFALLS

- Place a bite block in the mouth of the patient while in left lateral decubitus position with neck flexed forward.
- A stent should not be placed proximally across the UES as this can lead to significant discomfort.
- A stent across the LES may lead to increased reflux.

Suggested Readings

1. Doosti-Irani A, Mansournia MA, Rahimi-Foroushani A, Haddad P, Holakouie-Naieni K. Complications of stent placement in patients with esophageal cancer: a systematic review and network meta-analysis. *PLoS One*. 2017;12(10):e0184784.
2. Fugazza A, Repici A. Endoscopic management of refractory benign esophageal strictures. *Dysphagia*. 2021;36(3):504-516.
3. Kamboj AK, Hoversten P, Leggett CL. Upper gastrointestinal bleeding: etiologies and management. *Mayo Clin Proc*. 2019;94(4):697-703.
4. Poincloux L, Rouquette O, Abergel A. Endoscopic treatment of benign esophageal strictures: a literature review. *Expert Rev Gastroenterol Hepatol*. 2017;11(1):53-64.
5. Teh JL, Shabbir A, Yuen S, So JB. Recent advances in diagnostic upper endoscopy. *World J Gastroenterol*. 2020;26(4):433-447.

Chapter 47

Endoscopic Ultrasound, Endoscopic Mucosal Resection, and Endoscopic Submucosal Dissection

CHRISTINA L. COSTANTINO
KUMAR KRISHNAN
UMA M. SACHDEVA

Introduction

- Barrett esophagus (BE) is a risk factor for esophageal adenocarcinoma.
- Dysplastic BE is treated with mucosal ablative therapies.
- Endoscopic mucosal resection (EMR) is used as an adjunct with ablative therapy for nodular lesions in the setting of BE.
- Endoscopic ultrasound (EUS) is an important tool in determining esophageal cancer T and N stages, but has limited ability distinguishing T1a from T1b lesions.
- EMR serves to both stage and treat early-stage esophageal cancers limited to the mucosa and submucosa (T1a, T1b).
- Endoscopic submucosal dissection (ESD) is increasingly used for complete endoscopic resection of T1b esophageal cancers.

Endoscopic Ultrasound

Instruments and Equipment

- Standard 7.5 MHz radial EUS
  - Allows for assessment of esophageal wall depth in five layers

Or,

- High-frequency (>20 MHz) radial EUS
  - Allows for greater detail, revealing nine layers of esophageal wall
- Suction and insufflation capabilities
- Linear EUS for ultrasound-guided tissue sampling capabilities

Anesthesia and Patient Positioning

- Patient placed in left lateral decubitus position
- Moderate IV sedation, monitored anesthesia care, or potentially general anesthesia depending on the patient, provider, and comorbidities

Principles of Endoscopic Ultrasound

- EUS allows for assessment of lesion depth of penetration in order to guide therapy
  - EUS assessment of absence or presence of submucosal invasion (ie, T1a vs T1b, Figure 47.1) is less reliable so EMR is often used for staging of early lesions

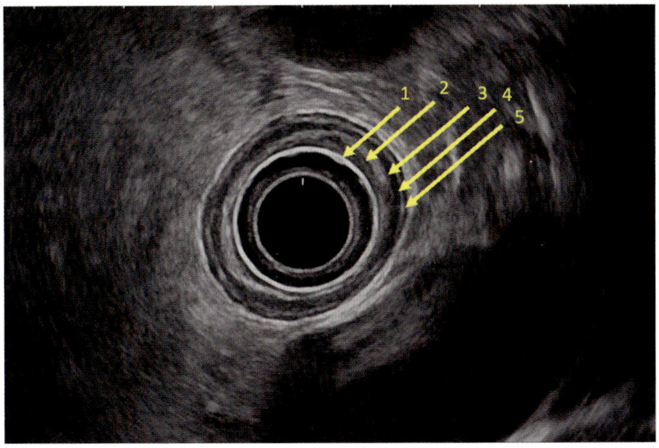

FIGURE 47.1 ▌ Endosonographic borders of lesion are well-defined by standard endoscopic ultrasound. 1, Superficial mucosal interface; 2, deep mucosa (lamina propria and muscularis mucosae), (hypoechoic, dark); 3, submucosa (hyperechoic, white); 4, muscularis propria (hypoechoic, dark); and 5, adventitia.

  - EUS is most optimal for determining T2-4 and N stages (Figure 47.2)
  - Able to delineate resectable and unresectable T4 tumors by level of invasion into mediastinal structures
- Periesophageal lymph nodes can be evaluated for shape, size, echogenicity, and irregularity (Figure 47.3)
  - Size: 1 cm in short axis is the upper limit of normal
  - Echogenicity: homogenous and hypoechoic is likely malignant
- Biopsy of the primary tumor and any identified lymph nodes can be performed concurrently with EUS

Endoscopic Mucosal Resection

Preoperative Considerations

- Nothing by mouth after midnight
- Anticoagulation including coumadin, Xarelto, Eliquis, and Plavix is held preoperatively. Aspirin 325 or 81 may be continued periprocedurally.
- EMR and ESD are for early-stage lesions (T1a, T1b); those who are T1bN0 may be considered for endoscopic resection if they are not good surgical candidates/frail/provider preference.

Anesthesia and Patient Positioning

- Induction of general anesthesia and intubation in supine position
- Turn patient to left lateral decubitus position

Instruments and Equipment

- Therapeutic upper GI endoscope with a 3.7-mm inner channel
- Dual-channel therapeutic upper endoscope with 2.8- and 3.7-mm inner channels

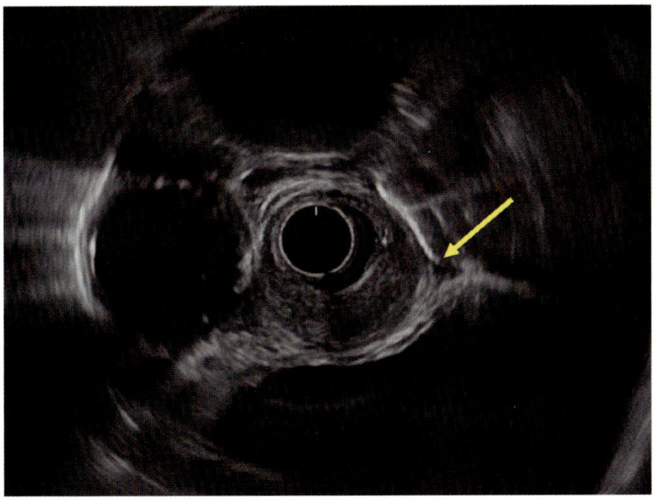

FIGURE 47.2 ▌ Hypoechoic mass (indicated by arrow) found in the lower third of the esophagus with irregular endosonographic borders, suggesting invasion into the adventitia, staged T3.

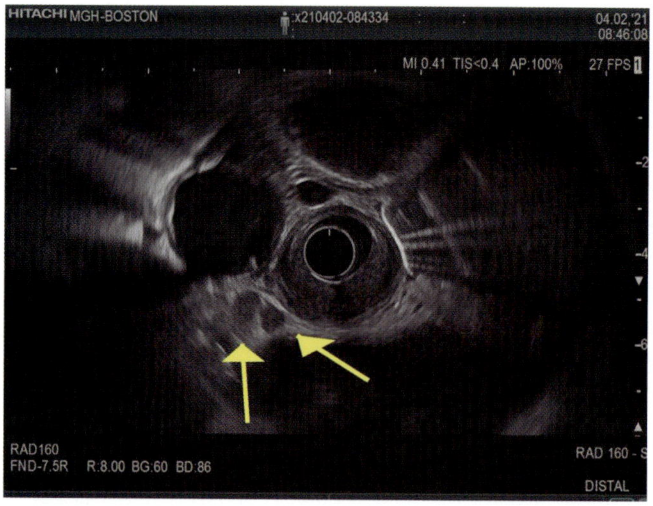

FIGURE 47.3 ▌ Several, subcentimeter, hypoechoic abnormal lymph nodes (indicated by arrows) adjacent to the esophageal tumor. WD/7278625.

- Band-assisted EMR
  - *Captivator EMR Device, Boston Scientific (Marlborough, MA)*
    - Six rubber bands attached to translucent cap, which contain tripwire/string that is passed through working channel and connected to a knob at the insertion of the working channel
    - Each band can be deployed by turning the knob at the working channel insertion
  - *Duette© kit from Cook Medical (Bloomington, MA)*
- Cap-assisted EMR
  - *Cap-assisted EMR kit from Olympus (Center Valley, PA)*
    - Standard gastroscope
    - Translucent cap that can accommodate a snare
- Endoscopically applied hemoclips or over-the-scope clips can be utilized in the event of full-thickness perforation or bleeding

Principles of EMR Technique

- For resection of lesions up to 2 cm in diameter
- Diseased mucosal tissue may be captured with a rim of submucosal tissue into the cap with suction applied to the endoscope creating a pseudopolyp configuration
- The muscularis propria should be left intact

Endoscopic Technique (Video 47.1)

- Irrigation of distal esophagus with N-acetylcysteine
  - To remove superficial mucous and more readily detect subtle changes in the mucosa
- Evaluate the lesion using chromoendoscopy facilitated by two modes of optical enhancement:
  - Chemical chromoendoscopy: methylene blue
  - Optical chromoendoscopy: narrow-band imaging (Figure 47.4)
    - Enhances mucosal and vascular surface pattern irregularities to identify areas of dysplastic BE
- Utilize tip of snare to apply cautery markings around periphery of lesion to ensure complete resection
- Goal of EMR is to capture mucosal and some submucosal tissue while leaving muscularis propria intact
- **Band-assisted EMR:** We utilize the Captivator© device from Boston Scientific (Marlborough, MA) (Figure 47.5).
  - Lesion of interest should be targeted in the center of the translucent cap
  - Apply suction to endoscope
    - Repositioning of the cap may be required to ensure entire lesion is suctioned into the cap
    - Areas that do not adequately lift into resection cap or appear ulcerated are indicative of more extensive submucosal fibrosis and will likely need surgical resection
  - Deploy band, creating a pseudopolyp

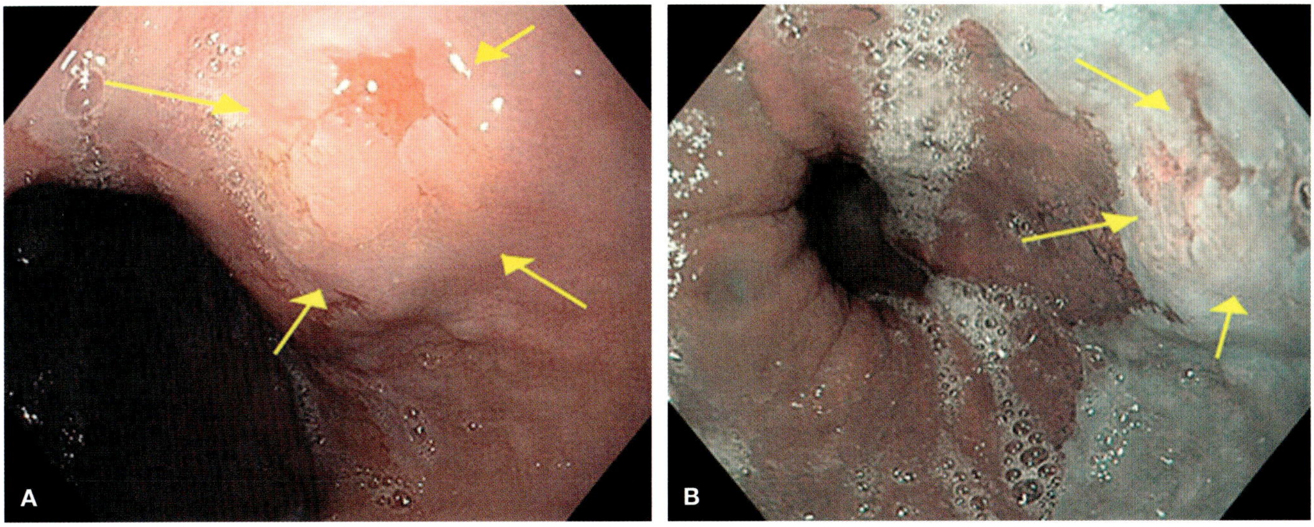

FIGURE 47.4 ▍ White light **(A)** and narrow band imaging of Barrett region **(B)** demonstrate that mucosal and vascular surface pattern irregularities help identify areas of dysplasia. Arrows show borders of dysplastic region.

- Advance snare through working channel and position around the pseudopolyp
- Snare can be placed either above or below the band
- Standard snare cautery (either coagulation or blended cut settings) is utilized to resect lesion at the base of pseudopolyp
- Evaluate the resection bed for bleeding and evaluate depth of resection
- Additional or neighboring areas can be resected using the same technique to ensure a wide resection margin
  - Additional second band can be deployed adjacent to resection base to create a larger resection area
- Remove resection specimens using endoscopic basket retrieval forceps

- **Cap-assisted EMR,** Olympus (Center Valley, PA)
  - Advantage is capturing slightly larger circumference of tissue over band-assisted technique
  - A small submucosal injection is performed to elevate the lesion.
    - Injection of indigo carmine or methylene blue dye can be helpful to determine the depth of resection.
    - Elevation helps protect from thermal injury to muscularis propria.
  - The lesion is centered within the cap and suction is applied bringing the lesion into the cap.
  - The snare is closed once an adequate amount of the tissue is captured.
    - Inspection of the tissue rim circumferentially indicates if adequate tissue is captured.
    - Gentle rotation of the snare, with pseudopolyp elevated in the cap, indicates whether muscle is also captured in the pseudopolyp.
  - Electrocautery is applied and the polyp is resected.
  - Assess the base of the resection to assess for full-thickness injury.
    - If blue dye is utilized with initial saline injection, the resection base should be stained uniformly blue, indicating that only mucosa and submucosa have been resected. Areas of white or yellow surrounded by blue submucosa can indicate full-thickness injury.

TIPS

- *Blue dye can be injected to elevate lesion and protect from thermal injury as well as to assess level of invasion.*
- *Goal is to trap mucosal lesion and submucosal margin while leaving the muscularis propria intact.*

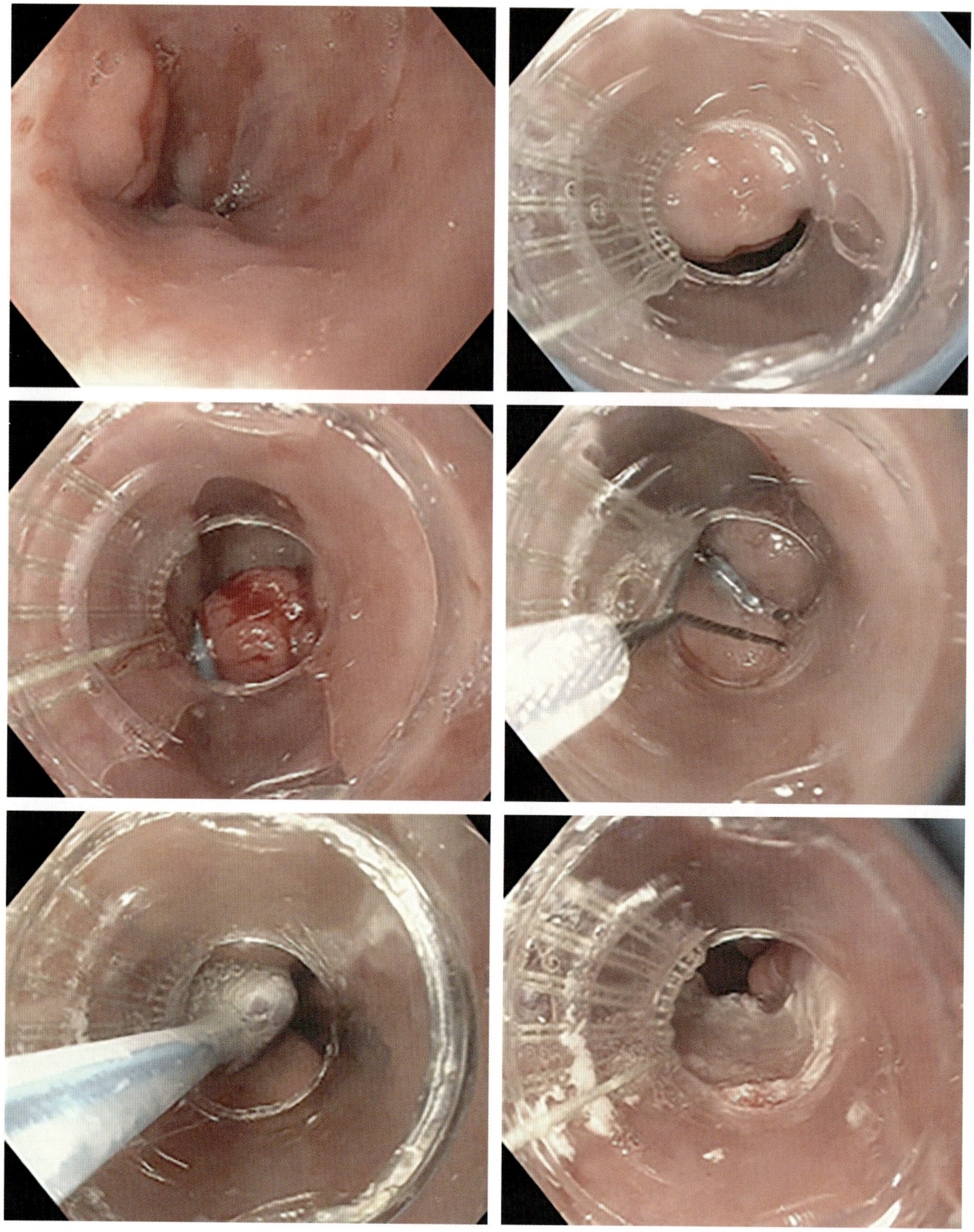

FIGURE 47.5 ▌ Endoscopic mucosal resection. Band-assisted endoscopic mucosal resection. Suction is applied over the lesion, which is then captured into the translucent cap, creating a pseudopolyp. Utilizing the Captivator© device (Boston Scientific, Marlborough, MA), a band is deployed around the base. A snare is then advanced around the lesion and below the band and electrocautery applied, separating the lesion from the esophagus. A Roth-Net retrieval device is utilized to capture the lesion. The resection bed is inspected to ensure complete resection and hemostasis.

Endoscopic Submucosal Dissection

- Utilized for lesions size 2 cm or greater, or invading the submucosa (T1b)

Instruments and Equipment

- Therapeutic endoscope with a 3.7-mm inner channel
- Injection needle (saline, glycerol solution, or sodium hyaluronate mixture)
- Endoscopic needle knife: hook knife, triangle-tip (TT) electrosurgery knife, or DualKnife *(Olympus Optical Co., Tokyo, Japan)*
- Endoscopic clips or hemoclips

Technique

- Use electrocautery hook knife or a TT knife to circumferentially mark the mucosa surrounding the lesion.
- Inject 5 to 10 mL of saline, glycerol solution, or sodium hyaluronate mixture into the submucosa to elevate the lesion away from the muscularis propria.
  - Addition of epinephrine (1:20,000) can be useful for hemostasis.
  - If the tumor does not appear to lift despite 5 to 10 mL of injection, it likely extends beyond the submucosa and will require surgical resection.
- Create a mucosal incision to allow access to the submucosal space using electrocautery.
- Suction is applied to the lesion in order to elevate it further.
- Dissection of the submucosal plane is achieved with a combination of insufflation and electrocautery until complete *en bloc* resection of the lesion with appropriate margin has occurred (Figure 47.6).

Postoperative Care

- Most common symptom postoperatively is chest pain secondary to iatrogenic ulcer created from resection base. This is usually self-limited.
- Diet: liquid diet for 24 hours, followed by soft diet for 1 week, then resume normal diet
- EUS and EMR patients may be discharged the same day as their procedure. ESD patients are often observed for 1 day in the hospital depending on the extent of resection.
- Medications:
  - Double-dose proton pump inhibitor
  - Sucralfate suspension × 1 week
  - Tylenol with codeine elixir can be considered as needed for pain.
  - Avoid nonsteroidal anti-inflammatory drugs.
  - Antiplatelet agents held for 48 hours post resection
- EMR patients undergo follow-up endoscopy in 2 months, while ESD patients undergo surveillance endoscopy depending on the pathology at 6 months to 1 year.

Early Potential Complications

- Bleeding: This can be treated immediately by centering the area of bleeding with the translucent cap and utilizing coagulation with hemostatic forceps
- Perforation: Hemostatic clips can be used for small perforations. Full-thickness perforations can result in mediastinitis, pneumomediastinum, and decompensation and may require esophageal stenting (see Chapter 42, Esophageal Perforation).

Late Potential Complications

- Extensive mucosal resections can result in stricturing and is related to the size of the resection bed.
  - A resection of >50% circumference will result in stricture formation and may require subsequent endoscopic dilations.

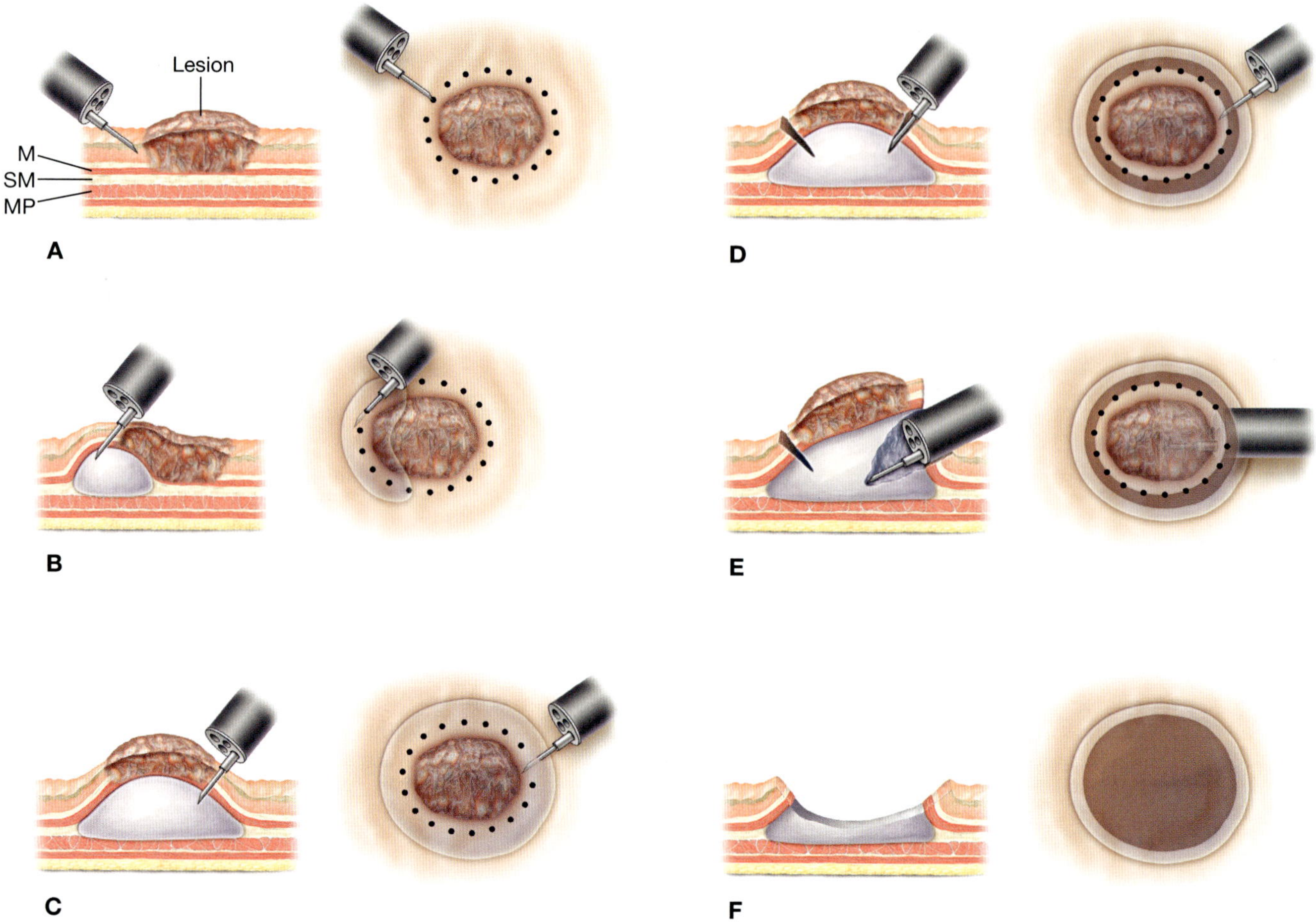

FIGURE 47.6 ▌ Representation of endoscopic submucosal dissection: **A.** electrocautery hook knife or a triangle-tip knife is utilized to circumferentially mark the mucosa surrounding the lesion; **B and C.** injection of 5 to 10 mL of normal saline, glycerol solution, or sodium hyaluronate mixture solution circumferentially elevates the lesion away from the muscularis propria; **D.** creation of mucosal incision with electrocautery allowing access to the submucosal space; **E.** dissection of the submucosal plane is achieved with a combination of insufflation and electrocautery; and **F.** complete en bloc resection of the lesion. M, mucosal; MP, muscularis propria; SM, submucosal. (From Hoppo T, Jobe BA. Endoscopic mucosal resection. In: Luketich JD, ed. *Master Techniques in Surgery: Esophageal Surgery*. Wolters Kluwer; 2014:378. Figure 33.5.)

PEARLS AND PITFALLS

- EMR and ESD can be used for resection of early stage lesions (T1a, T1b).
- Candidates for resection should not have any evidence of lymph node involvement on EUS.
- In order to complete endoscopic resection, the mucosa must be able to be lifted by injection into the submucosal space.
- If insufficient lifting of the submucosal space, there is increased risk for perforation and endoscopic resection should not be performed.

Suggested Readings

1. Krishnan K, Komanduri S. Endoscopic mucosal resection for Barrett's related neoplasia. In: Grams J, Perry K, Tavakkoli A, eds. *The SAGES Manual of Foregut Surgery*. Springer; 2019:359-365.
2. LoCicero J, Shields TW. Diagnostic studies of the esophagus. *Shields' General Thoracic Surg*. 2019;2019;1620-1637.
3. Luo RB, Jacobsen GR. Endoscopic management of benign submucosal tumors. In: Grams J, Perry K, Tavakkoli A, eds. *The SAGES Manual of Foregut Surgery*. Springer; 2019:615-621.
4. Ning B, Abdelfatah MM, Othman MO. Endoscopic submucosal dissection and endoscopic mucosal resection for early stage esophageal cancer. *Ann Cardiothorac Surg*. 2017;6(2):88-98.
5. Pech O, May A, Manner H, et al. Long-term efficacy and safety of endoscopic resection for patients with mucosal adenocarcinoma of the esophagus. *Gastroenterology*. 2014;146(3):652-660.e1.
6. Shim CS, Jung IS. Endoscopic removal of submucosal tumors: preprocedure diagnosis, technical options, and results. *Endoscopy*. 2005;37(7):646-654.

Chapter 48

Whole Lung Lavage for Pulmonary Alveolar Proteinosis

ANTONIA KRESO
COLLEEN M. KEYES
YOLONDA L. COLSON

Perioperative Considerations

- The goal is to lavage an entire lung with fluid to clear out alveoli that are filled with proteinaceous material.
- Sequential lavage of each lung with return trips to the operating room is encouraged.

Double-Lumen Endotracheal Tube Considerations

- Communication with the anesthesia team about endotracheal tube (ETT) positioning is critical.
- Double-lumen ETT is used in order to protect the side that is not getting lavage. Do not use a bronchial blocker as there is insufficient airway protection.
- It is critical to confirm ETT tube location after positioning to ensure proper seating of balloon and bronchial/tracheal lumens.
- Intubating one side with the bronchial lumen and inflating the balloon allows for a good seal on that side.
- It may be required to inflate the tracheal balloon to protect the fluid from pooling in the trachea.

Patient Positioning

- Before the patient goes to sleep, the inflatable vest is secured across the patient's chest (Figure 48.1).
- The patient is placed in lateral decubitus position with the side up that will get the lavage.
- Both arms are out with the arm that is on top draped over a pillow for support (Figure 48.2A).
- Joints are in physiologic position with bony parts padded.
- ETT position is confirmed with bronchoscope to ensure that the side not getting the lavage is protected with a balloon that is well positioned.
- Patient is secured to the table.
- The vest is attached to the chest physiotherapy apparatus that will perform high-frequency chest wall oscillation (Figure 48.2B).

Instruments and Equipment

- The chest percussion vest therapy includes the inflatable vest and the oscillatory system, which is set to 14 Hz, pressure of 6 mm Hg, and cycle length of 10 minutes (Figure 48.2B).
- Lavage fluid (0.9% normal saline, warmed to 42 °C)
- Fluid warmer

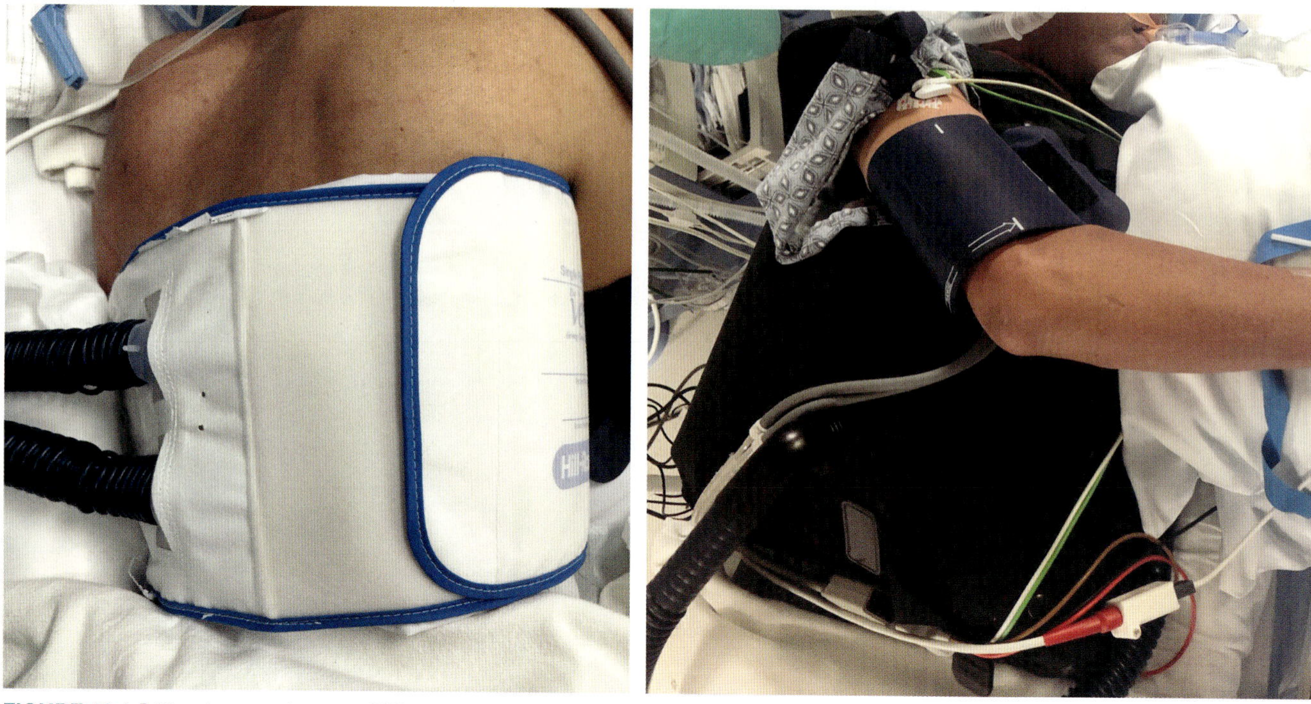

FIGURE 48.1 | Chest percussion vest. Different types of inflatable vests can be used, which are attached to tubing that functions to inflate the vest for percussion therapy.

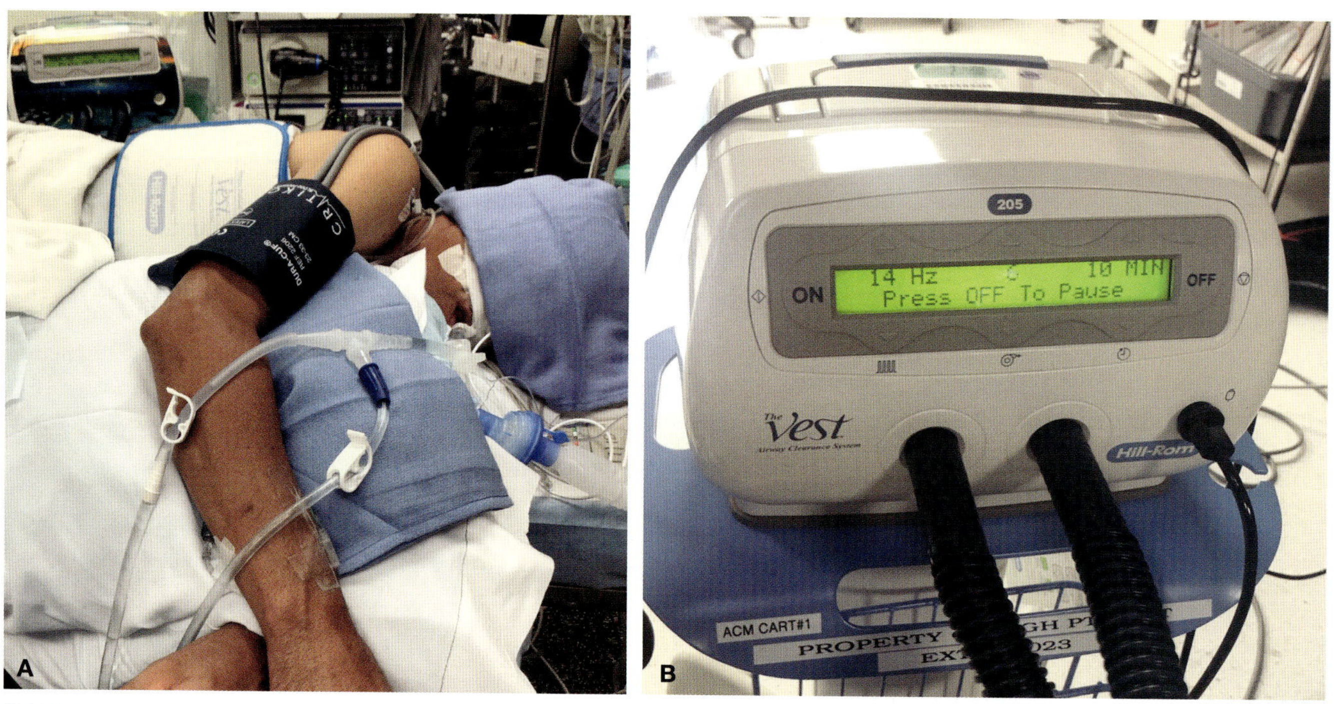

FIGURE 48.2 | **A:** Final patient positioning with the patient in lateral decubitus position with the side up that is to receive the lavage. The patient's arm is wrapped over several pillows. **B:** The oscillatory system with the machine set to 14 Hz, pressure of 6 mm Hg, and intervals of 10 minutes. Air hoses are shown in black and attach to the patient's vest.

- Tubing to connect the lavage fluid to the patient's ETT and tubing to suction away the fluid from the patient's chest (Figure 48.3)
- Each tubing should have a controllable lock on it that can regulate how much fluid gets instilled and how much suction is applied to drain the fluid (Figure 48.3).
- Multiple collection bags for collecting suctioned lavage fluid

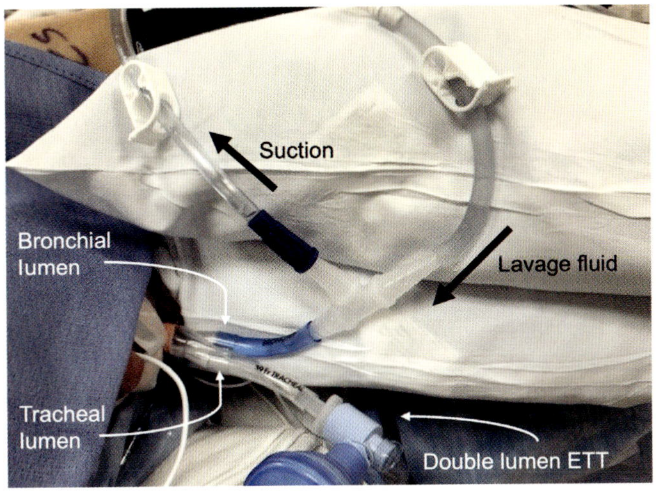

FIGURE 48.3 ▌ Tubing setup. The patient's double-lumen endotracheal tube (ETT) is shown. One lumen is connected to the ventilator circuit and the other lumen (tracheal lumen in this case) is connected to the inflow and outflow system for lavage and suctioning using a three-way connecting piece. Each tube has a white clamp that can be used to regulate lavage fluid and suction.

TIPS

- *An important step is protecting the opposite lung from filling with fluid during lavage.*
- *Repetitions on one side should be continued until the lavage fluid becomes clearer compared to the initial lavage.*
- *Positioning with the lavage lung up allows better V/Q match of the dependent (nonlavage) lung.*
- *It is helpful to transfer the patient to the recovery room on positive pressure BiPAP (5-10 mm Hg) and wean as tolerated.*

Technique

- After the patient is intubated, positioned, and the ETT position is verified, 1 L of warmed normal saline is instilled into the patient's chest.
- Chest percussion vest therapy is begun by turning on the oscillatory system to vibrate at 14 Hz for 10 minutes.
- During the vibrations, ETT output is monitored to ensure that there is no fluid flowing back through the lumen that is used for ventilation.
- After 10 minutes of chest percussion vest therapy, the saline inflow line is clamped and the suction tubing is unclamped. The wall suction is set to medium levels (100-125 mm Hg).
- A log is kept of how much fluid flows into the chest and how much is suctioned out after every liter of lavage. This allows one to keep a net volume that still remains in the patient's lungs. The aim is to have no more than 500 to 800 mL of fluid left in the chest.
- After no more fluid can be suctioned, the suction line is clamped, the irrigation line is unclamped, and another liter of warmed saline is instilled into the lung and the vibration machine is turned on for another cycle. This is repeated until the fluid that returns is significantly clearer (Figure 48.4).
- This is repeated with multiple liters of saline. Typically, we use 10 L to achieve good results (Figure 48.4).

Postoperative Care

- It is not uncommon that the patient requires transient positive pressure to maintain the alveoli open and allow for good gas exchange.
- Postoperative chest x-rays are useful to rule out pneumothorax and to have a new baseline of the radiographic appearance of the lung fields.
- Obtaining interval CT scans of the chest can determine the extent of clearance and help with planning for future lavage (Figure 48.5).

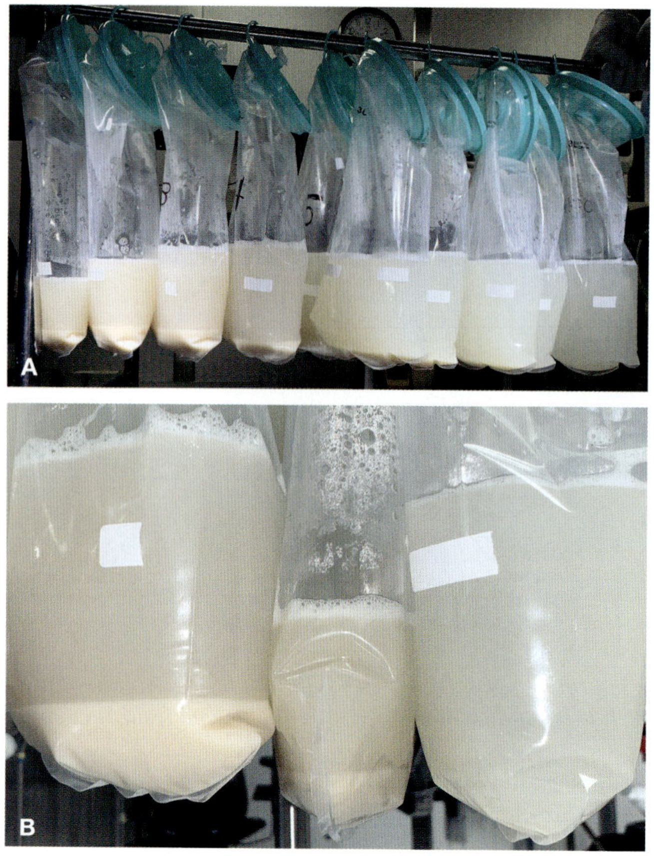

FIGURE 48.4 ▎ Comparison of fluid from the beginning of the lavage process to the final suctioned sample. **A:** Each bag contains the volume that was suctioned out after a liter of saline was instilled. The bags are lined up in order from initial lavage (left) to final lavage (right). In the illustrated example, 11 L of saline was used for lavage. **B:** Close-up of a washing where the initial return (on the left) and final return (on the right) are shown.

Troubleshooting

Patient's Oxygen Saturation Is Falling

- Check that the patient's pulse oximeter is attached appropriately.
- Communicate with the anesthesia team to determine if ventilator mechanics have changed: Is there a new loss of lung volume? Have peak pressures changed?
- Auscultate lung fields to ensure there is no large pneumothorax.
- Have bronchoscopy readily available and visualize the bronchial and tracheal lumens to ensure that the ETT is not malpositioned and that the balloon is getting a good seal.
- Fluid can be instilled into the operative side and using bronchoscopy, the protected lung can be observed to ensure no fluid is leaking around the balloon.
- The ventilated side can be suctioned with the bronchoscope to see if there is a plug that is preventing gas exchange.
- An intraoperative chest x-ray can be obtained if a pneumothorax is suspected.

Volume of Lavage Fluid Instilled Cannot Be Suctioned Out

- If the patient has thick mucus, instilling 1 L of fluid may not be enough to thin out the mucus, leading to difficulty suctioning out all of the fluid.
- In this instance, more fluid can be instilled, percussion therapy resumed, and more frequent checks can be done to see if additional fluid can be suctioned out.
- The amount of suction needs to be controlled as one can cause the alveoli to collapse with excessive suction, thereby trapping fluid within alveoli.
- Disconnecting the suction tubing intermittently can allow the system to reset and withdraw more fluid.
- Positioning the suction tubing to have gravity assistance can help with removing the lavage fluid.
- Typically, 500 to 800 mL of fluid is left within the patient after 10 cycles of lavage.

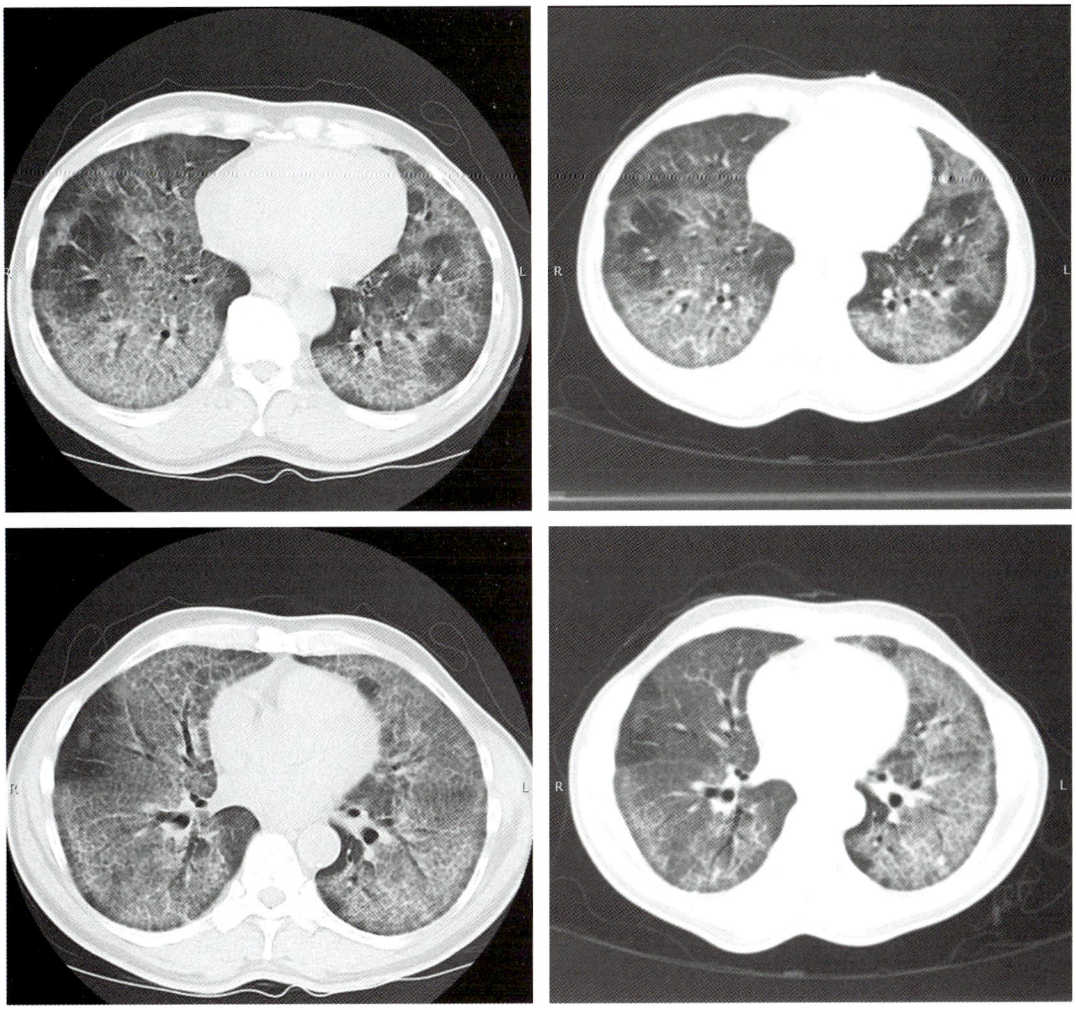

FIGURE 48.5 | CT images from before (on the left) and after (on the right) right-sided lung lavage.

PEARLS AND PITFALLS

- Bronchoscopy prior to the lavage may not show gross abnormalities.
- During oscillations, the ETT can become dislodged and can cause fluid to leak from the operative side to the side that is ventilated. This should be avoided.
- The ETT can also become dislodged preventing appropriate suctioning and removal of lavage fluid.
- Monitoring the patient's oxygenation status is critical during this procedure as any change should prompt the surgeon and anesthesia team to check the setup.
- Typically, 10 L of total fluid is used to lavage the lungs to get a good response (Figure 48.4). It is important to keep a running net volume that has not been suctioned out of the chest.
- With each cycle of lavage, more fluid should be suctioned out as the proteinaceous fluid becomes thinner. At the end of the repeated lavage cycles, we aim not to leave more than 500 to 800 mL of fluid within the lung.
- Consider prelavage placement of a Foley catheter given fluid absorption during lavage.

Suggested Readings

1. Michaud G, Reddy C, Ernst A. Whole-lung lavage for pulmonary alveolar proteinosis. *Chest*. 2009;136(6):1678-1681.
2. Trapnell BC, Whitsett JA, Nakata K. Pulmonary alveolar proteinosis. *N Engl J Med*. 2003;349(26):2527-2539.

Index

Note: Page numbers followed by *f* indicate figures, *t* indicate tables, and *b* indicate boxes.

U

V

Z